W0112539

# Daily Practical Sheet in Biochemistry

## (For MBBS Students)

# Daily Practical Sheet in Biochemistry

## (For MBBS Students)

**Simmi Kharb**

MBBS, MD

Professor, Dept. of Biochemistry,
Pt. BD Sharma Postgraduate Institute of Medical Sciences,
Rohtak (Haryana)

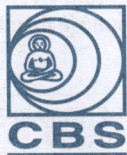

# CBS PUBLISHERS & DISTRIBUTORS PVT. LTD.

NEW DELHI • BENGALURU • CHENNAI • KOCHI • MUMBAI • PUNE

ISBN: 978-81-239-2428-1

**First Edition: 2015**
Reprint: 2015

Copyright © Publisher

All rights reserved. No part of this book may be reproduced or transmitted in any form or by any means, electronic or mechanical, including photocopying, recording, or any information storage and retrieval system without permission, in writing, from the publisher.

*Published by:*

Satish Kumar Jain for CBS Publishers & Distributors Pvt. Ltd.,
4819/XI Prahlad Street, 24 Ansari Road, Daryaganj, New Delhi - 110002
delhi@cbspd.com, cbspubs@airtelmail.in • www.cbspd.com
Ph.: 23289259, 23266861, 23266867 • Fax: 011-23243014

*Corporate Office:* 204 FIE, Industrial Area, Patparganj, Delhi - 110 092
Ph: 49344934 • Fax: 011-49344935
E-mail: publishing@cbspd.com • publicity@cbspd.com

*Branches:*
- *Bengaluru:* 2975, 17th Cross, K.R. Road, Bansankari 2nd Stage,
  Bengaluru - 70 • Ph: +91-80-26771678/79 • Fax: +91-80-26771680
  E-mail: cbsbng@gmail.com, bangalore@cbspd.com
- *Chennai:* No. 7, Subbaraya Street, Shenoy Nagar, Chennai - 600030
  Ph: +91-44-26681266, 26680620 • Fax: +91-44-42032115
  E-mail: chennai@cbspd.com
- *Kochi:* 36/14, Kalluvilakam, Lissie Hospital Road, Kochi - 682018
  Ph: +91-484-4059061-65 • Fax: +91-484-4059065
  E-mail: cochin@cbspd.com
- *Mumbai:* 83-C, Dr. E. Moses Road, Worli, Mumbai - 400018
  Ph: +91-9833017933, 022-24902340/41 • E-mail: mumbai@cbspd.com
- *Pune:* Bhuruk Prestige, Sr. No. 52/12/2+1+3/2,
  Narhe, Haveli (Near Katraj-Dehu Road Bypass), Pune - 411041
  Ph: +91-20-64704058/59, 32342277 • E-mail: pune@cbspd.com

*Representatives:*

- Hyderabad: 0-9885175004
- Nagpur: 0-9021734563
- Vijayawada: 0-9000660880
- Kolkata: 0-9831437309, 0-9051152362
- Patna: 0-9334159340

*Printed at*:
Neekunj Print Process, Delhi

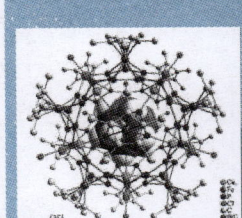

# Preface

When one opens a comprehensive textbook of biochemistry for the first time, it can be a daunting experience for him. One wonders to look at such a detailed material being presented that has to be mastered in one professional of MBBS. This book has been written to ease your entry into exciting world of biochemistry. The goal of the book is to help you revise the topic covered in a lecture along with suitable interpretation of clinical correlations.

**Dr. Simmi Kharb**

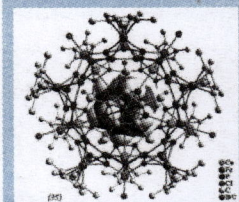

# Contents

# Introduction

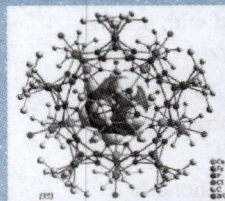

## CELL

While studying cell, we will discuss the following:

- Study of components of cells
- How they can be isolated
- Various functions of each component

### Key features of cell

1. Cell is structural and functional unit of life.
2. Most chemical reactions take place within cells.
3. Of two types:
   – Prokaryotic cell
   – Eukaryotic cell
4. Human body composed of $10^{14}$ cells.

### PROKARYOTIC CELL

- Lack well-defined nucleus
- Contain rigid cell wall

### EUKARYOTIC CELL

- Contain well defined nucleus
- Contain more complicated internal structure
- Cells are highly complex and organized.
- Cells possess a genetic program and the mean to use it.
- Cells are capable of producing more of themselves
- Cells acquire and utilize energy, carry out a variety of chemical reactions: metabolism.
- Cells engage in mechanical activity, able to respond to stimultion and capable of self regulation.

### Common features of prokaryotes and eukaryotes:

- Plasma membrane similar
- Genetic information:
  – Encoded in DNA, genetic code identical

| | **Comparison** | |
|---|---|---|
| **Sr. No.** | *Prokaryotic cell* | *Eukaryotic cell* |
| 1. Size | Small 1-10 μ | Large 10-100 μ |
| 2. Cell wall | Present | Extracellular matrix |
| 3. Cell membrane | Rigid cell wall | Flexible plasma membrane |
| 4. Sub-cellular organelle | Absent | Distinct organelle present |
| 5. Nucleus | Not well defined | Well defined, contain membrane |
| 6. DNA | Found as nucleoid | DNA associated with histones |
| 7. Histones | Absent | Present |
| 8. Nucleolus | Absent | Present |
| 9. Genome | Single, circular chromosome | Multiple chromosome |
| 10. Metabolism | Both aerobic and anaerobic | Aerobic |
| 11. Respiratory enzymes | Located in plasma membrane | Located in mitochondria |
| 12. Cell division | Cleavage, fission | Mitosis, meiosis |
| 13. Cytoplasm | Lack organelle and cytoskeleton | Contain organelle and cytoskeleton |

- Transcription, translation mechanisms similar
- Ribosomes similar
- Similar mechanism for synthesizing and inserting membrane proteins
- Metabolic pathways:
  - Similar pathways
  - Similar conservation of energy as ATP
  - Similar mechanism of photosynthesis (in cyanobacteria and green plants)
- Proteasomes similar (archaebacteria and eukaryotes)

### Features of eukaryote not found in prokaryotes

- Division of cell into cytoplasm and nucleus of nuclear membrane
- Complex chromosome composed of: DNA, associated proteins
- Cytoplasmic organelles: Golgi complex, lysosome, ER, peroxisome, mitochondria.
- Specialized organelle for aerobic respiration: mitochondria

- Flagella, cilia
- Cell division, sexual reproduction: mitosis, meiosis
- Presence of two genes per cell, one from each parent.

### CELL STRUCTURE

- Variable, closely related to function:
- Chief cell-large quantity of ER
- Macrophage-active lysosome
- Adipose tissue – large quantity of stored TAG.

### General features of cell structure:

Seven major compartments common to eukaryotic cells:

1. Cytosol
2. Mitochondria
3. Rough endoplasmic reticulum
4. Smooth endoplasmic reticulum
5. Lysosomes

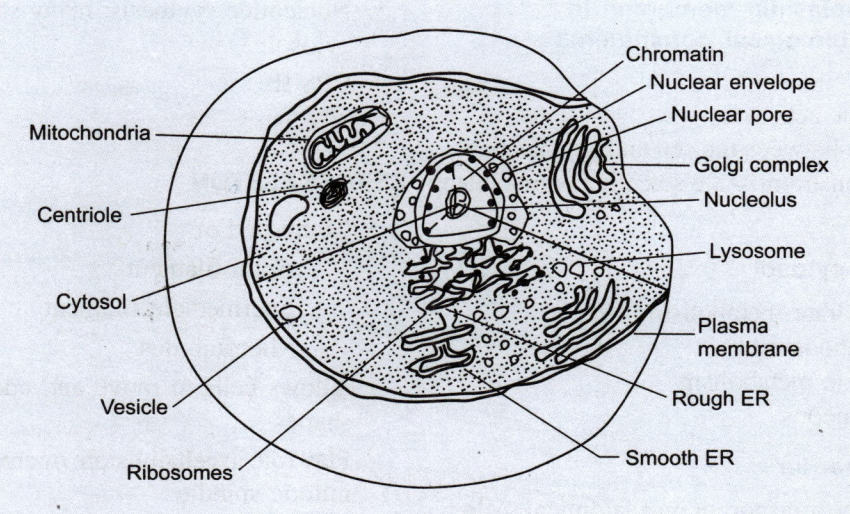

Fig. 1.1. Cell structure.

6. Peroxisomes
7. Nucleus

Throughout any discussion of medical biochemistry, you must try to recognize the relationship of a metabolic process to the organizational structure within the cell, and then it will be clear to you how metabolic pattern of eukaryotic cell is markedly affected by the presence of compartments namely, cytosol, and mitochondria.

## Cell specialization

Different activities of multicellular organisms are conducted by different types of specialized cells formed by differentiation, e.g. skeletal muscle cell contain a network of precisely aligned filaments of contractile proteins; cartilage cells; RBC become disk shaped stacks filled with a single protein Hb that transports $O_2$.

## Structure and biochemical functions of sub-cellular components

• Cell membrane (will be discussed in next chapter).

• Protoplasm (Cytosol, cytoskeleton, nucleoplasm)
• Nucleus
• Organelle

## CYTOSOL

• Fluid compartment
• Soluble part, viscous gel
• Represent 50-60% of total cell volume
• It is in contact with all sub-cellular organelle
• Contains: Enzyme, metabolites and salts.

## Composition of cytosol

1. Proteins:
   (i) Enzymes of:
       Carbohydrate metabolism
       Protein metabolism
       Fat metabolism
   (ii) Transporter, carrier proteins
2. Metabolites: Produced by carbohydrate and amino acid metabolism.
3. Other molecules: $Na^+$, $K^+$, $Ca^{+2}$, $Mg^{+2}$, $HCO_3'$, $Cl'$, $PO_4'$

## Role of cytoplasmic membrane in partitioning biological constituents of cells

Cell membrane acts as a:
 (i) Mediator between the cell and environment
 (ii) Shape constraint: As a selective permeable barrier

## Function of cytosol

- Carbohydrate metabolism
- Fat metabolism
- Nucleotide metabolism
- Miscellaneous

## Permeable barrier

- It could be transport or on anatomical scale.
- Helps in:
    - selective removal of wastes from blood in the kidney
    - blood-brain barrier
    - neurotransmission
- Act as a site for receptor
    - hormones
- Helps in cell to cell interaction:
    - contact inhibition
    - cell adhesion

## Metabolic pathways in cytosol

1. Carbohydrate metabolism
   Glycolysis
   PPP
   Glycogen
2. Fatty acid synthesis (*denovo*)
3. Amino acid metabolism
   Oxidation
   Deamination
   Decarboxylation
   Transamination
4. Initial step of:
   Heme synthesis
   Urea synthesis

5. Nucleotide synthesis: many steps occur in cytosol:
   CPS II
   ATCase

## CYTOSKELETON

- Composed of
    - Actin filament
    - Intermediate filament
    - Microtubules
- Allows cells to move and adopt different shapes
- Play role in cell division: microtubules form mitotic spindle
- Does not affect gene expression

### Microtubules

- 25 nm thick, hollow, composed of $\alpha$ and $\beta$ tubulin subunits.
- Also, microtubules transport materials in neuronal axons.
- In cilia and flagella, microtubules are arranged as a ring of pairs surrounding two central fibers.

### Intermediate filament

- Attach to desmosomes and hemidesmosomes.
- 10 nm thick

### Actin filament

- Attach to adherens junction
- 7 nm thick
- React with myosin filament in muscle cells to bring about contraction.

### Role: Cytoskeleton

- Cell movement
- Cell division

- Determining cell shape
- Axonal transport

Cilia: Move fluid over epithelial surfaces e.g. respiratory tract

Flagella of spermatozoa: used as means of propulsion

## Applied aspect

**Immotile cilia can cause Kartagener's syndrome:**

- Sinusitis
- Bronchitis
- Situs inverses

Immotile cilia caused by fault in motor protein dynein responsible for rhythmic movement of cilia and flagella.

## Myofibrils

- Contractile element of skeletal muscle cells
- Thick filament formed by *myosin*
- Thin filament formed by *actin*

## Cell junctions

Four classes of junctions: tight, adherens, desmosomes, gap junctions

i. **Tight junctions:**
   Form a seal between cells
   Occur in bands around cell
   Form barriers for certain molecules
   Restrict movement of membrane proteins to fixed areas of cell membrane (Fig. 1.2).

ii. **Adherens junctions**
   - Tether actin molecule of neighbouring cells.

iii. **Desmosomes**
   - Join intermediate filament networks of neighbouring cells
   - Confer mechanical stability to epithelial layer by interlinking cytoskeletons cells of the joint.

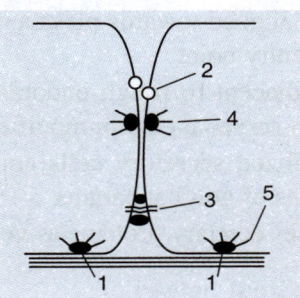

**Fig. 1.2.** Gap junctions.

- Do not allow passage of molecules between cells
- **Hemidesmosomes:**
  Anchor intermediate filament within a cell to the basal lamina

iv. **Gap Junctions**
   - Allow passage of small molecules from cytosol of one cell to another

## NUCLEUS

Large fragmental structure bounded by a double membrane and contains darker nucleolus.

- Cells in human body generally have a single nucleus.
- Skeletal muscle cells have many nuclei
- Mature RBCs have no nucleus
- Nucleus is primary store of DNA and mitochondria contain their own DNA

## GOLGI APPARATUS

- Flattened, membrane-bound organelle, disc-like membraneous cisternae
- Responsible for modification of lipid and proteins
- Sorts, modifies and transports them to targets
- Contain many distinct cisternae arranged in stacks
- Each stack has two faces:

Trans: aligned towards plasma membrane-serve entry point

Cis: adjacent to rough endoplasmic reticulum - serves as exit for modified proteins.

- Specialized secretory cells contain large amounts of golgi apparatus
- Release secretary proteins as vesicles.

## CGN: Cis Golgi network

Function as a sorting station that distinguishes between proteins to be shipped back to ER and those that are allowed to proceed to Golgi Station.

## Secretion of vesicles

They pass through plasma membrane to surrounding media e.g. Ig from plasma cells reach plasma membrane and form integral part of it forming secretory vesicle, where products are stored and released under appropriate stimuli e.g., Trypsinogen (pancreatic acinar cells), Insulin (β cells Langerhans). Targeted to lysosomes after tagging it to mannose of N-oligosaccharide.

## Endoplasmic Reticulum (ER)

System of membranes that enclose a lumen forming a network of flattened sacs (cisternae)

Two types:
- Smooth (SER)
- Rough (RER)

## SER

- Composed of tubular network throughout cytoplasm
- Also known as translational ER
- Involved in modification and detoxification of hydrophobic compounds.
- Hepatocytes have large number of SER.
- Predominates in cells specialization in lipid metabolism.

## RER

- RER is continuous with outer membrane of nuclear envelope
- Has grainy appearance on electron microscopy due to high concentration of membrane bound ribosomes.
- Involved in synthesis of proteins destined to be targeted to organelles or to function outside the cell.
- Disulphide bond formation and glycosylation occurs in RER.

## Sequence of events of protein modification in RER

Membrane-bound ribosomes in RER synthesize proteins

↓

Freed protein into ER lumen

↓

Direct protein to ER by sequence of hydrophobic amino acid residues

↓

Proteins are sorted by recognition of amino acid sequences

↓

Proteins get unfolded and pass into mitochondria and peroxisomes

## Applied aspects

Cells of pancreas, salivary gland have extensive RER.

## Functions of SER

- Synthesis of:
  Lipoprotein
  TAG
  Phospholipids
  Part of cholesterol
  Bile salts

- Steroid hormone synthesis
- Detoxification: of organic compounds: barbiturate, ethanol
- Conjugation reactions
- Sequester calcium ion

## Functions RER

- **Synthesis of proteins:**
  Mucoprotein, polypeptide hormone, insulin, glucagon, antibodies, plasma protein (albumin)
- Synthesis of integral membrane proteins other than those of mitochondria.

## MICROSOMES

When cells are fractionated, complex ER network is not isolated as a whole, but is disrupted in many places. These membranes automatically reassemble to form **Microsomes**.

### Cytochrome P$_{450}$ family

- System of oxygen transferring enzymes.
- Oxidize thousand of different hydrophobic compounds to more readily excretable hydrophilic derivatives.
- Sometimes convert harmless compounds into a potent carcinogen, e.g. benzo (a)pyrene activation
- Genetic variation of cytP$_{450}$ enzymes in humans is responsible for difference in response to many drugs in terms of effectiveness and side effects from person to person

## Cell Size

Cells and their organelle are defined in micrometers (μ):

Nucleus: 5–10 μ

Mitochondria: 2 μ

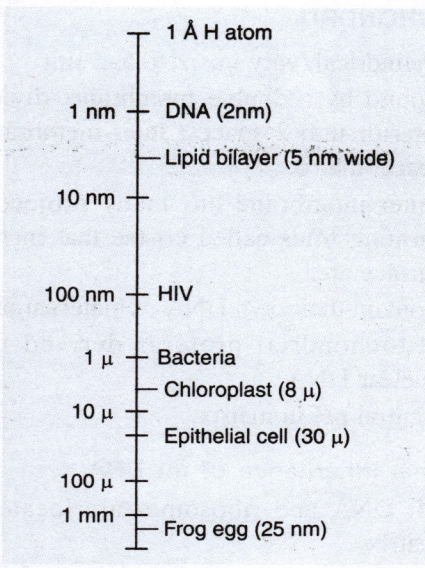

Fig. 1.3. Cell size.

Prokaryotic: Cells 1–5 μ
Eukaryotic Cell: 10–30 μ

### Fact file: Cell size

- Greater is cytoplasmic volume, longer it will take to synthesize number of messages required by that cell.
- With increase in cell size, surface area/volume ratio decreases
- Surface area determines ability of cell to exchange substances
- Cells specialized for absorption of solutes e.g. intestinal epithelium typically possesses microvilli that increase surface area for exchange.
- As cell size increases, time required for diffusion to move substances in and out of a metabolically active cell becomes longer.
- O$_2$ requires 100 microseconds to traverse a distance of 1 μm. Thus for a distance of 1 mm, it requires $10^6$ longer time.

## MITOCHONDRIA

- Cylindrical, vary in size 0.5–2 $\mu m$
- Bound by a double membrane, dividing interior into 2 spaces: inter membranous space, matrix
- Inner membrane has many projections forming folds called cristae that increase surface area.
- Contain their own DNA of maternal origin
- Mitochondrial proteins derived from nuclear DNA
- Neutral pH in matrix.

## Maternal inheritance of mt DNA

- Mt DNA and ribosomes are located in matrix
- Equipped with independent protein synthesizing machinery
- Supplies up to 35% of protein of mitochondria, rest come from nucleus
- Mitochondria have evolved from aerobic bacteria by endosymbiosis.

## Biochemistry of mitochondria

## Functions

- Power plant of cell
- Principal producer of ATP
- Operation of citric acid cycle and production of NADH
- β-oxidation of FA
- Oxidation of NADH by ETC is coupled with synthesis of ATP
- Storage of calcium ions

## E/M

Appear as sausage-shaped bodies.

## Distribution

- Liver or stomach: Distributed haphazardly
- Muscle: Packed systematically around myofibrils
- Adipocytes: Mitochondria surround large globules of TAG.

## NUCLEUS

- Largest cellular organelle
- Most prominent organelle of a cell
- All cells in body contain nucleus except RBCs
- In some cells, nucleus occupies most of available space, e.g. small lymphocyte, spermatozoa

| Enzymes/proteins in mitochondria compartment | | | | |
|---|---|---|---|---|
| OMM* | Intermembraneous | IMM+ | | Matrix |
| | | Outer | Inner | |
| MAO Acetyl CoA synthetase PLA$_2$ | Adenylate Kinase Creatine kinase Nucleotide metabolism | GA-3P DH Enzymes of respiratory chain β-OH butyrate deH | SDH | TCA β-oxidation Glutamate deH Cis aconitase Replication of mt DNA Protein synthesis Transport system: Pyruvate, malate |

* Outer mitochondrial membrane
+ Inner mitochondrial membrane

## Structure

- Bound by a double (each 8nm thick) membrane known as nuclear envelope
- Separated by 20-40nm perinuclear space
- Outer membrane (ONM) continuous with membrane of ER: dotted with ribosomes.
- ONM and inner nuclear membrane (INM) connected by nuclear pores arranged in hexagonal array of diameter: 60-90nm
- On inner side of INM lies nuclear lamina.

## Nuclear lamina

- Composed of fibrous network
- Made up of 3 major proteins: **Lamins**.
- Lamins get phosphorylated during mitosis causing break down of nuclear envelope.
- Nucleus contains DNA: repository of genetic information.
- DNA associated with histones forms: **Nucleosomes**.
- A single chromosome is composed of about a million nucleosomes

## CHROMATIN

- Assembly of nucleosomes constitute **Chromatin.**

## Components

- DNA, histone (basic proteins)
- Non histone proteins
- RNA

Humans have 46 chromosomes compactly packed in the nucleus.

Human haploid genome has $2.8 \times 10^9$ bp.

## Function

- Site of storage and replication of DNA, the genetic material

## Energy supply for nucleus

- Nucleus possesses entire glycolytic sequence of enzymes
- Some nuclei e.g. lymphocytes can carry out oxidative reactions of citric acid cycle.

## CLINICAL CONSEQUENCE

### NUCLEUS

Regulation of DNA repression and function is severally disturbed in serious pathological conditions e.g. cancer leading on to uncontrolled production of a particular hormone from normal gland or ectopic production.

### NUCLEOLUS

- Sub-cellular organelle located in nucleus
- Bead like structure
- Contain RNA particularly rRNA
- Directly reflects synthetic activity of cell
- Disappears during cell division at prophase
- Becomes associated with their satellite chromosomes

### Size

- 15 nm in diameter

### Functions

- Site of synthesis of most rRNA and where ribosome assembly begins
- Enzymes present:
  - RNA polymerase
  - Ribonuclease

### NUCLEOPLASM

Ground substance of nucleus, contains enzymes of:

- Glycolysis
- Citric acid cycle
- HMP shunt

## LYSOSOMES

- Membrane bound sacs that contain hydrolytic enzymes
- pH of lysosomal matrix: 5.0.
- Most abundant in macrophages, fewer in lymphocytes
- Lysosomes receive cellular and endocytosed proteins and lipids that need digestion and the resulting metabolites are transported either by vesicles or directly across the membrane

### Functions

- Control intracellular digestion of macromolecules
- All acid hydrolases in lysosomes are maintained at a pH 5.0 and are inactive in neutral pH of cytosol
- Suicide bag of cell

## LYSOSOMAL ENZYMES

### Features

- Protein in nature
- Synthesized in RER
- Receive n-linked oligosaccharide
- Transported to SER by pinching out as vesicle, transported to golgi complex, where mannose residue get phosphorylated and then directed to lysosomes

### Nature of lysosomal enzymes

Termed as hydrolases

**Cleave:** C-O
C-N
C-C covalent bonds

**Types:** 1. Hydrolase
2. Protease
3. Nuclease
4. Phosphatase
5. Lipid degenerating enzymes
6. Sulfatase

| Lysosomal enzymes | |
|---|---|
| *Enzyme* | *Types* |
| 1. Hydrolases | (Polysaccharide hydrolyzing enzyme) |
| | α-glucosidase |
| | β-galactosidase |
| | α-mannosidase |
| | Hyaluronidase |
| | Lysozyme (bacterial cell wall) |
| | Fucosidase |
| | Sialidase |
| 2. Protease (Protein hydrolyzing enzymes) | Cathepsin |
| | Collagenase |
| | Peptidase |
| 3. Nuclease | Acid ribonuclease |
| | Acid deoxyribonuclease |
| 4. Phosphatases | Acid phosphatase |
| | Acid phosphodiesterase |
| 5. Lipid hydrolyzing enzymes | Acid lipase |
| | Lipase |
| | Phospholipase |
| | Esterase |
| 6. Sulfatase | Iduronate sulfatase |
| | Heparan N-sulfatase |
| | β-galactosidase |

### Action of chloroquin

- Chloroquin inactivates lysosomal enzymes by neutralizing lumen of lysosomes
- In uncharged form chloroquin readily passes through lipid bilayer and enters lysosomes
- Then, chloroquin picks up proton, becomes charged and accumulates.
- Antiparasitic activity of chloroquin probably results from inhibition of parasites lysosomal hydrolases through neutralization of their lysosome.

## LIFE CYCLE OF LYSOSOMES

### Primary lysosome

- Synthesized in golgi apparatus as vesicles
- Spherical
- Do not contain particulate or membrane debris
- Here enzymes are not involved in digestive process

### Secondary lysosome

- Large irregularly-shaped vesicles in which digestion of material is underway
- Appear as a result of fusion of primary lysosomes with other membrane organelles
- Contain particles or membrane in the process of being digested
- Endocytic vesicles and phagosomes are fused with lysosomes to form secondary lysosomes

### Two pathways of life cycle of lysosomes

1. Heterophagy
2. Autophagy

## HETEROPHAGY

Endocytosis of ingested particle occurs in the form of an intracellular vesicle which fuses with a primary lysosome to form secondary lysosome. Here, active digestion of ingested particle by lysosomal enzyme occurs, amino acids or monosaccharide are released into cytoplasm for further metabolism.

Undigested material so remains forms tertiary lysosomes, which may be expelled by exocytosis.

## AUTOPHAGY

Similar to heterophagy, but the particle trapped in vacuole is usually another sub-cellular particle or organelle.

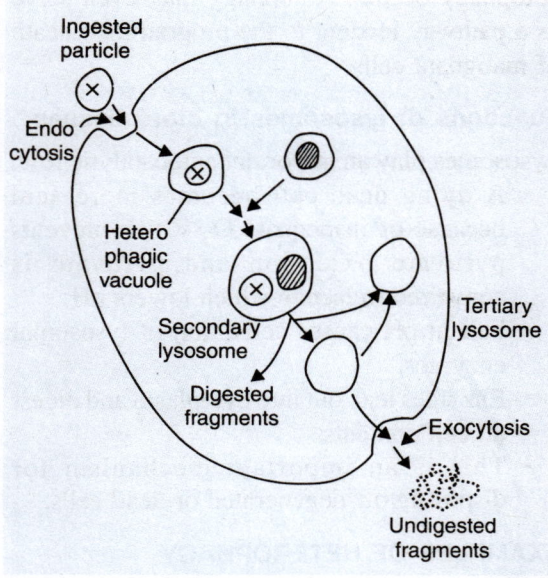

Fig. 1.4. Heterophagy.

One mitochondrion undergoes autophagy every 10min in a mammalian cell. If a cell is deprived of nutrients, a marked increase in

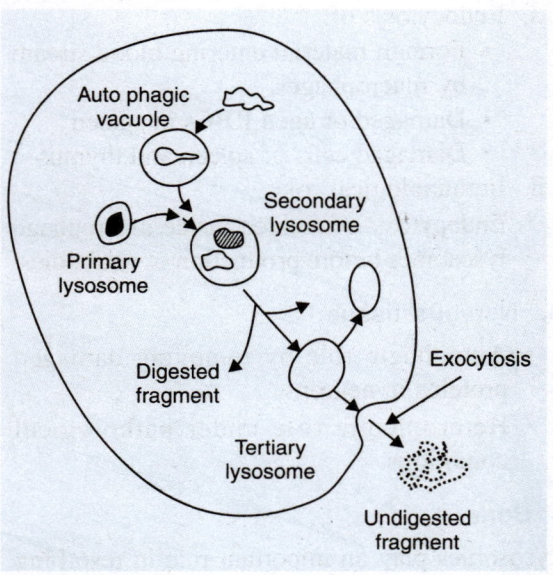

Fig. 1.5. Autophagy.

autophagy occurs. Autophagy may even serve as a pathway leading to the programmed death of malignant cells.

## Functions of lysosomes in other tissues

Lysosomes play an important autocatalytic role:
- A dying dead cell becomes more acid because of inadequate $O_2$ which prevents pyruvate oxidation and pyruvate is converted to lactate which lowers pH.
- Fall in pH causes activation of lysosomal enzymes.
- Enzymes leak out into cytoplasm and digest all cell contents.
- This is an important mechanism for disposing off degenerated or dead cells.

## EXAMPLES OF HETEROPHAGY

### 1. Kidney

Proximal tubule: albumin and Hb that have passed through glomerulus are absorbed into lysosomes, degraded by lysosomal cathepsins.

### 2. Lymphoid tissue: spleen and thymus:

  i. Endocytosis of:
   - Foreign material entering blood stream by macrophages.
   - Damaged or aged RBCs in spleen
   - Damaged cells of spleen and thymus
  ii. Immunological role:
   Endocytosis of antigen inside macrophage lysosomes before production of antibodies.

### 3. Nervous tissue

- Autophagic role by removing damaged proteins in neurons.
- Heterophagic role under pathological conditions.

### 4. Bone

Lysosomes play an important role in resorbing bone, remodeling the cells of bone by osteoclasts.

Enzymes are hyaluronidase, peptidase, and collagenase

### 5. Uterus

- Autophagy activity increases at the end of cycle
- Post partum involution of uterus occurs by both autophagy and heterophagy

### 6. Mammary gland

- Involution of mammary gland following cessation of lactation
- Autophagy reduce cytoplasmic content
- Heterophagy removes dead cell and milk

### 7. Other tissues

- Anterior pituitary
- Testis
- Prostate
- Spermatozoa (lysosomal hyaluronidase)

## CLINICAL APPLICATIONS

### 1. Gout

Phagocytosed urate crystals damage vacuole and release hydrolytic enzymes causing inflammation

### 2. Tumour metastasis

Certain cancer cells liberate cathepsins (which are normally restricted to interior of lysosomes) which:
- hydrolyze collagen and elastin
- degrade basal lamina
- tumor cells move out
- causing distant metastases

### 3. Lysosomal storage disease

  i. Tay Sach's $Gm_2$ gangliosidosis:
   Autosomal recessive
   Neurological problem
   Early death

ii. I-cell disease (inclusion cell disease):
Enzymes which phosphorylate mannose residue of glycoprotein in golgi complex to target it to lysosome are ABSENT
Severe neurological and bone deformity

## 4. Lysosomal acid lipase deficiency

- Autosomal recessive
- Deposition of TAG and cholesterol esters in tissues particularly liver
- Early onset of atherosclerosis

## 5. Apoptosis

- Lysosomes have a role in apoptosis

## 6. Glycogen storage disease type-II

- Acid maltase deficiency
- Glycogen particles taken up by autophagy
- Cannot be digested by autophagy and accumulate in lysosomes

## 7. Hurler's disease

- Deposition of GAG: dermatan sulfate
- L-iduronidase deficient in lysosomes

## PEROXISOMES

- All animal cells except RBCs contain peroxisomes
- Single membrane cellular organelles having fine granular matrix
- Also known as microbodies. 0.3–1.5 mm in diameter
- Prominent in WBCs and platelets, contain oxidative enzymes involving $H_2O_2$
- Contain enzymes that oxidize:
  – D-amino acid
  – Uric acid
  – Long chain FA (oxidation)

– Synthesis of glycerolipids and plasmalogens
- $H_2O_2$ produced in these reactions are detoxified by catalase.

## ZELLWEGER SYNDROME

- Absence of functional peroxisome
- Autosomal recessive
- Very long chain FA accumulate
- Bile acid synthesis abnormality
- Dying in one year

| Metabolic functions of subcellular organelles | |
|---|---|
| *Organelle* | *Functions* |
| Nucleus | DNA replication, transcription |
| ER | Biosynthesis of: proteins, gly-coproteins, lipoproteins |
| | Ethanol oxidation |
| | Drug metabolism |
| | FA desaturation |
| | Synthesis of cholesterol |
| Golgi apparatus | Maturation of synthesized proteins |
| Lysosome | Degradation of proteins, carbo-hydrates, lipids, nucieotides |
| Mitochondria | ET chain |
| | ATP generation |
| | TCA cycle oxidation |
| | FA, KB production |
| | Heme, urea synthesis (part) |
| Cytosol | Protein synthesis |
| | Glycolysis |
| | Glycogen metabolism |
| | HMP shunt |
| | Transamination |
| | FA synthesis |
| | Cholesterol synthesis (part) |
| | Purine, pyrimidine synthesis (part) |

**Other defects**

- Neonatal adrenoleukodystropy
- Infantile Refsum disease

**How we study cells**

- Microscopes provide windows to the world of the cell
- Cell biologists can isolate organelles to study their function.

## CELL FRACTIONATION

### Goal

To separate major organelles of the cells so that their individual functions can be studied

- Uses ultracentrifuge
- Fractionation begins with homogenization, gently disrupting the cell
- Mixture is spun in centrifuge to separate heavier pieces into the pellet
- At higher speed and longer durations, smaller organelles can be collected in subsequent pellets

**Use**

- Cell fractionation prepares quantities of specific cell components.
- Functions, and structure of organelle can be studied.

## SUB-CELLULAR FRACTIONATION (SCF)

Breaking open of a cell (by homogenization) and separation of organelles from one another by centrifugation.

### Steps

- Extraction
- Homogenization
- Centrifugation

  Then subject it to:
  - EM
  - Marker enzyme

### Application: SCF

- Major component of experimental approach
- Functions of organelles have been elucidated

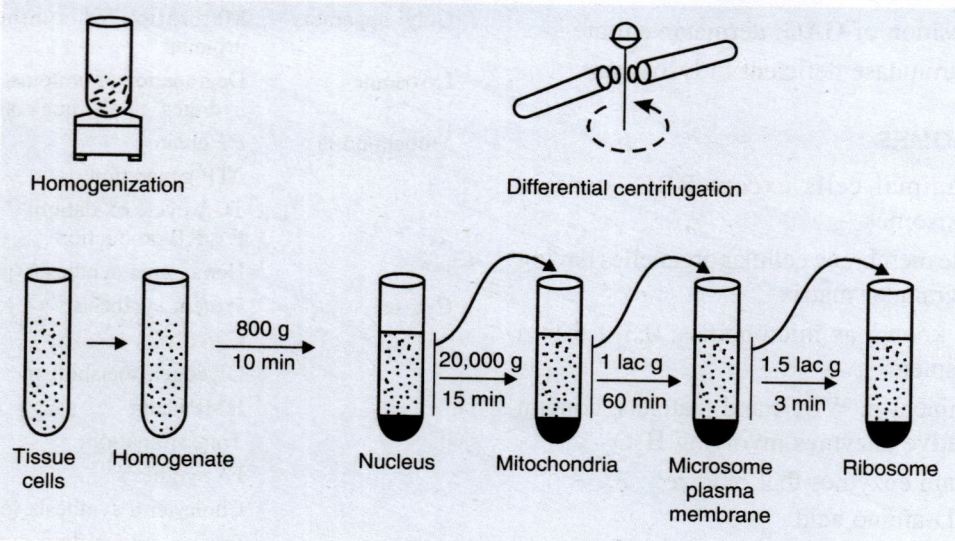

**Fig. 1.6.** Cell fractionation.

## Marker enzymes

A marker is a chemical or enzyme that is almost exclusively combined to one particular organelle.

| Organelle | Marker |
|---|---|
| Nucleus | DNA, RNA, Adenyl transferase |
| Mitochondria | MAO |
| OMM | Sulfite oxidase |
| Intermembraneous | Cyt c oxidase, SDH |
| IMM | Glutamate deH |
| Matrix | High content of RNA |
| Ribosome | Cathepsin, acid phosphatase |
| Lysosomes | Galactosyl transferase |
| Golgi apparatus | Catalase, uric acid oxidase |
| Peroxisome | D-amino acid oxidase |
| Cytosol Microsome (ER) | LDH, G-6-Pase, NADPH – cyt reductase |

## Marker enzymes of different membranes

| Membrane | | Enzyme |
|---|---|---|
| Plasma | | 5'NTD, Adenyl cyclase, $Na^+$, $K^+$ ATPase |
| ER | | G-6-Pase |
| Golgi | Cis | Glc NAc transferase I |
| | medial | Golgi mannosidase II |
| | trans | Galactosyl transferase |
| IMM | | ATP synthase |

## Whole cells can also be used to study biochemical processes

Applicable to:
- Blood cells can be purified easily
- Cells in tissue culture

## Methods

1. Purification of cells: on basis of density.
2. Flow cytometry: separates different cell types.
3. Fluorescence-activated cell sorter (FACS): can select one cell from thousands of other cells. E.g. WBC.

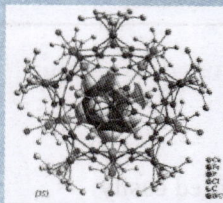

# Chemistry and Membrane Transport

## CHEMISTRY

## I. Carbohydrates: Structure and Function

### Features

- Widely distributed
- Most abundant biologic molecule
- Have structural and metabolic role
- Polyhydroxy aldehydes or ketones
- General formula: $(CH_2O)_n$, where $n \geq 3$

### Importance of Glucose

- Universal fuel for fetus
- Major fuel for all tissues, even microbes in our intestines
- Form structural component of membrane
- Form carbohydrate with specific function:

- Ribose – nucleotides
- Galactose – lactose in milk
- Glycolipid
- Glycoprotein.

### Classification

Monosaccharide, disaccharide, oligosaccharide, polysaccharide

### MONOSACCHARIDES

Formula: $(CH_2O)_n$

Based on number of carbon:
- with three carbons: triose
- with four carbons: tetrose
- with five carbons: pentose
- with six carbons: hexose

Based on functional groups:

Aldehyde: Aldose

Ketone: Ketose

## Classification

| Sr. No. | Class | Sub-class | Examples | |
|---------|-------|-----------|----------|---|
| | | | *Aldose* | *Ketose* |
| 1. | Monosaccharide | Triose | Glycerol | Dihydroxy acetone |
| | | Tetrose | Erythrose | Erythrulose |
| | | Pentose | Ribose | Ribulose |
| | | Hexose | Glucose | Fructose |
| 2. | Disaccharide (composed of two monosaccharide) | Maltose | 2glucose units $\alpha 1 \rightarrow 4$ glycosidic bond | |
| | | Sucrose | $\alpha$D glucose $+\beta$ D fructose $\alpha 1 \rightarrow \beta_2$ bond | |
| | | Lactose | $\alpha$D galactose $+ \beta$D glucose $1 \rightarrow \beta_4$ bond | |
| 3. | Oligosaccharide (composed of 2-10 monosaccharide units, O-linked) (attached to OH group) e.g. IgA<br><br>N-linked (attached to protein via N-glycosidic bond e.g. Aspartate side chain) e.g. dolichol phosphate | Malto-triose | Maltose and $\alpha 1 \rightarrow 6$ glucose | |
| 4. | Polysaccharide (10 or more monosaccharide unit) and their derivatives | –<br><br>– | Amylose<br>$\alpha$DG: $\alpha 1 \rightarrow 4$ bond<br>Amylopectin 24–30 monomers<br><br>($\alpha$D glucose) $1 \rightarrow 4$ linkage plus $\alpha 1 \rightarrow 6$ branching<br>**Homopolysaccharide**:<br>Contain only one kind of monosacharides<br>Starch: $\alpha 1 \rightarrow 4$ linkage and $\alpha 1 \rightarrow 6$ branching<br>Glycogen: 12-14 monomers of D-glucose $\alpha 1 \rightarrow 4$ linkage and $\alpha 1 \rightarrow 6$ branching | |
| | | | Cellulose | $\beta$D glucose<br>$\beta 1 \rightarrow 4$ bond |
| | | | Inulin | $\beta$D fructose |
| | | | Dextran* | $\alpha$D glucose linked at $\alpha 1 \rightarrow 6$ bond, with few branches |

\* Dextran: breakdown product of starch

Limit dextrin: formed when hydrolysis of starch reaches a branch point.

## Heteropolysaccharides

Composed of repeating units of monosaccharides, their derivative or proteoglycans.

| *Mucopolysaccharides  (Glycosamainoglycans)* | *Mucoprotein (Glycoprotein)* |
|---|---|
| Hyaluronic acid | Sialic acid |
| Chondroitin sulfate | Neuraminic acid |
| Dermatan sulfate | Gangliosides |
| Keratan sulfate | |
| Heparin sulfate | |

## GAG

| GAG | Repeating unit | Tissue distribution | Function |
|---|---|---|---|
| Hyaluronic acid | GlcUA and GlcNA<br>GlcUA $\xrightarrow{\beta1,3}$<br>GlcNAc $\xrightarrow{\beta1\rightarrow3}$ GlcUA | Synovial fluid | Vitreous body, eye, cartilage, loose connective tissue |
| Chondroitin | GlcUA<br>GalNAc | Cartilage | To maintain structure and function of tissues located at the site of calcification in endochondral bone |
| Dermatan sulfate | IdUA, GalNAc<br>IdUA $\xrightarrow{\beta1,3}$ GalNAc | Skin, valves, blood vessels lung, sclera | Sclera: maintain shape of eye ball |
| Keratin sulfate | GlcNAc, Gal<br>GlcNAc $\xrightarrow{\beta1,3}$<br>Gal $\xrightarrow{\beta1\rightarrow4}$ GlcNAc | Cornea bone, cartilage, horny structures, hair, nail | Corneal transparency |
| | Linked to protein via:<br>N-linkage (type1)<br>O-linkage (type 2) | Cornea<br>Loose connective tissue | Corneal transparency<br>Ground substance |
| Heparan sulfate | GlcN, GlcUA,<br>GlcN $\xrightarrow{\alpha1\rightarrow4}$<br>GlcUA$\rightarrow$ GlcN | Lung, muscle, liver, component of synapse, glomerulus, vesicles | Present on cell surface or bound to ECM, responsible for charge selectiveness |
| Heparin | GlcN, IdUA<br>IdUA $\xrightarrow{\alpha1,4}$ GlcN | Granules of mast cells, liver, lung, skin | Function as intracellular binding site, anticoagulant, bind to lipoproteins lipase causing LP release |

Key: GlcUA – glucuronic acid, GlcN – glucosamine, A – Acetyl

## Organ and site specific functions of GAG

| GAG | Organ | Site | Function |
|---|---|---|---|
| Heparin sulfate | Liver | Intracellular on cell surface | Anticoagulant |
| Heparan sulfate | Kidney | Renal basement membrane | Charge selectivity of glomerulus |
| Keratan sulfate<br>Dermatan sulfate | Cornea | In between collagen fibers | Corneal transparency |
| Heparin | Mast cells | Secretory granules | Inflammatory response |
| Heparin sulfate | Vascular wall | - | Anticoagulant activation of lipoprotein lipase |

## Disease associated with GAG

| GAG | Disease |
|---|---|
| Hyaluronic acid (HA) | Permit tumor cells to migrate through extracellular matrix<br>Tumor cells induce fibroblasts to synthesize increased amounts of HA, facilitating their own spread |
| Heparan sulfate | Tumor cells lack this GAG, results: lack of adhesiveness of these cells |
| HA, chondroitin sulfate, heparin sulfate, dermatan sulfate | Arterial smooth muscle cell proliferation in atherosclerotic lesions and plaque |
| GAG | Arthritis, Autoantigens |
| Chondroitin sulfate | Diminishes in cartilage with age, contributing to development of osteo-arthritis |
| HA, keratin sulfate | Increase in cartilage with age, causes osteoarthritis |
| GAG in skin | Characteristic changes of age occur in skin |

## Carbohydrate derivatives

| Sr. No. | Derivatives | Example | Location/constituent of |
|---|---|---|---|
| 1. | Amino sugar | Glucosamine<br>Galactosamine<br>Neuraminic acid | Chitin<br>Cartilage, chondroitin sulfate |
| 2. | Sugar acids | Ascorbic acid, glucuronic acid | Vitamin C, proteoglycan |
| 3. | Deoxy sugar | 2-deoxyribose | DNA |
| 4. | Sugar alcohol | D-sorbitol, D-mannitol | Minor pathway intermediates |
| 5. | Phosphoric acid esters | D-glucose-1-phosphate | Minor pathway intermediates |

## OXIDATION OF CARBOHYDRATES

### Oxidized forms

(a) Gluconic acid, 6 phosphogluconate
(b) Uronic acid, glucuronic acid

### Structure: Monosaccharides

All monosaccharides are optically active due to presence of atleast one asymmetric carbon.

### Asymmetric carbon

• Carbon atom bonded to four different atoms or groups of atoms is asymmetric carbon.

### Isomers

Presence of asymmetric carbon allows formation of isomers and the number of isomers of a compound depends on the number of asymmetric carbon atoms (n) and is equal to $2^n$, e.g. glucose has 4 asymmetric carbon atoms, thus $2^4 = 16$ isomers.

### Anomer

New carbon formed during cyclization is anomeric carbon, e.g. during hemiacetal and hemiketal formation (e.g. $C_1$ in glucose).

Depending on the size of ring formed,

## Blood group antigens

| Antigen | Structure |
|---------|-----------|
| O | Fucose – Galactose<br>\|<br>N-Acetyl glucosamine<br>\|<br>R |
| A | NAc Galactosamine<br>\|<br>Fucose- Galactose<br>\|<br>N-Acetyl glucosamine-R |
| B | Galactose<br>\|<br>Fucose-Galactose<br>\|<br>N-Acetyl<br>\|<br>glucosamine<br>\|<br>R |

## Isomerism

structure is designated pyranose, if it is 6-membered ring or furanose, if it is 5-membered ring. A six membered ring structure can adopt either a chair or boat configuration. D-glucose adopts a chair conformation.

## Mutarotation

$\alpha$ and $\beta$-forms equilibrate via the straight chain aldehyde form. This occurs due to opening of hemiacetal ring.

## Reducing sugar

Sugar possessing free anomeric carbon atom that is not involved in a glycosidic linkage is reducing sugar. The end containing free anomeric carbon is reducing end.

This free aldehyde or ketone group reduces alkaline copper sulfate, e.g. Lactose, maltose.

Sucrose is a non-reducing sugar, because glycosidic bond between anomeric carbon C1

| Sr. No. | Isomerism | Reasoning | Example |
|---------|-----------|-----------|---------|
| 1. | D-L isomerism (stereoisomer) | • Same chemical formula<br>• Differ in position of –OH group on one or more asymmetric carbon (e.g. C5 in glucose) Mirror images of each other | D, L glucose (Fig. 2.1) |
| 2. | Optical isomerism (Enantiomer) | Presence of asymmetric carbon rotate plane polarized light either to right [dextrorotatory, (+)] or to left [levorotatory (–)] | Enantiomer<br>(+) isomer<br>(–) isomer |
| 3. | Epimerism | Differ as a result of variation in configuration of –OH and –H glucose on C-2, 3 and 4 of glucose, galactose at $C_4$ and mannose at C-2 or conformation that differ only at one carbon atom | Mannose at C-2 (Fig. 2.2)<br>Galactose at C-4 |
| 4. | Anomerism | Differ in configuration at carbonyl or anomeric carbon | $\alpha$ anomer, $\beta$ anomer (Fig. 2.3)<br>$\alpha$:- OH on anomeric is below plane of ring,<br>$\beta$:- OH is above plane of ring |
| 5. | Aldose-ketose isomerism | Same molecular formula, but due to position of carbonyl carbon | Glucose: C-1 is aldehyde fructose (Fig. 2.4). C-2 is keto (Fig. 2.5) |

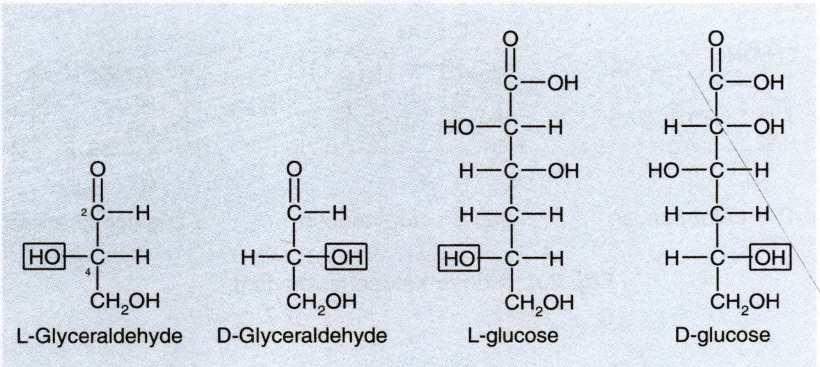

**Fig. 2.1.** D-L isomerism (Glyceraldehyde).

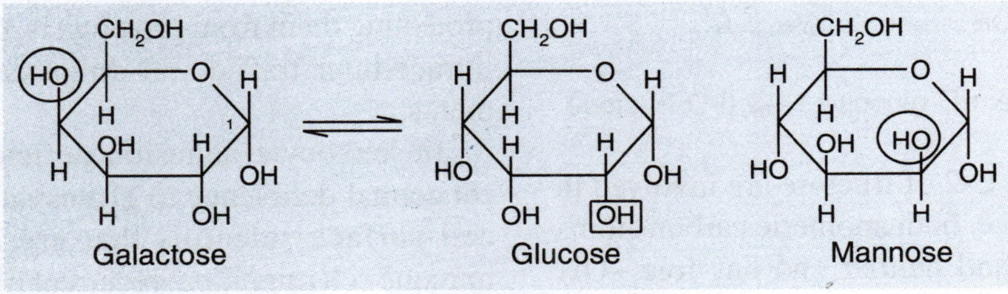

**Fig. 2.2.** Epimerism.

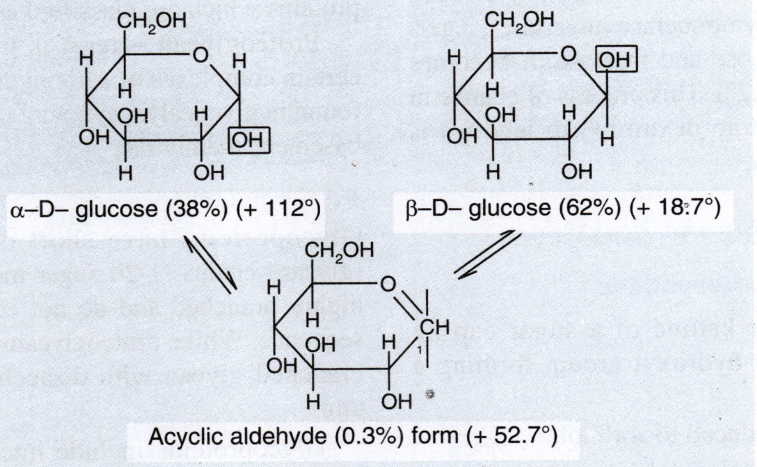

**Fig. 2.3.** Mutarotation (Anomerism).

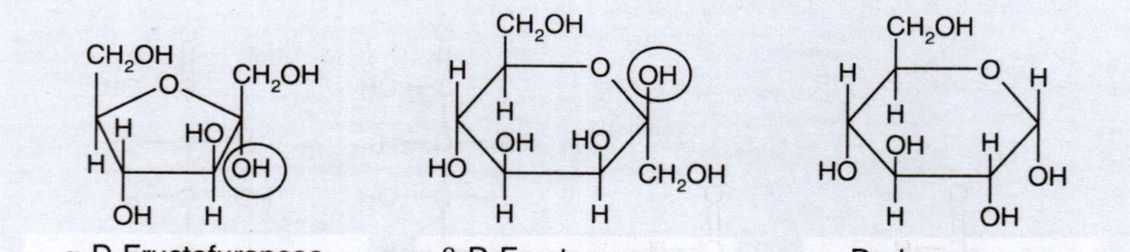

**Fig. 2.4.** Aldose-ketose isomerism.

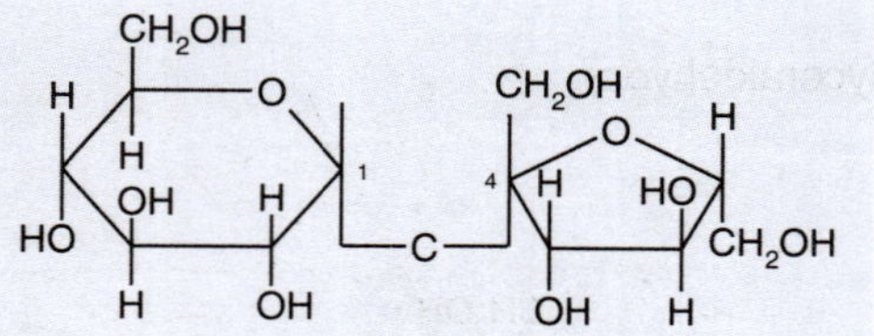

**Fig. 2.5.** Sucrose: αD glucose 1→2 β-D fructose.

of a glucose and C-2 of fructose are involved in bond formation i,e. both anomeric carbon atoms are substituted and neither end has free –OH group (Fig. 2.5).

### Inversion of sugar

Sucrose is dextrorotatory (+66.5°) and on hydrolysis by enzyme sucrase (invertase), it gets converted to glucose and fructose. It becomes levorotatory (–28.2°). This process of change in optical rotation from dextro (+) to levo (–) is inversion of sugar.

## TESTS FOR REDUCING SUGARS

### Reduction of carbohydrates

- Aldehyde or ketone of a sugar can be reduced to a hydroxyl group, forming a polyol.
- Glucose is reduced to sorbitol
- Galactose to galactitol
- Sorbitol does not readily diffuse out of cells

and accumulates in cells causing osmotic damage to neurons and cataract.

### Glycosylation of proteins

This can alter protein and modify their function, protecting them from proteolysis, directing their intracellular traffic and direct cellular movements.

In leukocyte adhesion deficiency (LAD), congenital deficiency to glycosylate ligands for cell surface selectins that are required for immune cell migration; recurrent life threatening infections are common in such patients.

### Glycoproteins (Mucoproteins)

Carbohydrate is found attached to many globular proteins which are classified as glycoproteins.

Proteoglycan – term is used to describe certain complexes of carbohydrate and proteins found in glycocalyx, synovial fluid of joints and basement membrane.

### Proteoglycans

Glycoproteins have short oligosaccharide (glycan) chains (1-20 sugar moiety in length), highly branched and do not contain repeating sequence. While, proteoglycans are long, linear, branched glycan with disaccharide repeating units.

Glycoproteins include integral membrane proteins that function as receptors for hormones or other molecules.

## Functions of glycoprotein

| Function | Example |
|---|---|
| Structural | Component of plasma membrane |
| Lubricant | Component of mucus |
| Receptor | Hormone, other molecules |
| Hormone | hCG, thyrotropin, erythropoietin |
| Immune system | Immunoglobulin, complement, interferon |
| Transport | Recognition signal |
| Cell-cell interaction | Mediate cell to cell interaction |
| Stabilization | Stabilize protein against denaturation, proteolysis |

## Protein carbohydrate linkages

Protein carbohydrate linkages are of two types:

- O-linkage
- N-linkage

**O-linkage:** Sugar is attached via –OH group of a serine or threonine residue.

**N-linkage:** Sugar is attached via amide $-NH_2$ group of asparagine residue.

## O-linked Oligosaccharides

Proteins in mucous secretions contain oligosaccharides linked by a glycosidic linkage

## Glycoprotein structure and function

| | |
|---|---|
| **Collagen** | Glycosyl-galactose disaccharide linked to hydroxylysine residue. **In tendon:** collagen is less glycosylated, form ordered fibrous structure **In basement membrane:** Collagen is heavily glycosylated, form meshwork structure |
| **Mucin** | O-linked oligosaccharides containing sialic acid, galactose and GalNAc mainly, sometimes GlcNAc and fucose **Salivary mucin:** contain unusually large number of serine or threonine residues glycosylated with a sialic acid-galactose GalNAc trisaccharide. O-linked oligosaccharides are negatively charged (due to presence of sialic acid), repel each other to prevent protein folding and assume an extended state, yielding a highly viscous (mucous) solution |
| **LDL receptor** | Found in plasma membrane of smooth muscle cells and fibroblasts Contain two N-linked biantennary complex chains in addition to a cluster of O-linked chains attached to membrane Attached to hydrophobic amino acid region which keep LDL in extended state **Biantennary:** Terminal trisaccharide sequences, one attached to each mannose |
| **Protein folding** | N-linked oligosaccharides help in protein folding in ER |
| **Cell-cell interaction** | Provide specific cell recognition and is a key factor in fertilization, inflammation, development and differentiation, virus infectivity |
| **Targeting of lysosomal enzymes** | Lysosomal enzymes are n-linked glycoproteins and sorted by exposing Man-6-P structures (by hexosaminidase) which are recognized by Man-6-P receptor in golgi |
| **Protein stability and solubility** | Proteins secreted from cells such as plasma proteins are conferred increased solubility and stability by oligosaccharide chains |

## Mucopolysaccharidosis

| Genetic defects of proteoglycan metabolism | | |
|---|---|---|
| *Syndrome* | *Defect* | *Products accumulated in lysosome* |
| I Hurler | α-1-iduronidase[4] | Heparan sulfate (HS), Dermatan sulfate (DS) |
| II Hunter | Iduronate sulfatase[3] | HS, DS |
| III Sanfilipino A | Heparin sulfatase | HS |
| Sanfilipino B | NAc glucosaminidase | |
| Sanfilipino C | NAc Gln-6-sulfatase[1] | |
| IV Morquio's | Galactose-6-sulfatase | KS |
| V Maroteaux-Lamy | NAc Gal-4-sulfatase | DS |
| VI Sly | β-glucuronidase | DS, HS |

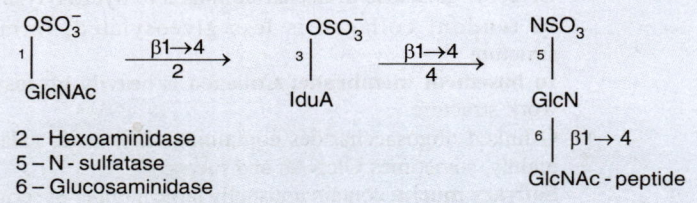

2 – Hexoaminidase
5 – N - sulfatase
6 – Glucosaminidase

**Fig 2.6.** Lysosomal degradation of HS.

between N-acetyl galactosamine (GalNAc) and hydroxyl group of serine or threonine residues.

### N-linked oligosaccharides

Always attached by glycosylamine linkage of N-acetyl glucosamine (GlcNAc) to amide nitrogen of asparagine residue; characteristic of plasma and membrane proteins; Mucopolysaccharidosis.

### Clinical features of lysosomal storage disease

- Skeletal deformity
- Mental retardation
- Early death in severe cases

### Diagnosis

- Urine GAG
- Leukocyte/fibroblast assay for specific enzymes

# II. Lipids: Structure And Function

## LIPID CHEMISTRY

Lipids of major physiologic significance are fatty acids, their ester, cholesterol and steroids.

## Fact file: Lipids

- Hydrophobic
- Insoluble in water, soluble in polar solvents.

- Composed of saturated or unsaturated long chain hydrocarbons with a carboxyl group at end of chains.
- Important dietary constituent.
- Serve as:
  - Source of energy
  - Thermal insulator
  - Important component of cell membrane
  - Lipoprotein serves transport function
  - Storage: TAG, stored in adipose tissue
  - Precursor for steroid hormones

## General formula

Saturated fatty acid:

$$CH_3 - [CH_2]_n - COOH$$

N = number of methylene groups

Systemic name gives number of carbons followed by acid suffix.

- anoic for saturated FA
- enoic for unsaturated FA
  e.g. Palmitic acid, 16C: hexadecanoic acid.

## Important points

- Carbons are numbered from carboxyl carbon (carbon no. 1).
- Carbon adjacent to it is carbon no. 2 ($\alpha$-carbon).

- Terminal methyl carbon is $\omega$-carbon or n-carbon.
- Position of double bond:
- $\Delta^9$: double bond between C9 and 10
- $\omega^9$: double bond on 9th carbon

## Fatty acids

- Exist as free or esterified to glycerol.
- Humans have FA with even number of carbon atoms: 16-20 carbon in length, saturated or unsaturated. The aliphatic chain may be saturated or unsaturated (containing one or more double bonds).

## Neutral lipids

Being uncharged, acyl glycerols, cholesterol and cholesterol esters are termed neural lipids.

## CLASSIFICATION

- Simple
- Complex
- Precursor and derived lipids

## 1. Simple lipids

Esters of FA with alcohol:

i. Fats – esters of FA with glycerol
ii. Waxes – esters of FA with higher molecular weight alcohols.

| Name | No. of carbon atom | Systemic name | Double |
|------|--------------------|---------------|--------|
| Lauric acid | 12 | Dodecanoic acid | - |
| Myristic acid | 14 | Tetradecanoic acid | - |
| Palmitic acid | 16 | Hexadecanoic acid | - |
| Stearic acid | 18 | Octadecanoic acid | - |
| Palmitoleic acid | 16 | Cis-Hexadecenoic acid | 1:9 ($\omega$9) |
| Oleic acid | 18 | Cis-Octadecenoic acid | 1:9 ($\omega$9) |
| Elaidic acid | 18 | Trans-octadecenoic acid | 1:9 ($\omega$9) |
| Linoleic acid | 18 | Cis-9, 12 octadecoidenoic acid | 2:9, 12 ($\omega$6) |
| Linolenic acid | 18 | Cis-9, 12, 15 octadecatrienoic acid | 3:9, 12, 15 ($\omega$3) |
| Arachidonic acid | 20 | Cis 5, 8, 11, 14 Eicosatetraenoic acid | 4:5, 8, 11, 14 ($\omega$6) |

## 2. Complex lipids

Esters of FA with alcohol and containing an additional group

i. **Phospholipids:**
Esters of FA with alcohol and phosphoric acid residue.
Alcohol can be glycerol : glycerophospholipids.
Alcohol can be sphingosine: sphingophospholipids.

ii. **Glycolipids (Glycosphingolipids):**
Esters of FA, contain sphingosine and a carbohydrate

iii. **Other complex lipids:**
Sulfolipids, aminolipids, lipoproteins

## 3. Precursor and derived lipids

Include fatty acids, glycerol, steroids, alcohol in addition to glycerol and sterols, fatty aldehydes, and ketone bodies, hydrocarbons, lipid-soluble vitamins and hormones.

## Unsaturated fatty acid

May contain one or more double bonds
- Mono unsaturated: One double bond
- Polyunsaturated: Two or more double bond
- Eicosanoids: Prostanoid, leukotriene, prostacyclin, thromboxane

## Isomerism in unsaturated fatty acid

- Naturally occurring unsaturated FA have cis double bonds.
- Display geometric isomerism

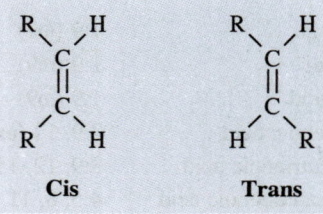

**Cis**          **Trans**

- In cis configuration, molecule bent at 120° in double bond and produces kinks.
- In trans configuration, molecule remains straight at double bond.
- With increase in chain length, melting point of even- numbered fatty acids increases and it decreases with unsaturation.

## Triacylglycerol

- Ester of fatty acid and glycerol
- Naturally occurring fat, storage form of fat

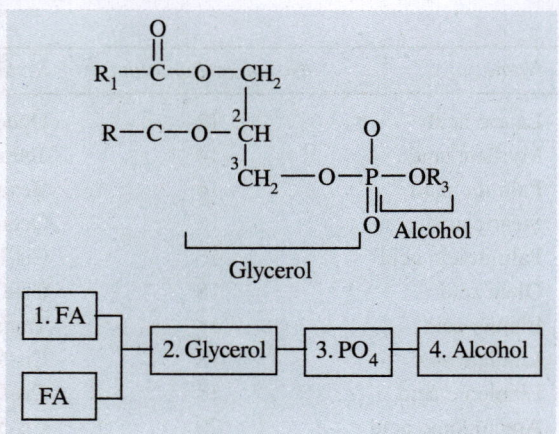

$R_1$ and $R_3$: saturated FA
$R_2$: unsaturated

## 1. Glycerophospholipids (GPL)

- Major class of membrane lipids
- Abundant in all biological membrane.

## Phospholipid

1. Fatty acid
2. Platform back bone with FA attached
3. $PO_4$
4. Alcohol attached to $PO_4$

FA components provide hydrophobic barrier and remainder is hydrophilic

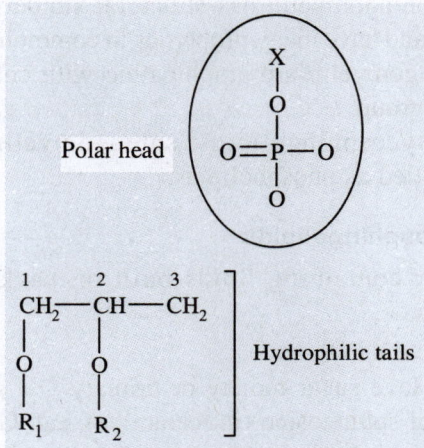

Thus GPL contain:

– phosphorylated head
– 3-C glycerol back bone
– 2 hydrocarbon fatty acid chains

Simplest GPL is phosphatidic acid or diacylglycerol

GPL include:

• Phosphatidylcholine (PC)
• Phosphatidyl ethanolamine (PE)
• Phosphatidyl serine (PS)
• Phosphatidylcholine glycerol
• Phosphatidylcholine inositol
• Diphosphatidyl glycerol (Cardiolipin):

Present exclusively in inner mitochondrial membrane.

GPL contain two fattty acyl groups esterified to C-1 and C-2 of glycerol.

| | $C_1$ | $C_2$ |
|---|---|---|
| PC | Palmitic/stearic acid | Oleic, linoleic, linolenic acid |
| PE | Contains palmitic acid on $C_1$ or oleic acid | Arachidonic acid |

Usually, on C-1, saturated FA is found: e.g. palmitic, stearic acid and on C-2, unsaturated FA is present e.g. oleic, linoleic, linolenic acid.

Designation of GPL does not specify which FA is present as seen in case of P.C. and P.E.

Saturated FA: is a straight chain.

Unsaturated FA: can be trans, however, usually cis occurs naturally and produces a kink.

There is a high degree of coiling of hydrocarbon chain in a glycerophospholipid that is disrupted by a double bond.

### Glycerol ether phospholipids

• α-β unsaturated.
• Plasmalogen is ethanolamine ether/ choline esterified to $PO_4$.

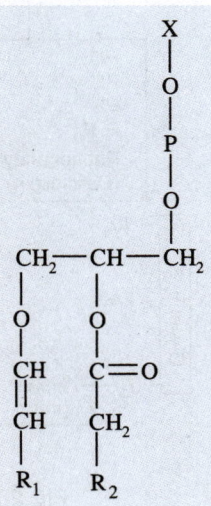

Ethanolamine plasmalogen – abundant in nervous tissue and heart.

Thus, glycosphingolipids are amphipathic, contains:

- Polar end or head group because of charged $PO_4$ and substitution on $PO_4$
- Non-polar tail due to hydrophobic carbohydrates chains of fatty acyl groups.

Every tissue and cellular membrane has a distinct composition of GPL and a definite pattern of FA composition.

## 2. Sphingolipids

In sphingomyelin, terminal OH group of sphingosine is esterified to phosphorylcholine, so that its polar head similar to P.C. (Fig. 2.7).

- 2nd major class
- Contains sphingosine back bone rather than glycerol

- Sphingosine (amino alcohol) is basis of sphingolipids
- Sphingosine is linked to FA by amide bond forming CERAMIDE
- Sphingomyelin has P.C. esterified to 1-OH group: Most abundant sphingolipid in mammalian tissues.

Sphingomyelin has structural similarity to GPL and have many properties in common, e.g. Sphingomyelin are amphipathic with charged head group.

Glycosphingolipids, sphingomyelin are classified as phospholipids.

## Glycosphingolipids

Sugar containing lipids built on backbone ceramide.

- Lack $PO_4$
- Have sugar moiety or primary OH group of sphingosine (in ceramide), e.g. Gluco-cerebroside –present in non neuronal tissue

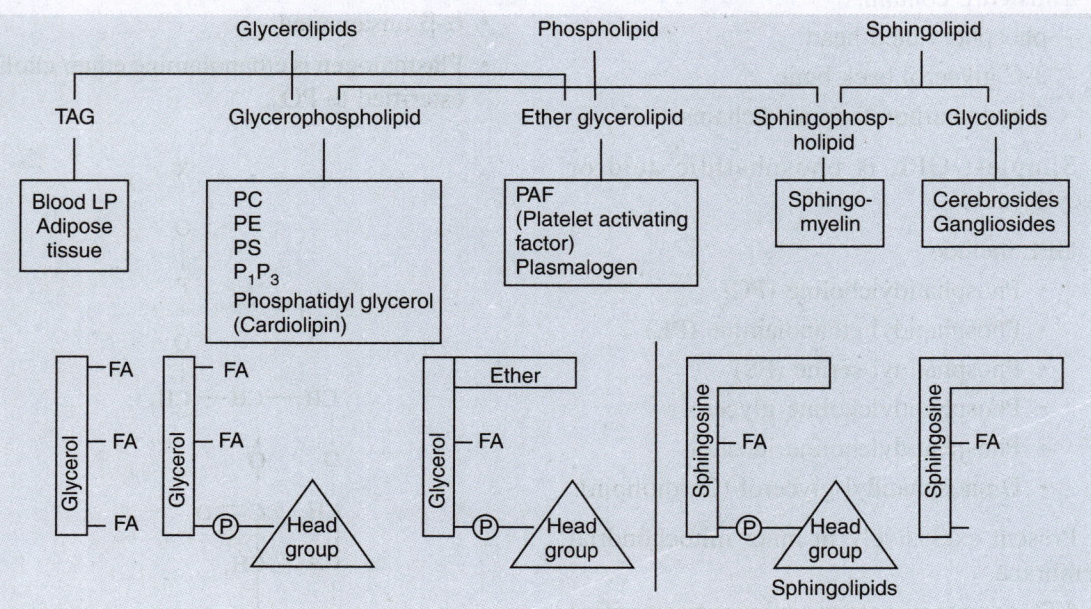

**Fig 2.7.** Types of glycolipids and sphingolipids.

- Galactocerebroside – present in brain and nervous tissue
- Ganglioside contain sialic acid residue in head groups. Present in brain (represent 5-8% of total lipid in brain).

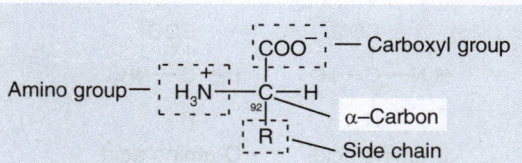

Fig. 2.8. General structure of amino acid chain.

# III. Proteins: Structure and Function

## PROTEINS

| Table 2.1. Functions of proteins |
|---|
| Structural: make up cytoskeleton to provide structure and strength to cells |
| * Component of:    – Collagen<br>                 – Elastin<br>                 – Keratin |
| Enzyme catalysis |
| Transport |
| Storage |
| Hormone |
| Blood coagulation |
| Immunity |
| Control of gene expression |

There are about 300 amino acids present in nature and only 20 $\alpha$-amino acids coded by genetic code appear in proteins. Additional amino acids occur in specific protein by "post translational" modifications of these 20 common amino acids, e.g. Peptidyl proline-4-hydroxy proline, Peptidyl lysine-5 hydroxy lysine, Peptidyl glutamate-$\gamma$-carboxy glutamate.

### Amino Acids

Amino acids are functional units of proteins. Amino acids are composed of two **functional groups** – amino ($-NH_2$), carboxyl ($-COOH$); a hydrogen atom ($-H$) and a **distinctive side**-chain ($-R$), attached to a central carbon termed $\alpha$-**carbon**.

Except for glycine, all acids contain at least one asymmetric carbon atom ($\alpha$-carbon atom).

$$H_2N - \underset{\underset{R}{|}}{\overset{\overset{H}{|}}{C}} - COOH$$

Fig. 2.9. Structure of amino acid.

- $NH_2$ = amino group (basic)
- $COOH$ = carboxyl group (acidic)
- R = side chain

Of these 20 amino acids, only **proline** is an imino acid ($-NH-$), and not an $\alpha$-amino acid.

### Optical Activity

Due to tetrahedral orientation of four different group about $\alpha$-carbon atom, amino acids exhibit optical isomerism. (i.e. ability to rotate plane polarized light).

These isomers are non-superimposable mirror images and referred to as **enantiomers**.

The two amino acid configuration (based on configuration of D and L-glyceraldehyde) are D-(dextro or right) and L-(levo or left) (Fig. 2.10).

**Only L-$\alpha$-amino acids** occur in proteins.

### Amphoteric properties of amino acids

Amino acids have two ionizable weak acid groups, $-COOH$ and an $NH_3^+$. In aqueous solution, amino acids exist as **Zwitterions** i.e., they have both positive and negative charges.

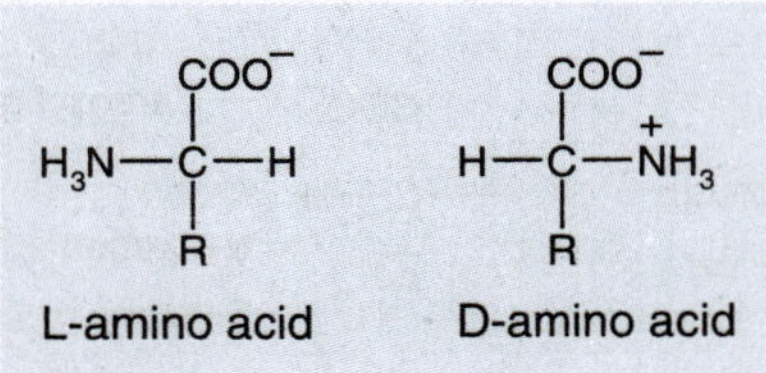

**Fig. 2.10.** Amino acid configuration.

The α-carboxyl group is negatively charged and α-amino group is positively charged and overall molecule is **electrically neutral**. At **low pH**, amino acid is positively charged (cation) and at **high pH**, amino acid is negatively charged (anion). The pH at which a molecule exists as a Zwitterion (electrically neutral) is termed **isoelectric pH** and is electrically neutral.

## Classification of amino acids

### (a) Based on Structure

On the basis of side chain (–R) attached to α-carbon atom, amino acids can be divided into polar and non polar amino acids.

### Table 2.2.

| Polar (hydrophilic) | Non polar (hydrophilic) |
|---|---|
| Glycine | Alanine |
| Serine | Leucine |
| Threonine | Isoleucine |
| Cysteine | Valine |
| Arginine | Methionine |
| Histidine | Proline |
| Lysine | Tyrosine |
| Aspartate | Phenylalanine |
| Asparagine | Tryptophan |
| Glutamate | |
| Glutamine | |

### (b) Based on side chain

Polar amino acids are exposed on surface of proteins and non-polar one are buried in hydrophobic core of a protein.

### Table 2.3. L-/α-amino acids

| Amino acid | Structure of R moiety |
|---|---|
| **Aliphatic amino acids** | |
| Glycine [Gly, G] | H |
| Alanine [Ala, A] | $CH_3$ |
| Valine [Val, V] | $CH$ with two $CH_3$ |
| Leucine [Leu, L] | $CH_2-CH$ with two $CH_3$ |
| Isoleucine [Ile, I] | $CH-CH_3-CH_3$ with $CH_3$ |
| **Neutral amino acids** | |
| Serine [Ser, S] | $CH_2-OH$ |
| Threonine [Thr, T] | $CH-OH$ with $CH_3$ |
| Asparagine [Asn, N] | $CH_2-C$ with $=O$ and $NH_2$ |
| Glutamine [Gln, Q] | $CH_2-CH_2-C$ with $=O$ and $NH_2$ |
| **Acidic amino acids** | |
| Aspartic acid [Asp, D] | $CH_2 - COOH$ |
| Glutamic acid [Glu, E] | $CH_2 - CH_2 - COOH$ |
| **Basic amino acids** | |
| Histidine [His, H] | 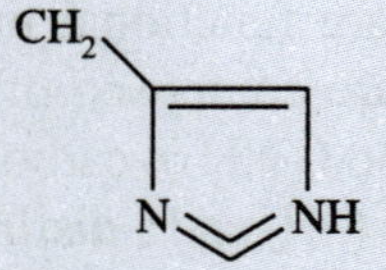 $CH_2$ imidazole ring (N, NH) |

*(Contd.)*

| Amino acid | Structure of R moiety |
|---|---|
| Lysine [Lys, K] | $CH_2-CH_2-CH_2-CH_2-NH_2$ |
| Arginine [Arg, R] | $CH_2-CH_2-CH_2-NH-C-NH_2$ |

**Sulfur-containing amino acid**

| | |
|---|---|
| Cysteine [Cys, C] | $CH_2-SH$ |
| Methionine [Met, M] | $CH_2 - CH_2 - S- CH_3$ |

**Imino acid**

| Proline (Pro, P) | 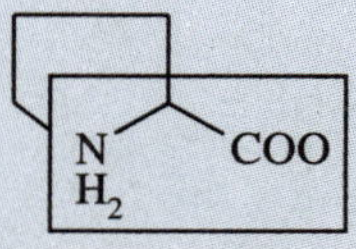 |
|---|---|

## c. Based on nutritional requirement

(i) Essential Amino acid

(ii) Non-essential Amino Acid

(i) **Essential amino acids:** Amino acids that cannot be synthesized by body and must supplied in diet are called essential amino acids. They are ten in number and include the following.

Methionine, Arginine, Threonine, Trypto-phan, Valine, Isoleucine, Leucine, Phenyl-alanine, Lysine, Histidine

(ii) **Non-essential amino acids:** Amino acids that can be synthesized by the body to meet its demands. They include-glycine, alanine, serine, cysteine, aspartate, asparagine, glutamate, glutamine, tyrosine, proline.

## d. Based on their metabolic fate

Amino acids can be classified based on fate of their carbon skeletons

| Glycogenic | | Ketogenic | Both |
|---|---|---|---|
| Ala | Met | Leu | ILe |
| Arg | Pro | | Lys |
| Asp | Ser | | Phe |
| Cys | Thr | | Trp |
| Glu | Val | | Tyr |
| Gly | | | |
| His | | | |

# IV. Nucleic Acid

## STRUCTURE AND METABOLISM

### Nucleotide

• Combination of heterocyclic amine, a pentose and phosphoric acid

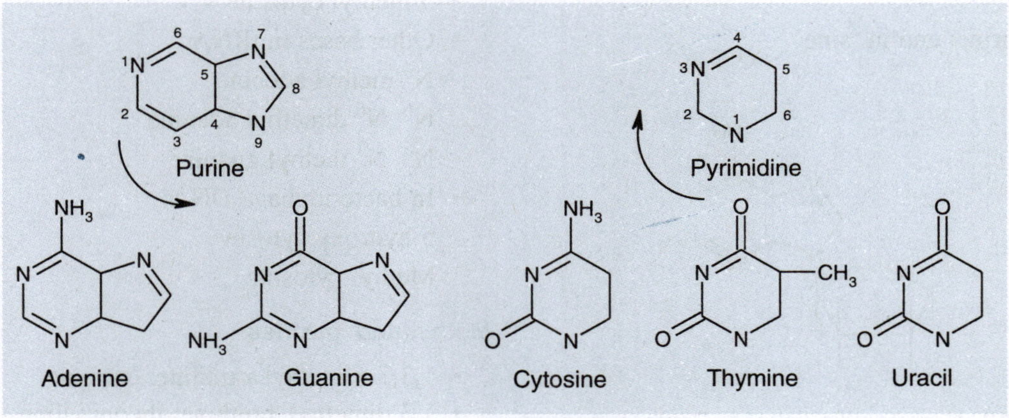

**Fig. 2.11.** Structure of bases.

- Monomeric unit of nucleic acids
- Purine and pyrimidines supply building blocks of nucleic acid
- Also, they are high energy intermediates
- Form part of coenzyme: FAD, NAD, NADP, CoA, SAM
- Have regulatory function: signal transduction, second messenger (cAMP, cGMP).

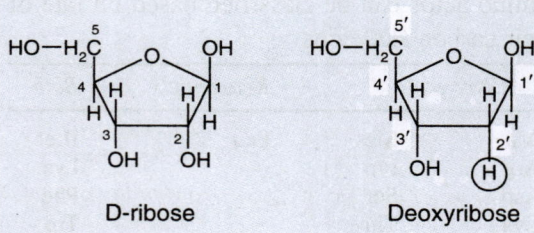

Fig. 2.12. Numbering of sugars is primed.

## Nucleoside (Fig. 2.12)

## Nucleotides

Linking one or more phosphates with a nucleoside onto 5′ end of molecule through esterification

## NAMING-CONVENTIONS

### Nucleoside

- Purine: end in 'sine'

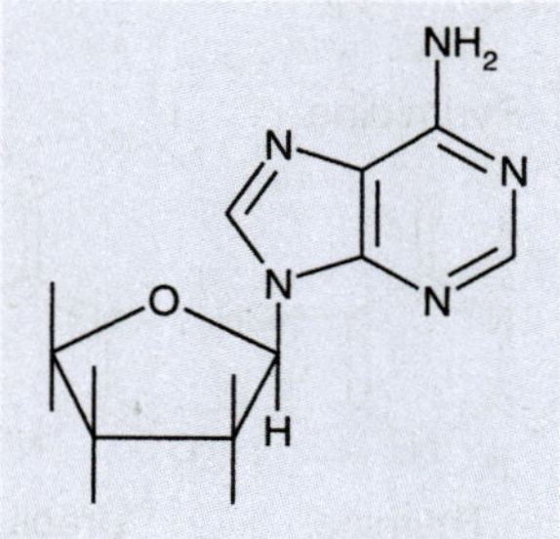

NH₂ structure

Fig. 2.13. N glycosidic linkage. Pentose sugar added to $N_9$ or $N_1$ by N–glycosidic bond.

Adenosine, guanosine
- Pyrimidine end in 'dine'
Thymidine, cytidine, uridine

## Nucleotides

Start with nucleotide name and add mono-, di-, or triphosphate to it.

- Adenosine monophosphate
- Deoxythymidine diphosphate

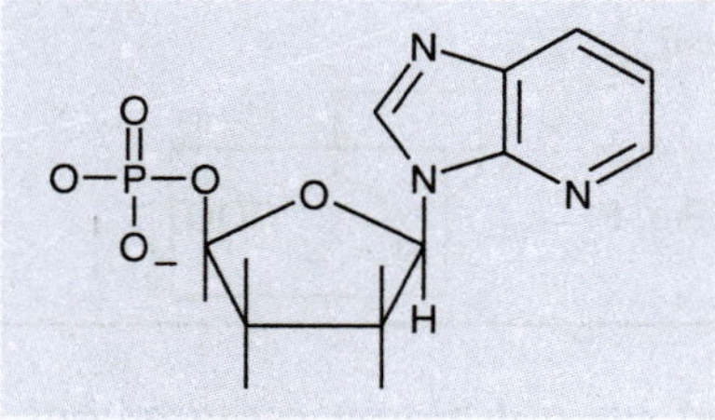

Fig. 2.14. Nucleotides.

## PSEUDOURIDINE

### TMP

- Contains ribose rather than deoxyribose
- Arises when UMP of preformed tRNA is methylated by SAM

## UNUSUAL BASES OR MINOR BASES

- 5 methyl cytosine
- Other bases in tRNA:
$N^6$ methyl adenine
$N^6$, $N^6$ dimethyl adenine
$N^6$, $N^7$ methyl guanine
- In bacteriophage DNA:
5 hydroxy cytosine
Methyl cytosine

## Methylated purines

- 1,3,7 trimethyl xanthine: caffeine
- 1,3 dimethyl xanthine: theophylline
- 3,7 dimethyl xanthine: theobromine

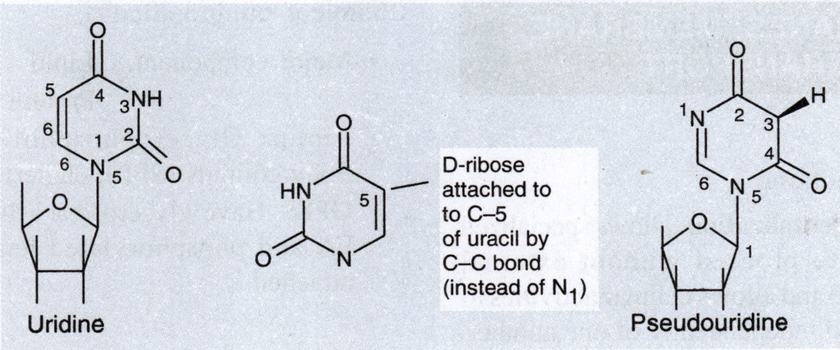

**Fig. 2.15.** Pseudouridine.

## Free nucleotides

Xanthine, hypoxanthine, uric acid.

| Nucleotide | Function |
|---|---|
| **I. Nucleotide** | |
| 1. Adenosine nucleotides | |
| ATP | Source of energy |
| cAMP | Second messenger |
| Active sulfate (adenosine 3'phosphate 5'phospho sulfate PAPS) | Sulfur donor (proteoglycans) Sulfur conjugation of drugs |
| Active methionine (5-adenosyl methionine SAM) | Methyl donor, source of propylamine, in polyamines |
| 2. Guanosine derivative | |
| GDP | Coupled to substrate level phosphorylation |
| GTP | Allosteric regulation, energy source |
| cGMP | Intracellular signal second messenger (NO) |
| 3. Hypoxanthine IMP | Purine salvage pathway |
| 4. Uracil UDP-G | Glycogen synthesis Glycoprotein synthesis |

*(Contd.)*

| Nucleotide | Function |
|---|---|
| UDP-Gln | Glucuronide conjugation reaction of bilirubin, drugs |
| 5. Cytosine | |
| CTP | Phosphoglycerate synthesis |
| CDP | CDP choline: formation of sphingomyelin with ceramide |
| **II. Coenzyme** | NAD, FAD, NADP, CoA, SAM |
| **III. Monomeric precursors** | Monomeric unit of RNA, DNA |
| Energy metabolism | ATP, muscle contraction, active transport, ion gradient, phosphate donor |
| Monomeric unit | NTP, dNTP (for RNA, DNA) |
| Physiological mediators | Adenosine (coronary blow flow), cAMP, cGMP (second messenger), signal transduction (GTP binding protein) |
| Precursor function | GTP (mRNA capping) |
| Activate intermediates | UDP-G (glycogen), CDP-choline (phospholipid), SAM (methylation), PAPS (Sulfation) |
| Allosteric affects | ATP (negative for PFK), AMP (positive for phosphorylase B), dATP (negative effector RNP reductase) |

# MEMBRANES, MEMBRANE TRANSPORT

## MEMBRANES

### Membrane functions

1. **Compartmentalization**: allows specialized activities to proceed without external interference and allows cellular activities to be regulated independently of one another.
2. **Frame work for biological activities**: Provide frame work within which components can be ordered for effective interaction.
3. **Provide selective permeability barrier**: To prevent unrestricted exchange of molecules from one side to the other.
4. **Transport of solutes:** From one side of membrane to another e.g. sugar, amino acids, ions.
5. **Signal transduction**: Membrane possess receptors to which various ligands can bind to generate a signal that stimulates or inhibits internal activities.
6. **Cell to cell interaction.**
7. **Energy transduction.**

### Biological membranes

- Highly viscous and plastic structures, form boundaries around cell and sub-cellular compartments.
- Acts as selective permeability barrier
- Involved in signaling processes
- Contain varying amount of lipid and protein and carbohydrates
- Thickness 60-100 Å..
- Dynamic structures
- Thermodynamically stable, metabolically active
- Show chemical asymmetry: two faces of biological membrane differ from one another

### Chemical composition

- Major component:   Lipid
                      Protein
- Lipids: Glycerophospholipids (GPL), Sphingolipids (SPL), cholesterol
- GPL:  Have glycerol back bone to which FA and phosphorylated head group are attached

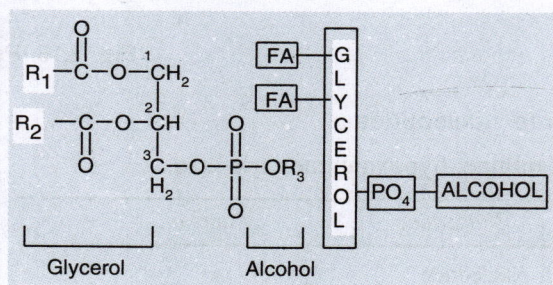

**Fig. 2.16.** Glycerophospholipid.

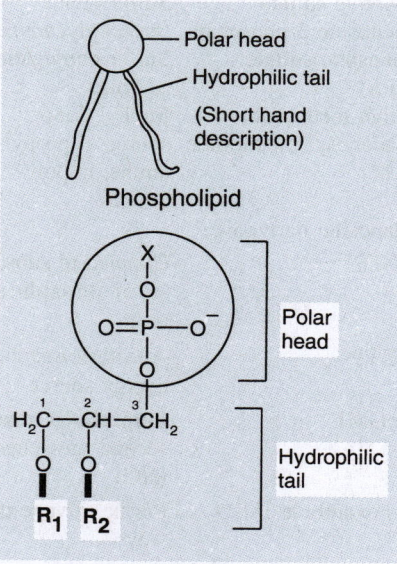

**Fig. 2.17.** Glycerophospholipid.

Phosphatidate, phosphatidylcholine, phosphatidylethanolamine, phosphatidylglycerol, phosphaditylinositol, phosphatidyl-serine, and diphosphatidyl glycerol.

Present exclusively in IMM.

GPL contain two fatty acyl groups esterified to C-1 and C-2 of glycerol:

- C1: Usually saturated FA is found e.g. palmitic, stearic acid and form a straight chain.
- C2: Unsaturated FA is present e.g. oleic, linoleic, linolenic acid; usually cis and produces a kink.

| $C_1$ | | $C_2$ |
|---|---|---|
| PC | Palmitic/Stearic acid | Oleic, linoleic, linolenic acid |
| PE | Palmitic/oleic acid | Arachidonic acid |

## Plasminogen

- Ethanolamine, ether/choline esterified to phosphate
- Abundant in nervous tissue and heart.

Every tissue and cellular membrane has a distinct composition of GPL and a definite pattern of FA composition (Fig. 2.18).

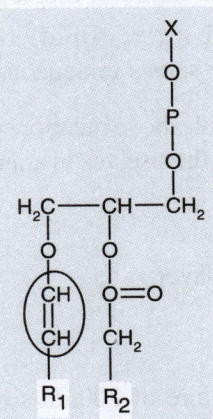

**Fig. 2.18.** Plasmalogen (α-β unsaturated ether).

## SPL

In sphingomyelin, terminal-OH group of sphingosine is esterified to phosphorylcholine, so that its polar head is similar to PC.

### Features

- Contain sphingosine back bone
- Sphingosine amino alcohol
- Sphingosine linked to FA by amide bond forming ceramide
- Sphingomyelin has PC esterified to 1-OH group
- Most abundant sphingolipid in mammalian tissues
- Lack phosphate, have sugar or primary group of sphingosine

### Similarities between GPL and SPL

- Amphipathic with charged head group
- Both are classified under phospholipids

| SPL | Location |
|---|---|
| Glucocerebroside | Present in non-neuronal tissue |
| Galactocerebroside | Present in brain and nervous tissue |
| Ganglioside | Contain sialic acid in head groups, present in brain |

### Cholesterol in membrane

- Most common sterol in membrane
- Also found in golgi apparatus, mitochondria and nuclear membrane
- Intercalates among PL with its OH group at interface and remainder in leaflet
- Amphipathic
- Ring system gives rigidity to membranes

### Lipid composition varies in different membranes

- Highest concentration of neutral lipids and SPL in plasma membrane

- Myelin membrane rich in SPL and GPL
- Intracellular membrane contain primarily GPL
- In mitochondria, nucleus and RER lipid composition is similar
- Cardiolipin present exclusively in IMM
- Phosphatidylcholine, SPL predominant and ethanolamine, GPL are second.
- In mitochondria, there is no sphingosine
- Golgi apparatus has high concentration of neutral lipids especially cholesterol

## Carbohydrates in membrane

- Oligosaccharides covalently attached to
  - Proteins to form glycoproteins
  - Lipids in lesser amount to form glycolipids

Sugar in glycoprotein and glycolipid: glucose, galactose, mannose, fructose, n-acetyl glucosamine (NAc Gln), n-acetyl galactosamine (NAc Galn), Sialic acid.

## Location

Carbohydrates are located on:
- External side of plasma membrane
- Luminal side of ER.

## Role

- Cell-cell recognition, adhesion, receptor action
- Carbohydrates of glycolipids of RBC plasma membrane determine whether person's blood type is A, B, AB or O.

## Amphipathic nature of membrane lipids

- Membrane lipids contain hydrophobic and hydrophilic regions termed: **Amphipathic.**
  - Polar head of phospholipids and –OH group of cholesterol are:
    Hydrophilic: favor contact with water
    Hydrophobic tail: Saturated fatty acids straight chain
- Unsaturated FA – make kinked tails.

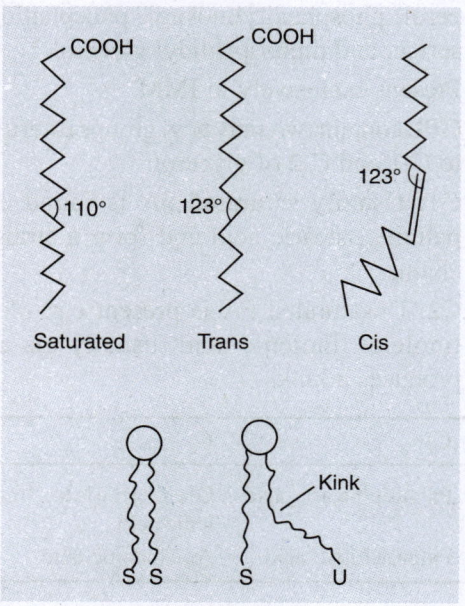

**Fig. 2.19.** Saturated and unsaturated FA in phospholipidds.

## Role of kinking

Unsaturated FA make kinked tails and as more kinks are inserted in tails, membranes become less tightly packed and becomes more fluid.

- Membrane formation is consequence of amphipathic nature of molecules
- PL and GL (glycolipid) readily form bimolecular sheets in aqueous media.

Molecules with above mentioned preferences can thus arrange themselves in aqueous solution in two ways:

- Micelle
- Lipid bilayer

## Micelle

A globular structure of 200nm size with polar head surrounded by water and carbohydrate tails sequestered inside.

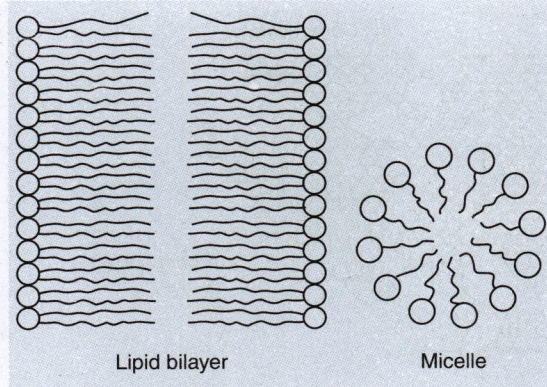

**Fig. 2.20.** Phospholipids and glycolipids form bi-molecular sheets in aqueous media.

## Lipid bilayer

Lipid bilayer in formed due to hydrophilic and hydrophobic moieties of membrane lipids resulting in hydrophobic interior and hydrophilic exterior interacting with aqueous medium on each side of the bilayer.

### Formation of lipid bilayer

- Self assembly process
- Rapid and spontaneous in water
- Dividing force is hydrophobic interactions.

### Permeability

- Steroids traverse bilayer more readily than electrolytes
- Non lipid soluble molecules can't pass through bilayer and require pores and channels for them

### Liposomes

- They are lipid vesicles with aqueous compartments enclosed by a lipid bilayer.
- Produced by suspending phospholipids (PC) in aqueous medium and sonicating to give closed vesicles of 500Å.
- Important experimental and clinical tool

### Uses

1. To study effect of varying lipid composition on certain membrane functions.
2. Drugs, antibodies or isolated gene/DNA can be entrapped inside them to target them to specific tissues

## Biological membrane structure

### Fluid mosaic model

Proposed by Singer Nicolson (1972), widely accepted.

According to this model, membranes are two dimensional solutions of oriented lipids and globular proteins (Fig. 2.21)..

### Role of biological membrane

- Permeability barrier
- Solvent for integral membrane proteins

### Translational diffusion

PL undergoes redistribution in the plane of biological membrane, termed **translational diffusion**. It is several mm/sec.

Flippases-proteins that allow phospholipids to flip from one membrane surface to the other.

### Transverse diffusion

A transition of molecule from one membrane surface to other is transverse diffusion or flips flop.

The characteristics of lipid bilayer explain many of the observed cellular membrane properties:

- Fluidity
- Flexibility
- Ability to self anneal
- Impermeability
- The model continues to undergo modification and refinement. It allows lateral movement, but not rotation.

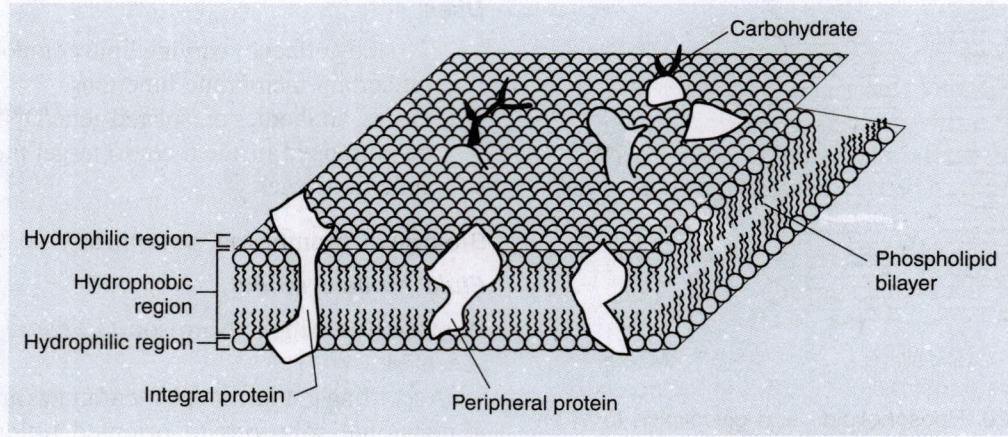

**Fig. 2.21.** Membrane structure.

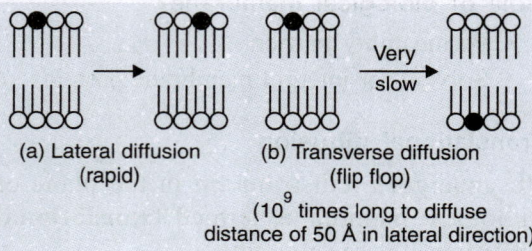

**Fig. 2.22.** (a) Lateral diffusion, (b) Transverse diffusion.

## Membrane fluidity

Depends on:

- Temperature
- Composition
- Lipid composition
- Ordered/disordered
- Rigid/fluid

Lipids with short or unsaturated FA chain undergo phase transition.

When transition temperature ($T_m$) raised above melting temperature, rigid to fluid state occurs.

$T_m$ depends on length of fatty acyl chain, degree of unsaturation.

## Facts

- Saturated FA favor rigid membrane
- Double bond produces bend in hydrocarbon chain interferes high ordered packing and lowers $T_m$.
- Higher $T_m$ required to increase fluidity
- Longer, saturated FA chains increase $T_m$, decrease fluidity; cis unsaturated bond lowers $T_m$ and increase fluidity
- Cholesterol insertion in bilayer limits fluidity owing its rigid ring.

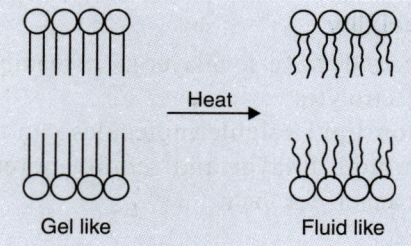

**Fig. 2.23.** Effect of temperature on membrane fluidity.

## Lipid rafts and caveolae

The presence of the lipid ordered micro domains in cells has transformed fluid mosaic model into more complex system.

## Lipid rafts

- Dynamic assembly of proteins and lipids that float freely in lipid bilayer.
- Dynamic areas of exoplasmic leaflet of lipid bilayer enriched in cholesterol, SPL

## Caveolae

- Small surface invaginations seen in many cells and postulated to be formed by rafts on cell surface.
- Serves to store and down regulate raft proteins or acts as reservoir of rafts
- Several groups of pathogens, bacteria, virus, prion, parasites hijack lipid rafts for their purposes
- Lipid rafts play a role in signal transduction.

## Fluidity of membrane affects its functions

- As membrane fluidity increases, its permeability to water and hydrophilic molecules increases
- Membrane fluidity can control activity of membrane bound enzyme, membrane functions such as phagocytosis and cell growth.

- Examples
  - RBCs in spur cell anaemia have a high cholesterol content, also seen in cirrhotic liver and premature RBC destruction in spleen
  - Insulin receptor: Increased unsaturated FA concentration in membrane increases fluidity and alters the receptor to bind more insulin.
  - Calcium ions decrease fluidity causing decrease in repulsion between polar groups and increasing packing of lipid molecules, thus decreasing fluidity.

## Asymmetry

- Occurs in membrane bilayer
- Important for function of biological membranes
- Established during its biosynthesis
- Have different components and enzyme activities on both the surfaces
- Maintained throughout the lifetime of protein.

For example RBC membrane: SPL and PC on outer leaflet and PE, PS on inner leaflet and cholesterol on both leaflets.

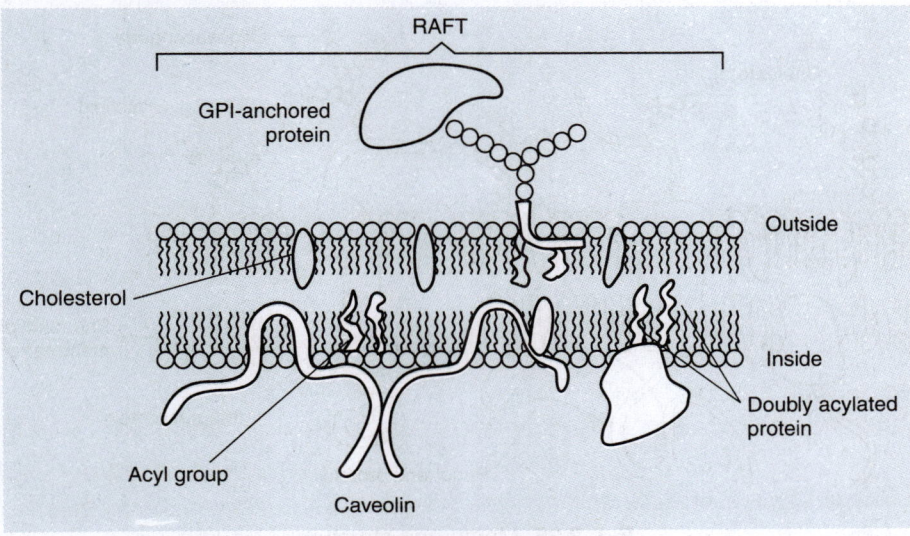

**Fig. 2.24.** Membrane raft group.

## Regional asymmetries

- Villous border of mucosal cells
- Gap junction, tight junction, synapses occupy much smaller regions of membrane and generate local asymmetry
- PL: have inside-outside asymmetry (transverse asymmetry)
- PC, SM: outer leaflet
- PS, PE: Inner leaflet

## GP and GL

- Abundant in RBC membrane
- Absent in mitochondrial membrane

## Membrane proteins

- Features of proteins in membrane: myelin has low protein content (18%)
- Mitochondria has higher protein content (75%)
- Plasma membrane has intermediate protein content.

## Function of proteins in membrane

1. Form a permeability barrier
2. Associated with bilayer as membrane proteins (integral and peripheral)

## Proteins in membrane

Proteins in membrane are classified as:

- Peripheral (extrinsic)
- Integral (intrinsic)

## Integral membrane proteins

- Span the lipid bilayer
- Present in membrane
- Amphipathic and globular e.g. transporter, receptors, G protein
- Distributed asymmetrically across bilayer
- May span bilayer many time
- Require detergents for their release

## Peripheral proteins

- Bound to membrane by electrostatic and H-bond interaction with the head groups of lipids and integral proteins
- Do not interact with PL of bilayer
- Do not require detergents for their release
- Can be bound on cytosolic or extracellular side of membrane
- May be anchored to bilayer

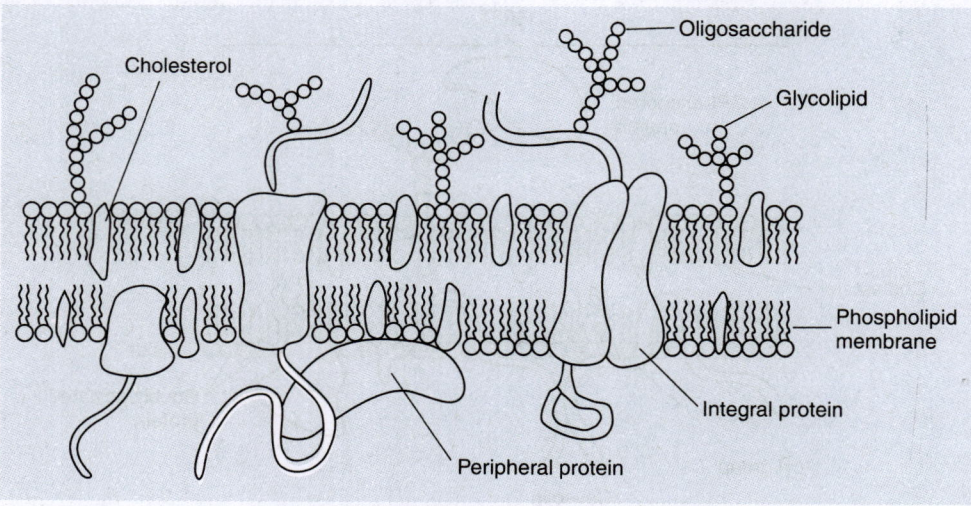

**Fig. 2.25.** Membrane structure.

## Interaction of proteins with membrane

- Membrane-spanning: α-helices: most common
- Channel forming: β-strands: porin protein
- Bound to other membrane protein
  For example, Ankyrin: peripheral protein is bound to spectrin (a cytosolic structure) to maintain biconcave shape of RBC
- $PGH_2$ synthase :
  Lies along outer surface of membrane
  Bound by a set of α-helices
  Integral protein

Its localization is crucial for its function, as arachidonic acid, a substrate generated by hydrolysis of membrane lipids and reaches the enzyme through a hydrophobic channel.

Aspirin, ibuprofen block this channel, thus inhibiting PG synthesis.

## MEMBRANE TRANSPORT

### Membrane permeability

Plasma membrane is:

- Selectively permeable
- Water, gases ($O_2$, $CO_2$) can pass directly through it
- Other molecules (sugar, amino acid, ions etc.) require presence of transporter
- Permeability is conferred by two classes of membrane proteins: pumps and channels.

### Types of transport

1. Passive transport
2. Active transport

### Passive transport

- Molecules move from a higher to lower concentration
- Movement of molecules across a membrane does not require energy.

- Permeability property of membrane ensures that:
  - Essential molecules such as glucose, amino acids, and lipids readily enter the cell
  - Metabolic intermediate remain in cell
  - Waste compounds leave the cell, allowing cell to maintain a constant internal environment.

### Simple diffusion

- Type of passive transport
- Does not require transport protein e.g. Water, gases, urea, ethanol
- Rate of diffusion is directly proportional to concentration gradient
- Not saturable

### Terminology

#### Transporter

Translocation of molecule or ion across membrane by binding or physically moving the substance.

#### Group translocation

Involves movement as well as chemical modification of substrate, e.g. uptake of glucose by cell and its phosphorylation before its release into cytosol.

#### Pores

Tertiary and quaternary structures of intrinsic membrane proteins create an aqueous hole that permits diffusion of substrate through membrane in direction of a lower concentration.

### Site of transporters

- Epithelial lining of all body cavities
- Stomach secrete acid
- Intestine secrete glucose, amino acid to blood
- Urinary bladder
- Skin

## Membrane translocations

| Type | Class | Example |
|---|---|---|
| Channel (pores) | Voltage regulated | Na channel |
| | Agonist regulated | AcH ® |
| | cAMP regulated | Cl channel |
| | Others | pressure, stretch, heat sensitive |
| Transporter | Facilitated diffusion | G-transporter |
| | Active, mediated by: | Respiratory chain |
| | (i) Primary ATPase | Na/K ATPase Multidrug resistance |
| | ATP binding cassette | Na dependent G-transporter |
| | (ii) secondary | |
| Group translocation | - | Amino acid translocation |

## Channel and pores in membrane function differently

Membrane channels and pores are intrinsic membrane proteins and are differentiated based on their degree of specificity for molecules moving across the membrane.

## Channel

Selective for inorganic ions and anions, while pores are not. They are:
- Specific
- Amphipathic
- α-helical

## Common modification

- Amphipathic, α helices of associated protein sub units or domains within a single polypeptide
- Create an aqueous space

*Exception:* Porin in gram negative bacteria: β-sheet:
- Transport proteins are specific for particular molecule or group of structurally similar molecule
- Display Michalis-Mentin type of binding kinetics: $V_{max}$, $K_m$ influenced by pH,

| Comparison | |
|---|---|
| *Pore/channel* | *Transporter* |
| 1. Substrate move/drive down hill in direction of low concentration. Can conduct millions of ions per second | 1. Uphill can move only hundreds to thousands molecules per second |
| 2. Do not bind molecule ion to other side of membrane | 2. Translocate ion/molecule by binding and physically moving the substance |
| 3. Can be inhibited | 3. Inhibited: Competitive Non-completive Defined reaction kinetics |
| 4. Some degree of specificity | 4. Specific to substrate |
| 5. Rate faster: $10^7$ ion s$^{-1}$ | 5. $10^2$–$10^3$ molecule s$^{-1}$ |
| 6. Activity can be modulated | 6. Activity can be modulated |
| 7. Different drugs for specific channels have been developed | 7. Different drugs for specific transporters have been developed |

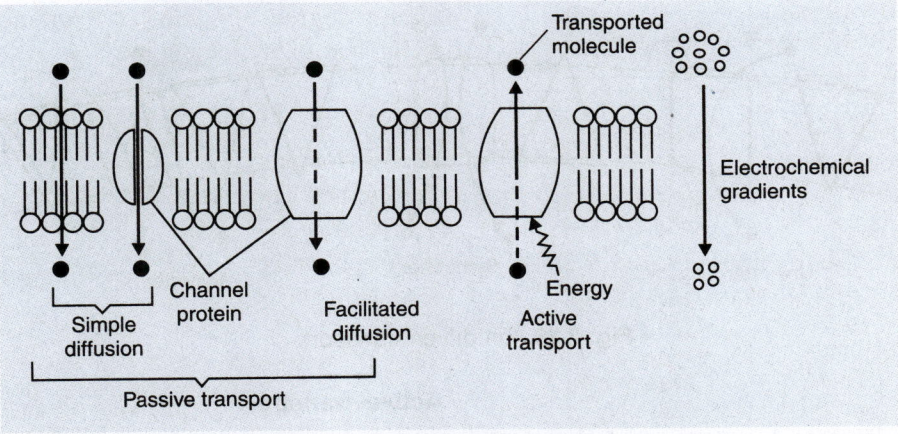

**Fig. 2.26.** Membrane transport.

temperature, inhibitor molecule in similar manner to enzyme.

## Facilitated diffusion (or passive mediated transport)

- Facilitated diffusion is translocation of solutes through cell membrane without expenditure of energy.
- It requires presence of specific integral membrane protein to facilitate movement of molecules known as **uniport**.

## Uniport system

- Moves one type of molecule bidirectionally
- Molecule binds to protein on one side of membrane, protein undergoes conformational change and transports molecule across the membrane and releases it on the other side.

## Ping pong mechanism explains facilitated diffusion

Protein carrier in lipid bilayer associates with a solute undergoes a conformation change (pong to ping) and discharges solute on the other side. Empty carrier then reverts to original conformation (ping to pong) to complete the cycle.

### Features

- Reversible
- Regulated by hormones

### Role of hormones in facilitated diffusion

By changing the number of transporter available.

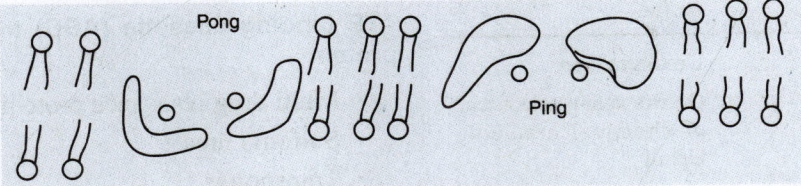

**Fig. 2.27.** Ping Pong mechanism.

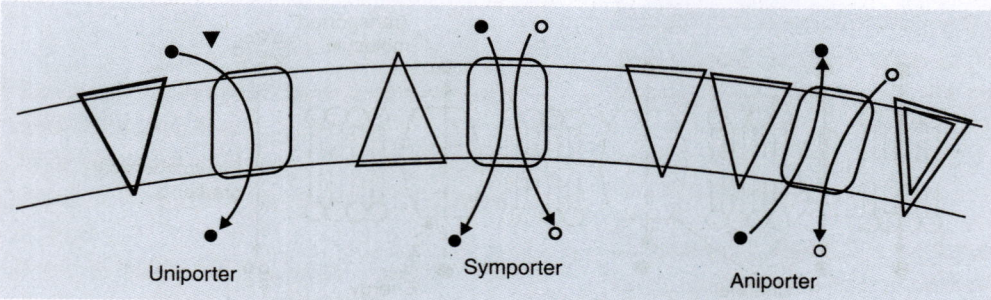

**Fig. 2.28.** Ion driven transport.

## Examples

i. Insulin: increase transport of glucose and fat in muscle

ii. Glucocorticoids: enhance amino acid transport in all cells

iii. Estrogen: increase amino acid transport in liver

## Facilitative vs active transport

### Similarities

Both have:

- Specific binding sites for solute
- Carrier is saturable
- Carrier follows enzyme kinetics
- No covalent interaction occurs
- There is $K_m$ (binding constant) for the solute
- Transport can be blocked by competitive inhibitors

### Differences

| Facilitative | Active |
|---|---|
| Bidirectional | Unidirectional |
| Occurs down hill | Occurs against electrical or chemical gradient-Uphill |
| Does not require energy | Requires energy |

## Active transport

Requires an input of metabolic energy that comes from ATP hydrolysis or light.

i. ATP driven ions:

$Na^+$, $K^+$, $Ca^{+2}$, $H^+$

Uses $Na^+/K^+$ ATPase.

- Provides energy required for transport of molecule across membrane
- Maintains $Na^+/K^+$ gradient and membrane electrical potential across plasma membrane: all cells maintain a high internal concentration of $K^+$ and low concentration of $Na^+$.

ii. Ion driven active transport

$Na^+/K^+$ ATPase

- Tetramer: $2\alpha$, $2\beta$ subunits.
- Integral membrane protein
- Coupled to ATP hydrolysis
- 2 $Na^+$ ions pumped out and 3 $K^+$ ions pumped inside.

## ATP binding cassette (ABC) transport protein

- Multi drug resistance protein
- Sulfonyl urea
- Transporter
- Xenobiotics

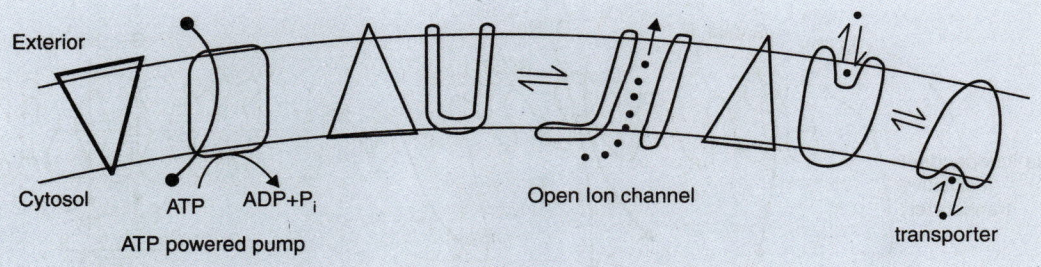

**Fig. 2.29.** Pumps, channels and transporter.

## Glucose transport

- Glucose transport is facilitated transport
- Five glucose transporters have been reported: GLUT 1-5.
- GLUT1 has 12 hydrophobic segments in transporter region.
- GLU2 - Exports glucose from liver cells.

Rest of the transporters are responsible for movement of glucose into cell.

| Transporter | Location |
|---|---|
| GLUT 1 | Muscle, heart, blood brain barrier |
| GLUT 2 | Liver, Pancreas, intestine, kidney |
| GLUT 3 | Neuron, kidney |
| GLUT 4 | Muscle, adipose tissue, heart (insulin-sensitive) |
| GLUT 5 | Muscle, sperm |

## SGLT-1

- Sodium-dependent glucose transporter-1
- Secondary active transport of glucose
- Binds sodium and glucose at separate sites and transports them through plasma membrane of intestine
- Inhibited by Ouabain, phlorhizin
- The movement of $Na^+$ and glucose across the cell sets up a difference in osmotic pressure causing water to follow simple diffusion. This forms the basis of *glucose rehydration therapy*.

## Ion driven active transport

It is movement of molecule across a membrane coupled with movement of ion, e.g. $Na^+$, $K^+$

## Types

### i. Symport

- Both molecule and ion move in same direction, e.g. $Na^+$/glucose transporter SGLT-1
- Cl/$HCO_3$ exchange transporter
- RBC band 3 anion transporter

### ii. Antiport

- Ions move in opposite direction
- Concentration gradient of one compound can drive the movement of other solute, e.g. Cl/$HCO_3$ exchanger: in RBC, kidney
- In RBC: adjust $HCO_3$ concentration in arterial and venous blood
- In Kidney: responsible for base ($HCO_3$) efflux to balance ATP-driven $H^+$ efflux.
  - ATP-ADP transporter antiport: in inner mitochondrial membrane
  - $PO_4$-$H^+$ symport
  - Dicarboxylate carrier: exchanges malate for phosphate

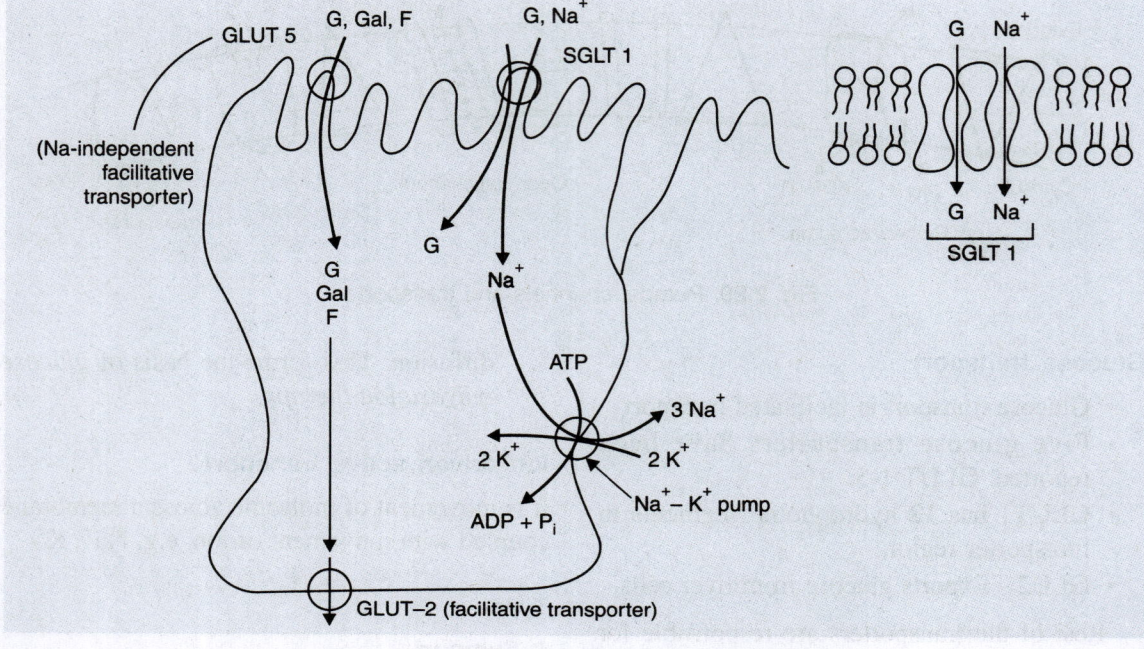

Fig. 2.30. Glucose transporters.

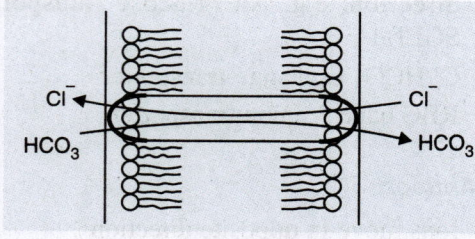

Fig. 2.31. Cl⁻/HCO₃ exchange.

– Glutamate transport: exchange of aspartate

## CALCIUM TRANSLOCATION

### Ca$^{+2}$ transporting ATPase

• This movement is coupled with ATP hydrolysis along concentration gradient.
• Ca is present in membranes of ER where it transports calcium ions out of the cytosol into lumen of ER.

## CFTR

Cystic fibrosis trans membrane conductance regulator (CFTR)

• Type of ABC transporter
• Serves as both conductance regulator and chloride channel.

## H⁺/K⁺ ATPase

• Present in epithelial lining of stomach (parietal cells)
• Secretes a solution of concentrated acid into stomach chamber
• At resting state, these pump molecules are situated in cytoplasmic membrane of parietal cell and are non-functional.
• When food enters stomach: a hormone message is transmitted to parietal cells. Causing pump containing membranes to move to

| Sr. No. | Solute | Mechanism | Tissues |
|---|---|---|---|
| | **Transport mechanisms of various solutes** | | |
| 1. | Sugars | | |
| | Glucose | Passive, active symport with $Na^+$ | Widespread, renal tubules, small intestine |
| | Fructose | Passive | Intestine, liver |
| 2. | Amino acids | | |
| | Amino acid specific transporter | Active transport with $Na^+$ | Intestine, kidney, liver |
| | All amino acid except proline | Active group translocation | Liver |
| | Specific amino acids | Passive | Intestine |
| 3. | Dicarboxylic acid | Active symport with $Na^+$ | Kidney |
| 4. | Lactate and monocarboxylic acid | Active symport with $H^+$ | Widespread |
| 5. | Neurotransmitter: GABA, norepinephrine, glutamate, dopamine | Active symport with $Na^+$ | Brain |
| 6. | Urea | Passive | RBC, kidney |
| 7. | Inorganic ions | Active | Mitochondria |
| | $H^+$ | Active | Lysosome, endosome, golgi complex |
| 8. | $Na^+$ | Passive | Distal tubular |
| 9. | Na, $H^+$ | Active, antiport | PCT, small intestine |
| 10. | $Na^+$, $K^+$ | **Active ATP driven** | All cell plasma membrane |
| 11. | Ions: | | |
| | $Ca^{+2}$ | Active ATP driven | Plasma membrane and ER |
| | $Ca^{+2}$, $Na^+$ | Active antiport | Widespread |
| | $H^+$, $K^+$ | Active antiport | Gastric, parietal cell |
| | $Cl^-$, $HCO_3^-$ | Passive antiport | RBC, tissues |

apical cell surface, where they fuse with plasma membrane and begin acid secretion.

• Drugs:
 – Prilosec inhibit $H^+/K^+$ ATPase to prevent heart burn
 – Zantac, Pepcid and Tagomet: 
 – Block receptor on surface of parietal cell stopping cell from getting activated by hormone
 – Does not inhibit $H^+/K^+$ ATPase pump.

## Types: Active transport

• Primary
• Secondary

### Primary

• Requires ATP as energy source
• 3 types: P-, V-, F- type

**P-type:** Protein is phosphorylated and dephosphoryated during transport. Eg. $Na^+$-$K^+$ translocation

| Diseases due to loss of membrane transport system | |
|---|---|
| *Sr. No.* *Transport defect* | *Outcome* |
| 1. Glucose-galactose transport | Decreased uptake in intestine |
| 2. Fructose transport system alteration | Fructose malabsorption |
| 3. Decreased neutral amino acids in epithelial cells | Hartnup disease symptoms in intestine and kidney |
| 4. Cystinuria | Renal absorption of cysteine and basic amino acid arginine is abnormal, cystine renal stones. Tryptophan deficiency: pellagra-like syndrome |
| 5. Hypophosphatemia | Vitamin-D resistant rickets: renal absorption of phosphate abnormal |
| 6. Cystic fibrosis (CF) | cAMP regulated Cl channel affected increasing viscosity of body secretions |

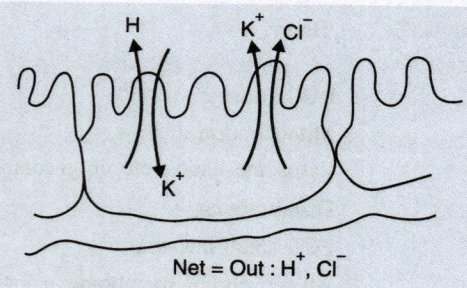

Fig. 2.32. $H^+/K^+$ ATPase in gastric mucosal cell.

**V-type:** Responsible for acidification (proton pumps) of:
- Interior of lysosome
- Endosomes
- Golgi apparatus
- Vesicles

**Secretary vesicle:**
- Utilize energy of ATP without forming a phosphorylated protein
- Cause active transport of hydrogen
- V pumps are present in plasma membrane of kidney tubules: to maintain acid-base balance by secreting proton into urine.

**F-type:**
- Involved in ATP synthesis
- Present in mitochondria ($F_1/F_0$ ATPase or ATP synthase)

### Secondary

For translocation of solutes transmembrane chemical gradient of $Na^+$ or $H^+$ is required, e.g. sugar, amino acids

### Ionophores

- Certain bacteria synthesize small organic molecules, ionophores that function as shuttles for movement of ions across membranes.
- They contain hydrophilic centers that bind specific ions and are surrounded by hydrophobic regions
- Each ionophore has definite ion sensitivity

### Types

1. **Mobile carriers:** These readily diffuse in a membrane and can carry an ion across the membrane.
2. **Channel former:** These create a channel that traverses the membrane through which ions can diffuse.

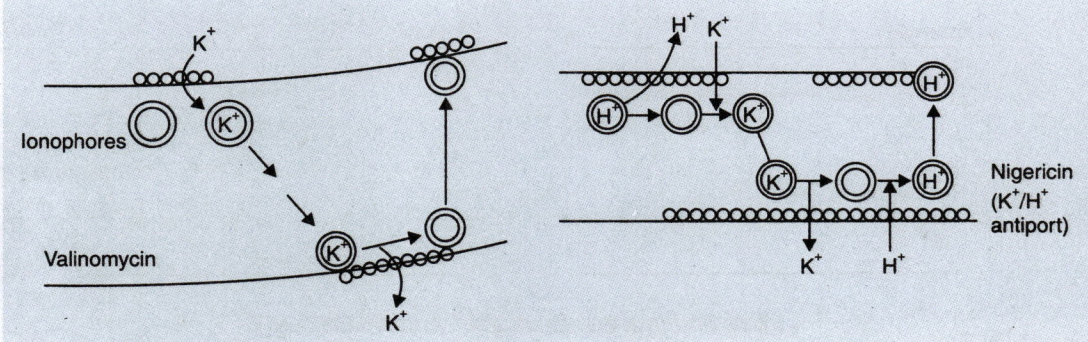

**Fig. 2.33.** Ionophores.

## Examples

### Valinomycin K⁺ uniport:

- 1000 times more affinity for $K^+$ than $Na^+$
- 10 times more affinity for $Ca^{+2}$ than $Mg^{+2}$.

### A23187:

- $Ca^+/2H^+$ antiport

### Nigericin:

- $K^+/H^+$ antiport (neutral)

### Gramicidin:

- $H^+$, Na, $K^+$, $Rb^+$ forms channels

### Alamethicin:

- $K^+$, $Rb^+$ forms channels

Ionophores are valuable experimental tools studying ion translocation in biological membranes and manipulation of ionic composition of cells.

## Aquaporins (AP)

- Proteins that form water channels in certain membrane e.g. RBC, collecting ducts in kidney.
- Tetramer transmembrane proteins.
- Mutation in gene coding AP-2 causes diabetes insipidus.

### Movement of large molecules

Large molecule can enter or leave cells through mechanisms such as exocytosis and endocytosis

### Cotransport (Coupling active transport to existing ion gradient)

$Na^+$, $K^+$, $H^+$ ions produce concentration gradient by which free energy can be stored in a cell, e.g. glucose.

Its movement across apical plasma membrane is against concentration gradient and occurs by a cotransport with sodium.

$Na^+$ concentration is kept very low in the cell by primary active transport ($Na^+/K^+$ ATPase).

Tendency of $Na^+$ to diffuse back into cell down the concentration gradient is tapped by plasma cells to drive glucose into cells against concentration gradient termed as secondary active transport with help of sodium/glucose cotransporter.

# Enzymes

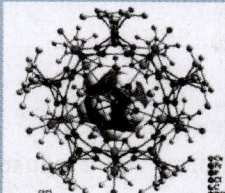

## Definition

Biological polymers synthesized by living cells catalyzing chemical reactions. They are:

- Biological catalysts.
- Neither consumed not produced.
- Do not alter equilibrium constant of reaction, but, increase rate of reaction.

## Enzymes are constituted by proteins

- Enzymes fold into a stable tertiary structure under conditions required for catalysis.
- Some enzymes catalyze reaction without prosthetic groups: using amino acids in active site.
- Others require a cofactor or prosthetic group:
  - Inorganic ions (metal ions)
  - Organic and/or metalloorganic molecules (coenzymes)

## Features

- Catalyst for biological reactions
- Control almost every metabolic reaction in living organisms
- Most are proteins
- Lower activation energy
- Increase rate of reaction
- Activity lost if denatured

## Function

- Essential for breakdown of nutrients to supply energy
- Chemical building block formation
- Conversion of building blocks into protein, DNA; membrane, cells and tissues require/involve energy
- Supply 'E' for cell motility, muscle contraction

## Practical applications of enzyme

- Many human genetic diseases result from mutation in one enzyme (resulting its malfunctioning or complete absence).
- **Diagnostic tool:** level (and/or activity) of enzyme in blood and tissues are often used in detection of some diseases.
- **Action of drugs** are commonly exerted through binding and inhibition of enzyme.
- Ideal candidates for biotechnology, chemical industry, food processing industry and agriculture.
- Used as drugs, in gene therapy.

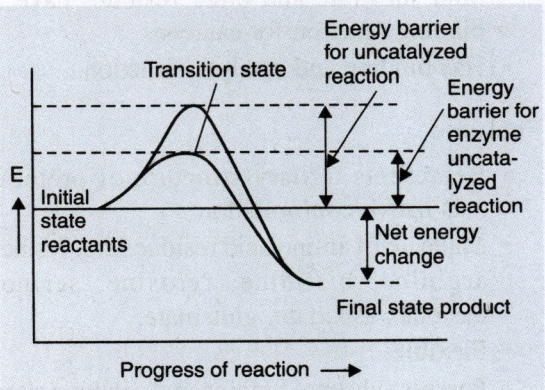

**Fig. 3.1.** Free energy of activation and action of typical enzyme.

## Factors affecting enzyme activity

### Enzyme concentration

Velocity of a reaction (v) increases with enzyme concentration [E], if the substrate concentration [S] is constant.

At $V_{max}$, all active sites of enzyme are saturated with substrate.

## Clinical correlation

1. **ATT drug:** Isoniazid, antitubercular (AT'T) drug is activated by n-acetyl transferase

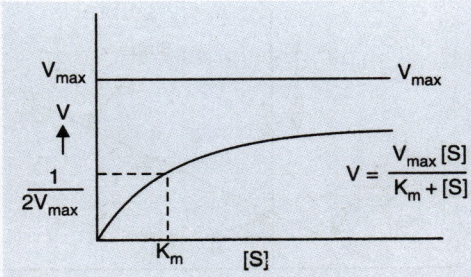

**Fig. 3.2.** Plot of velocity (v) and substrate (s) concentration.

$$V = \frac{V_{max}[S]}{K_m + [S]}$$

Two polymorphisms of this enzyme exist:

i. Fast acetylators: clear drug from blood about 300% faster than 2nd group

   $K_m$ normal, $V_{max}$ three times the normal.

ii. Slow acetylators: slow acetylation of drug

   Result in presence of drug for longer period

   Causes: hepatotoxicity and neuropathy.

2. **Hypersensitivity to alcohol:** Alcohol is metabolized to acetaldehyde by alcohol dehydrogenase:

$$\text{Alcohol} \xrightarrow[\text{Dehydrogenase}]{\text{Alcohol}} \text{Acetaldehyde}$$

Aldehyde dehydrogenase exists in two forms:

i. High affinity (low km)

ii. Low affinity (high km)

People sensitive to alcohol lack high affinity form, resulting in excess acetaldehyde, causing vasodilatation, facial flushing and tachycardia.

Linear plot for determining $V_{max}$; Double reciprocal plot of 1/V versus 1/[S].

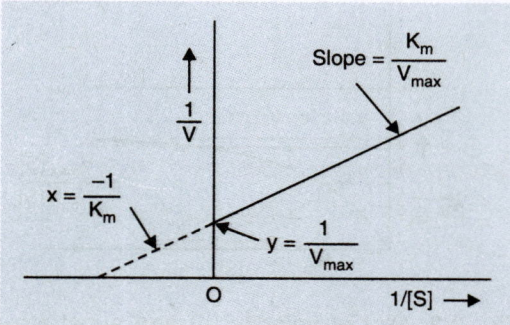

**Fig. 3.3.** Lineweaver Burk plot.

## Regulation of enzyme activity by post-translational (covalent) modification

Enzyme activity may increase or decrease after covalent addition of chemical group.

**Phosphorylation affects enzymes**: Enzymes inhibited by phosphorylation:

– Pyruvate dehydrogenase
– Glycogen synthase

Enzymes inhibited by phosphatase: glycogen phosphorylase.

Enzyme stimulated by phosphorylation:

– Glycogen phosphorylase

**Removal of peptide:** Pro-enzyme (zymo-

gen) have an additional peptide attached, removal of which results in active enzyme, e.g.:

– Proinsulin: C-peptide links insulin A and B chains
– Procarboxypeptidase to carboxypeptidase
– Chymotrypsinogen to chymotrypsin
– Trypsinogen to trypsin

## ACTIVE SITE

**Active site**: Site involved in binding of substrate and catalysis:

• Region of enzyme in which side chains of some amino acid residues are tailored to bind substrate and other residues have a binding function for catalysis
• Has binding and catalytic function.

### Features

• Represents tertiary structure of protein: 3-D native conformation
• Made up of amino acid residues e.g. lysine, arginine, histidine, tyrosine, serine, cysteine, aspartate, glutamate.
• Flexible
• Possess substrate binding and catalytic sites

### Enzyme specificity

Enzymes have high specificity:

• Many enzymes recognize only a single compound as substrate
• Digestive enzymes e.g. proteases are less specific
• Exhibit three types of specificity:

### i. Stereo specificity

Optical specificity: Act only on one isomer, e.g.:

• Hexokinase - D-Hexose
• Glucokinase - D-glucose
• L-amino acid oxidase - L-amino acids

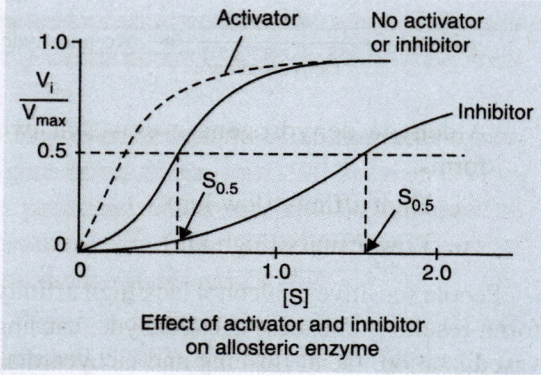

**Fig. 3.4.** Effect of activators and inhibitors on allosteric enzyme.

**Remember:** isomerases do not exhibit stereo specificity, as they interconvert isomers.

### ii. Reaction specificity

Specific for type of reaction they catalyze, e.g.:

- Decarboxylation
- Transamination
- Oxidative deamination
- Catalyzed by different enzyme

### iii. Substrate specificity

Depend on specific group or bond, e.g.:

- Glucokinase acts on glucose only
- Trypsin acts on linkages formed by basic amino acids.

### Defective enzyme

Defective enzyme can result from:

- Genetic defect
- Nutritional deficiency
- Toxins

## CLASSIFICATION OF ENZYMES (Table 3.1)

### 1. Oxidoreductase

### Oxygenase

- Catalyze direct transfer and incorporation of oxygen into a substrate molecule.
- Involved in both synthetic and degradation reactions

It is of two types:
- Mono-oxygenase
- Di-oxygenase

### Dioxygenase

- Incorporate both atoms of molecular oxygen, e.g.
  - Homogentisate oxidase
  - 3OH anthranilate oxidase
  - L-tryptophan pyrrolase

### Monooxygenase

Examples:

- Mixed function oxidase
- Hydrolase
- Cyt $P_{450}$ family

### CytP$_{450}$ super family

- Heme containing monoxygenases form cytP$_{450}$ superfamily
- Over 1000 such enzymes are known
- Require both NADH and NADPH as reducing equivalents for reduction of these cytochromes.

### Microsomal cytP$_{450}$

- Has important role in detoxification, e.g.
  - Benzpyrene
  - Aminopyrene
  - Aniline
  - Morphine
  - Benzphetamine

**Table 3.1.** Classification of enzymes

| Class | Reaction | Enzyme |
|---|---|---|
| Oxidase | Use oxygen as acceptor | L-and D-amino acid oxidase |
| Dehydrogenase | Use molecules other than oxygen as 'e' acceptor | Alcohol dehydrogenase |
| Oxygenase | Directly incorporate oxygen into substrate | Oxygenase, mono and dioxygenase, cyt oxidase |
| Peroxidase | Use $H_2O_2$ as 'e' acceptor | GSHP$_x$ |

- Hydroxylated and solubility increases and it gets excreted
- Induced by phenobarbital

## Mitochondrial cytP$_{450}$

- Found in steroidogenic tissues:
  - Adrenal cortex
  - Testis
  - Ovary
  - Placenta
- Biosynthesis of :
  - Steroid hormones
  - Bile acids
- Catabolism of vitamin D:
  - 1α hydroxylase
  - 24α hydroxylase
- Catabolism of cholesterol
  - 7α hydroxylase

## Cytochrome oxidase

- Hemeproteins (other examples of heme-proteins: Mb, Hb, other cyt)
- Present in ETC in mitochondria
- Contain copper

## Dehydrogeases (deH)

- Do not use oxygen as 'H' acceptor
- Use NAD or NADP
- May depend on riboflavin (FMN, FAD)
- NAD linked deH: Catalyze oxidative reactions of:
  - Glycolysis
  - TCA
  - Respiratory chain
- NADP-linked deH: Involved in reductive synthesis:
  - FA synthesis
  - Steroid hormone
  - PPP

- FMN/FAD-dependent deH:
  - Succinate deH
  - Acyl CoA deH
  - Glycerol 3P-deH
  - Dihydrolipoyl deH
  - Electron-transferring flavoproteins

## Hydroperoxidase

- Use $H_2O_2$ or organic peroxides as substrate
- Two enzyme:
  - Catalase
  - Peroxidase

**Peroxidase:** Reduce peroxides using 'e' acceptor

**Prosthetic group:** Protoheme
$$H_2O_2 + AH_2 \rightarrow 2H_2O + A$$
e.g. GSHP$_x$

## Catalase:

- Uses $H_2O_2$ as 'e' donor
- Uses one mole of $H_2O_2$ as an oxidant or 'e' acceptor.
$$2H_2O_2 \rightarrow 2H_2O + O_2$$

## Sources of $H_2O_2$:

- Mitochondrial ETC system
- Microsomal ETC system
- Xanthine oxidase

## 2. Transferases

| Class | Reaction | Enzyme |
|---|---|---|
| Methyl transferase | Methyl/1-C | Transmethylase |
| Amino transferase | NH$_2$ from amino acid to keto acid | Transaminase |
| Kinase | PO$_3'$ (ATP to substrate) | Hexokinase |
| Phosphorylase | PO$_3'$ (Pi to substrate) | Phosphorylase |

## 3. Hydrolase

| Class | Reaction | Enzyme |
|---|---|---|
| Protease | Cleave amide bonds in proteins | Trypsin, Pepsin, Renin |
| Phosphatase | Remove phosphate | ALP |
| Phospho-diesterase | Cleave phospho-diesterase bond | Phospho-diesterase |

## 4. Lyase

| Class | Reaction | Enzyme |
|---|---|---|
| Aldolase | Elimination reaction to produce aldehyde group | Aldolase |
| Decarboxylase | Elimination of $CO_2$ | Carbonic anhydrase Fumarase |
| Synthase | Linkage of two molecules without involvement of ATP | HMG CoA synthase |

## 5. Isomerase

| Class | Reaction | Enzyme |
|---|---|---|
| Mutase | Transfer of groups within a molecule | Epimerase, Cis-trans isomerase, Retinol isomerase |
| Racemase | Interconvert L- & D-stereoisomer | Racemase |

## 6. Ligase

| Class | Reaction | Enzyme |
|---|---|---|
| Carboxylase | Use $CO_2$ as substrate | Pyruvate carboxylase, Acetyl CoA carboxylase |
| Synthetase | ATP-dependent condensation of two molecules | Glutamine synthetase |

**Remember:**

Synthetase     use ATP
Synthase      use no ATP

*Caution*: Synthases could be lyases

### Apo Enzyme

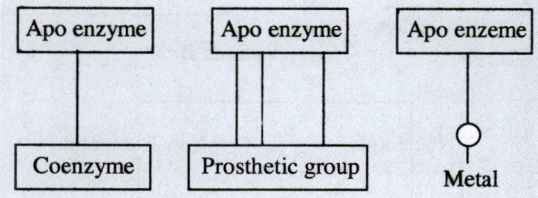

The entire complex is holoenzyme i.e.:

Apo enzyme     – protein part
Cofactor        – coenzyme
Prosthetic group   – metal-ion-activator

### Coenzyme

- Low molecular weight
- Dialyzable
- Non-protein organic substance
- Serve as substrate shuttles or group derived from vitamin

For example, NAD, biotin, PLP, THF

| Coenzyme | Vitamin | Clinical group attached |
|---|---|---|
| TPP | Thiamin | Aldehyde |
| FAD | Riboflavin | Electrons |
| NAD | Nicotinate | Hydride ions |
| Pyridoxal phosphate | Pyridoxal phosphate | Amino group |
| Biotin | Biotin | $CO_2$ |
| THF | Cobalamin ($B_{12}$) | H atom and alkyl group |
| Lipoate | - | 'e', acyl group |

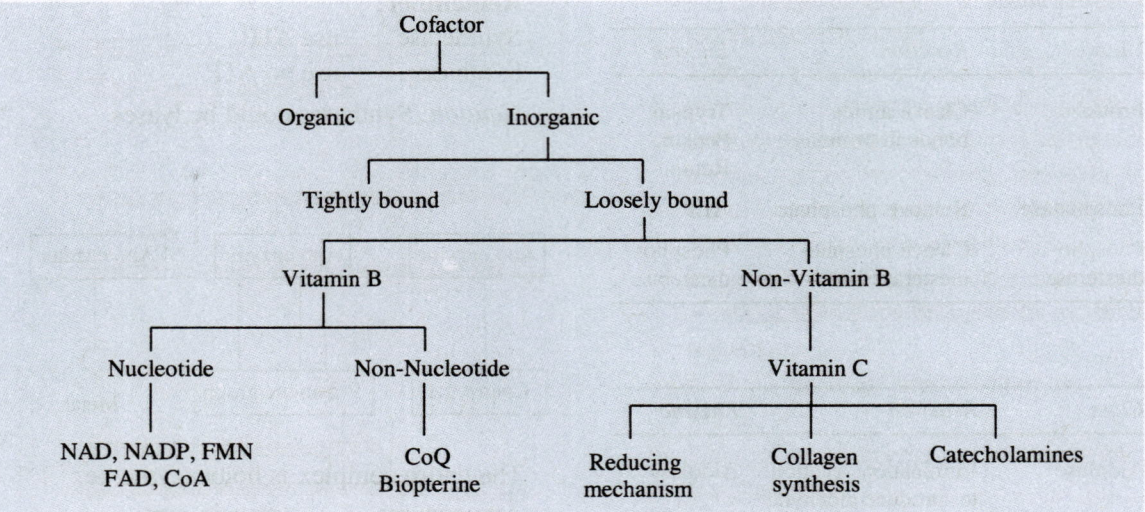

## ROLE OF METAL IONS IN OXIDATION AND REDUCTION

- Cu, Fe: can accept or donate 'e' in oxidation reduction reaction
- Na, K, Ca, Zn, Mg: do not participate in redox reaction

## Fe-S proteins

- Non-heme protein
- Unique class of metalloenzyme
- Centre has 1 or more clusters of sulfur – bridged iron chelates
  'S' can come from cysteine or cystine and free ionic sulfur
- Have low reducing potential
- Function in electron transport reaction

## MECHANISM OF ENZYME CATALYSIS

### How do enzymes work

- Enzyme catalyzed reactions are reversible and rate of reaction depends on concentrations
- Enzymes don't affect the point of equilibrium
- Enzymes only change the time of equilibrium
- Reactions will always go forward

## ENERGY CHANGES DURING A REACTION

- During a chemical reaction, bonds must be broken and new bonds are remade to form products.
- Breaking bonds require energy: **Endergonic**
- Making bonds releases energy: **Exergonic**

## Anabolic reactions

Large complex molecules are build up from smaller ones.

## Catabolic reactions

- Break down large complex molecules into smaller, simpler one
- Exergonic

All reactions begin by breaking bonds which requires activation energy to start.

## ENZYMES WORK BY LOWERING ACTIVATION ENERGY

- Done by enzyme substrate (ES) complex
- E-S complex lower activation energy
- Make the reaction proceed quicker and easier
- Without enzyme, activation energy is too high for reaction to occur

## TYPES OF ENZYME CATALYSIS

1. General acid base catalysis
2. Covalent catalysis
3. Metal catalysis

### Acid base catalysis

- Unstable charged intermediate are formed that transform proton to form molecule
- Water acts as proton donor, e.g. HIV protease
- Aspartatic acid as acid-base catalysis

### Covalent catalysis

- Enzyme form covalent bond with substrate.

### Metal catalysis

- Oxidation-reduction reaction by donating-accepting 'e'
- Provide stabilizing energy by electrostatic interaction

## ENZYMES FAMILIES

- Serine protease
- Aspartate protease

### Serpins

Serine Protease Inhibitors (endo peptidase) family of proteins of medical importance.
- Their dysfunction causes:
  Blood clotting disorders

Emphysema

Cirrhosis
- Members of serpins:
  - $\alpha$-1 antitrypsin (AT):
    Inhibit elastase
  - Antithrombin:
    Inhibit thrombin

## MECHANISM OF ACTION

### Suicidal inhibitors

- Involves initial formation of a complex between serpin and protease, followed by a cleavage inhibitor-serpin complex so that serpins are destroyed as a result of their action.

## ENZYME INHIBITION

### Inhibitors

- Cause a loss of catalytic activity
- Change the protein structure of an enzyme
- May be competitive or non competitive
- Some effects are irreversible

### Reversible vs. Irreversible inhibition

**Reversible:** Interact with enzyme via non covalent association

**Irreversible:** Interact with enzyme via covalent association

### $K_m$

- $K_m$ of $10^{-7}$ M implies 'S' has great affinity for enzyme than if $k_m$ is $10^{-3}$ M.
- Smaller the $K_m$, tighter is interaction between E and S
- Hexokinase ($K_m = 0.1$mM) has greater affinity for glucose than glucokinase ($K_m = 5$ mM)
- Unit = molar i.e., per mol, M

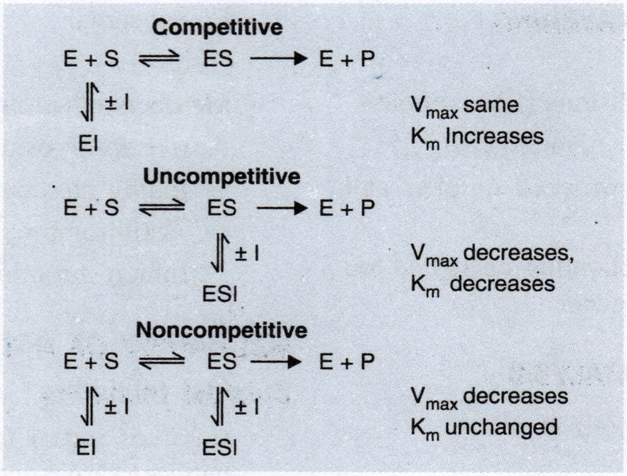

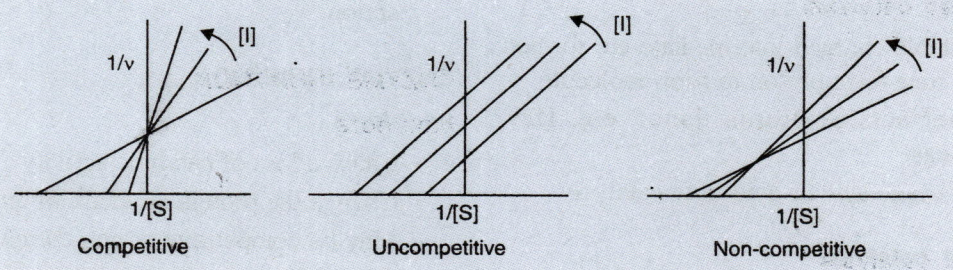

**Competitive**

$$E + S \rightleftharpoons ES \longrightarrow E + P$$

$$\Updownarrow \pm I$$

$$EI$$

$V_{max}$ same
$K_m$ Increases

**Uncompetitive**

$$E + S \rightleftharpoons ES \longrightarrow E + P$$

$$\Updownarrow \pm I$$

$$ESI$$

$V_{max}$ decreases,
$K_m$ decreases

**Noncompetitive**

$$E + S \rightleftharpoons ES \longrightarrow E + P$$

$$\Updownarrow \pm I \qquad \Updownarrow \pm I$$

$$EI \qquad ESI$$

$V_{max}$ decreases
$K_m$ unchanged

**Fig. 3.5.**

**Fig. 3.6.** Enzyme inhibition: If inhibitor and substrate compete for same enzyme, the inhibition is **competitive**. If no, the inhibition is either **non-competitive** or **uncompetitive** depending on whether or not inhibitor can affect the velocity at low substrate concentration.

## Michaelis-Menton equation

Hyperbolic kinetics, saturation kinetics where [s] = substrate concentration.

Describes the way in which velocity of an enzyme reaction depends on substrate concentration (Fig. 3.7). $V_{max}$ is velocity approached at a saturating concentration of substrate.

At high [s], v does not change much when [s] changes:

$$V = \frac{V_{max}[s]}{(K_m + [s])}$$

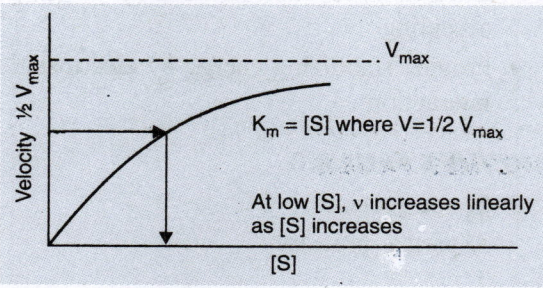

**Fig. 3.7.**

## Measure of catalytic activity - Kcat

**Kcat**: turnover number

Number of substrates converted to product

per enzyme molecule per unit time, when 'E' is saturated with 'S'.

$$K_2 = Kcat = V_{max}/Et$$

- Value of Kcat ranges from less than 1/sec to many millions per sec.

## Turnover (Kcat)

Unit = time$^{-1}$

- No. of molecules of 'S' converted to 'P' per unit time per mole of enzyme.
- Large Kcat, faster is reaction

For example:

| Enzyme | Kcat (sec$^{-1}$) |
|---|---|
| Catalase | 40,00,000 |
| Chymotrypsin | 100 |
| Lysozyme | 0.5 |

## Enzyme activity

- Usually expressed as initial rate ($v_o$) of reaction being catalyzed
- Unit $v_o$ = μmol/min by enzyme.
- Where 1 μmol/min = IU = 16.67 nanokat unit (U) or Katal

**Activity:** refers to total units of an enzyme in a sample

**Specific activity:** number of units per mg of proteins (unit/mg)

## Specific activity

- Number of units per mg of protein
- Measure of purity of an enzyme
- During purification of enzyme, its specific activity increases and value of specific

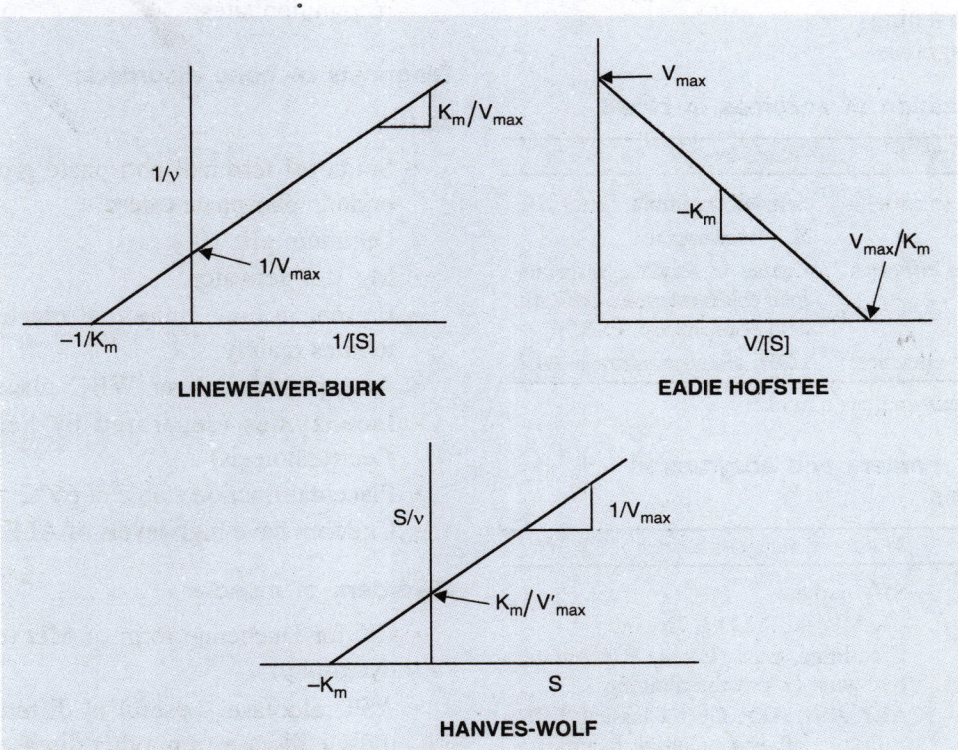

LINEWEAVER-BURK

EADIE HOFSTEE

HANVES-WOLF

**Fig. 3.8.** Instead of curved plots, Michaelis-Menton equation can be rearranged to give a straight line from where $K_m$ and $V_{max}$ can be calculated. Lineweaver-Bluk plot is useful in showing effect of inhibitor.

activity becomes maximal and constant when enzyme is pure.

## Enzyme units

Amount of enzyme which will catalyze transfer of 1 μmol of 'S' per minute at 25°C under optimal condition for that enzyme.

Katal is accepted SI unit.

## Information obtained from enzyme measurements in serum

- Presence of disease
- Organ (s) involved
- Etiology/nature of disease: different diagnosis
- Extent of disease – more damaged cells – more 'leaked' enzymes in blood
- Time – course of disease (recovery/ worsening)
- Prognosis

## Classification of enzymes in blood

| Classification | Example |
|---|---|
| Plasma specific enzymes | Serpins, thrombin, factor XII, X, plasminogen |
| Secreted enzymes | Lipase, α amylase, trypsinogen, cholinesterase, prostatic acid phosphatase, PSA* |
| Cellular enzymes | LDH, aminotransferase, ALP |

* not an enzyme, but a marker

## Plasma markers and enzymes in diagnosis

| Organ | Marker in serum or urine |
|---|---|
| Brain | S100 protein |
| Heart | CK-MB, AST, LDH, Troponin |
| Kidney | Creatinine, urea (U): ALP, NAcGln, lysozyme U: protein: albumin |
| Liver | ALT, AST, ALP, GGT Classical LFT: Bilirubin, albumin, clotting factors |
| Pancreas | Amylase, lipase |
| Skeletal muscle | CK (MM), AST, Mb, Aldolase |

## Enzymes that facilitate diagnosis of genetic disease

- Many disease result from alteration in an individual's DNA
- Tools for detection of genetic mutation are available
- Rely on catalytic efficiency and significance of enzyme catalysis
  For example,
  PCR – uses ability of enzyme to serve as catalytic amplifier to analyze DNA in samples (thermostable DNA poly-merase).
- RFLP – for prenatal diagnosis of hereditary disorders, involve cleavage of ds DNA by restriction endonuclease which can detect subtle alteration in DNA that affect their recognition sites.

## Diagnosis of bone disorders:

### ALP

- Splits off terminal phosphate group from organic phosphate esters.
- Optimum pH: 10
- $Mg^{+2}$ as activator
- Present in bone, intestinal mucosa, renal tubules mainly
- Also, present in liver, WBC, placenta
- Isoenzymes (separated by heating or electrophoresis)
- Placental fraction stable at 65°C
- Children have high levels of ALP

## Disorders of muscle

- CK for Duchenne form of MD (muscular dystrophy)
- AST, aldolase – useful in differentiating muscle disease from other diseases.

## AST or SGOT

- Found in all tissues

- Highest concentration in cardiac and skeletal muscle disorders
- Rises 6-12 hrs post MI, peaks at 24-48 hrs, normal by day 4-6

## DIAGNOSIS OF PROSTATE CANCER

### ACP (Acid Phosphatase)

- Same mode of action as ALP
- High in prostate
- Tartarate inhibition
- Also present in kidney, platelets, RBC, bone, spleen
- Optimum pH<6
- Used in diagnosis, treatment, follow up
- PSA better screening/diagnostic tool

## PANCREATIC ENZYMES

- Diagnosis of acute pancreatitis:
  – Amylase: S and P isoenzymes (S = salivary, P = pancreatic)
  – Lipase
- Non pancreatic abdominal disease, appendicitis and peritonitis cause hyperamylasemia

## GENETIC DISORDERS

Pseudo cholinesterase:

- Inability of hydrolyze succinyl choline
- Exposure to organophosphorus, insecticides decrease its activity

G6PD deficiency

Galactose-1-P uridyl transferase deficiency

## DIAGNOSIS OF LIVER DISORDERS

- AST
- ALT:
  Diagnosis of liver disease
  More sensitive to hepatocellular damage
- In hepatitis: ALT/AST > 1

ALT usually higher than AST in most of liver disease, exception: Alcoholic hepatitis: where AST higher than ALP
- ALP
- GGT: Located in canaliculi of hepatocytes Elevated in all hepatocellular disorders Useful in:
  – Detecting hepatic injury caused by Alcohol
  – Hepatic metastasis in an icteric patient
- Management of infections hepatitis:
  – Better prognosis if returns to normal
  – Later increase indicates exacerbation of disease
- Bile duct obstruction

## CARDIAC ENZYMES

- Creatine kinase
- CK MB
- Lactate dehydrogenase (LDH)
- Aspartate aminotransferase (AST)

## MYOGLOBIN

- Found in skeletal, cardiac muscle
- Small size allows early detection rapid clearance
- Not specific for cardiac muscle

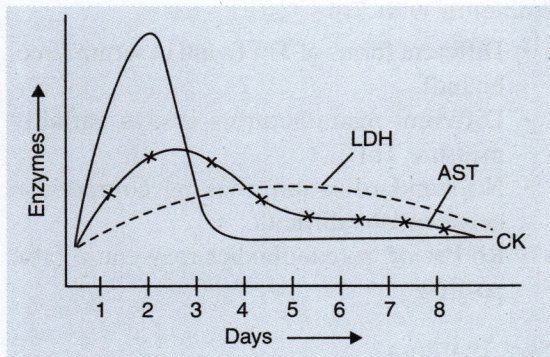

**Fig. 3.9.** Diagnostic enzymes in MI.

## TROPONIN

- Formed only in muscle
- Predominantly bound to myofibers: small fraction free
- For TnI and TnT, difference is between cardiac and skeletal muscle forms
- Release from fibrils causes high levels for many days

### Troponin T

- Cardiac-like form, found in fetal, skeletal muscle
- About 6% cytosolic, detectable earlier than $T_nI$
- Second generation assay detects less damage than $T_nI$

### Troponin I

- Found only in cardiac muscle
- About 2% cytosolic
- Later detection than $T_nT$

### Tn in renal failure

- Elevated TnT are seen commonly in renal failure (up to 50%)
- High TnI seen occasionally
- Patients with Tn have high likelihood of cardiac death in year after detection

### Problems with TnI

- Different forms of TnI found in serum (free, bound)
- Different manufacturers assays variably measure TnI
- No standardization, making comparison between labs difficult
- Rh Factor, autoantibodies may cause false positive

### Ideal markers?

- TnI, TnT currently considered equivalent

- Rapid change markers such as myoglobin required to detect reinfarct

### New markers

- Ischemia modified albumin (IMA)
- Glycogen phosphorylase B
- Fatty acid binding protein (FABP)

## REGULATION OF ENZYME ACTIVITY

In metabolic pathways, the end products often feed back inhibit the committed step to prevent build up of intermediates and unnecessary use of metabolites and energy!

**Importance:**

1. Many human diseases including cancer, diabetes, cystic fibrosis, Alzheimer's disease are characterized by regulatory dysfunctions triggered by pathogenetic agents or genetic mutations.
2. Many oncogenic viruses elaborate tyrosine kinases that modify regulatory events that control pattern of gene expression, contributing to initiation and progression of cancer.

**Remember**: Knowledge of factors that control rate of enzyme catalyzed reactions is essential to the understanding molecular basis of disease!

## REGULATION OF ENZYME QUANTITY

In humans, alterations in levels of specific enzymes can be affected by a change in rate constant for overall process of synthesis ($K_s$) and degradation ($K_{deg}$) or both.

## CONTROL OF ENZYME SYNTHESIS

- Enzyme synthesis depends on: presence of inducers

**Inducible enzymes:**

Examples

Tryptophan pyrrolase

Threonine dehydratase

Enzymes of urea cycle

HMG CoA-R

Cyt $P_{450}$

- Conversely, an excess of metabolite may curtail synthesis of its cognate enzyme via repression.

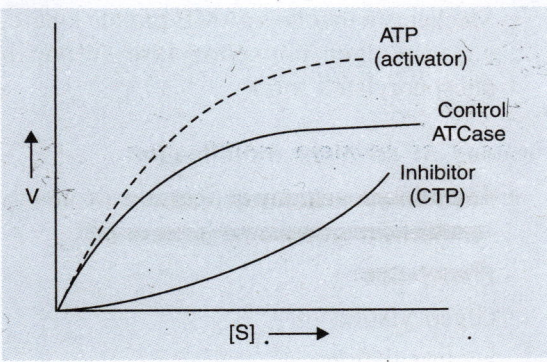

**Fig. 3.10.** ATCase activity.

## MECHANISM OF CONTROL OF ENZYME SYNTHESIS

Induction and repression involve:

- Cis-elements
- Specific DNA sequences located upstream of regulated genes and trans-acting regulatory proteins

## CONTROL OF ENZYME DEGRADATION

- Enzyme are degraded by ubiquitin proteasome (Ub) pathway
- Dysfunction of Ub-proteasome pathway contributes to accumulation of aberrantly folded protein species, characteristic of severe neurodegenerative disease.

## REGULATING CATALYTIC ACTIVITY

- Allosteric regulation
- Covalent modification

## ALLOSTERIC INHIBITOR

It changes the conformation of enzyme, distorting the active site and reducing the ability to catalyze the reaction

**Example:**

**ATCase**

- Aspartate transcarbamoylase
- Committed step of pyrimidine synthesis
- 6 catalytic subunit, each with active site
- 6 regulated units to which allosteric effectors: CTP, ATP bind
- ATCase feed-back inhibited by end-product CTP, activator is ATP
- Gives sigmoidal curve on plot of V against [S]
- High levels of ATP signal cell that 'E' is available for replication, so ATCase gets activated causing pyrimidine synthesis
- When pyrimidine is abundant, high level of CTP inhibit ATCase, preventing pyrimidine synthesis.

## COVALENT MODIFICATION

Covalent modification is of two types:

- Partial proteolysis
- Phosphorylation

### Phosphorylation

- Addition or removal of P groups to and from enzyme

- Mechanism involves cAMP, protein kinase, e.g. glycogen phosphorylase active in phosphorylated form

### Process of covalent modification

- Introduces structural features to newly synthesized proteins by process of:
  Prenylation
  Glycosylation
  Hydroxylation
  FA acylation
- Protein functions can be regulated by:
  Methylation
  Adenylation
- Phosphorylation/dephosphorylation- most common
- Targets for protein kinase: his, lys, arg, asp

### Protein phosphorylation

- Side chain – OH groups of ser, thr, tyr can form phosphate esters, catalyzed by protein kinase
- Phosphorylation by ATP can activate enzyme, e.g. Glycogen phosphorylase
- Addition/removal of phosphate group causes changes in tertiary structure of enzyme that alters its catalytic activity.

### PROTEIN KINASE

Reside on target enzyme:

It is of three types:

- Ser/Thr protein kinase: cAMP dependent protein kinase
- Tyr protein kinase
- Calmodulin dependent protein kinase: when calmodulin binds $Ca^{+2}$, an activator of number of ser/thr protein kinases

### PROTEIN PHOSPHATASE

### Catalyze hydrolysis of phosphate group

It is of two types:

- Class I: Enzyme specific for ser/thr phosphates
- Class II: Enzyme that hydrolyze tyr phosphates.

### Enzymes active in dephosphorylated form

- HMG CoA-R
- Acetyl CoA carboxylase (ACC)
- Glycogen synthase
- Pyruvate dehydrogenase (PDH)

### Reversible covalent modification

- Phosphorylation/dephosphorylation
- Adenylation: transfer of adenylate from ATP
- ADP ribosylation: transfer of ADP-ribosyl moiety from NAD

### Clinical implications of covalent modification

- Cyclic nucleotides and protein phos-phorylation:
  Cholera toxin: Causes persistent activation of cAMP
- Phosphodiesterase inhibited by:
  - Theophylline: bronchodilators
  - Sildenafil citrate (Viagra)
- Protein kinase and phosphatase are important targets for drugs, e.g. Gleevac: tyrosine kinase inhibitors

### Proteolytic activation of enzymes

Some enzymes are synthesized as large inactive precursors known as **zymogens** or **proenzymes.**

- Zymogens are activated by irreversible hydrolysis of one or more peptide bonds. For example:

  Trypsinogen → Trypsin

  Chymotrypsinogen → Chymotrypsin

  Proelastase → Elastase

## Zymogen activation

- It does not require ATP
- Zymogen activation is not reversible, once activated, enzyme stays active!

## Purpose of synthesis of enzyme as zymogens

- Synthesis and secretion of proteases as catalytically inactive proenzyme protects the tissue of origin from auto digestion, e.g. Pancreas.
- Enzymes required intermittently but, rapidly are often secreted in an initial inactive form. Since secretion or synthesis of required protein might be insufficiently rapid for response to a pressing patho-physiological demand such as loss of blood.

## Zymogen: Examples

Proteins synthesized as proproteins include:

- Insulin
- Pepsin
- Trypsin
- Chymotrypsin
- Factors of blood coagulation and blood clot dissolution
- Collagen

## Regulation of enzyme synthesis and break down:

Amount of a particular enzyme present in a cell or tissues changes according to rate of its synthesis and degradation.

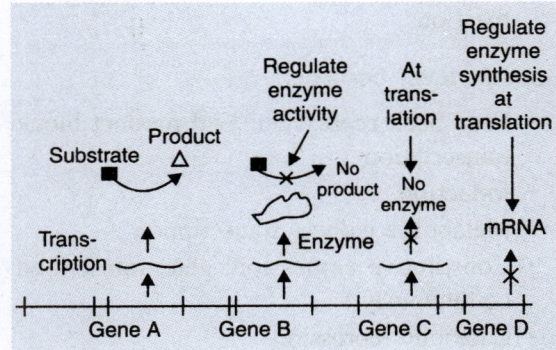

Fig. 3.11. Regulation of enzyme activity and synthesis.

## Need for regulation?

Metabolic events must meet the requirement for an organism to survive. Metabolic activity is often controlled by:

- Release of hormone and other messenger molecules, triggered by changes in level of 'S' in blood or by signals from nervous system
- Cellular activity might by controlled directly by changes in cell environment.
- Maintenance of tissue health involves constant cycle of cell death and regeneration.

## Types of control of reaction in the cell:

- Genetic level (control of transcription)
  - Controlling amount of enzymes
  - Common in prokaryotes
- Enzymatic level (control of product formation)
  - Controlling activities of enzymes
  - Most common in eukaryotes

## Enzymatic level control

- Enzymes are transcribed and translated
- Feed back inhibition of allosteric enzymatic reactions

## Genetic level control

- Feed back repression: End product block transcription
- Induction
- Metabolite induces transcription
- Constitutive expression: gene transcribed continuously
- Catabolic repression
- Several operons influenced by presence of glucose:

If glucose is present, most operons for other sugar metabolism are regulated off

## DIFFERENCE

### Enzyme level control

- Fast
- Quick to reverse
- Inefficient

### Genetic level control

- Slow
- Slow to reverse
- Efficient for longtime control

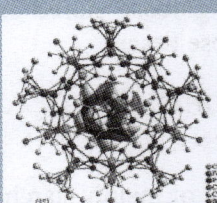

# Metabolism

## 1. CARBOHYDRATE METABOLISM

### INTRODUCTION

Overview of human metabolism (Fig. 4.1):

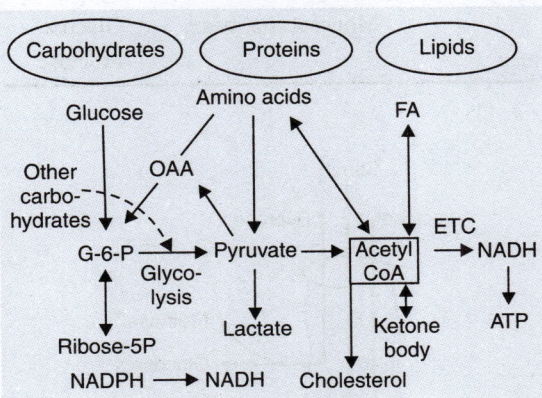

**Fig. 4.1.** Overview of human metabolism.

### Carbohydrate metabolism: Fact file

- Primary metabolite: glucose

- Fructose and galactose enter the pathways at various points
- All cells can utilize glucose for energy production
  - Glucose uptake from blood to cells usually mediated by insulin and transporters
- Liver is central site for carbohydrate metabolism:
  - Glucose uptake independent of insulin
  - The only exporter of glucose

### Compartmentalization

| Compartment | Metabolic pathway |
|---|---|
| Cytosol | Glycolysis |
| | PPP |
| | FA synthesis |
| Mitochondrial matrix | TCA |
| | FA oxidation |
| | KB production |
| | Oxidative phosphorylation |
| In both | Urea cycle |
| | GNG |

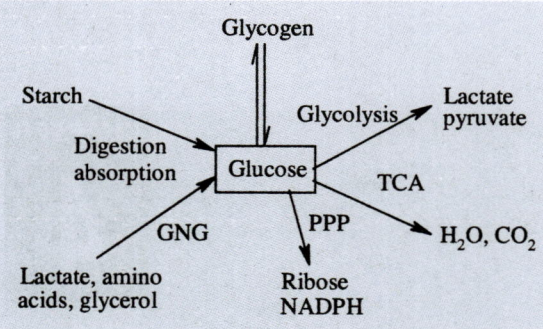

## FATE OF GLUCOSE

### Fed state

- Storage as glycogen in:
  Liver
  Skeletal muscle
- Storage as lipid in:
  Adipose tissue

### Fasting state

- Metabolized for energy
- New glucose synthesized

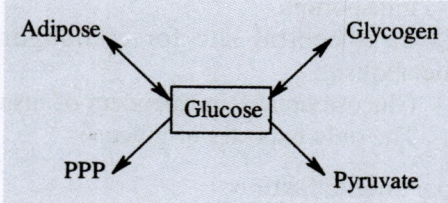

## FOUR MAJOR METABOLIC PATHWAYS OF GLUCOSE

- Immediate source of energy via glycolysis and TCA
- PPP
- Glycogen synthesis in liver/muscle
- Precursor for TAG synthesis.

Energy status of body regulates pathway to get energy.

## FATE OF ABSORBED GLUCOSE

| Ist priority | Glycogen storage |
|---|---|
|  | Liver |
|  | Muscle |
| 2nd Priority | Provide energy: |
|  | Oxidized to ATP |
| 3rd Priority | Stored as fat: |
|  | Only excess glucose stored as TAG in adipose tissue |

## (i) DIGESTION OF CARBOHYDRATES

### Outline

Dietary carbohydrates consist of mainly starch, sucrose, lactose and glucose.

| Dietary carbohydrates | | |
|---|---|---|
| Include: | Polysaccharides | Starch |
|  |  | Glycogen |
|  | Disaccharides | Sucrose |
|  |  | Lactose |
|  |  | Maltose |
|  | Monosaccharides | Glucose |
|  |  | Fructose |

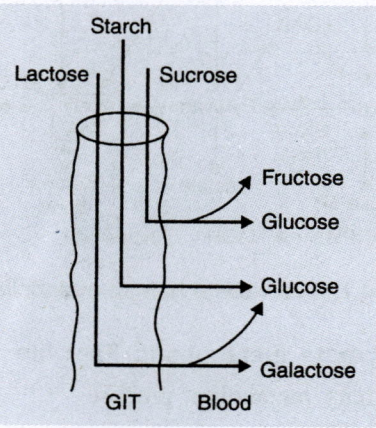

**Fig. 4.2.** Overview of carbohydrate digestion.

### Main dietary components

| Carbohydrate | Food |
| --- | --- |
| Starch (Amylose) | Potato, rice, bread |
| Amylopectin | Potato, rice, bread, muscle, liver |
| Sucrose | Table Sugar, sweets |
| Lactose | Milk (dairy products) |
| Glucose | Fruit, honey |
| Fructose | Fruits, honey |

### Dietary disaccharides

| Sugar | Dietary source | Components |
| --- | --- | --- |
| Sucrose | Cane/beet sugar | Glucose-fructose |
| Lactose | Milk sugar | Galactose-glucose |
| Maltose | Malt sugar | Glucose-glucose |
| Isomaltose | | Glucose-glucose (1-6) |
| Trehalose | Synthesized by bacteria fungi | Glucose-glucoside |

### Site of digestion

- Mouth
  - Amylase
- Esophagus
  - Peristalsis
- Stomach
  - No digestion of carbohydrates
- Pancreas
  - Amylase
- Small intestine
  - Amylase
  - Absorption
- Large intestine
  - Egestion

### Digestion of carbohydrates (Fig. 4.4a)

- Begins in the mouth
  - α-amylase
    Optimum pH 6.7
    Range 6.6-6.8
    Breaks α 1-4 glycosidic bond

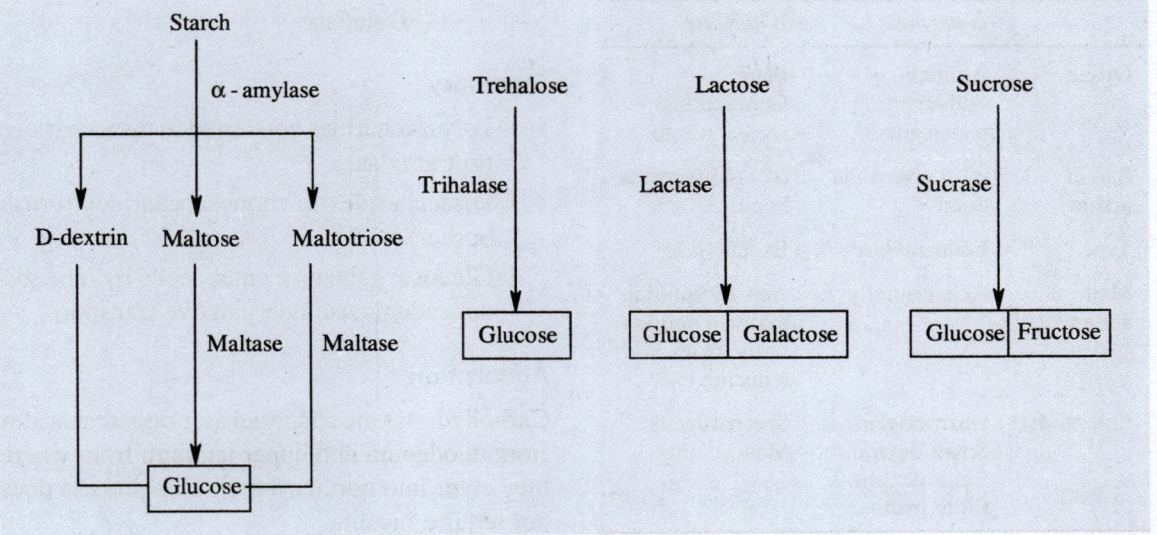

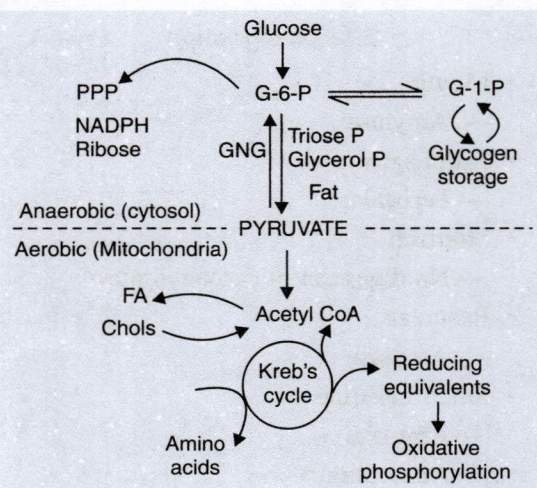

**Fig. 4.3.** Glucose metabolism summary.

- Result:
  - Maltose
  - Maltotriose
  - Limit dextrin
  - Salivary α-amylase: α1-4 endogluco-sidase.

**Table 4.1.** Comparison

|  | *α-amylase* | *β-amylase* |
|---|---|---|
| Origin | Animal: Salivary pancreatic | Plant: Germinating seeds, potato |
| Site of action | α1-4 glycosidic bond | α1→4 glycosidic bond |
| Type | Endoamylase | Exoamylase |
| Mode of action | Acts centrally | Acts by splitting maltose sequentially from non-reducing end |
| End product | Dextrinogenic Small dextrin Limit dextrin Little maltose | Saccharogenic Maltose only |

## STOMACH

- Not much carbohydrate digestion
- Acid and pepsin unfold proteins
- Due to high acidity pH 3.0 in stomach, carbohydrate digestion halts in stomach.

## PANCREAS

Pancreas secretes:

- Bicarbonate: to neutralize acid
- α-amylase: to continue carbohydrate digestion (Fig. 4.4b)

## SMALL INTESTINE

- Pancreatic enzyme: α-amylase (Fig. 4.5).
- Final digestive process occurs at mucosal lining of jejunum
- Declines as it proceeds down
- Enzymes:
  - Oligosaccharidases
  - Disaccharidases:
    - Maltase
    - Sucrase – Isomaltase
    - Lactase
    - Trehalase

## Summary

- Polysaccharides converted to disaccharides (gut amylase)
- Disaccharides to monosaccharides (brush border)
- Glucose, galactose enters cells by: energy-dependent, secondary active transport.

## Absorption

Carbohydrates are absorbed as monosaccharides from duodenum and upper jejunum from where they enter into portal system. This process does not require insulin.

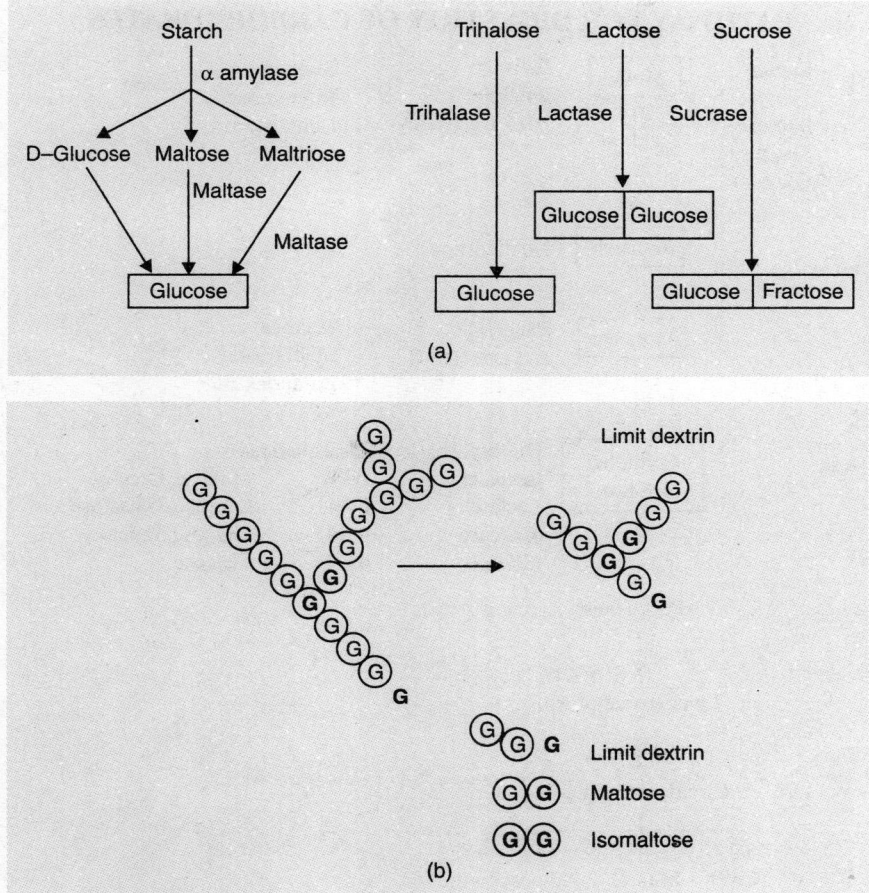

**Fig. 4.4.** (a) & (b). Action of α-amylase.

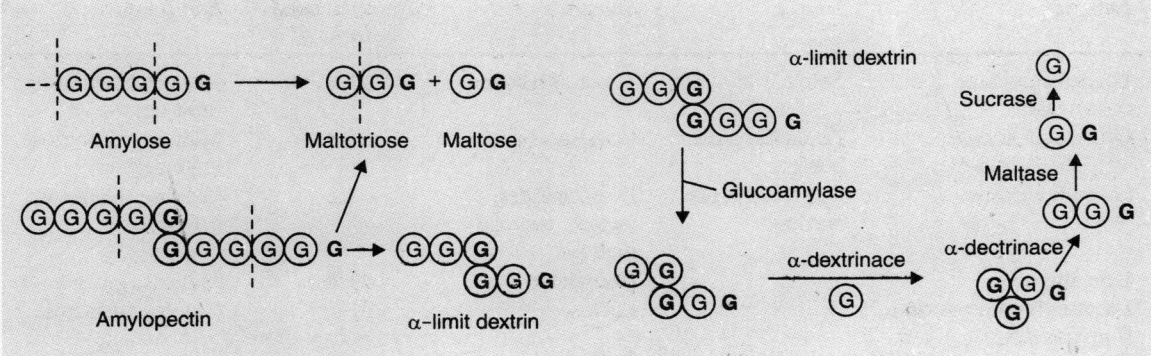

**Fig. 4.5.** Digestion of carbohydrates.

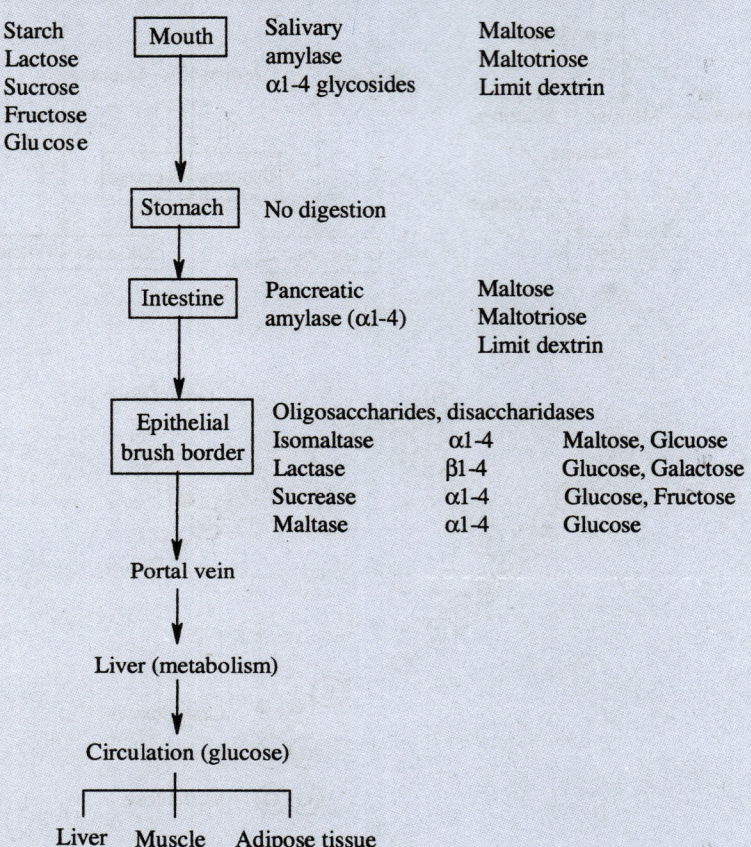

## PATHWAY FOR DIGESTION OF CARBOHYDRATES

Starch    [Mouth]    Salivary      Maltose
Lactose          amylase       Maltotriose
Sucrose          $\alpha$1-4 glycosides    Limit dextrin
Fructose
Glucose

[Stomach]    No digestion

[Intestine]    Pancreatic      Maltose
          amylase ($\alpha$1-4)    Maltotriose
                        Limit dextrin

[Epithelial brush border]    Oligosaccharides, disaccharidases

| | | | |
|---|---|---|---|
| Isomaltase | $\alpha$1-4 | Maltose, Glcuose |
| Lactase | $\beta$1-4 | Glucose, Galactose |
| Sucrease | $\alpha$1-4 | Glucose, Fructose |
| Maltase | $\alpha$1-4 | Glucose |

Portal vein

Liver (metabolism)

Circulation (glucose)

Liver    Muscle    Adipose tissue

**Table 4.2.** Enzymes of carbohydrate digestion

| Enzyme | Source | Substrate | Glycosidic bond hydrolyzed | End product |
|---|---|---|---|---|
| Polysaccharidase $\alpha$-amylase | Saliva, pancreas | Starch, glycogen | $\alpha$1-4 | Maltose, maltotriose, limit dextrin |
| Oligosaccharidase | Epithelial brush border | Oligosaccharides | $\alpha$1-4 | Maltose, maltotriose, limit dextrin |
| Disaccharidases | Epithelial brush border | Disaccharides, lactose, sucrose maltose | $\alpha$1-4 | Glucose, Galactose, Fructose |
| Isomaltase | | Isomaltose | $\alpha$1-6 | Maltose, glucose |
| Lactase ($\beta$-galactosidase, $\beta$-glycosidase) | | Lactose | $\beta$1-4 | Glucose, galactose |
| Sucrase ($\alpha$-glycosidase) | | Sucrose | $\alpha$1-4 | Glucose, fructose |
| Maltase | | Maltose | $\alpha$1-4 | Glucose |

## Site

- Duodenum
- Upper jejunum

## Insulin not required

## Mechanism

- Simple diffusion
- Facilitated transport
- Active transport

### Monosaccharides are absorbed by:

- Glucose: Active transport
  - Sodium dependent active transporter: SGLT-1
  - Require 'E': linked to $Na^+/K^+$ ATPase pump
- Galactose:
  - SGLT-1
  - GLUT5
  - Absorbed more rapidly than glucose
- Fructose
  - Na independent facilitative transporter
  - GLUT5
  - Does not require energy ('E')

GLUT2:
Moves glucose, galactose, fructose into blood

## Disaccharidases

- Brush border enzymes
- Maltase
- Sucrase-Isomaltase
- Lactase
- Trehalase

## Absorption of glucose by intestinal mucosal cells

- Transporter or carrier system has a high degree of specificity

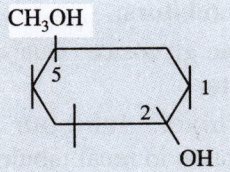

- −OH group at C2 should have the same configuration as glucose
- A pyranose ring should be present
- A methyl or substituted methyl group should be present at C-5

## Rate of absorption

Galactose > glucose > fructose.

## Transport of carbohydrates across brush-border membrane

Transport of Glucose, Galactose: SGLT-1
  - Carrier mediated diffusion: Fructose, Mannose
  - Down the concentration gradient: Fructose, sugar alcohol
  - Simple diffusion: pentose

### SGLT-1:

  - Coupled to $Na^+$–$K^+$ pump.
  - Allows glucose and galactose to be transported against concentration gradient.
  - SGLT-1 has separate sites for glucose and $Na^+$ binding.
  - $Na^+$ is transported down its concentration gradient causing the carrier to carry glucose against its concentration gradient.
  - Hydrolysis of ATP is linked to sodium pump which provides energy for active transport.
  - Three $Na^+$ ions are expelled from the cell in exchange for two $K^+$ ions.

**SGLT-1 Inhibitors:**

- Cardiac glycoside: Ouabain: Na pump inhibitor
- Phlorhizin: Inhibitor of glucose absorption in renal tubules
- Cholera toxin: (–) NaCl absorption but not facilitative transport of Na and glucose

ORS (oral rehydration solution) provide

| 110 mM | Glucose |
|--------|---------|
| 99 mM | $Na^+$ |
| 74 mM | $Cl^-$ |
| 39 mM | $HCO_3^-$ |
| 4 mM | $K^+$ |

Since SGLT-1 not inhibited by cholera toxin and presence of glucose allows uptake of Na to replenish stores.

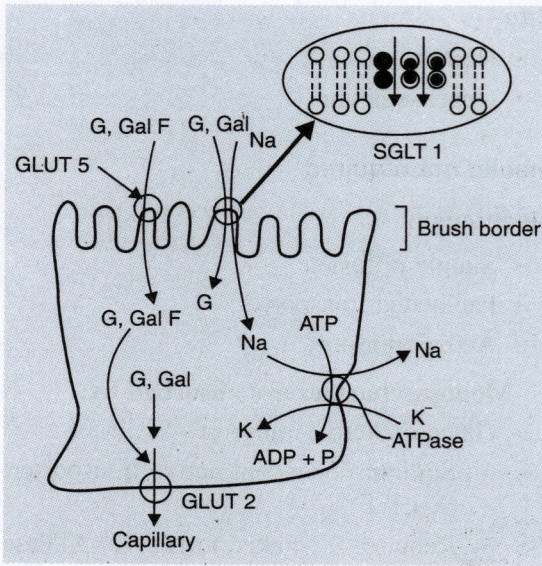

Fig. 4.7. Glucose transporters.

**GLUT 5:**

Na independent facilitative transporter, allow glucose, galactose, fructose to be transported with their concentration gradient.

**Non-digestible carbohydrates or dietary fiber**

Dietary carbohydrates include refined carbohydrates such as sucrose and fruit juices and complex carbohydrates such as starch.

Fiber consists of carbohydrates indigestible by gut lumen and includes cellulose, hemicellulose, lignin pectin, gums, pentosans and betaglucan.

The main role of fiber is to regulate gut transit and mobility. Also, they aid in water retention during passage of food along gut, producing larger and softer feces. Cellulose and lignin in wheat bran are beneficial for colonic function. Gums and protein in legumes and fruits are most soluble fibers that lower blood cholesterol levels and are beneficial in diabetes.

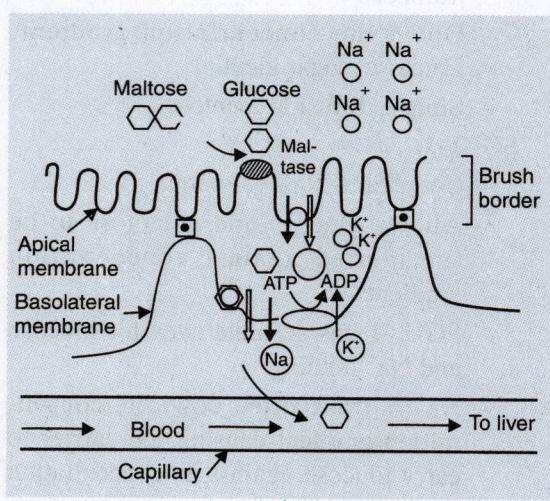

Fig. 4.6. Absorption of glucose.

**GLUT-2:**

Exit of all sugar from cell is via GLUT 2 facilitative transporter

## Defects in enzymes of carbohydrate digestion

- Intestinal disaccharide deficiencies
- Lactose intolerance
- Decline in lactase with age
- Lactose gets fermented in large intestine to produce gas and volatile fatty acid.
- Water retention causes diarrhoea, bloating.

## Lactase deficiency

- Congenital absence of lactase
- Acquired lactase deficiency

## Symptoms

- Distension
- Abdominal bloating
- Nausea
- Cramping pain
- Diarrhoea

## Mechanism

- Lactase enzyme absent in brush border.
- Lactose draws water into lumen (osmotic effect).
- Bacterial action causes lactic acid production which draws water into lumen causing watery diarrhoea and malabsorption of other nutrients.

## Diagnosis

- Intestinal biopsy

- Lactose loading test
- $^{14}C$ lactose breath test
- Hydrogen breath test

## Hydrogen breath test

Give 50 g lactose orally and collect hydrogen from breath. In lactose deficiency hydrogen breath increased due to bacterial action.

## Treatment

- Lactose free diet.

## Sucrase deficiency

- 2% incidence in North America.

## Symptoms

- Infant: Colic
- Adult: Abdominal fullness, distension, nausea, cramps, watery diarrhea

## Cause

Low or detectable sucrase.

## Mechanism

Same as lactase deficiency.

## Types

- Congenital
- Acquired: Secondary to intestinal disease, e.g. Tropical sprue

## Diagnosis

Hydrogen breath test.

| | Condition | Defect | Clinical feature |
|---|---|---|---|
| 1 | Lactose intolerance Inherited lactase deficiency Secondary lactase deficiency | Lactase deficiency | Abdominal discomfort Cramps, diarrhea Intolerance to milk |
| 2. | Sucrase deficiency | Inherited | Same as lactase deficiency |
| 3. | Disacchariduria | Disaccharidases deficiency | Fructose, sorbitol malabsorption |
| 4. | Monosaccharide malabsorption | Defect in SGLT-1 | Fructose, sorbitol malabsorption, watery diarrhea |

## GLUCOSE, GALACTOSE MALABSORPTION

### Symptoms

- Severe diarrhea
- Dehydration
- Sugar in stool
- Glucose in urine

### Defect

- Glucose carrier protein defect
- Defect in glucose binding site

### Diagnosis

- Stools contain glucose, galactose
- Glucose in urine.
- No rise in glucose after meals.

### Treatment

Eliminate glucose from diet.

## (i) Glycolysis

### Importance

- Principal route for glucose metabolism
- Main pathway for fructose and galactose
- RBCs is unique among all cells of body tissues. It uses glucose and glycolysis as sole source of energy.
- Provide ATP to skeletal muscle in absence of oxygen.
- Enzymes of this pathway demonstrate stereospecificity for naturally occurring D-isomers.
- RBCs lack mitochondria and are completely reliant on glycolysis as source of energy.

### Conditions where glycolysis is affected

- Myocardial infarction: poor glycolytic activity
- Hemolytic anaemia: pyruvate kinase deficiency
- Fatigue: PFK deficiency in muscle

- Cancer: glycolysis proceeds at a much higher rate than citric acid cycle
- Lactacidosis : PDH deficiency

### Site: Cytosol

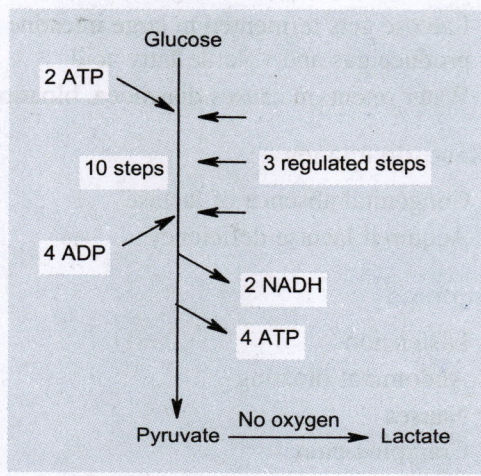

Summary: Glycolysis.

### Transport of glucose into cells

- Glucose travels across cells membrane via transport protein
- Insulin stimulates glucose transport into muscle and adipose cells by causing GLUT4 within the cells to move to cell membrane
- Insulin does not significantly stimulate transport of glucose into tissues such as liver, brain and RBCs

**BPG mutase:** Bifunctional enzyme.
Both mutase and phosphatase activity

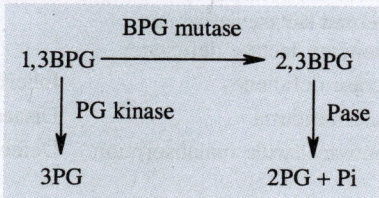

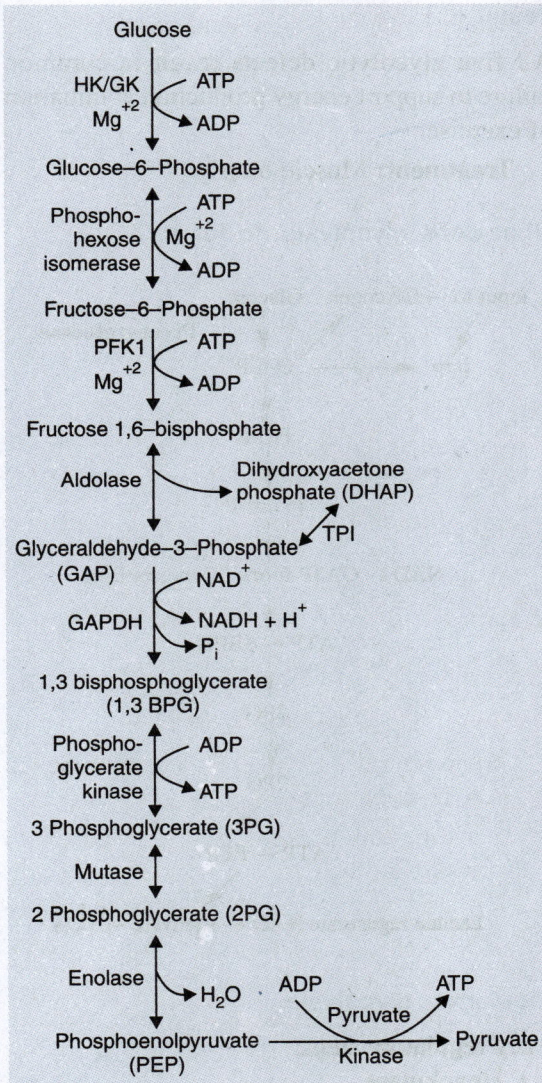

**Fig. 4.8.** Reactions of glycolysis.

PG kinase step bypassed by:

- BPG mutase and free energy released as heat
- Important for economy of RBC
- Allows glycolysis to proceed when need for ATP is minimal

## 2,3 BPG pathway in RBCs

**2,3 BPG:** Major phosphorylated intermediate in RBC, present at even higher concentration than ATP or iP.

- In glycolysis 10-20% of glycolytic intermediate 3BPG is diverted to synthesis of 2,3BPG

**HbF:** Composed of $2\alpha$ and $2\gamma$ subunits

- Has low affinity for 2,3 BPG than HbA.
- So, HbF has high affinity for $O_2$.
- This difference facilitates unloading of $O_2$ at the maternal fetal interface (i.e., placenta)

## Oxygen shortage/hypoxia

Raises 2,3 BPG levels. 2,3 BPG is allosteric effector of $O_2$ affinity of Hb.

## Adaptation to high altitude

- Increases number of RBCs
- Increases Hb concentration
- Lowers affinity of Hb for $O_2$
- Increases ability of Hb to unload $O_2$ to tissues.
- Glycolysis ends in lactate production.
- Some cells at times undergo glycolysis for lactate production despite their capacity for oxidative metabolism, e.g. Muscle during oxygen debt, phagocytes in poorly perfused tissues or in pus.

## Anaerobic glycolysis

- Under aerobic conditions, most of pyruvate metabolized via TCA
- Under anaerobic conditions and in RBCs under anaerobic condition, pyruvate gets converted to lactate by LDH

## Energetics

| Reaction | Enzyme | ATP gain/loss |
|---|---|---|
| G→G6P | GK, HK | –1ATP |
| F6P→F1,6BP | PFK | –1 ATP |
| GA3P→1, 3BPG | GAPDH | +2NADH = + 6ATP |
| 1,3 BPG→3BPG | PGK | +2 ATP |
| PEP→Pyruvate | PK | +2 ATP |

Net ATP = 10-2ATP = 8ATP

## Anaerobic glycolysis

Pyruvate → Lactate (LDH)

2NADH = –6ATP

Net ATP = 8 ATP–6ATP = 2ATP

Absence of **Aldolase** (in RBC, muscle): presents with hemolytic anaemia.

TPI deficiency has neonatal **hemolytic** anaemia as well as progressive **neurological** involvement and cardiomegaly later on.

## DISORDERS OF GLYCOLYSIS CAUSING EXERCISE INTOLERANCE

### Types

1. Myophosphorylase deficiency (GSD V)
2. PFK deficiency
3. PGK deficiency: X-linked recessive
4. PGM deficiency.
5. LDH deficiency.

Types 1, 2, 4, 5: Autosomal dominant (AD).

### Clinical features

- Exercise intolerance
- Raised serum creatinine
- No lactate rise on forearm exercise test
- Myoglobinuria

Signs and Symptoms begin in adolescent.

## Result

All five glycolytic defects result in common failure to support energy production at initiation of exercise.

**Treatment:** Muscle biopsy.

## What does glycolysis do for us?

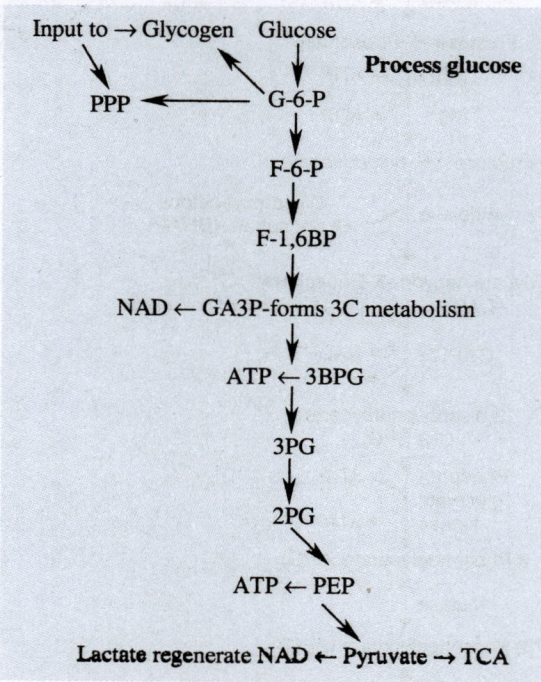

## Regulation glycolysis

3 key regulatory steps:
- Hexokinase
- Phosphofructokinase (PFK)
- Pyruvate kinase

PFK-1
- Pacemaker of glycolysis.
- Glucostat
- Rate limiting step:
  - Committed step: Ensures that reactions proceeds to completion

- Enzyme regulated by:
  Covalent modification
  Allosteric regulation

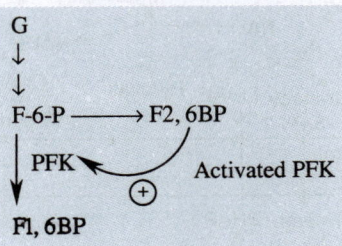

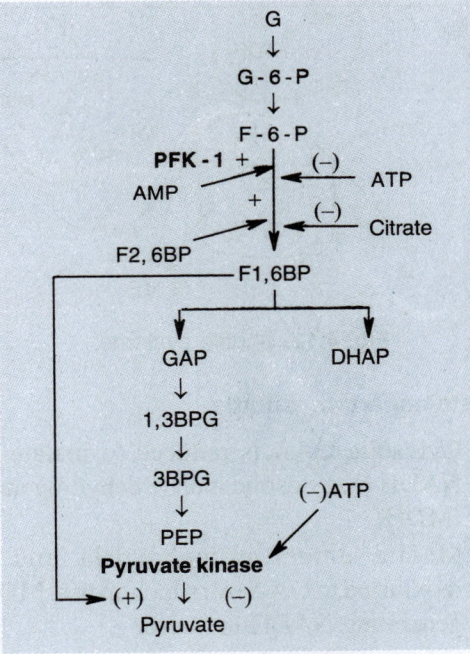

**Fig. 4.9.** Control points in glycolysis.

## Pyruvate kinase

Allosteric regulation:
- F1, 6 BP allosteric activator
- ATP, alanine in liver: inhibitor

Covalent modification:
- Phosphorylated by glucagon via cAMP and PKA
- Inhibited by phosphorylation

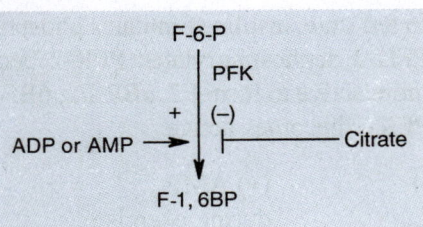

**Fig. 4.10.** Allosteric regulation of glycolysis

Pyruvate kinase:
- Activated by F1, 6P
- In fed state inhibited in liver (not muscle) by phosphorylation
- Inhibited by alanine
- Phosphorylation (during fasting when glucagon is high).

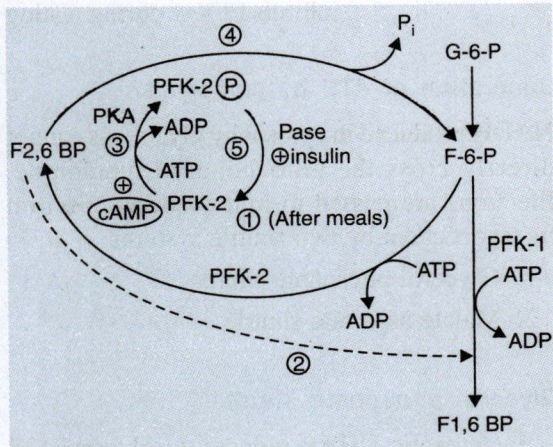

**Fig. 4.11.** Enzyme regulation after meals and during fasting.

1. After meals: F2, 6BP formed from F-6-P by PFK-2.
2. F2, 6-BP activates PFK-1, glycolysis stimulated.
3. In fasting state, PFK-2 phosphorylated by PKA which is activated by cAMP.
4. PFK-2 converts F2, 6BP to F-6-P and F2, 6BP levels fall, PFK-1 less active.

5. In fed state, insulin stimulates phosphatase, PFK-2 dephosphorylated PFK-2 becomes more active to form F2, 6BP. F2, 6BP rises, PFK-1 becomes active.

| PFK-1: | (+) AMP<br>during exercise<br>AMP high<br>ATP low |
|---|---|
| Glycolysis promoted by FPK to generate more ATP | (–) by ATP, citrate when ATP high, cell does not need ATP, glycolysis inhibited. High citrate indicate more substrates entering TCA: glycolysis shows down |

Insulin: increases PFK-1 in fed state glucagon inhibits PFK-1 during fasting

## Generation of ATP by glycolysis

NADH produced in cytosol by glycolysis cannot directly cross the mitochondrial membrane. Electrons are passed to mitochondrial electron transport chain by two shuttle systems:

1. Glycerol phosphate shuttle
2. Malate aspartate shuttle

## Glycerol phosphate shuttle

- Cytosolic DHAP reduced to glycerol -3P by NADH
- Glycerol 3-P reacts with FAD-linked dehydrogenase in IMM
- DHAP is regenerated and reenters cytosol.
- Each mole of $FADH_2$ produced generates 2 moles of ATP via oxidative phosphorylation.
- Because, glycolysis produces 2 moles of NADH per mole of glucose, 6 moles of ATP are produced by the shuttle

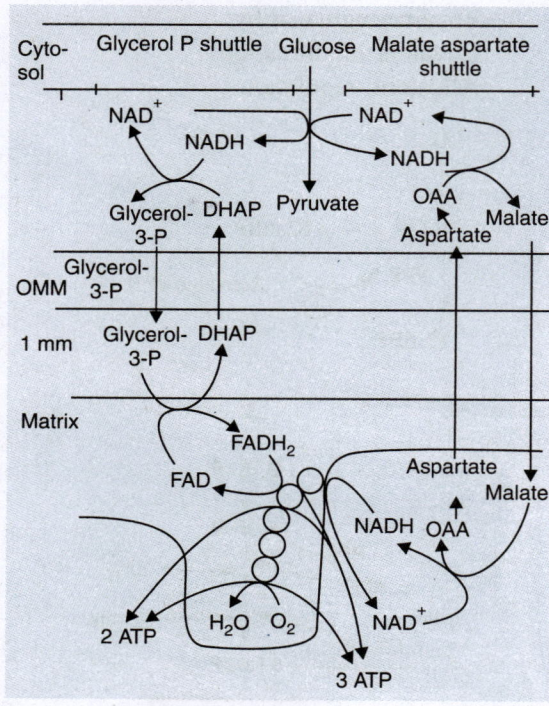

**Fig. 4.12.** Shuttle systems.

## Malate-aspartate shuttle

- Cytosolic OAA is reduced to malate by NADH by cytosolic malate dehydrogenase (MDH)
- Malate enters mitochondria and is reoxidized to OAA by mitochondrial MDH, generating NADH in matrix
- OAA cannot cross mitochondrial membrane, gets transaminated to aspartate, which can be transported into cytosol and reconverted to OAA by another transamination reaction.
- In mitochondrial matrix, each mole of NADH generates 3 moles of ATP via oxidative phosphorylation
- Thus, glycolysis produces 2 moles of NADH per mole of glucose, and 6 moles of ATP produced by this shuttle.

## Metabolism of glucose in RBC: Fact file

- RBC represent 40-45% of blood volume
- RBC is structurally and metabolically the simplest cell in the body
- During its maturation, RBC loses all its subcellular organelles
- With ribosomes or ER: it cannot synthesize or secrete protein or oxidize fats
- RBC relies exclusively on blood glucose as a fuel
- Metabolism of glucose in RBC is entirely anaerobic.
- Glucose enters RBC by facilitative diffusion via insulin dependent GLUT1
- A 70 kg adult with 5L blood volume has (2L) of RBCs
- These RBCs constitute 3% body mass, consume 20 g (0.1 mole) of glucose/day, representing about 10% of total body glucose metabolism
- In RBC, 90% glucose (~18 g or 0.1 mole) is metabolized via glycolysis, yielding ~0.2 mole of lactate (18 g/d), generating 0.2 mole ATP per day.
- 10-20% used for synthesis of Hb 2,3 BPG.
- 10% glucose is diverted to PPP to protect to against oxidative damage and other constituents

## Why a ten step pathway of converting glucose to lactate is required, can't it be done in fever steps?

- Glycolysis is central pathway
- Most glycolytic intermediates serve as branch points to other metabolic pathways i.e., fat, protein and nucleic acid and other pathways of carbohydrate metabolism.

## Clinical aspects of glycolysis

- Arsenite*, Mercuric ions: Bond SH group of lipoic acid, hence inhibit PDH enzyme
- Fluoride: Inhibit enolase
- Inherited PDH deficiency: Lactacidosis
- Hemolytic anaemia
  - Aldolase A deficiency
  - PK deficiency
- Exercise intolerance
  - PFK (muscle): common
  - PGK, PGM, LDH

## What is energetics for anaerobic glycolysis in arsenate poisoning?

- Zero.
- Because no substrate level phosphorylation occurs

**Explanation:** Arsenate is used by GAPDH producing 1 arsenato-3-phosphoglycerate (instead of 1,3 BPG). This acyl arsenate bond hydrolyzes and no ATP is generated by substrate level phosphorylation.

## METABOLISM OF LACTATE

### Lactate:

- Produced by:
  - RBCs as end product of glycolysis
  - Exercising muscle
- In white muscle, when muscular activity is so great that amount of NADH produced exceeds the capacity of muscle mitochondria to oxidize it anaerobic oxidation.
- Lactate produced in muscle is taken up from blood by liver and used as a substrate for gluconeogenesis.

---

* Also, hemolytic anaemia, type-V GSD and muscle cramping result.

## What happens to lactate in RBC?

Lactate diffuses out into blood; this lactate in blood has two fates:

1. Plasma membrane of some cells, particularly cardiac muscle contain lactate carrier and lactate enters the cells, gets reverted back to pyruvate and enters TCA and oxidative phosphorylation to form ATP, thus **sparing glucose** for muscle cells.

2. Excess lactate, enters liver and converted to pyruvate and enters GNG to form glucose.

   **Cori cycle**: LDH enzyme oxidizes lactate to pyruvate which is used by heart as fuel.

## Glycolysis and different physiologic status

**After carbohydrate rich diet:**
Glycolysis increased to metabolize excess dietary glucose.

**During fasting:**
- Glycolysis reduced in most tissues.
- Tissues cover their energy needs by oxidation of fatty acids and other alternative substrates.

## Glycolytic pathway interconnects lipid and protein metabolism (Fig. 4.13)

## $CO_2$ producing cycles

- TCA
- HMP
- Uronic acid pathway

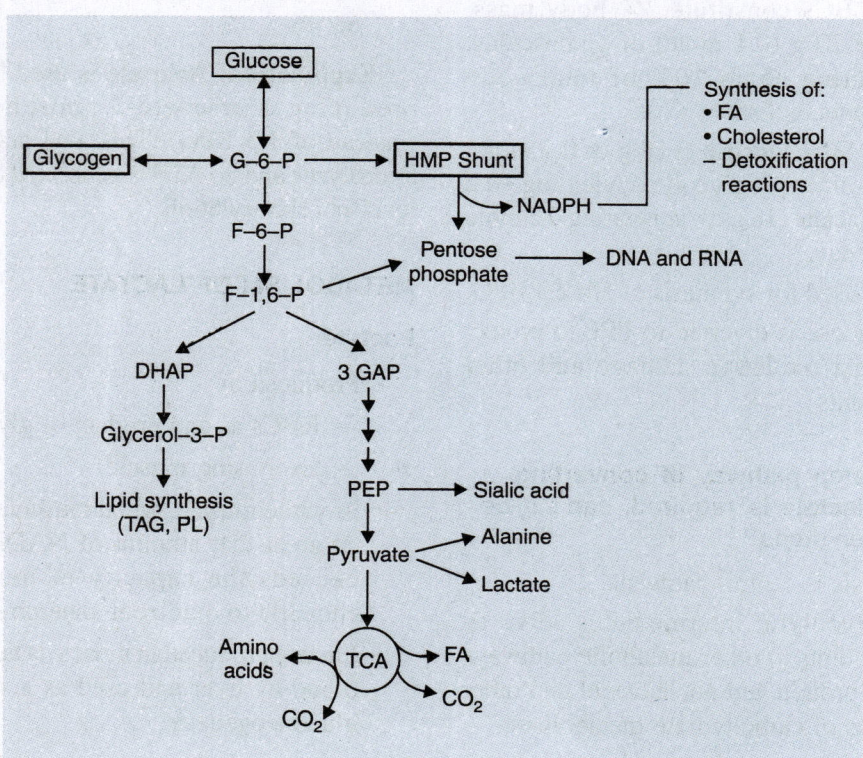

**Fig. 4.13.** Interaction of glycolysis with other metabolic pathway.

# (ii) Krebs Cycle (TCA Cycle)

Citric Acid Cycle (TCA) or Tricarboxylic acid cycle or Krebs cycle:

## Features

- Occurs in mitochondria
- Strictly aerobic process
- Converts acetyl CoA to $CO_2$
- Functions both catalytically (starts and ends at OAA) and amphibolically (catabolism or anabolism)

## PDH COMPLEX

## TCA plays a pivotal role in metabolism

- GNG
- Transamination
- Deamination
- FA synthesis
- Both oxidative and synthetic processes

## Importance: TCA

- Final common pathway for oxidation of carbohydrates, fats and proteins
- Major role in GNG, transamination, deamination, FA synthesis

- Principal organ: liver
- Abnormalities of its enzymes are incompatible with life.

## PDH complex deficiency

Without mitochondrial oxidation, pyruvate is reduced to lactate by PDH enzyme. The ATP yield from anaerobic glycolysis is less than a tenth of that produced from complete oxidation of glucose via TCA.

## Diagnosis

- Elevated lactate
- Normal lactate/pyruvate ratio
- No evidence of hypoxia

## Treatment

- Ketogenic diet
- Restrict: protein (<15%) and Carbohydrate (<5%)
- Plus Pantothenic acid, riboflavin and nicotinamide supplements.

## Fluoroacetate

- Inhibitor of aconitase (competitive)
- Suicide substrate
- Converted to fluoroacetyl CoA and finally fluorocitrate

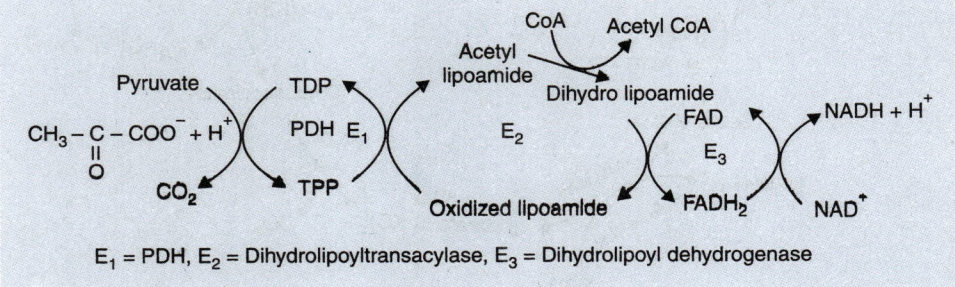

$E_1$ = PDH, $E_2$ = Dihydrolipoyltransacylase, $E_3$ = Dihydrolipoyl dehydrogenase

**Fig. 4.14.** Mechanism of action of PDH complex.

**Table 4.3.** Component of PDH complex

| 5 cofactors | 3 enzymes | 4 vitamins |
|---|---|---|
| TPP | PDH | Thiamin (TPP) |
| Lipoamide | Dihydrolipoyl | Riboflavin (FAD) |
| FAD | trans acylase | Nicotinamide ($NAD^+$) |
| CoA | Dihydrolipoyl | Pantothenic acid |
| $NAD^+$ | dehydrogenase | (CoA) |

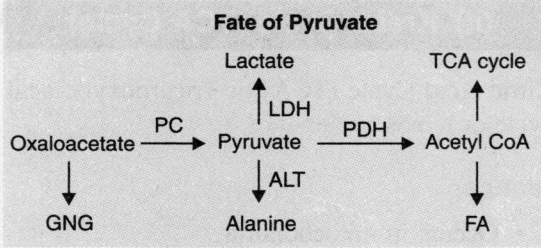

Fate of Pyruvate

**Fig. 4.14a.** Fate of pyruvate.

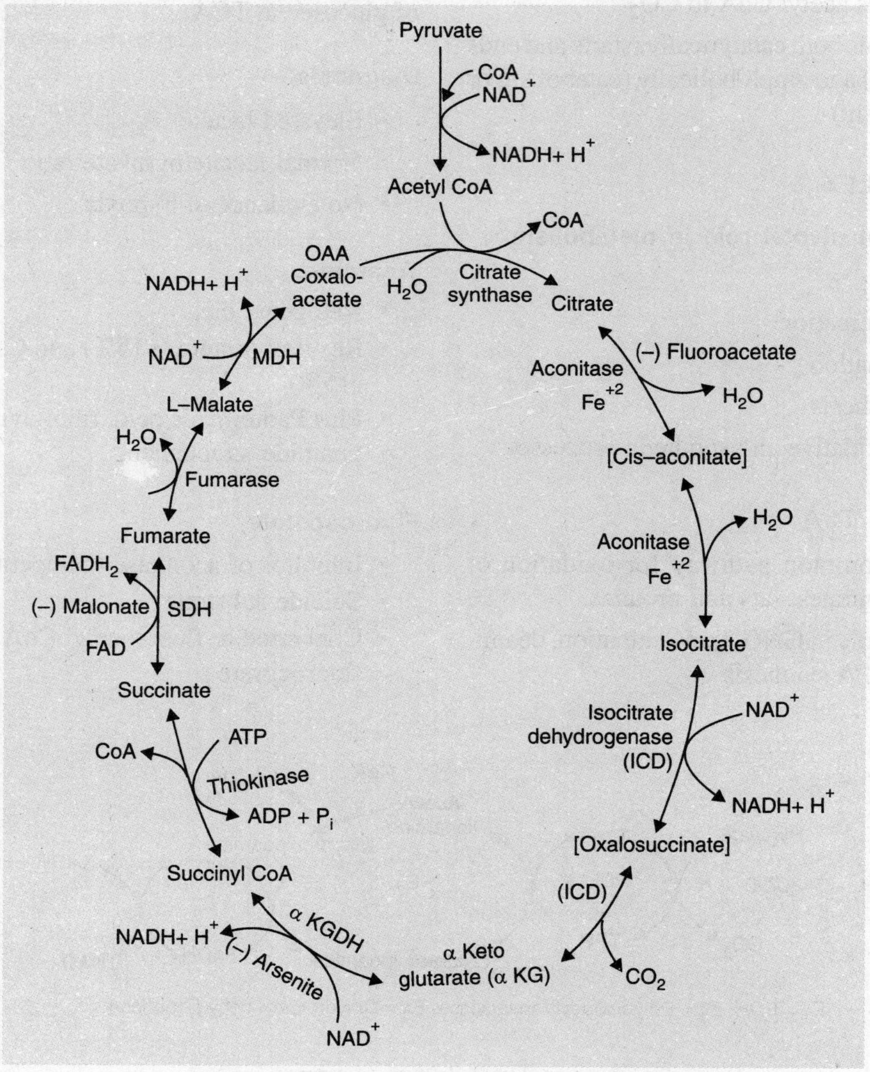

**Fig. 4.15.** Citric acid cycle.

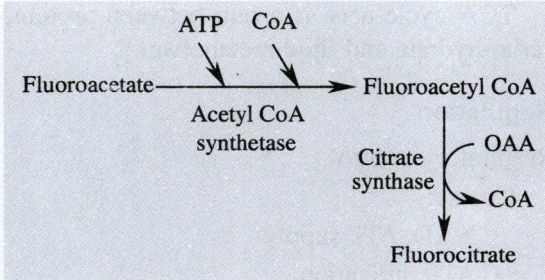

- Fluorocitrate inhibits aconitase enzyme and hence TCA cycle

## Malonate block

**Malonate:**

- 3-carbon dicarboxylic acid homologue of succinate
- Competitive inhibitor of succinate dehydrogenase (SDH)

## Regulation of TCA

Regulated by cell's need for energy in form of ATP

Determinants of regulation:
  - NAD/NADH
  - ATP/ADP
  - Acetyl CoA/CoA ratio

TCA is activated when fuel are consumed, generating ATP and NADH, presence of OAA.

**High ADP:** That is cell needs energy, reactions of ETC accelerated:

- NADH rapidly oxidized – TCA speeds up
- ADP allosterically activates ICD.

**High ATP:** That is cell has adequate energy ETC slows:

- NADH builds up – allosterically inhibits ICD.
- TCA inhibited.

Isocitrate accumulates and citrate concentration rises inhibiting citrate synthase:

- High NADH slows the cycle
- OAA converted to malate when NADH is high, so less substrate available for citrate synthesis.

### Amino acids producing intermediates of TCA

- **Glutamate:**
  - Converted to αKG:
  - Formed from glutamine, proline, arginine, histidine
- **Aspartate:** Transaminated to OAA
- **Valine, isoleucine, methionine and threonine:** Produce propionyl CoA which is converted to methyl malonyl CoA and finally succinyl CoA
- **Phenylalanine, tyrosine, aspartate:** Form fumarate.

### Shuttling of citrate from mitochondria: Results in:

- Conversion of cytosolic NADPH to NADH required for FA synthesis
- Citrate is shuttled back into mitochon-dria to regenerate OAA

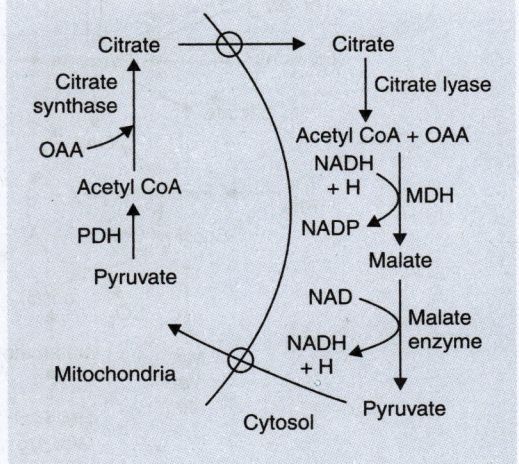

**Fig. 4.16.** Shuttling of citrate from mitochondria.

– Acetyl CoA is generated from citrate in cytosol.

## Amphibolic nature of the cycle

TCA cycle plays a role in both oxidative (catabolic) and synthetic (anabolic) processes i.e. it is **Amphibolic**. Gluconeogenesis, transamination, deamination and fatty synthesis are linked to TCA cycle.

## OAA

### Catalytic role of OAA in TCA

**Fasting:**

FA oxidation increases ATP and NADH in mitochondria

- This increase in NADH shifts malate: oxaloacetate towards malate
- Malate exported to cytosol for GNG
- Acetyl CoA from FA oxidation directed towards KB formation due to lack of OAA.

TCA cycle acts as a hub between protein, carbo-hydrate and lipid metabolism.

## Regulation

Respiratory control

Coarse:

- NAD, ATP supply
- ATP utilization
- [ATP]/[ADP]
  [NADH]/[NAD]

Regulated at steps catalyzed by:

| | |
|---|---|
| Citrate synthase ⎤ | (+) ADP |
| ICD | (–): via feed back |
| αKGDH ⎦ | inhibition by: |
| | ATP |
| | Citrate |
| | NADH |
| | Succinyl CoA |

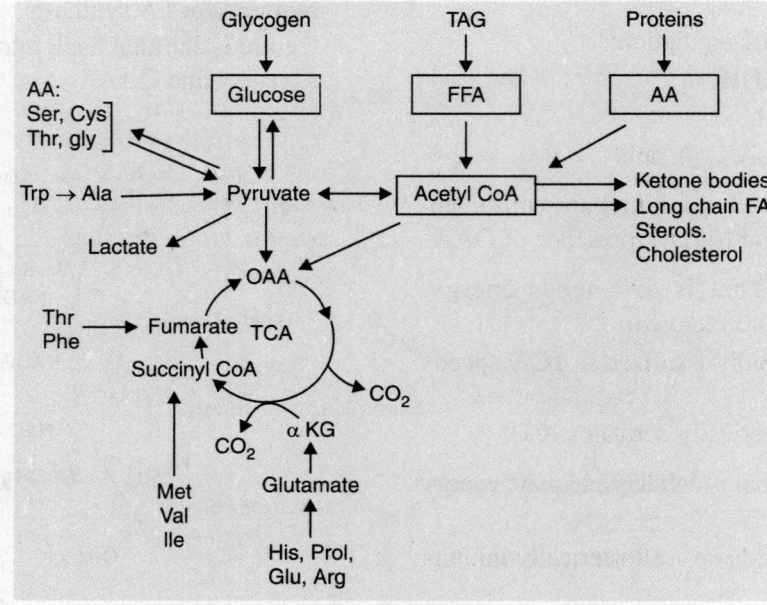

**Fig. 4.17.** Amphibolic nature of TCA cycle.

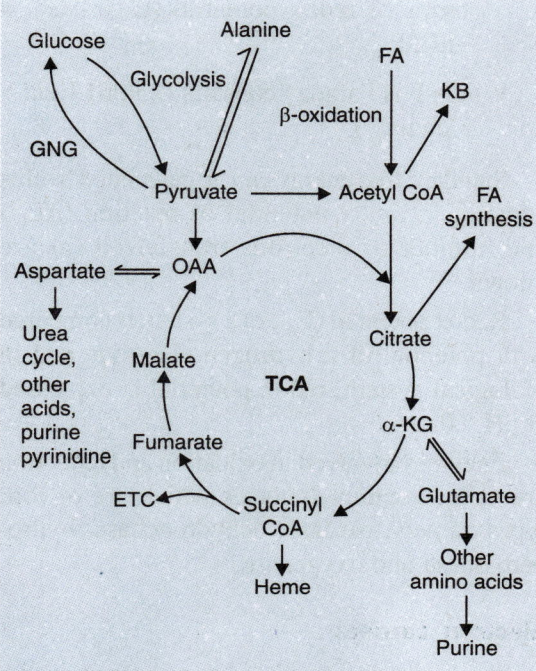

**Fig. 4.18.** TCA cycle interconnects protein carbohydrate and metabolism.

**PDH:**

- (–) acetyl CoA, NADH
- (–) NADH/NAD,
- (–) Acetyl CoA/CoA

**SDH**: (–) OAA, ↑ ATP/ADP

### (iii) ETC, Oxidative Phosphorylation, Reactive Oxygen Species (ROS)

### BIOENERGETICS

It is the study of energy changes occurring during biochemical reactions.

All chemical reactions, including those catalyzed by enzymes follow laws of thermodynamics and one of these laws defines a property known as free energy (also called Gibb's free energy).

Free energy is associated with every chemical compound and is the amount of useful work that can be obtained. Free energy of compound is equal to free energy per mole time, the number of moles of that component.

### Standard state

- pH 7
- Temperature: 25°C (298°K)
- Solutes at 1M (molar concentration)
- Gases at 1 standard atmosphere (atm) pressure

### Enthalpy (H)

It is the heat content of a body.

### Entropy (S)

It is the degree of randomness or disorder of a system. Greater is degree of disorder, higher the value of S.

Change in free energy $\Delta G = \Delta H - T\Delta S$

Free energy change ($\Delta G$) of reaction is difference between total free energy of reactants and those of the products.

### Standard free energy (G°)

It is equal to free energy of component at unit activity level (1 mol l$^{-1}$)

$G_1 = G_1° + Rl\ In\alpha_1$

R = gas constant (1.987 × 10$^{-3}$ kcal mol$^{-1}$ deg$^{-1}$)

T = temperature (°C + 273)

In = natural log (converted to log$_{10}$ by multiplying by 2.303)

$a_1$ = activity of i$^{th}$ component.

At equilibrium, $\Delta G = 0$, (free energy of both sides are equal)

If $\Delta G$ is negative reaction will proceed in reverse direction until equilibrium is reached.

## Exergonic reaction

If change in free energy is less than zero ($\Delta G < 0$), reaction proceeds spontaneously with release of energy.

## Endergonic reaction

If change in free energy is more than zero ($\Delta G > 0$), reaction cannot proceed spontaneously unless there is input of energy to drive reaction forward.

## High energy phosphate compounds

All organisms obtain supply of their free energy from their environment to maintain their living processes. ATP is principal donor of free energy in biological system and serves as "universal currency" for energy in cells.

ATP has intermediate value of group transfer potential:

$$ATP \rightarrow ADP + Pi; \Delta G^\circ = -7.3$$
$$ATP \rightarrow AMP + PPi; \Delta G^\circ = -7.7$$

## High energy phosphates

They include ATP, creatine phosphate. In humans, amount of ATP formed approximates body weight and is broken down every 24 hours. Creatine phosphate provides energy in muscles and is regenerated during resting phase at the expense of ATP. Other high energy phosphates include GTP, CTP, and UTP.

## Oxidation-reduction reactions

These reactions involve electron transfer.

Oxidation is loss of electron and reduction is gain of electrons.

- A (oxidized) + B (reduced) $\leftrightarrow$ B (oxidized) + A (reduced).
- Free energy changes can be expressed in

terms of redox potential ($E'^\circ$). $\Delta G^{\circ\prime} = -nF\Delta E_o{}'$.

Where F is Faraday constant (23.061 Kcal $\times$ volt$^{-1} \times$ equiv$^{-1}$).

Standard free energy can be calculated by this equation if redox potential of reaction ($\Delta E_o{}'$) and number of electrons transferred (n) are known.

Redox potential ($E_o{}'$) of a system is compared with potential of a hydrogen electrode and in biological system, redox potential is expressed at pH 7.0.

Enzymes involved in oxidation and reduction are called **oxidoreductases** which are of four types namely, oxidase, dehydrogenase, hydroperoxidase and oxygenase.

## Electron carriers

In aerobic system, molecular oxygen is the ultimate acceptor of electrons derived from the fuel molecules. Electrons are first transferred from metabolites to specialized electron carriers and then to molecular oxygen via mitochondrial electron transport chain.

NAD, NADP, FAD, FMN are common electron carriers.

## Oxidative phosphorylation

All the energy released from oxidation of carbohydrate, fat and protein is made available in mitochondria as reducing equivalents (–H or e$^-$) and these are funneled into respiratory chain form water with oxygen.

## Electron transport chain (ETC)

Enzymes of electron transport chain are embedded in inner mitochondrial membrane (IMM) in association with the enzymes of oxidative phosphorylation.

## Overview of ETC

1. **NADH and FADH$_2$:** Reduced form of NAD and FAD, produced by:
   - Glycolysis
   - β oxidation of fats
   - TCA cycle
   - Pass electrons to components of ETC located in IMM
   - NADH freely diffuses from matrix to membrane
   - FADH$_2$ tightly bound to enzymes that produce it within IMM
2. Transfer of electrons from NADH to oxygen: Occurs in three stages.
3. Each complex uses energy from electron transfer to proton pump to cytosolic side of IMM.
4. Proton-motive force (an electrochemical potential) is generated and when proton enter back into matrix through ATP synthase complex and ATP is produced. Also, some energy is lost as heat during transfer of electrons through ETC.
5. ETC has a large negative $\Delta G^\circ$, so electrons flow from NADH (FADH$_2$) towards O$_2$.

**Table 4.4.** Enzyme/compounds in mitochondria

Outer membrane:
   Acyl CoA synthetase
   Glycerol phosphate acyl transferase
Inter membrane space:
   Adenyl kinase
   Creatine kinase
Inner membrane:
   Respiratory chain enzymes
   Cardiolipin
   ATP synthase
   Membrane transporters

### Organization of ETC (Fig. 4.19)

1. **Complex I:** NADH-CoQ oxidoreductase:
   - Entry point for electrons from NADH.
   - CoQ (ubiquinone) or Q is electron acceptor and FMN and Fe-S centers are prosthetic groups.
   - Rotenone and barbiturates inhibit electron transfer from NADH to CoQ.
2. **Complex II:** Succinate-Q reductase:
   - Entry point of electrons from succinate into ETC.
   - FAD, Fe-S centers and heme (cyt b$_{560}$) are prosthetic groups and coenzyme Q is electron acceptor.
   - Carboxin inhibits complex II.
3. **Q (coenzyme Q):** Accepts electrons from complex I and complex II.

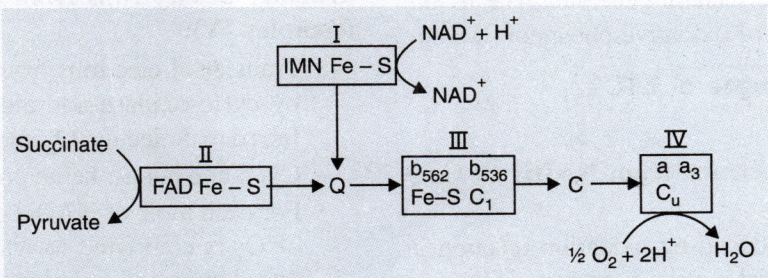

**Fig. 4.19.** Mitochondrial electron transport chain.

4. **Complex III:** Q-cytochrome c oxido-reductase:
   - It passes electrons onto cytochrome c.
   - Heme (cytochrome b and $c_1$), Fe-S centers are the prosthetic groups and cytochrome c is electron acceptor.
   - Antimycin A is inhibitor of complex III.
5. **Cytochrome C:** It is the *only soluble protein* (with heme as prosthetic group) of ETC and transfers electrons from complex III to complex IV.

**Table 4.5.** Sources of NADH production

| |
|---|
| αKGDH |
| ICD |
| MDH |
| PDH |
| β-oxidation of fatty acids |

6. **Complex IV:** Cytochrome c oxidase:
   - It is electron acceptor for cyt c and its prosthetic groups are copper and cyt a, $a_3$.
   - Electrons are accepted by molecular oxygen to form water.
   - Electrons are transferred from cyt c to $Cu^{2+}$, then to cyt a, cyt $a_3$ and then to $O_2$.
   - Carbon monoxide, azide, cyanide and hydrogen sulfide are inhibitors of electron transfer from cyt c to $O_2$.
   - The flow of electrons through the respiratory chain generates ATP by the process of oxidative phosphorylation.

### Three major stages of ETC

*Stage I*

**Transfer of electrons from NADH to CoQ (complex I):**

- NADH produced by oxidation reaction in mitochondrial matrix diffuses to IMM and passes its electrons to FMN.

- FMN passes electrons through a series of Fe-S protein complexes to CoQ. CoQ accepts one electron at a time forming semiquinone and ubiquinone.
- Energy produced by these electron transfers is used to pump protons to cytosolic side of IMM.

*Stage 2*

**Transfer of electrons from CoQ to cyt c:**

- CoQ passes electrons via Fe-S centers to cyt b and cyt $c_1$ (complex III) which transfers electrons to cyt c by cyt c reductase.
- **Pecularities of cytochrome:**
  - cyt contains heme as prosthetic group
  - $Fe^{3+}$ (ferric) state of heme iron accepts one electron and gets reduced to $Fe^{2+}$ (ferrous)
  - Cyt carry one electron at a time and CoQ acts as an adaptor between electron transfers to complex I and III.
- Protons are pumped across IMM by using electron transfer from CoQ to cyt c.
- Proton move back via ATP synthase complex into matrix to drive ATP synthesis.
- Complex II: Electrons from $FADH_2$ enter ETC at CoQ level. Electrons are produced by succinate dehydrogenase reaction.

*Stage 3*

**Transfer of electrons from cyt c to cyt $aa_3$ (complex IV):**

- Transfer of electrons from cyt c to cyt $aa_3$ by cyt c oxidase and electrons are transferred to molecular $O_2$, reducing it to water.
- Cyt a and cyt $a_3$: heme proteins
- For each mole of NADH oxidized, ½ mole of $O_2$ is converted to water. Energy produced by transfer of electrons from cyt c to $O_2$ is used to pump protons across IMM.

## ATP production:

- As electrons pass through ETC from complex I to IV, proton-motive force is generated which consists of both membrane potential and pH gradient.
- Cytosolic side has higher $[H^+]$ than matrix, proton reenter matrix through ATP synthase complex, generating ATP.
- Remember:
  - IMM is permeable to protons.
  - $F_o$ component forms a channel through ATP synthase complex, through which protons flow.
  - $F_1$ is ATP synthesizing head connected to $F_1$ stalk projecting into matrix.

## Applied

### Fetal infantile mitochondria myopathy

- Occurs due to decreased activity of respiratory chain complex I, III and IV.
- Patients present with early progressive liver failure, hypoglycemia, increased lactate in body fluids and neurological abnormalities.

## Melas

- Acronym for: mitochondrial encephalopathy, lactacidosis and stroke.
- Caused by mutation in mitochondrial gene encoding complex I (NADH: Ubiquinone oxidoreductase)

## Leber's hereditary optic neuropathy (LHON)

- Point mutation in gene for cyt reductase
- Results in loss of central vision by age of 20 to 30 years.

## Kearns-Sayre syndrome

- Mutation in complex II of ETC
- Patients manifest with short stature, external ophthalmoplegia, retinopathy, ataxia, cardiac conduction defects.

## Leigh disease

- Mutation in cyt oxidase
- Lactacidemia, developmental delay, hypotonia, seizures.

## Energetics

- For every mole of NADH oxidized:
  - ½ mole of $O_2$ reduced to water
  - 3 moles of ATP produced
- For every mole of $FADH_2$ oxidized:
  - 2 moles of ATP produced

## ATP-ADP antiport

ATP produced in mitochondria is transported to cytosol in exchange with ADP via a transport protein in IMM called ATP-ADP antiporter (ANT, adenine nucleotide transferase).

## Uncouplers of ETC

- Compounds that allow normal function of ETC without producing ATP.
- They cause leakage or transport of H+ across membranes, collapses proton gradient before it can be used for ATP synthase.
- Energy is released as electrons are transferred down the transport chain, but is not trapped as ATP, but released as heat.
- Examples of uncoupler:
  - 2,4 dinitrophenol
  - Dicumarol
  - Chlorocarbonyl cyanide phenylhydrazine (CCCP)
  - Bilirubin.

## Oxidative phosphorylation

- It is the main source of energy in aerobic cells where free energy released along ETC is coupled to formation of ATP.

- According to chemiosmotic theory, flow of electron and generation of ATP are coupled by a proton gradient across the inner mitochondrial membrane (Fig. 4.20).

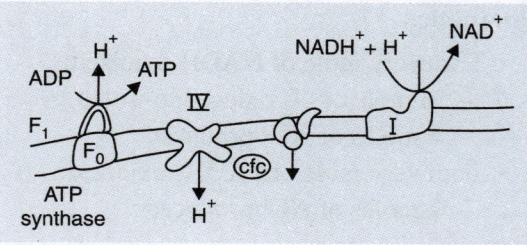

**Fig. 4.20.** Chemiosmotic potential drives oxidative phosphorylation.

- This proton motive force drives the mechanism of ATP synthesis and complexes I, III and IV act as proton pumps (Fig. 4.21).
- ATP synthase in inner mitochondrial membrane causes $H^+$ to pass through the membrane into matrix.

## Coupling sites for ATP synthesis

- Energy released by electron transfers catalyzed by three coupling sites: complex I, III and IV to form 1 mole of ATP each.

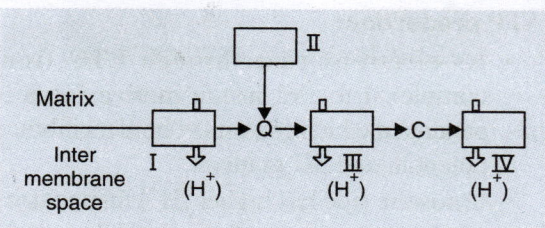

**Fig. 4.21.** Three respiratory chain complexes act as proton pumps.

- Electrons that enter chain from NADH form 3 mole of ATP and from $FADH_2$ form 2 moles of ATP.
- ATP synthase consists of two major complexes known as $F_0$ spans the membrane $F_0$ and $F_1$. $F_0$ has seven subunits and $F_1$ has five different types of subunits, three each of $\alpha$ and $\beta$ and one each of $\gamma$, $\beta$ and $\epsilon$, making nine in all. The core of $F_1$ complex consists of $\gamma$ subunit surrounded by six $\alpha$ and $\beta$ subunits arranged alternately.
- The dissipation of energy that occurs as protons pass down the concentration gradient to matrix drives the phosphorylation of ADP to ATP by the synthase.

| Table 4.6. Inhibitors of ETC | | |
|---|---|---|
| *Component* | *Substance* | *Mechanism* |
| Complex I | Rotenone | Inhibit NADH dehydrogenase |
| Complex II | Amytal | Blocks complex I |
| Complex III | Cyanide, carbon monoxide | Combine with cyt oxidase and electron transfer to $O_2$ blocked |
| Complex III | 2,4 dinitrophenol | Ionophore, uncouple allows proton to reenter matrix without going through ATP synthase |
| ATP synthase | Oligomycin | Binds to ATP synthase, acts as uncoupler |
| ATP-ADP antiporter | Atractyloside | Deplete mitochondria of ADP |

# (iv) Free Radicals

Any species capable of independent existence that contains one or more unpaired electrons.

Radicals can be formed by:
- Loss of a single electron from a non-radical, or by gain of a single electron by a non-radical
- Breakage of covalent bond 'homolytic fission'

### Biomedical importance

- Free radicals are formed in the body under normal conditions
- They cause damage to nucleic acids, proteins, and lipids in cell membranes and plasma lipoproteins
- This can cause cancer, atherosclerosis and coronary artery disease and autoimmune disease
- Epidemiological studies have shown protective role of antioxidant nutrients namely, selenium, vitamin C and E, β carotene, polyphenol.
- International trials show little benefit of antioxidant supplements.

### Nomenclature

- Free radical is denoted by a superscript dot to oxygen (or carbon)
  $HO^{\bullet}$, $NO^{\bullet}$, $CH_3^{\bullet}$
- If free radical is a charged species, dot is put and then the charge $O_2^{\bullet-}$

### Role of free radicals in biological systems

- Enzyme – catalyzed reactions
- Electron transport system in mitochondria
- Signal transduction and gene expression
- Activation of nuclear transcription factors
- Oxidative damage of molecules, cells, tissues
- Antimicrobial actions
- Aging and disease

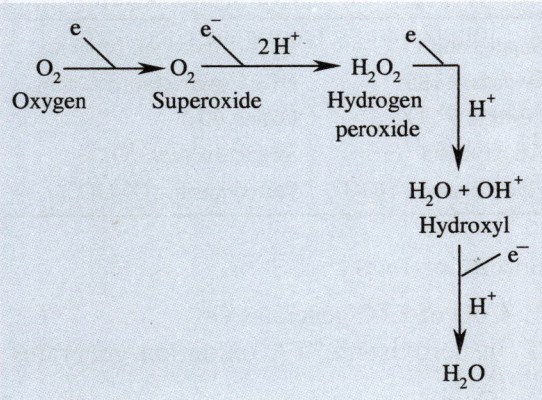

### Lifetime of free radical

Short life: $10^{-10}$ seconds.

### Oxygen radicals

- Molecules with extra electrons on oxygen
- Produced as byproduct of normal metabolic pathways of oxidative metabolism

### Reactive oxygens species

- Radicals – Hydroxyl (OH)
- Molecule – Hydrogen peroxide ($H_2O_2$), hydroxyl anion ($OH^-$)
- Ions – Hypochlorite ($OCl^-$)
- Superoxide anion ($O_2^{\bullet-}$) or ($O^{2-}$)

### Types of free radicals

1. Oxygen-centered radical
   Singlet oxygen, superoxide, hydroxyl radical
   - Sulfur-centered radicals
     Thiyl radical ($RS^{\bullet}$)
   - Carbon-centered radicals
     $CCl_3^{\bullet}$, $CH_2^{\bullet}$, $CHOH$
   - Nitrogen-centered radicals
     $NO^{\bullet}$, $R_2NO^{\bullet}$

**Table. 4.7.** ROS (Reactive oxygen species)

| Radicals | Non Radicals |
|---|---|
| Superoxide $O_2^{\cdot-}$ | $H_2O_2$ (hydrogen peroxide) |
| Hydroxyl $HO^\cdot$ | $HOCl$ (hypochlorous acid) |
| Peroxyl $ROO^\cdot$ | Ozone $(O_3)$ |
| Alkoxyl $RO^\cdot$ | Singlet oxygen $(O)^-$ |
| Hydroperoxyl $HOO^\cdot$ | Peroxynitrite $(ONOO^-)$ |

## Sources of ROS

1. CoQ of ETC generates $O^{2-}$
2. In peroxisome: FA oxidation generates $H_2O_2$
3. Cyt $P_{450}$ monoxygenase:
   - In detoxification of drugs, $e^-$ transported from NADPH to $O_2$.
   - Leakage of electrons during these conversions
4. NADPH oxidase: Enzyme is present in phagolysosome, in immune cells, $e^-$ transfer from $O_2$ to form $O^{2-}$.
5. Myeloperoxidase (MPO) in neutrophils catalyze formation of HOCl from $H_2O_2$
6. Ionizing radiation.

## Superoxide radicals

- **Generation of superoxide ($O^{2-}$):**
  The addition of a single electron to the ground-state molecule ($O_2 + e^- \rightarrow O^{2-}$).
- **Biological generation of $O^{2-}$ occurs in:**
  - Mitochondrial ETC
  - Enzymatic reduction of oxygen
  - Xenobiotic metabolisms (redox cycling)
  - Respiratory burst (phagocytes)
- **Mitochondrial ETC:**
  - Most important source of $O^{2-}$
  - Oxidation of NADH, $FADH_2$
  - β oxidation of FA

- ETC in IMM
- Energy released is used for ATP synthesis
- **Enzymatic reduction of oxygen:**

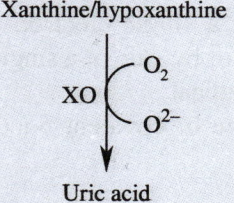

XO: Xanthine oxidase

- **Respiratory burst:**
  - Myeloperoxidase:
    Oxidizes $Cl^-$ to hypochlorous acid
    Chronic granulomatous disease
  - NADPH oxidase:
    Enzyme catalyzes:
    $NADPH \rightarrow NADP^+ + H^+$
    Electron is transferred from $NADPH_2$ to $O_2$, resulting in formation of $O^{2-}$.

## Hydroxyl radical ($HO^\cdot$)

Highly reactive oxygen species, formed from:
- Ionizing radiation
- Reaction of metal ions with hydrogen peroxidase
- Ozone

## Reactions of hydroxyl radical

- Hydrogen atom abstraction
- Addition
- Electron transfer

## Fenton reaction

A mixture of hydrogen peroxide and iron (II) salt causes formation of hydroxyl radical.

$$Fe^{2+} + H_2O_2 \rightarrow Fe^{3+} + OH^+ + HO^-$$
$$Fe^{3+} + H_2O_2 \rightarrow Fe^{2+} + O^{2-} + 2H^+$$

Haber-Weiss

$$Fe^{+2} + H_2O_2 \rightarrow Fe^{+3} + OH^- + HO^{\cdot}$$
$$Fe^{+3} + O^{2-} \rightarrow Fe^{2+} + O_2$$

Net reaction

$$O^{2-} + H_2O_2 \xrightarrow{\text{metal}} O_2 + HO^{\cdot} + OH^-$$

## NITROGEN-CENTERED RADICALS

### Nitric oxide (NO)

- Endothelial derived-relaxing factor (EDRF)
- Generated from conversion of arginine by nitric oxide synthase (NOS) enzyme

### Functions

Vascular function, platelet aggregation, immune response neurotransmitter, signal transduction, cytotoxicity

$$NO + O^{2-} \rightarrow ONOO^- \text{ (highly toxic)}$$

### Oxygen radicals in the body

- 1.5 mol of reactive oxygen species produced daily
- 3-5% of daily consumption of 30 mol of oxygen by an adult human being rather than undergoing complete reduction of water is converted to:
  - Singlet oxygen
  - Hydrogen peroxide
  - Superoxide
  - Perhydroxyl
  - Hydroxyl radicals

### Sources of oxygen radicals in body

### Multiple sources

- Ionizing radiation (X-ray, Uv)
- Transition metal ions, including $Cu^{+2}$, $Co^{+2}$, $Ni^{+2}$, $Fe^{2+}$.
- Nitric oxide (EDRF) itself is a radical

- Respiratory burst of activated macrophages
- Mitochondrial and microsomal ETC

### Types of sources of free radicals

| *Exogenous* | *Endogenous* |
|---|---|
| Ionizing radiation | Oxidative metabolic transformation |
| UV radiation | |
| Ultrasound | Mitochondrial ETC |
| Chemicals | Oxygen (respiratory) burst |
| Tobacco smoke etc. | during phagocytosis |
| | Eicosanoid synthesis |
| | Enzymatic reactions (oxygenase, oxidase) |
| | Xenobiotic metabolism |

### Oxidative stress

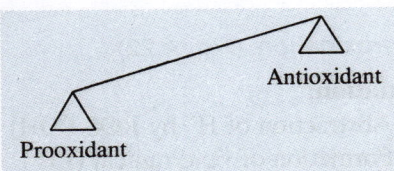

- Imbalance between prooxidants and antioxidant
- Oxidative damage: Damage caused by free radical/reactive oxygen species

### Cellular damages occur at various levels

- Membrane proteins, DNA etc and lead on to cell death, tissue injury
- Reduction of antioxidants
- Prevented by reduction of free radicals, inhibition of free radical formation
- Its not clear whether it is cause or consequence

### Free radical reactions are self-perpetuating chain reactions

- Being highly reactive molecular species with an unpaired electron.
- Persisting for a very short time ($10^{-9}$–$10^{-12}$ sec) before they collide with another

molecule and either abstract or donate an electron in order to achieve stability.

- They generate a new radical from the molecule with which they collide
- By terminating this chain reaction, free radicals can be quenched

### Damaging effects of free radicals

- Most damaging radicals in biological system are: oxygen radical ($O^{2-}$, $OH^\bullet$, $^\bullet OOH$)
- Oxidative damage: tissue damage caused by oxygen radicals
- Antioxidants are factors that protect against oxygen radical damage.

### Free radical damage to DNA, protein, and lipid

### Lipid peroxidation (Fig. 4.22)

- **Initiation:**
  - Abstraction of $H^+$ by ROS ($^\bullet OH$)
  - Formation of lipid radical ($LH^\bullet$)
  - Formation of peroxyl radical ($LOO^\bullet$, $ROO^\bullet$)

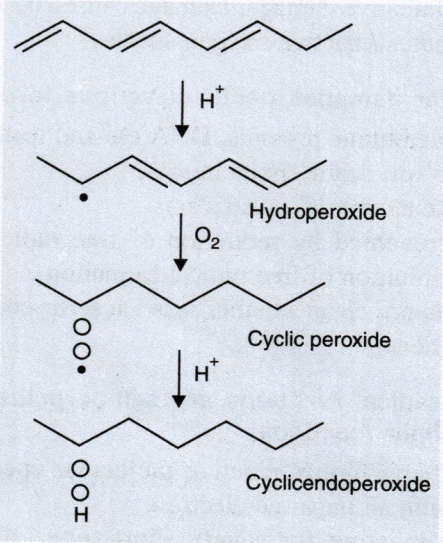

**Fig. 4.22.** Lipid peroxidation.

- **Propagation:** $H^+$ abstraction by lipid peroxyl radical ($LOO^\bullet$)
- **Termination:** Radical interaction, producing non radical product.

### Isoprostane (PGF$_{2a}$)

- Group of PG-like compounds produced by non-enzymatic free radical induced peroxidation of arachidonic acid
- Serves as reliable marker of oxidative stress *in vivo*

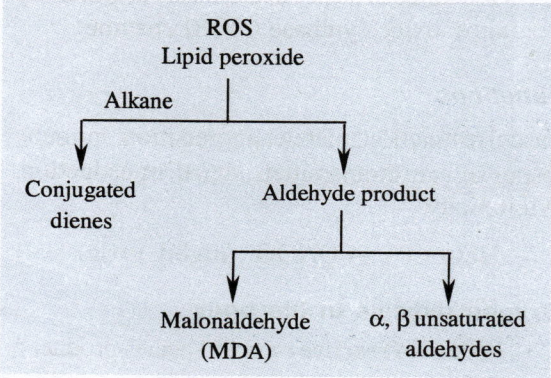

- Specific product of lipid peroxidation
- Stable compound
- Detectable in biological sample
- During oxidative injury, its levels increase
- Formation is modulated by antioxidants
- Not affected by lipid contents in diet.

### Deleterious effects of ROS

- ROS Chemically modify various biomolecules with in cell causing deleterious effects and cell death
- Damage to lipids, proteins, DNA.

### Oxidative DNA damage

- There is correlation between cancers, various diseases and oxidative DNA damage.

- Oxidative lesions of DNA occurs by:
  - Direct attack
  - Indirect activation of endonuclease enzymes
- Oxidative modification of bases result in mutation
- Oxidative modification of sugar moieties result in DNA strand break
- Abstraction of $H^+$ atom from carbon atoms of sugar molecules
- Disproportionation and rearrangements lead to C-C bond fragmentation and DNA strand break
- GC $\rightarrow$ TA transversions frequently detected in p53 gene and *ras* protooncogene

### DNA damage products

- 8-hydroxyguanine (8-OH Gua)
- 2-hydroxy adenine (2-OH-Ade)
- 8-hydroxy adenine (8-OH-Ade)
- 5-hydroxy cytosine (5-OH-Cyt)
- 5-hydroxy uracil (5-OH-Ura)

## PROTEIN OXIDATION

### Protein targets

- Receptors, transport proteins, enzymes etc.
- Secondary damage – autoimmunity

### Protein oxidation products

- Protein carbonyl group, 3-nitrotyrosine, other oxidized amino acids
- Most susceptible amino acids: Tyrosine, histidine, cysteine, methionine

### Oxidative protein degradation

- Result in modification of:
  - Amino acid chain
  - Prosthetic group of enzymes

- Resulting in:
  - Protein aggregation
  - Protein fragmentation
  - Activation of protease enzymes

### Measurement of total body radical burden

It can be estimated by measuring products of lipid peroxidation.

- Ferrous oxide in xylenol orange (FOX) assay.
- Dialdehydes formed from lipid peroxides can be measured by TBA reaction (TBARS)
- Measured in exhaled air:
  - Pentane (peroxidation of n-6 PUFA)
  - Ethane (peroxidation of n-3 PUFA)

### Measurement of oxidative stress

- Oxygen consumption
- Oxidative markers:
  - TBARS, lipid hydroperoxides
  - 8-OH Guanine protein hydroxylation products (nitrosation products)
- Free radical detection:
  - Single photon counting
  - Chemiluminiscence
  - Fluorescent probe
  - Electron paramagnetic resonance spectroscopy (EPR)

### Free radical and diseases

- Cancer
- Inflammation/infection
- Ischemia-reperfusion injury
  - Cardiac ischemia – reperfusion injury
  - Cerebral ischemia – reperfusion injury
- Neurodegenerative diseases
- Cardiovascular diseases
- Aging
- Others: Drug, chemical-induced toxicity etc.

## Oxidative DNA damage

- Point mutation
- Chromosomal aberrations
- DNA strand breaks
- Oxidation modification of DNA
- Base modification
- Sequence change
- Activation of kinases
- Activation of protooncogenes
- Inactivation of tumor suppressor genes

## Oxidative DNA damage and cancer

- ROS can attack deoxyribose, purine, and pyrimidine bases in DNA resulting in DNA strand breaks.
- DNA strand breaks cause deletions and point mutations.

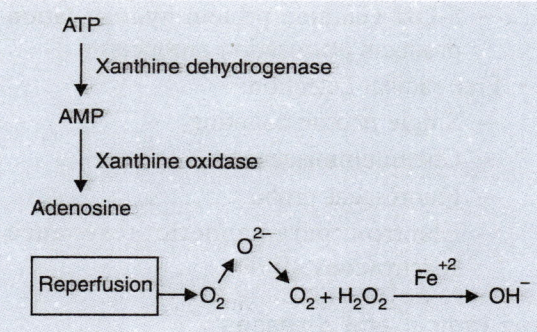

**Fig. 4.23.** Tissue injury.

## Ischemia – reperfusion injury

- Ischemic – reoxygenation injury occurs in: cerebral, cardiac ischemia (Fig. 4.23)
- Tissue damage is caused by excessive production of free radicals
  - High concentration of oxygen
  - Low levels of antioxidants
- Prevented by antioxidant supplementation

## Formation of oxidized LDL

- Direct action: foam cell formation
- Indirect action: down regulates the base excision repair pathway leading to higher level of 8-OH Gua.

## Atherosclerosis: Events

- Oxidized LDL stimulates monocyte chemotaxis, monocytes internalize ox-LDL forming foam cells.
- Oxidized LDL (ox-LDL) inhibits monocyte migration from the vascular wall
- Ox LDL causes endothelial dysfunction and injury
- Lipids engorged macrophages infiltrate blood vessel endothelium and are killed. This occurs in development of athero-sclerotic plaque which can occlude a blood vessel.
- Ox-LDL causes foam cell necrosis resulting in release of lysosomal enzyme and necrotic debris.

## Free radical theory of aging

- Aging: Cumulative consequence of free radical reactions
- Life-span experiments:
  - They explain the elationship between anti-oxidants, redox-sensitive trans-cription factors and free radical levels
  - Age-related decline in activation threshold of transcription factors and its normalization by antioxidants

## Radical damage

**Radical damage** may cause mutation, cancer, autoimmune disease and atherosclerosis.

- Radical damage to DNA can occur in:
  - Germ-line cells in ovaries and testes and can result heritable mutation

- Somatic cells and the result may be initiation of cancer
- Dialdehyde formed (as a result of radical – induced lipid peroxidation in cell membrane) can also modify bases in DNA
- Chemical modification of amino acids in proteins: leads to proteins that are recognized as non-self by the immune system: resultant antibodies cross-react with normal tissue proteins initiating autoimmune disease.

### Mechanisms of protection against radical damage

### Antioxidants

Compound that can delay the start or slow the rate of lipid oxidation reaction.

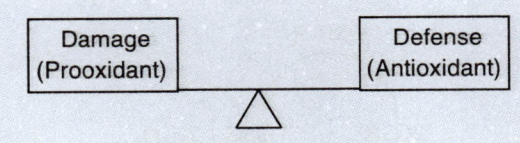

**Fig. 4.24.** Oxidant – antioxidant balance.

### Cellular defense mechanisms

- Isolation of generation sites of ROS
- Inhibition of propagation phase of ROS
- Scavenging of ROS
- Repair of damage caused by ROS

### Protection against ROS damage

- Direct protection against ROS:
  SOD, GSHPx, catalase
- Non-specific reduction system:
  GSH, vitamin C
- Protection against lipid peroxidation:
  GSH Px, vitamin E, β carotene

- Sequestration of metals: Transferrin, lactoferrin, ferritin, metallothionine
- Repair systems:
  DNA repair enzymes, metalloproteinases, GST

## ANTIOXIDANT DEFENSE SYSTEM

### Antioxidant enzymes

- SOD (superoxide dismutase)
- CAT (catalase)
- GSHPx (Glutathione peroxidase)

### Endogenous non-enzymatic antioxidants:

- GSH (glutathione)
- Bilirubin

### Exogenous antioxidant molecules

- α tocopherol – prevents oxidation of FA
- Carotenoids: β-carotene, lycopene-destroy a particularly damaging form of singlet oxygen.
- Ascorbic acid – radical scavenging, recycling of vitamin E
- Riboflavonoids – potent antioxidant activity.

### Superoxide dismutase (SOD)

$$2O^{2-} + 2H^+ \rightarrow H_2O_2 + O_2$$

- Only enzyme known to react with radical
- Presence of SOD implies $O^{2-}$ produced in cell during normal metabolism
- SOD is a primary antioxidant enzyme

### Catalase (CAT)

- Neutralizes $H_2O_2$
- $2H_2O_2 \rightarrow 2H_2O + O_2$
- Prevents lipid peroxidation and protein oxidation

## GSH cycle (Glutathione cycle)

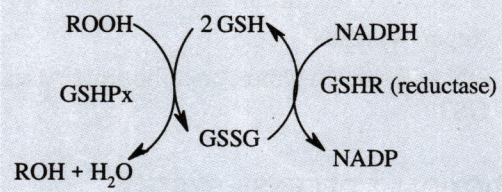

## GSHPx: function

Removes $H_2O_2$ and ROOH
$$ROOH + 2GSH \rightarrow ROH + H_2O + GSSG$$
- Deficiency in GSHPx leads to oxidative hemolysis
- Protects against lipid peroxidation

## Ascorbic acid

- Donate $1e^-$ to form semi dehydroascorbate
- DHA + 2GSH $\rightarrow$ ascorbate + GSSG (dehydroascurbate)

## Tocopherol

- Chain breaking antioxidant
- Scavenging peroxy radical
- Inhibits chain reaction of lipid peroxidation

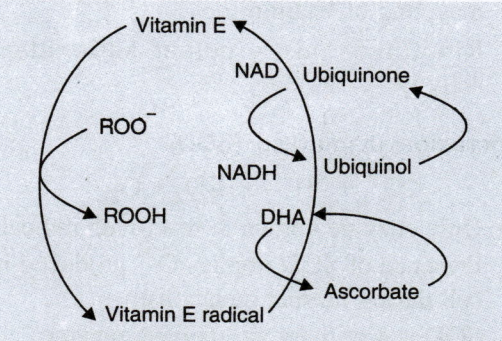

**Fig. 4.25.** Antioxidant network.

## BIOLOGICAL PROPERTIES OF NATURAL ANTIOXIDANT

## Natural antioxidants

- Polyphenol, carotenoid, lycopene

## Electron donor property

- Ability of antioxidant to donate an electron to a species – reducing property
- Antioxidant remains stable

## Preventive antioxidants

Include:
- SOD
- CAT
- GSHPx
- Singlet oxygen quencher
- Transition metal chelators (EDTA)

Preventive antioxidants minimize the formation of initiating radicals

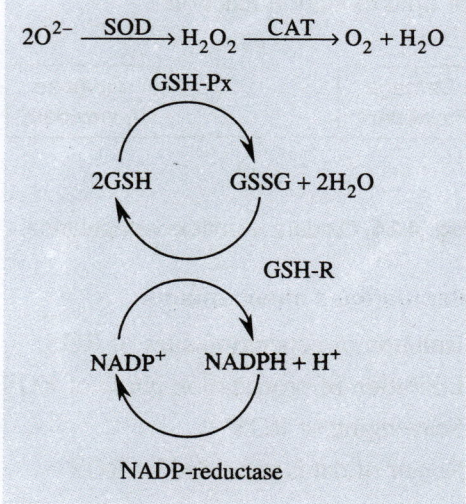

## Water soluble antioxidants

- Uric acid
- Ascorbate

## Lipid soluble antioxidant

- Ubiquinone
- Carotene

## ANTIOXIDANTS CAN ALSO BE PRO-OXIDANTS

### Ascorbate

### AOX role

- Ascorbate + $*O_2 \rightarrow H_2O_2$ + monodehydro-ascorbate

### Provident role

- Ascorbate + $O^{2-} \rightarrow$ +monodehydroascorbate
- Ascorbate + $Cu^{+2} \rightarrow Cu^+$ + monodehydro-ascorbate

## (v) Glycogen

### Structure

- Branched polymer of αD glucose
- Linkage α1-4 except at branch points: α1-6
- Branching more frequent in interior of molecule and less frequent at periphery.
- α1,6 branch is at every 8 to 10 residue.
- One glucose unit located at the reducing end of each glycogen molecule is attached to glycogenin.
- Glycogen molecules branches like a tree and has many non reducing ends where addition and release of glucose occurs during its synthesis and degradation.

## GLYCOGEN SYNTHESIS

### Fact file

- Occurs mainly in liver and muscle
- Process of glycogen synthesis for storing glucose in a rapidly mobilizable form.

1. Synthesis of UDPG

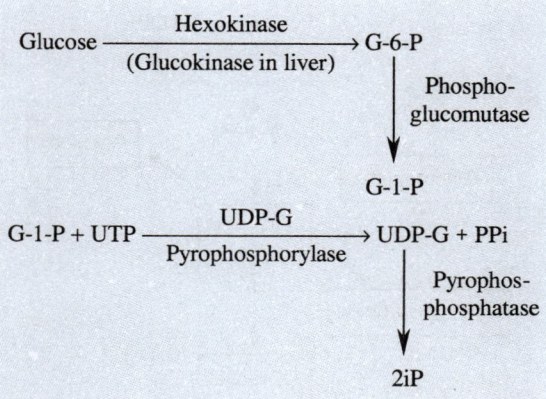

2. Action of glycogen synthase:
   Key regulatory enzyme.
   Transfers glucose residues from UDP-G to non-reducing end of glycogen
   UDP is released and converted back to UTP by ATP.

3. Formation of branches: When a chain contains 11 or more residues and oligomer of 6-8 residues in length is removed from non reducing end and reattached via α1-6 linkage to a glucose residue with α1-4 linked chain.

   **Enzymes:** Branching enzyme:
   Amylo $(1 \rightarrow 4) \rightarrow (1-6)$ trans glucosidase.
   Glucosyl 4-6 transferase

   New branch points are atleast 4 residues and average of 7-11 residues from previously existing branch points.

## UDP GLUCOSE

### Why glucose stored as polysaccharides?

- Rapid mobilization
- Support anaerobic metabolism
- Humans can't convert fats to glucose precursors

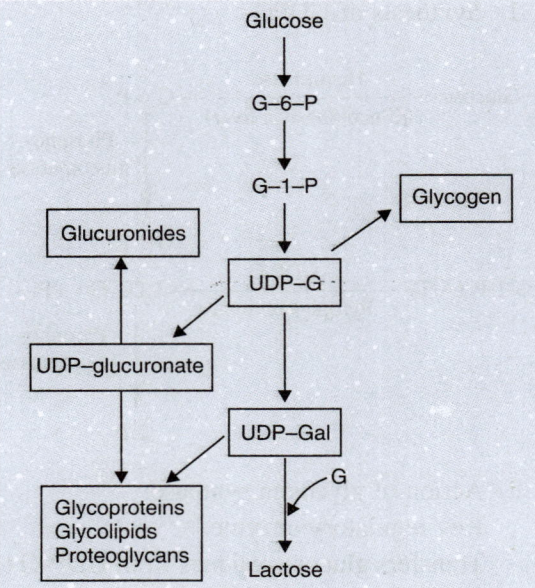

**Fig. 4.26.** Products derived from UDP-glucose.

- Glucose is osmotically active and still draw lots of water inside the cell.

## Osmotic problem of polymers

About 55,000 glucose residues are there in a molecule of glycogen of 21 nm diameter and molecular weight $10^7$.

## Biomedical importance of glycogen

- Liver glycogen is 450 mM after a meal, falling to 200 mM after overnight fast, after 12-18 hrs of fasting, liver glycogen is totally depleted.
- Glycogen storage diseases (Fig. 4.27):
  - Group of inherited disorders
  - Characterized by deficient mobilization of glycogen or deposition of abnormal forms of glycogen, causing:
    - Liver enlargement
    - Muscle weakness
    - Can be fatal

## Rules for branching

- Main chain must be atleast 11 monomer long
- 7 monomer units are transferred from main chain to branch point (Fig. 4.27a)
- Branch point must be at least 4 units from an existing branch
- Branching is accomplished using branching enzyme
- $\alpha1$-4 bond is broken on main chain and branch is made using $\alpha1$-6 bond (Fig. 4.27b).

## GLYCOGENOLYSIS (Fig. 4.27)

### Debranching (Fig. 4.28)

### Glycogenolysis: Glycogen degradation

Not reverse of glycogenesis, but it is a separate pathway.

### Glycogen phosphorylase

- Rate limiting step
- Causes phosphorylysis of $\alpha1$-4 linkages of glycogen to release G-1-P
- Requires pyridoxal phosphate as cofactor

| Comparison | |
|---|---|
| *Glycogenesis* | *Glycogenolysis* |
| Addition of $\alpha1$-4 linkages to non-reducing ends | Cleavage of $\alpha1$-4 linkages at non-reducing ends |
| 1 ATP per linkage used | Phosphorylysis (Pi in place of $H_2O$) |
| Branching enzymes | Debranching enzyme |
| Inactivated by cAMP | Activated by cAMP |

## Glycogenolysis in muscle and liver

Glycogen stores serve different functions in skeletal muscle cells and liver. In muscle,

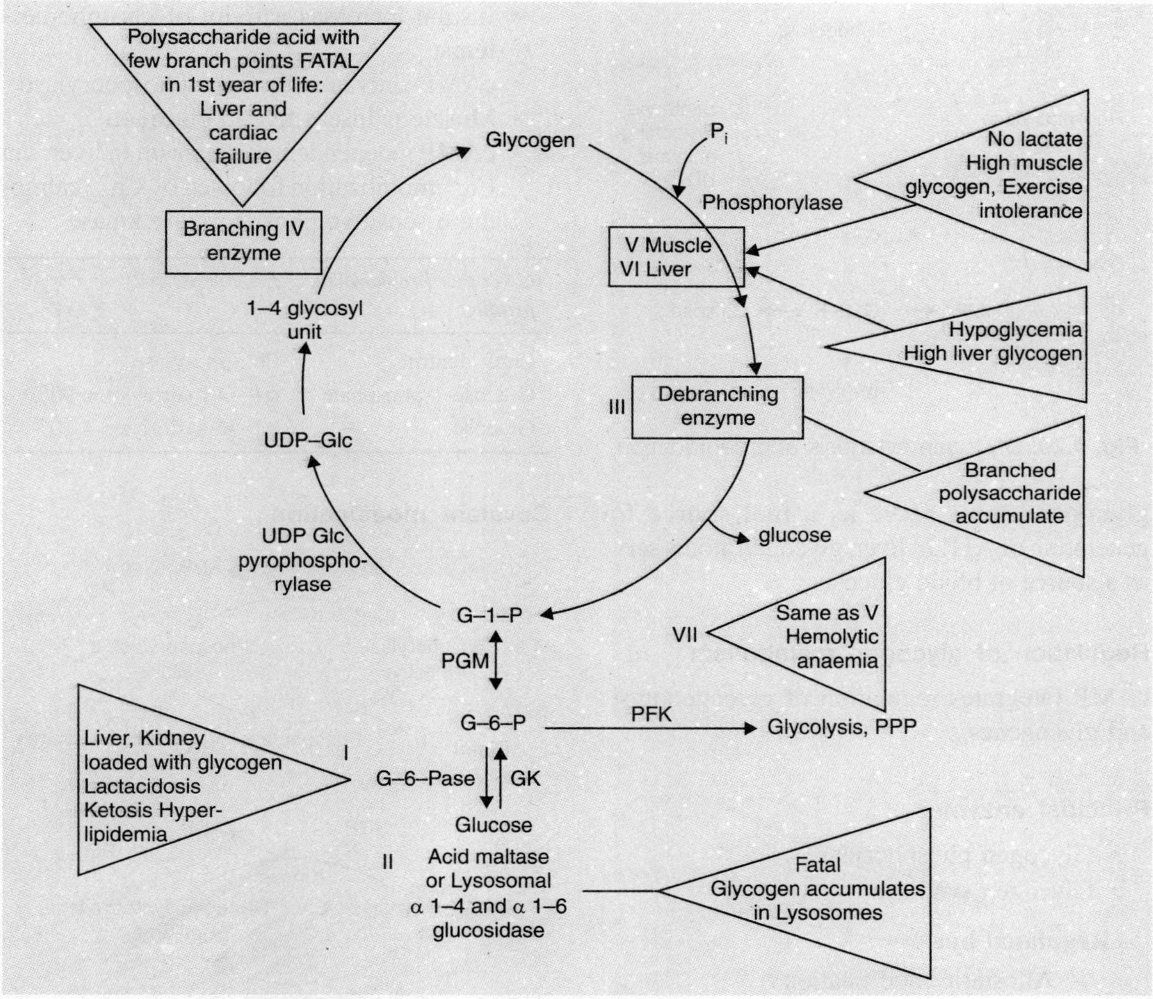

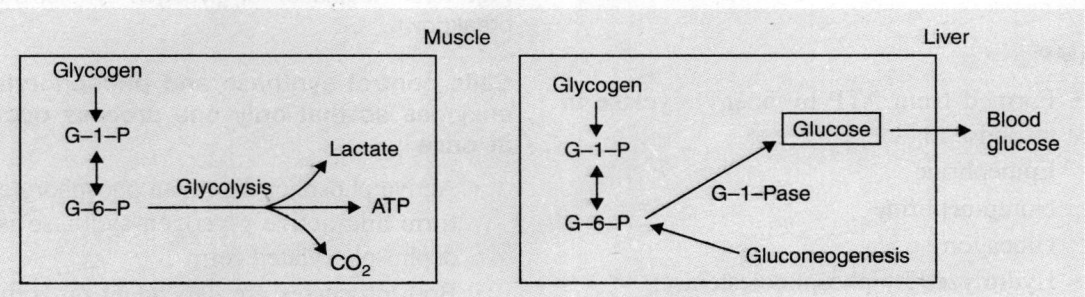

**Fig. 4.27.** Glycogen storage disease (GSD).

**Fig. 4.28.** Glycogenolysis.

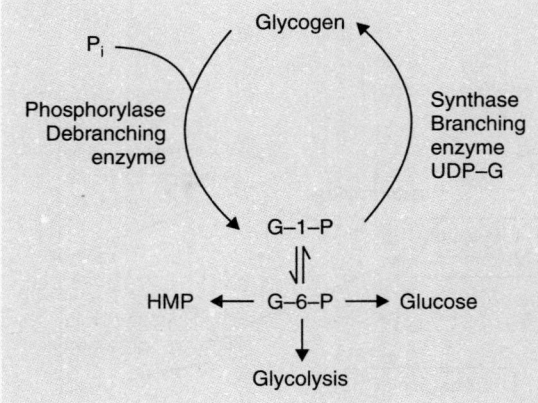

**Fig. 4.29.** Glycogen synthesis and degradation.

glycogen atoms serve as a fuel source for generation of ATP. In liver, glycogen atoms serve as a source of blood glucose.

## Regulation of glycogen metabolism

cAMP integrates regulation of glycogenolysis and glycogenesis

### Principal enzymes

- Glycogen phosphorylase
- Glycogen synthase

**Regulated by:**

- Allosteric modification
- Covalent modification in response to insulin action

### cAMP

- Formed from ATP by adenyl cyclase in response to:
  Epinephrine
  Norepinephrine
  Glucagon
- Hydrolyzed by phosphodiesterase:
  Terminating hormone action in liver

- Insulin increases activity of phosphodiesterase
- cAMP activates glycogen phosphorylase
- Muscle is insensitive to glucagon
- cAMP independent mechanism in liver: via $Ca^{2+}$ mobilization followed by $Ca^{+2}$/calmodulin sensitive phosphorylase kinase.

| Glycogen breakdown product | Enzyme activity |
|---|---|
| Limit dextrin | Phosphorylase |
| Glucose-1-phosphate | $\alpha1 \rightarrow 4$ hydrolysis = 90% |
| Glucose | $\alpha1 \rightarrow 6$ hydrolysis = 10% |

## Covalent modification

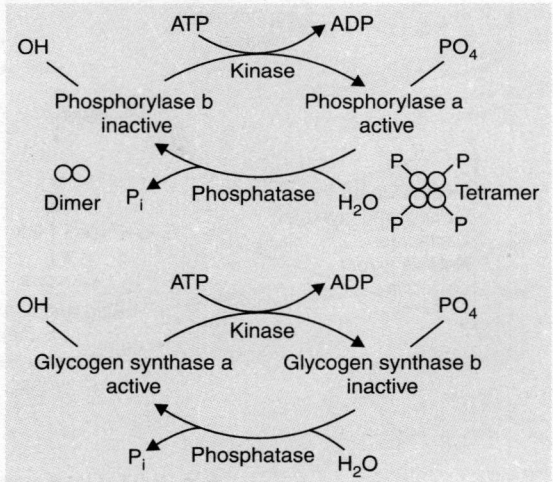

**Fig. 4.30.** Regulation of glycogen synthesis and breakdown.

## Cells control synthase and phosphorylase enzymes so that only one process occurs at once

- Active phosphorylase is in phosphorylated form and active glycogen synthase is in dephosphorylated form
- Both processes are dependent on activity of cAMP dependent protein kinase.

| Enzyme (active form) | Stimulated by | Inhibited by |
|---|---|---|
| Glycogen phosphorylase (phosphorylated) | Glucagon Epinephrine, cAMP, $Ca^{+2}$, AMP phosphorylation | Insulin ATP Glucose |
| Glycogen synthase (dephosphorylated) | Insulin G-6-P | Glucagon Epinephrine, cAMP, $Ca^{+2}$, AMP Phosphorylation |

## (vi) HMP Shunt

Hexose monophosphate shut, also known as pentose (pathway PPP)

### Functions of NADPH

1. Fatty acid synthesis
2. To reduce glutathione:
   - For oxidative damage to cells by reducing $H_2O_2$.
   - For transporting amino acids across the certain cells by γ-glutamyl cycle.
3. Generation of ribose 5-phosphate:
   - When NADPH low, oxidative reactions of the pathway can be used to generate ribose-5-phosphate for nucleotide biosynthesis.
   - When NADPH levels are high, reversible non oxidative portion of pathway can be used to generate ribose-5-phosphate for nucleotide biosynthesis from fructose-6-P and glyceraldehyde 3-phosphate (Fig. 4.31).

### Tissues absolutely requiring blood glucose for energy metabolism

RBCs and brain consume about 80% of 200 g of glucose consumed in the body per day and have

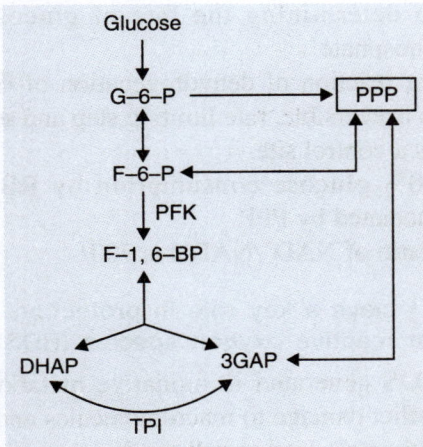

**Fig. 4.31.** HMP is a shunt.

absolute requirement for blood glucose for energy metabolism.

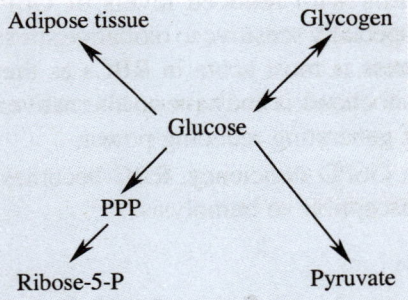

### Pathways requiring NADPH

- FA synthesis
- Cholesterol biosynthesis
- Neurotransmitter biosynthesis
- Nucleotide biosynthesis
- Detoxification
- Reduction of oxidized glutathione
- Cytochrome $P_{450}$ mono oxygenases

### Metabolism of G-6-P by PPP is coordinated with glycolysis

- Concentration of $NADP^+$ plays a key role

in determining the fate of glucose-6-phosphate.

- 1st reaction of dehydrogenation of G-6-P is irreversible, rate limiting step and serves as a control site.
- 10% glucose consumption by RBC is mediated by PPP.
- Ratio of $NAD^+/NADH$ is 700

### G-6-PD plays a key role in protection against reactive oxygen species (ROS)

- ROS generated in oxidative metabolism inflict damage to macromolecules and can ultimately lead to cell death.
- GSH combats oxidative stress by reducing ROS to harmless forms and itself gets oxidized (GSSG). Oxidized GSH (GSSG) is reduced back by NADPH.
- Cells with reduced levels of G6PD are especially sensitive to oxidative stress. This stress is most acute in RBCs as they lack mitochondria and have no alternative means of generating reducing power.
- In G6PD deficiency, RBC becomes more susceptible to hemolysis.

### Favism

RBCs are lysed within 24-48 hours after ingestion of fava beans.

### Clinical features

- Jaundice
- Kidney failure
- Primaquine and fava beans generate $H_2O_2$ and superoxide.

### Chronic granulomatous disease

Genetic deficiency of NADPH oxidase:

### Comparison Glycolysis & PPP

**Common**: G-6-P is common to both.

### Difference

|  | *PPP* | *Glycolysis* |
|---|---|---|
| $1^{st}$ reaction | NADP utilized | NAD and $CO_2$ utilized |
| NAD | Not produced at all | NADH produced |
| ATP | Not generated | Generated |
| Ribose-5-P | Generated | Not generated |

### Remember

- NADH: Oxidized by respiratory chain to generate ATP via oxidative phosphorylation.
- NADPH: Used for biosynthetic reactions which require reductive power.
- NADH and NADPH are not metabolically interchangeable.

Cells must carry out a set of reaction (PPP) that must specifically create NADPH.

### Uronic acid pathway

- In liver, it converts glucose to:
  - Uronic acid
  - Ascorbic acid (except in humans: due absence of enzyme L-gulonolactone oxidase)
  - Pentose
- It is alternative oxidative pathway for glucose, *no ATP produced*:
  - Occurs in liver
  - Cytoplasm
  - Starts with G-6-P
  - Ends with glucuronic acid, ascorbic acid and pentoses

Used:

- As part of proteoglycans
- For reactions of substrates such as steroid hormones, bilirubin
- Drugs excreted in urine or bile as glucuronide conjugate

## HMP in liver

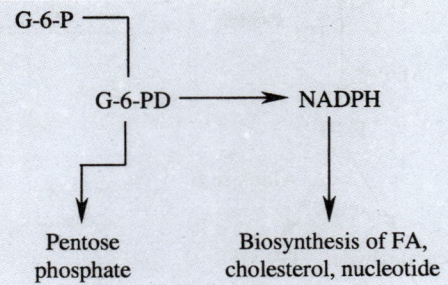

## HMP in neutrophil

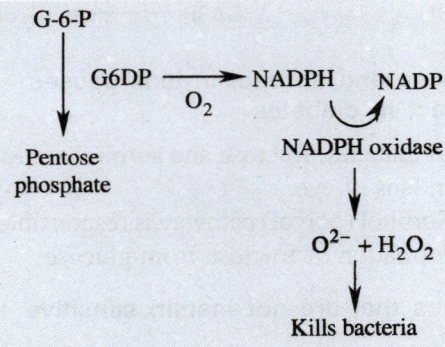

## In RBC

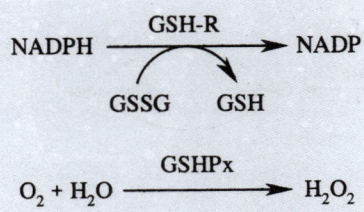

$H_2O_2$ accumulation causes Hb denaturation (Heinz bodies) and membrane damage (hemolytic anaemia).

## CLINICAL CORRELATION

### 1. Essential pentosuria

- Deficiency of reductase needed to convert L-xylulose to xylitol

- Accumulation of L-xylulose leads to its increased levels in the urine.

### 2. G6PD deficiency

- Causes drug induced hemolytic anaemia
- Mediterranean and Afro Caribbean in origin.
- Increased susceptibility to oxidants Primaquine, sulphonamide, aspirin, and fava beans.

### Functions: GSH

- Serves as a reluctant
- Conjugates to drugs making them water soluble
- Involved in amino acid transport across cell membrane
- Cofactor in some enzymatic reactions arrangement of protein disulfide bonds.
- SH of GSH is used to reduce peroxides (ROS) during oxygen transport.

ROS damage macromolecules (DNA, RNA and protein) and ultimately cell death. The resulting oxidized form of GSH is two molecules linked by a disulfide bridge (GSSG).

$$H \quad NADPH^+H^+ \quad GSSG \quad 2H_2O$$
$$FAD \quad GSH\text{-}R \quad GSHPx$$
$$NADP^+ \quad 2GSH \quad H_2O_2$$

## (vii) Fructose And Galactose Metabolism

### Fructose

- Fructose floods pathways in liver
- Increases FFA synthesis
- Increases esterification of FA

- Increases VLDL secretion
- Raises serum TAG
- Raises LDL-C

## FRUCTOSE METABOLISM (Fig. 4.32)

### Fructokinase

- Does not act on glucose
- Unlike glucokinase, its activity is not affected by fasting or by insulin
- Thus, fructose is cleared from blood of diabetic patients at a normal rate

### Fructose metabolism in extrahepatic tissues

- Hexokinase (HK) catalyzes phosphorylation of most hexoses including fructose
- Glucose inhibits phosphorylation of fructose: since it is a better substrate for HK.
- Fructose can be metabolized in adipose tissue and muscle
- Fructose found in seminal fluid
- Aldose reductase is responsible for synthesis of sorbitol.

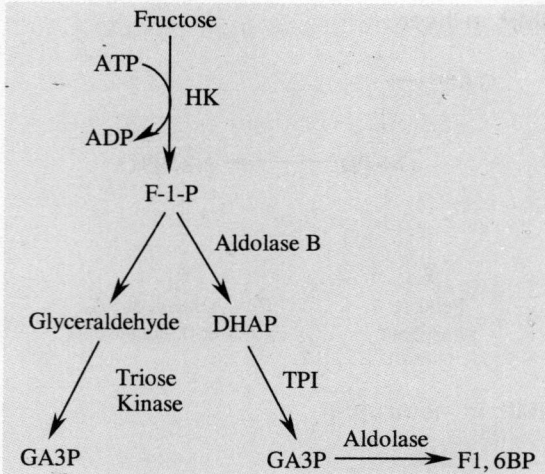

### Fructose and sorbitol in lens causes cataract in diabetes

- In diabetes, fructose and sorbitol are found in lens of eye.
- Sorbitol (polyol) pathway is responsible for formation of fructose from glucose.

### Tissues that are not insulin sensitive

- Lens
- Peripheral nerves
- Renal glomerulus

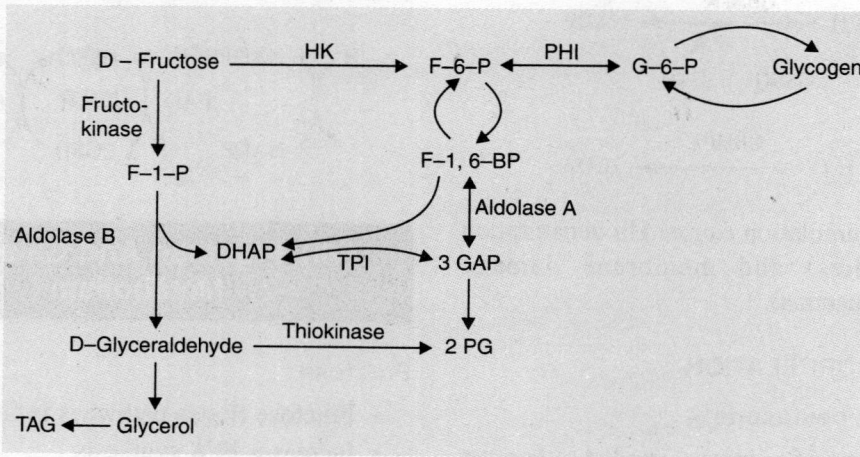

**Fig. 4.32.** Major pathways of fructose metabolism.

## Production of fructose from glucose

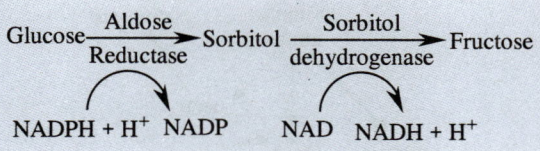

$$\text{Glucose} \xrightarrow[\text{Reductase}]{\text{Aldose}} \text{Sorbitol} \xrightarrow[\text{dehydrogenase}]{\text{Sorbitol}} \text{Fructose}$$

$$\text{NADPH} + \text{H}^+ \quad \text{NADP} \qquad \text{NAD} \quad \text{NADH} + \text{H}^+$$

**Aldose reductase** is found in Retina, Schwann cells, liver, kidney, RBC, seminal vesicles, placenta, and ovary.

## Sorbitol

- Does not diffuse through cell membrane its accumulation causes osmotic damage.
- Myoinositol levels also fall.
- Accumulates in retina, lens, kidney and nerve cells.

## Galactose

- Forms a small part of carbohydrate intake
- Present in diet in form of lactose in milk
- Important constituent of:
  - Lactose
  - Glycoprotein
  - Glycolipid
- Uptake of galactose by cells is insulin-independent
- Galactose does not stimulate insulin secretion

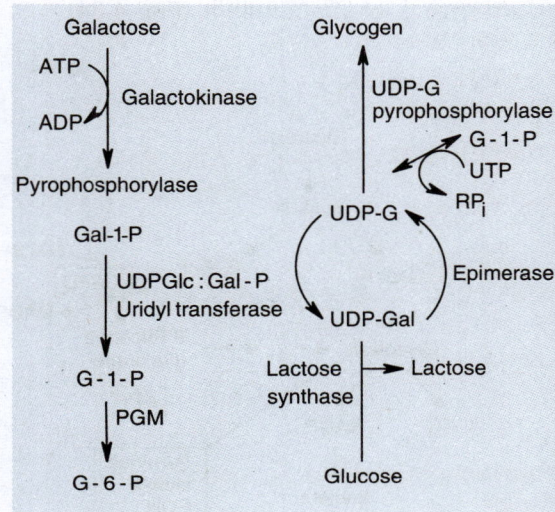

**Fig. 4.33.** Galactose metabolism.

- Galactose is required in body for:
  - Formation of lactose
  - As a constituent of:
    - Glycolipid
    - Glycoprotein
    - Proteoglycan

## Galactosemia

### Diagnosis

- Low blood glucose (hypoglycemia)
- Gal-1-P uridyl transferase activity low
- Urine: galactose, galactose-1-P

| Defect | Enzyme deficiency | Features |
|---|---|---|
| Galactosemia | Galactokinase 4 Epimerase | Accumulation of galactose in blood and tissues. In lens, galactose is reduced to dulcitol causing osmotic imbalance forming cataract |
| Classic galactosemia | Uridyltransferase | Cataract, mental retardation, liver cirrhosis |

## Inborn errors of metabolism (Fig. 4.34)

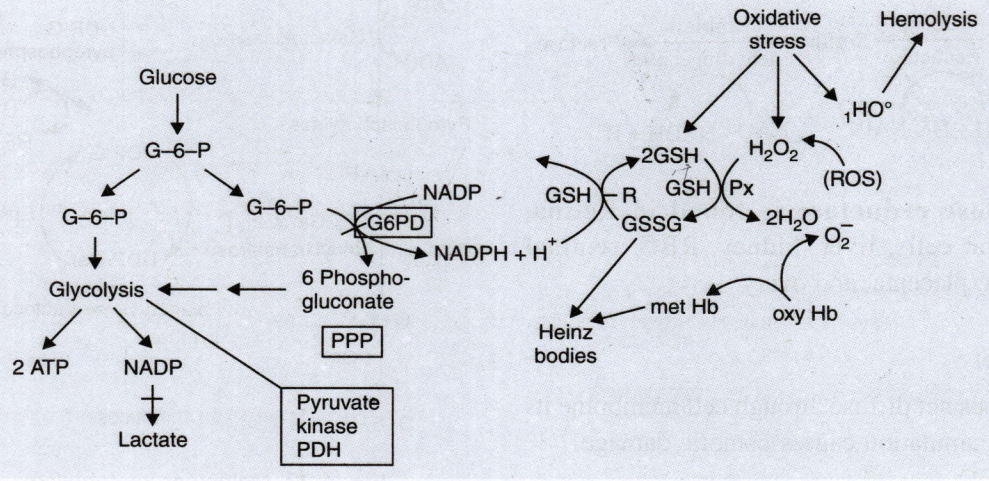

Fig. 4.34. Hemolysis by enzyme defect in glucose metabolism.

# (viii) GNG (Gluconeogenesis)

## Requirements for GNG

- Source of energy
- Source of carbons for formation of back bone of glucose molecule

**Energy** is provided by metabolism of FA released from adipose tissue

**Carbon skeleton** provided by:
– Lactate
– Amino acid (glucogenic)
– Glycerol
– Glycogen

Location:
– Liver 85-95%
  Epithelial tissue, small intestine, 5%.
  During starvation: kidney, 50%

**Requirement for GNG:**
– Source of energy
– source of carbons for formation of back bone of glucose muscle

Energy is provided by:
– Metabolism of FA released from adipose tissue

Carbon sksletons provided by:
– Lactate
– Amino acids (glucogenia)
– Glycerol
– Glycogen

## Why do we need glucose in our body?

- Tissues that synthesize glucose: Liver, kidney
- Tissues that use glucose as their primary energy source: Brain, muscle, RBC, testes.

## Situations in which we need GNG

- Normal physiological situation:
  – Between meals, during sleep
  – Exercise/work
- After heavy exercise or work (recycling of lactate)

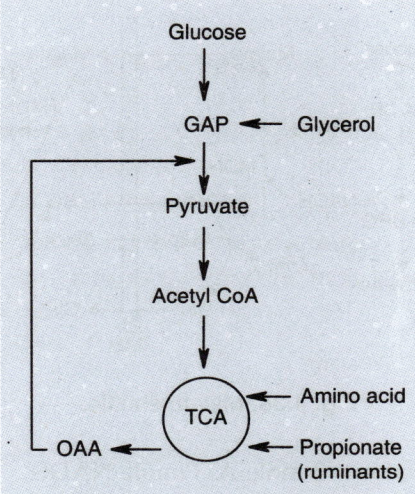

**Fig. 4.35.** GNG precursors

- After protein-rich diet (glucogenic amino acids)
- Starvation (glucogenic amino acids)

## Fact file: GNG

- Glucose is important fuel for CNS, RBC
- Brain is 100% dependent on glucose for energy
- Liver can store glycogen to last about 12 hours
- Thus, synthesis of new glucose called **gluconeogenesis** is carried out in liver and to some degree in kidney
- Not simply a reversal of glycolysis
- Insulin and glucagon are primary regulators
- Daily glucose requirement for human being: 160 g (120 g brain)
- Glycogen can provide 190 g.
- GNG accounts for up to 96% of total glucose production.

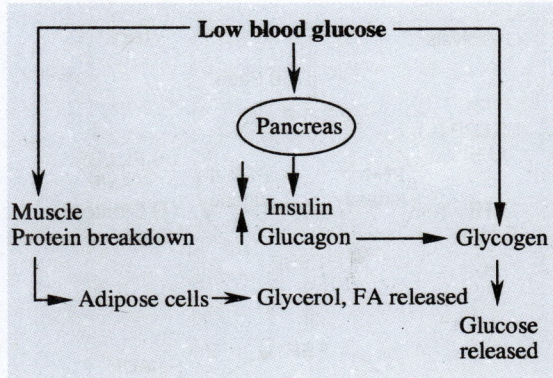

## Energetics GNG

Conversion of two mole of pyruvate to one mole of glucose requires:

- 4 moles of ATP
- 2 GTP
- 2 NADH

## Location of enzymes of GNG

- Pyruvate carboxylase: mitochondrial
- G-6-Pase: ER
- All other enzymes are cytoplasmic

## Function: GNG

- During starvation/period of limited carbohydrate intake: to maintain adequate blood glucose levels.
- During extended exercise: to use lactate in glycolysis and glycerol from lipolysis
- Metabolic acids: allows excretion of protons
- Allows use of dietary proteins in carbohydrate pathway

## GNG REQUIRES TRANSPORT BETWEEN MITOCHONDRIA AND CYTOSOL

### Glycerol shuttle

- Functions in muscle, brain
- Produces 2 moles ATP/mol NADH

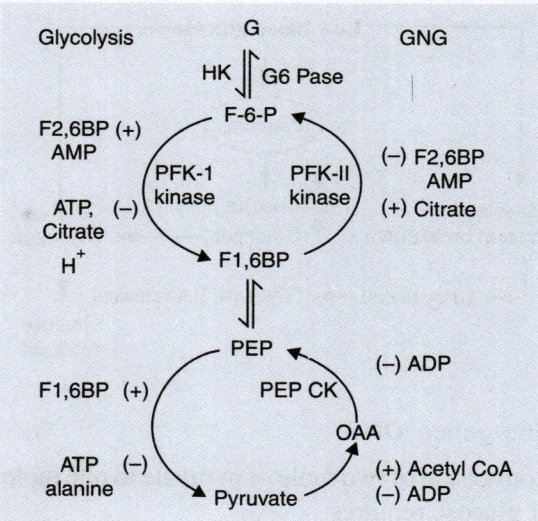

**Fig. 4.36.** Comparison of glycolysis and gluco-neogenesis.

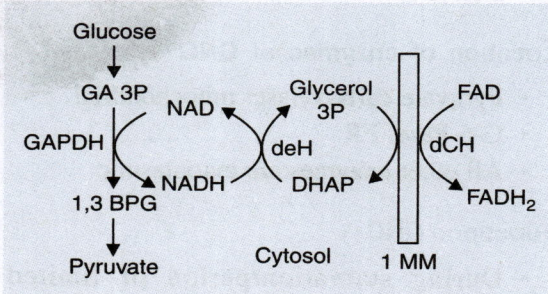

**Fig. 4.37.** Glycerol shuttle.

- Cytoplasmic NADH used to catalyze: DHAP to Glycerol 3P.
- Glycerol 3P enters mitochondria and oxidized to DHAP by FAD.
- $FADH_2$ transformed, supports the synthesis of 3 moles of ATP via ETC.
- DHAP formed, returns to cytosol to continue shunt.

## Malate shuttle

- Functions in heart, kidney, liver

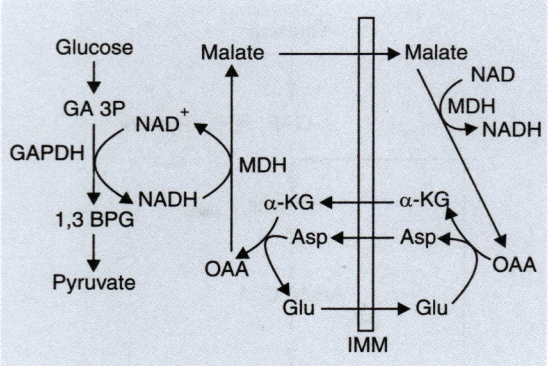

**Fig. 4.38.** Malate shuttle.

- Produces 3 mole ATP/mole NADH
- Cytosolic NADH catalyzes conversion of OAA to malate
- Malate enters mitochondria, oxidized back to OAA using mitochondrial NAD by MDH.
- NADH forms 3 moles of ATP
- OAA transported across IMM in form of aspartate
- OAA converted into aspartate in mitochondria which get transported to cytosol.
- In cytosol, aspartate is converted into OAA to complete the cycle.

## ATP production and electron shuttles:

- 6ATP/glucose (glycerol phosphate shuttle)
- 8ATP/glucose (malate shuttle)

## PRECURSORS FOR GNG

### 1. Lactate

**Source:**
- RBC
- Muscle
- Cori cycle

**Cori cycle:** Lactate is converted to pyruvate in liver

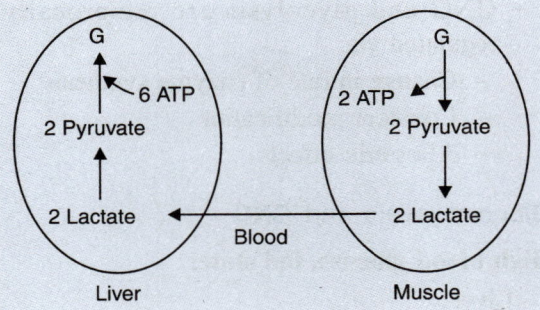

**Fig. 4.39.** Energetics of CNG.

- Pyruvate is formed from glucose in muscle, RBC and get converted to lactate by LDH
- Lactate enters liver via circulation to be converted by pyruvate

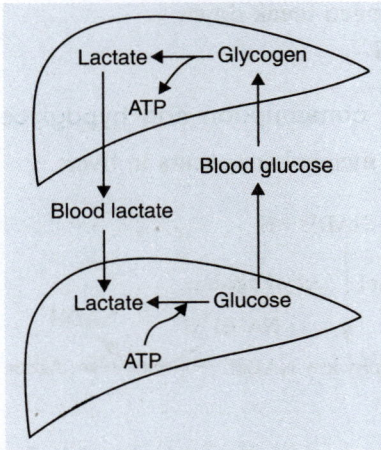

**Fig. 4.40.** Cori cycle.

- Pyruvate converted to glucose via GNG, released into circulation and serves as a source of 'E' for muscle
- Costs 6 ~ P (six high energy phosphate) in liver for every 2~P made available in muscle, net cost is 4~P.
- Although costly in ~P bonds, allows organism to accommodate large

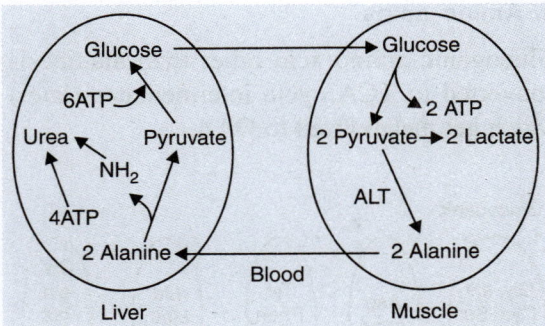

**Fig. 4.41.** Glucose-alanine cycle.

fluctuations in energy needs of skeletal muscle between rest and exercise.

## 2. Alanine and other amino acids

- Transamination of pyruvate to alanine
- Pyruvate derived from glycolysis or from amino acid degradation.
- Alanine cycle
- Glucose-alanine cycle

### Glucose alanine cycle

Alanine brings both carbon and nitrogen from muscle to liver

### Common features for Cori & glucose-alanine cycle

These mechanisms allows muscle cells to produce ATP with high rates at the expense of regenerating glucose from lactate and alanine in liver.

## 3. Glycerol

- Derived from adipocyte lipolysis
- Hepatic glycerol kinase
- Glycerol is released into blood and enters liver, where it gets converted to 3PG via 1, 3 BPG and GAD 3P to glucose via GNG

## 4. Amino acids

Glucogenic amino acid other than alanine is converted to TCA cycle intermediates (later) which get metabolized to OAA.

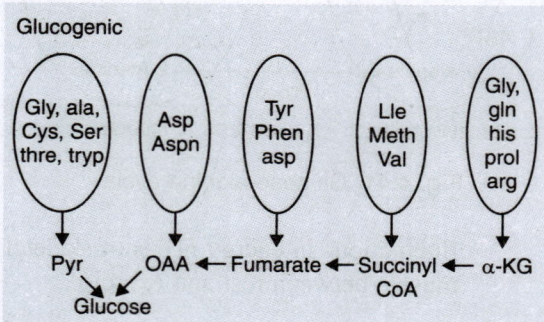

**Fig. 4.42.** Metabolic fate of carbon skeletons of amino acid .

## 5. Propionate

- End product of odd chain FA oxidation
- Converted to succinyl CoA and enters TCA and then GNG.
- Major source of glucose in ruminants.

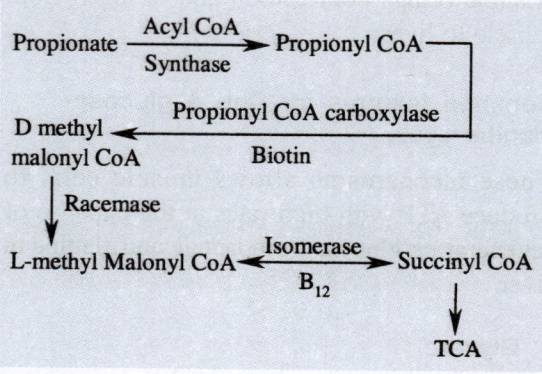

## 6. Glycogen

- Glucose-1-phosphate is released from glycogen by phosphorylase

  G-1-P → G-6-P → G

- GNG and glycolysis are reciprocally regulated via:
  - Change in rate of enzyme synthesis
  - Covalent modification
  - Allosteric effects

## Glucose levels and GNG

### High blood glucose, fed state:

Liver:

- Fuel conservation
- Glycogen synthesized
- Glycolysis activated
- PDH activated
- FA biosynthesis and fat storage occurs

### Low blood glucose fasting state:

Energy generation
Glycogen break down
GNG

## Alcohol consumption and hypoglycemia

Alcohol metabolism occurs in liver:

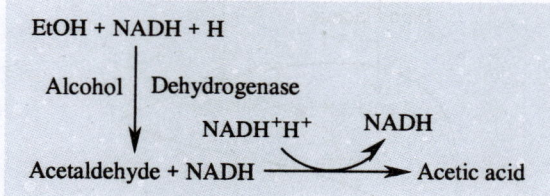

## Two step metabolism of alcohol: Features

- Relatively unregulated
- Leads to rapid rise in hepatic NADH
- Alcohol metabolism:

  Increase in hepatic NAD shift the equilibrium of LDH reaction towards lactate, limiting gluconeogenesis from pyruvate (derived from lactate or alanine)

- Also, shifts cytosolic OAA from TCA intermediates, reducing GNG

- Shifts DHAP towards glycerol 3P, reducing GNG from glycerol.
- Thus, redox imbalance produced by alcohol consumption leads to a large increase in NADH in cytoplasm, inhibiting flux of all major substrates into GNG.

## GNG

- Fairly efficient
- Liver can make 1 kg/d by GNG
- Does so in poorly controlled DM.

## Clinical correlates: GNG

1. G-6Pase deficiency (Von Gierke's disease) GSD I presents with severe hypoglycemia
2. PEP CK deficiency:
   Severe rare metabolic defect
   Severe cerebral atrophy
   Optic atrophy
   Fatty infiltration of liver
   Kidney
   Hypoglycemia
3. F1, 6 bisphosphatase deficiency:
   Neonatal hypoglycemia
   Acidosis
   Hepatomegaly
4. LDH deficiency:
   Muscle cramps
   Myoglobinuria after intense exercise.

## Energy requirements for GNG

1. From pyruvate
   $$\text{Lactate} \xrightarrow{\text{LDH}} \text{Pyruvate} \xrightarrow{\text{PC}} \text{OAA}$$
   Require 1 mole ATP

2. $$\text{OAA} \xrightarrow{\text{PEPCK}} \text{PEP}$$
   Require 1 mole ATP

3. $$\text{3PG} \xrightarrow{\text{Kinase}} \text{1, 3 BPG}$$
   Require 1 mole ATP

4. Since 2 moles of pyruvate are required to form 1 mole of glucose, 6 moles of high energy phosphate are required for synthesis of one mole of glucose.
   6ATP are hydrolyzed to synthesize glucose from pyruvate and only two molecules are generated in glycolysis in conversion of glucose to lactate. Thus, extra cost of GNG is 4 high phosphoryl transfer potential molecules.
   Thus, an extra four ATPs per glucose are required for reverse glycolysis.

## Regulatory enzymes of GNG

Under fasting conditions, glucagon is elevated and stimulates enzymes of GNG

1. PDH
2. Pyruvate carboxylase – activated by acetyl CoA
3. PEP carboxy kinase – inducible enzyme
4. PK: Glucagon via cAMP and protein kinase A causes PK to be phosphorylated and get inactivated.
5. PFK-1: Inactive, because its activators AMP, F2, 6BP are low and its inhibitor ATP is high due to oxidation of FA.
6. F1, 6B Pase: F2, 6BP low, so this enzyme is active
7. Glucokinase: Inactive glucose concentration is low.

## (ix) Regulation of Blood Glucose

### MAINTENANCE OF BLOOD GLUCOSE LEVELS

### In fed state

**Changes in insulin and glucagon levels:**

- After a meal, blood insulin levels increase following rise in blood glucose

- Glucose enters pancreatic β-cells via GLUT-2 (insulin independent), stimulates release of preformed insulin and promotes synthesis of new insulin.
- Additionally, amino acids (arginine and leucine) cause release of preformed insulin from β cells of pancreas.

**Depending on content of meal, blood glucagon changes:**

- A high carbohydrate meal causes glucagon to decrease.
- A high protein meal causes glucagon to increase.
- On normal fixed diet, glucagon remains fairly constant and insulin increases

**FATE OF DIETARY GLUCOSE IN LIVER**

- Glucose enters hepatocytes via GLUT2
- Glucose is oxidized for energy

- Excess glucose is converted to glycogen and to TAG of VLDL.
- GK has high km for glucose (about 6 mM), thus, its velocity increases after a meal when glucose levels are elevated on a high-carbohydrate diet, glucokinase is induced.
- Glycogen synthesis is promoted by insulin which stimulates the phosphatase, thus increasing the activity of glycogen synthase.
- Synthesis of TAG is also stimulated.

**FATE OF DIETARY GLUCOSE IN PERIPHERAL TISSUES**

- All cells oxidize glucose for energy
- Insulin stimulate transport of glucose into adipose and muscle cells
- In muscle, insulin stimulates the synthesis of glycogen
- Adipose cells convert glucose to the glycerol moiety for synthesis of TAG

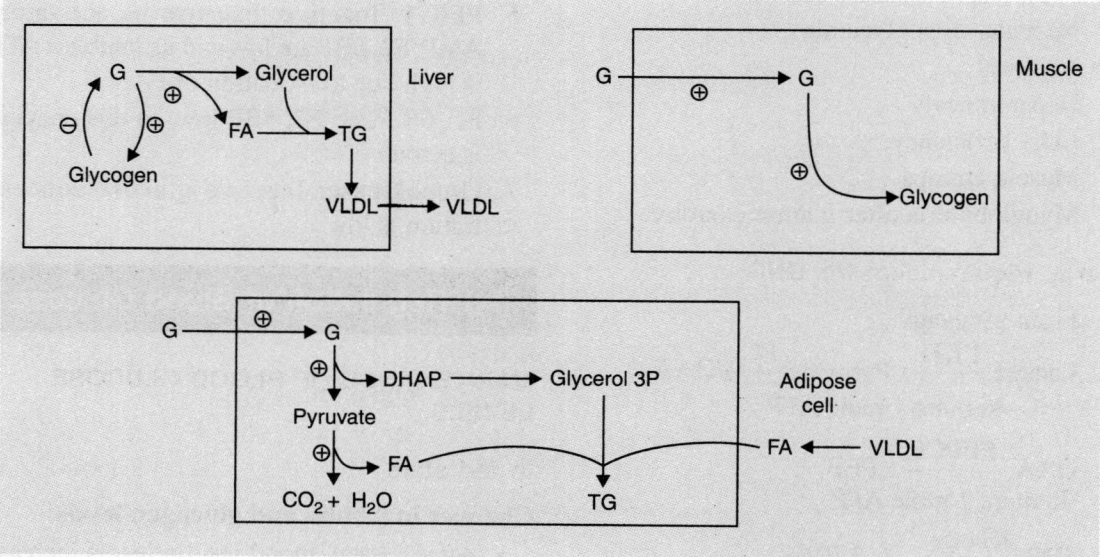

**Fig. 4.43.** Influence of insulin on glucose metabolism in various tissues.

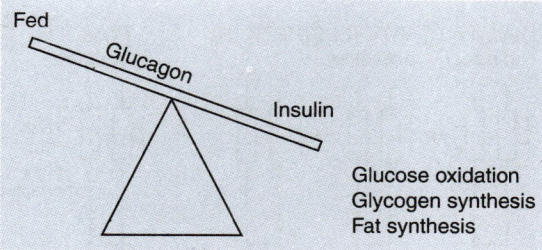

**Fig. 4.44.** Fate of glucose after meals.

## RETURN OF BLOOD GLUCOSE TO FASTING LEVELS

- Uptake of dietary glucose by tissues: (liver, adipose and muscle): causes blood glucose to decrease.
- After 2 hours of taking meal: blood glucose return to fasting level: 80-100 mg/dl.

### In fasting state

1. Changes in insulin and glucagon levels:
   Insulin levels decrease
   Glucagon level increase

### Result

- Glycogenolysis promoted
- GNG promoted to maintain blood glucose levels
- Lipolysis stimulated, FA oxidized and converted to ketone bodies.
  Glycogenolysis: Main source of blood glucose for 8-12 hours
  Gluconeogenesis: Stimulated within 4 hours, supplies large share of blood glucose as fasting state persists
  After 16 hours, GNG and glycogenolysis are about equal source of blood glucose.
- As glucagon stores are depleted, GNG predominates.
- After 30 hours, GNG is the only source of blood glucose.

### Prolonged fasting

- Changes in fuel utilization by various tissues occur to prevent blood glucose levels from decreasing abruptly during prolonged fasting.
- Level of ketone bodies rise in blood, brain uses ketone bodies for energy, decreasing its utilization of blood glucose.

### During exercise

- Exercising muscle uses ATP which is regenerated initially using creatine phosphate.
- Muscle glycogen is oxidized to produce ATP.
- Epinephrine causes production of cAMP which stimulates glycogen breakdown.
- Following increased blood flow to the exercising muscles, blood glucose and fatty acids are taken up and oxidized by muscle.
- As blood glucose levels begin to decrease, liver GNG and glycogenolysis maintain blood glucose levels.

## GLUCOSE HOMEOSTASIS

### Islets of langerhans

- 1 million islets
- Each islet containing 2500 cells
- β cell secrete insulin
- α cells secrete glucagon

## INSULIN

- Hormone of nutrient abundance
- Consists of two amino acid chains linked by disulfide bond.
- Synthesized as proinsulin (86 AA):
  - Functional insulin (51 AA)
  - C-peptide (29 AA)

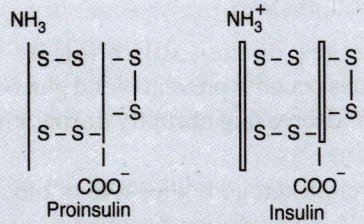

**Fig. 4.45.** Structure of insulin.

Functional insulin: Two chains:
– A chain: 21 AA
– B chain: 30 AA
   3 disulfide bonds

Insulin gene encodes a large precursor of preproinsulin. During translation, signal peptide cleaved (proinsulin). During packaging in granules by golgi, proinsulin is cleaved into insulin and C peptide.

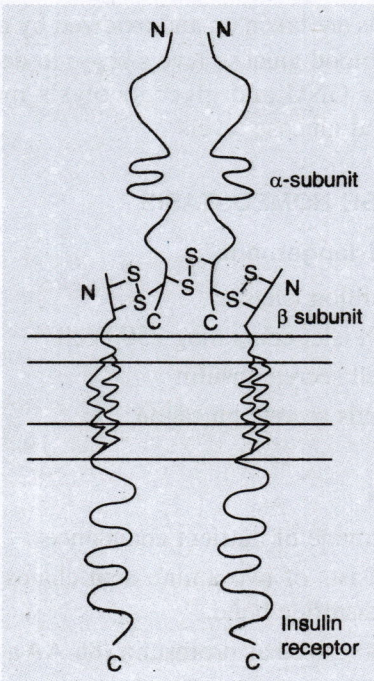

**Fig. 4.46.** Insulin receptor.

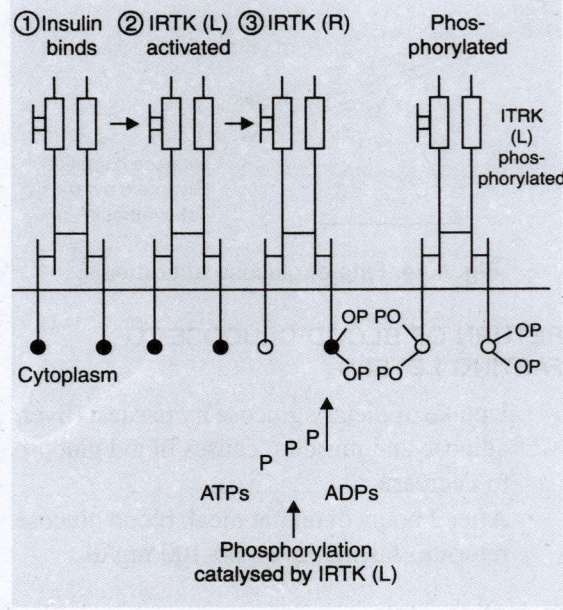

**Fig. 4.47.** Insulator receptor mechanism.

## Insulin synthesis

- Insulin synthesis is:
  - Stimulated by glucose or feeding
  - Decreased by fasting
- Threshold of glucose – stimulated insulin secretion is 100 mg/dL.
- Glucose rapidly increase translation of insulin mRNA and slowly increases transcription of insulin gene.

## Insulin receptor (IR)

- Tyrosine kinase
- Tetramer
  - Two α subunits
  - Two β subunits

. Insulin binding to α-chain transmits a signal through trans membrane domain to β-chain to activate tyrosine kinase activity.

## Insulin regulates by glucose transport by GLUT4

- Glucose uptake into myocytes and adipocytes is mediated by GLUT4
- Between meals, some GLUT4 is present in plasma membrane
- In response to high blood, insulin is released, which triggers movement of intracellular vesicles to plasma membrane. Thus exposing GLUT4 molecules on outer cell surface
- When blood glucose levels return to normal insulin release slows.
  GLUT4 molecules removed from plasma membrane and stored in vesicles.

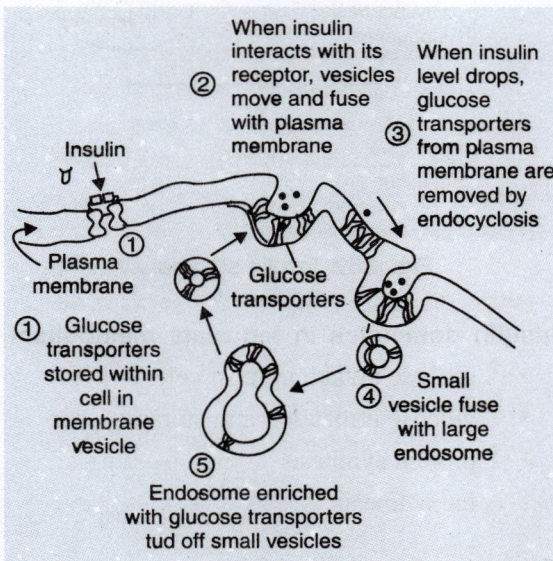

**Fig. 4.48.** Insulin synthesis.

### Mechanism

Following rise in blood glucose levels, insulin acts in muscle to:

- Increase glucose transport into cells by recruiting GLUT4 to plasma membrane
- Induce synthesis of hexokinase (HK).

- Activate glycogen synthase by covalent modification.
- Increase in GLUT4 transporter and hexokinase synthesis increases flux of glucose through pathway.

At rest, $K_{ATP}$ channel open, β cells secrete insulin. $K_{ATP}$ channels close, trigger endocytosis of insulin.

When blood glucose rises, GLUT2 transporter carry glucose into cells:

$$G \xrightarrow[GK]{HK} G6P \rightarrow \text{Enters glycosis}$$

When blood glucose level is high, active metabolism of glucose increases

### Sequence of events (Fig. 4.48)

- Intracellular ATP increase
- Closing of $K^+$ channels
- Change in membrane potential
- Voltage-gated $Ca^{+2}$ channels in plasma membrane open, $Ca^{+2}$ flows into cell, cytosolic $Ca^{+2}$ trigger insulin release by exocytosis.

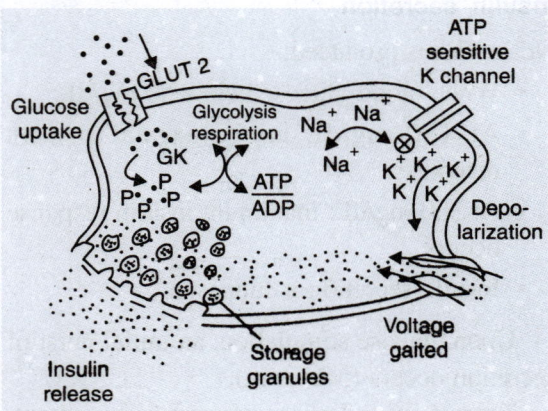

**Fig. 4.49.** Insulin release mechanism.

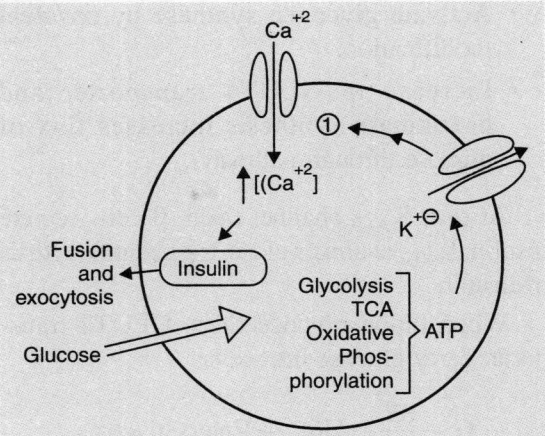

Fig. 4.50. Sequence of events in insulin release.

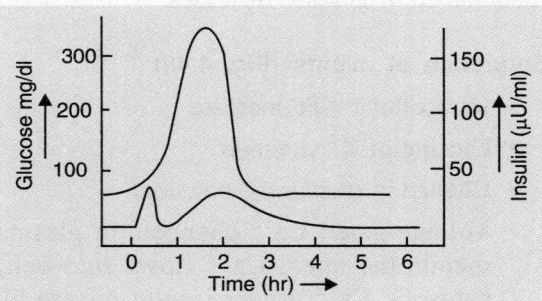

Fig. 4.51. Blood glucose and insulin level.

## Insulin secretion

No insulin is produced:

- When blood glucose below 50 mg/dL
- At 150 mg/dL half maximal insulin response
- At 300 mg/dL: maximum insulin response occurs.
- Insulin secretion is biphasic.

Upon glucose stimulation, an initial burst of secretion occurs (5-15 min).

Then, a second phase of gradual increment, that last for as long as blood glucose is high.

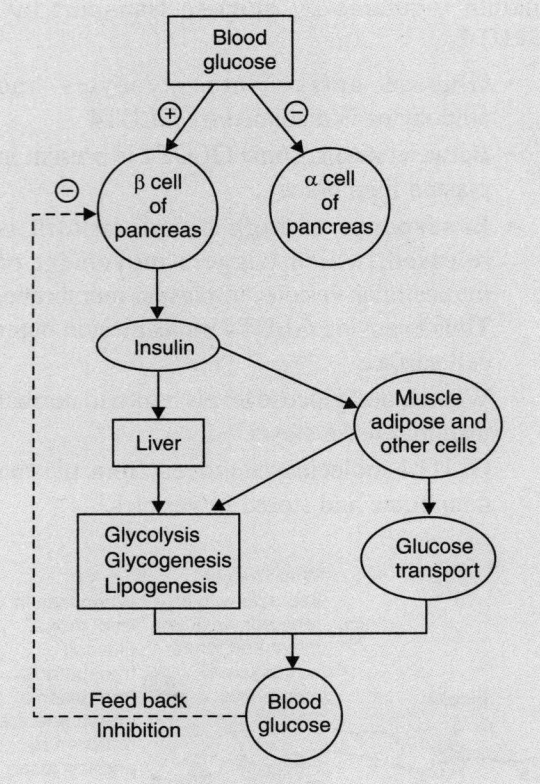

Fig. 4.52. Insulin summary.

## Insulin dominates in fed state metabolism

- ↑ glucose uptake in most cells
- ↑ glucose utilization and storage
- ↑ protein synthesis
- ↑ fat synthesis

## Glucagon (Fig. 4.53, 4.54)

## Physiological role of insulin

Maintenance of normal plasma glucose inspite of large changes due to food intake.

## Rapid uptake of dietary glucose

- Stimulation of glucose transport
- Stimulation of glucose utilization

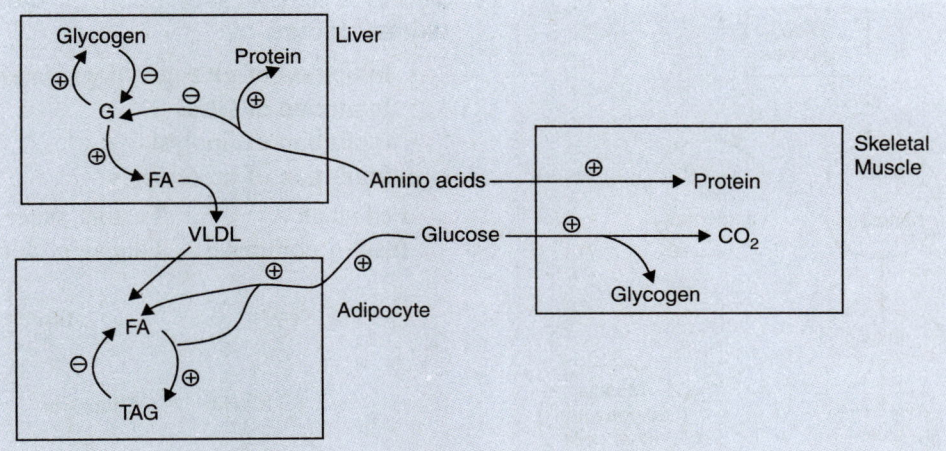

**Fig. 4.53.** Major sites of action of insulin.

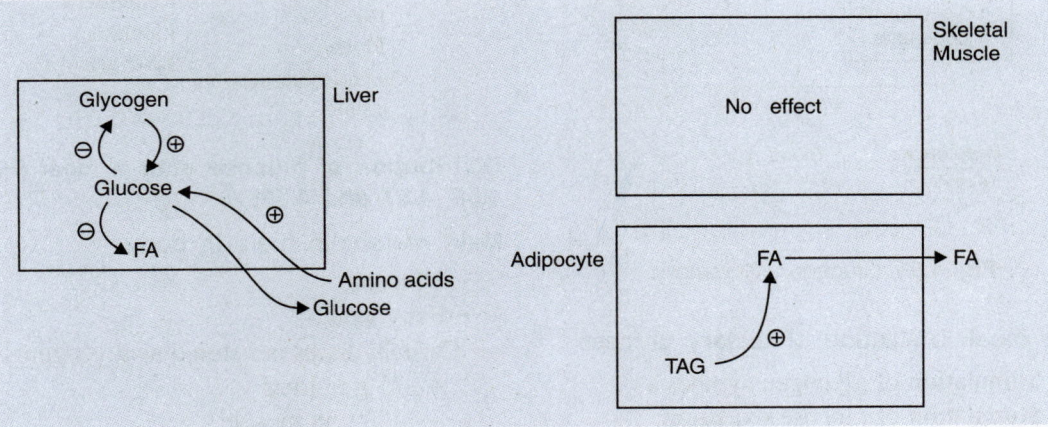

**Fig. 4.54.** Major sites of action of glucagon.

**Table 4.8.** Hormonal regulation of metabolism

|  | Lipolysis | Protein degradation | Glucose synthesis | Liver glycogen | Plasma glucose |
|---|---|---|---|---|---|
| Insulin | ↓ | ↓ | ↓ | ↑ | ↓ |
| Cortisol | ↑ | ↑ | ↑ | ↑ | ↑ |
| Glucagon | ↑ | – | ↑ | ↓ | ↑ |
| Growth hormone | ↑ | ↓ | ↑ | ↓ | ↑ |
| Catecholamines | ↑ | – | ↑ | ↓ | ↑ |
| Leptin | ↑? | – | – | – | ↑ |

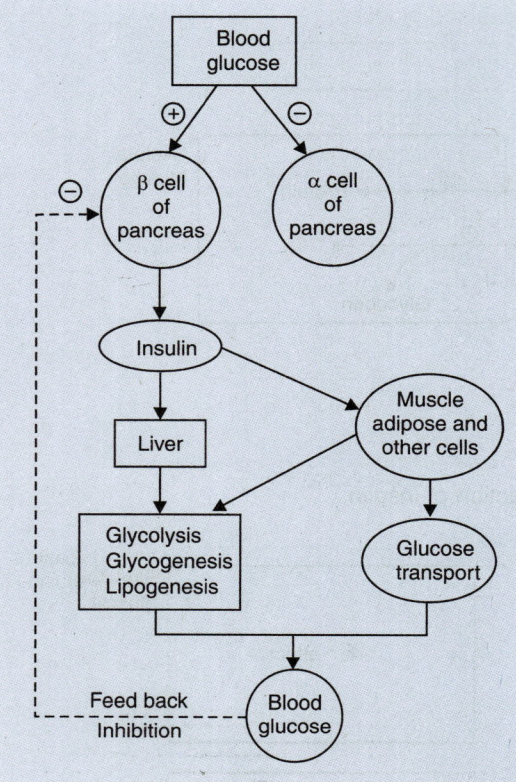

**Fig. 4.55.** Glucagon: Summary.

## After meal: Utilization of dietary glucose

- Stimulation of glycogen synthesis
- Stimulation of glucose oxidation
- Stimulation of lipid synthesis

## During a fast: Preservation of energy stores, occurs by:

- Inhibition of glycogen degradation
- Inhibition of GNG
- Inhibition of lipolysis
- Inhibition of proteolysis

Fed state:  Fasting state:
Insulin dominates  Glucagon dominates

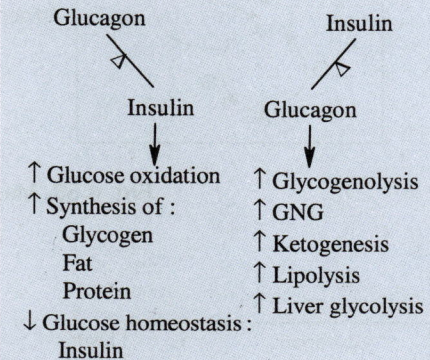

## Distribution of glucose after a meal (Figs. 4.56, 4.57 and 4.58)

## Main metabolic fuels in body

- Glucose
- Fatty acid

Carbohydrates are stored as glycogen:
- 75 g in liver
- 400 g in muscle
- Giving 1900 kcal, lasting for 16 h

| **Table 4.9.** Effect of insulin of blood glucose | |
|---|---|
| *Metabolic effect* | *Target enzyme* |
| ↑ glucose uptake (muscle, adipose tissue) | ↑ Glucose transporter GLUT 4 |
| ↑ Glucose uptake (liver) | ↑ Glucokinase |
| ↑ Glycogen synthesis (liver, muscle) | ↑ Glycogen synthase |
| ↓ Glycogen breakdown | ↓ Glycogen phosphorylase |
| ↑ Glycolysis, acetyl CoA production | ↑ PFK-1, PDH |
| ↑ Fatty acid synthesis (liver) | ↑ Acetyl CoA carboxylase |
| ↑ TAG synthesis | ↑ Lipoprotein lipase |

## Table 4.10. Effect of glucagon on blood glucose

| Metabolic effect | Target enzyme |
|---|---|
| ↑ Glycogen breakdown (liver) | ↑ glycogen phosphorylase |
| ↓ Glycogen synthesis (liver) | ↓ glycogen synthase |
| ↓ Glycolysis (liver) | ↓ PFK-1 |
| ↑ GNG (liver) | ↑ FBPase-2 |
| | ↓ Pyruvate kinase |
| | ↑ PEP carboxy kinase |
| ↑ Fatty acid mobilization | ↑ TAG lipase |
| ↑ Ketogenesis | ↑ Acetyl (CoA carboxylase) |

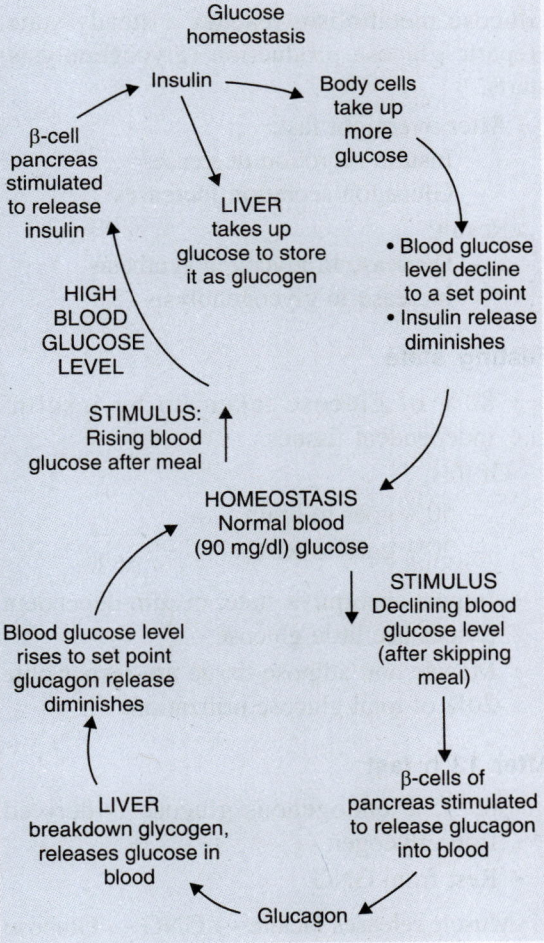

Fig. 4.56. Glucose homeactasis.

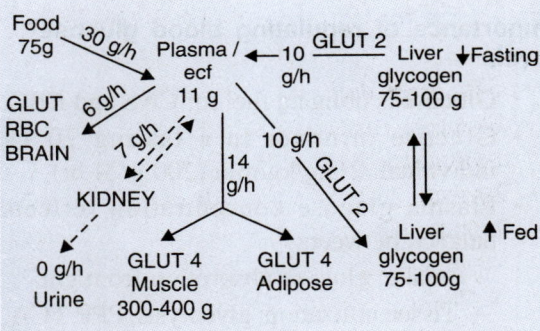

Fig. 4.56. Distribution of glucose after meals.

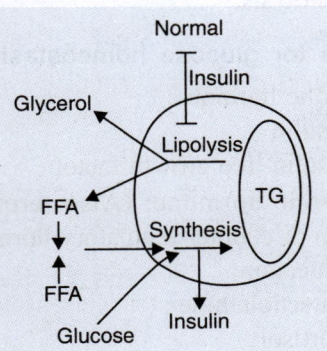

Fig. 4.58. Metabolism in diabetes.

Glycerol and long chain FA:
- Caloric value of fats: 9 kcal/g
- Body has unlimited capacity for accumulation of fats.

- 70 kg man has 15 kg fat as adipose tissue.
- This TAG store can give 1, 30,000 kcal

## Source of blood glucose

- Diet
- GNG
- Glycogenolysis

In 70 kg person: fuel reserves are:
- 1600 kcal in glycogen
- 24,000 kcal in mobilized protein
- 1,35,000 kcal in TAG

## Importance of regulating blood glucose levels

- Glucose is obligate fuel for CNS and RBC.
- Glucose turnover in a fasting 70 kg individual: 2 mg/kg/min (200 g/24 hr)
- Plasma glucose concentration reflects balance between:
  - Intake: glucose absorption from gut
  - Tissue utilization: glycolysis, PPP, TCA, glycogenesis.
  - Endogenous production: GNG, glycogenolysis.

## Hormones for glucose homeostasis

- Anabolic hormone:
  - Insulin
  - Insulin-like growth factor
- Catabolic hormone: (Also termed anti-insulin or counter regulatory hormones)
  - Glucagon
  - Catecholamine
  - Cortisol
  - GH

## Post prandial (absorptive) state

Following a meal:
- Insulin release stimulated
- Glucose release inhibited

This changes metabolism of:
- Liver
- Adipose tissue
- Muscle

Result:
- (+) Glucose oxidation
- (+) glycogen synthesis
- (–) lipolysis

Also, increase glucose uptake in insulin-dependent tissues, mainly skeletal muscle.

## Post-absorptive (fasting) state

Glucose metabolism reaches a steady state. Hepatic glucose production (glycogenolysis) starts.

After overnight fast:
- Insulin secretion decreases
- Glucagon secretion increases

Result:
- Decrease in glycogen synthesis
- Increase in glycogenolysis

## Fasting state

- 80% of glucose taken up by insulin-independent tissues

Of this:
- 50% goes to brain
- 20% goes to RBCs

- In post-absorptive state, insulin-dependent tissues use little glucose.
- Muscle and adipose tissue are responsible 20% of total glucose utilization.

## After 12 h fast

- 65-75% endogenous glucose is derived from glycogen
- Rest from GNG

Muscle releases lactate → GNG → Glucose → Skeletal muscle: **Cori cycle**.

Low insulin level stimulate proteolysis releasing alanine and glutamine: **Glucose alanine cycle**.

Alanine (muscle) → GNG (liver) → pyruvate.

## DIABETES

### Importance of insulin

Without insulin, glucose transport into the cells will be insufficient

- In absence of glucose, cells have to rely on protein and fat catabolism for fuel.
- When there is not enough insulin, excess glucose cannot be stored in liver and muscle.
- Glucose accumulates in the blood above normal levels, termed **hyperglycemia**.
  Normal blood glucose: 80-90 mg/dL
  Diabetic patient: 110-140 mg/dL
  **After meals:**
  Normal 120-140 mg/dL
  Diabetic patient <200 mg/dL

**What goes wrong when glucose concentration decrease too far:** Hypoglycemia.

**Symptoms of low blood glucose:** Tiredness, confusion, dizziness, headache, mood swings, muscle weakness, shaking.

### Diabetes mellitus

Insulin deficiency.
  Symptoms:
  - Hyperglycemia (high blood glucose)
  - Glycosuria (glucose in urine)
  - Polyuria (passage of copious urine)
  - Polydypsia (drinking large amount of water)
  - Polyphagia (increased appetite)
  - Weight loss

- Acids and ketones in blood from lipid breakdown
- Coma, if ketones build-up

### Excess blood glucose

- Exerts high osmotic pressure in ecf (extra cellular floud) causing dehydration.
- Excess of glucose begins to be lost from body in urine: GLYCOSURIA

### Glycosuria

Excess glucose in glomerular filtrate acts as an osmotic diuretic, inhibiting water reabsorption resulting in **Polyuria**:
  - Huge urine output
  - Decreased blood volume
  - Dehydration

Dehydration stimulates hypothalamic thirst centers, causing POLYDYPSIA: excess thirst

### Polyphagia

Excessive hunger, although there is plenty of glucose in blood, it cannot be used by cells and cells begin to starve for glucose.

### Effect of insulin deficiency on fat metabolism

- Deficiency of insulin accelerate breakdown of body's fat reserves for fuel.
- FFA becomes main energy substrate for all tissues except brain.
- Increased lipolysis resulting in production of ketones in liver.
- Ketone bodies lower pH, causes acidosis and KB are excreted in urine: **Ketonuria complications of ketosis**.
- Electrolyte loss
- Ketone body are negatively charged and carry positive ions with them

- Na, K are also lost from body
- Because of electrolyte imbalance, person gets abdominal pain, vomiting.
- Can result in coma, death

### Complications of diabetes

1. Reduction in blood flow to feet causing tissue death, ulceration, infection, loss of toe or feet.
2. Nephropathy – kidney damage
3. Retinopathy – damage to blood vessel of retina
4. Others: Cataract, skin infection, periodontitis, and neuritis

### Glucose intolerance

- Type I diabetes mellitus (DM)
- Type II DM
- Gestational diabetes
- Maturity onset diabetes of young (MODY)
- Insulin resistance

| | *Type I diabetes* | *Type II diabetes* |
|---|---|---|
| Age at onset | <40 | >40 |
| Body weight | Thin | Overweight |
| Symptoms | Appear suddenly | Appear slowly |
| Insulin production | None | Too little or it is ineffective |
| Insulin requirement | Must take insulin | May require insulin |
| Other name | Juvenile onset diabetes | Adult onset diabetes |

**Table 4.11.** Type I vs. Type II diabetes

### Causes of diabetes

1. Hereditary
2. Obesity
3. Age
4. Viruses
5. Physical trauma to pancreas
6. Drugs
7. Pregnancy

## IMPACT OF DIABETES ON METABOLISM

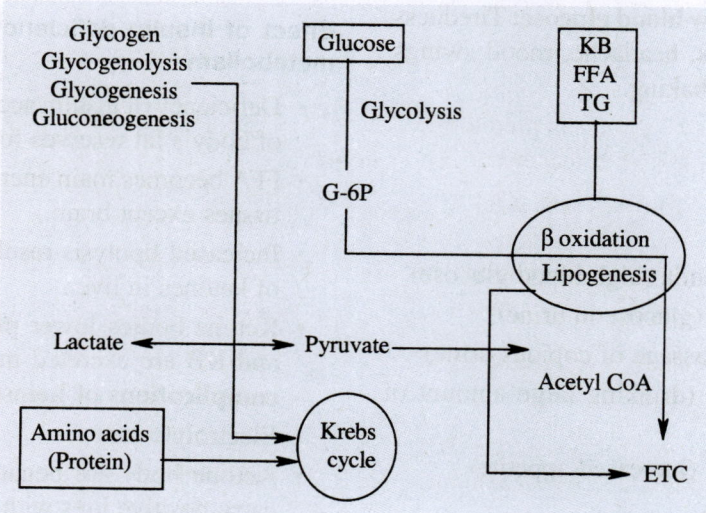

## Clinical features of DM

| Table 4.12. | |
|---|---|
| *Features* | *Biochemical reasoning* |
| Hyperglycemia | Decreased utilization and increased formation of glucose Increased glycogenolysis Increased gluconeogenesis |
| Glycosuria | Hyperglycemia exceeding renal threshold |
| Polyuria and polydypsia | **Osmotic diuresis:** Excessive loss of water and electrolytes: refractive errors of vision **Thirst:** Hyperosmolar state **Ketone bodies: (KB)** Increased FA oxidation and KB production. **Weight loss:** Loss of : Water Glycogen Fat Protein **Muscle weakness:** Muscle protein break down Loss of potassium |

## Diabetes mellitus

### Testing

**Fasting blood glucose:**
- 100-125 mg/dL, signals prediabetes
- >126mg/dL, signals diabetes

**Oral glucose tolerance test (OGTT):**
- Tested for 2 hours after glucose-rich drink
- 140-199 mg/dL signals prediabetes
- >200 mg/dL signals prediabetes

### Glycated hemoglobin test (HbA1c).

### Metabolic syndrome

Closely linked to insulin resistance and fatty liver, raised fibrinogen, hyperuricemia are associated features.

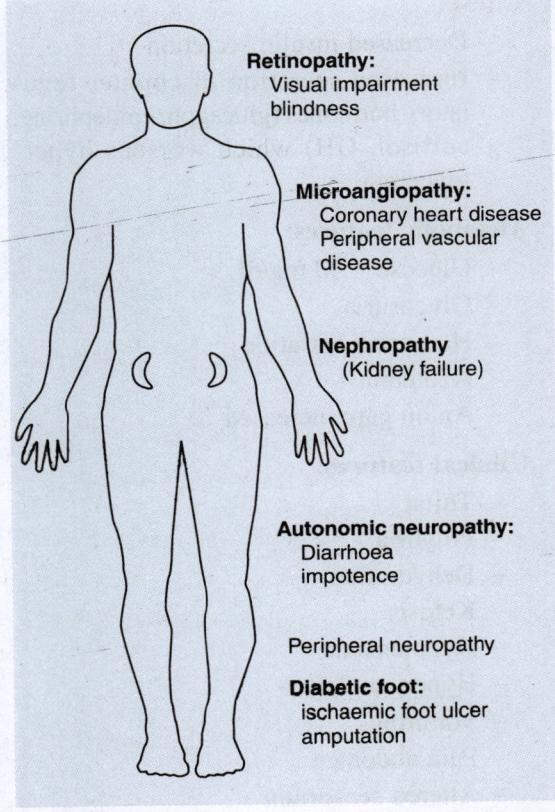

**Fig. 4.59.** Long term complications of diabetes.

Presence of three or more of the following features constitute metabolic syndrome:
1. Abdominal obesity
2. Fasting TG > 250 mg/dL
3. Fasting HDL < 38.6 mg/dL (M)
   <50 mg/dL (F)
4. Blood pressure ≥ 130/85 mmHg
5. Fasting blood glucose > 99 mg/dL.

### Diabetic ketoacidosis

Feature common in type I DM.

May be precipitated by:
- Stress
- Infection
- Trauma

**Cause:**
– Decreased insulin secretion
– Increased secretion of counter regulatory hormones (glucagon, epinephrine, cortisol, GH) which worsens hyperglycemia

**Metabolic features:**
– Glucose > 30 mg/dL
– Glycosuria
– Hemoconcentration
– Azotemia
– Anion gap: increased

**Clinical features:**
– Thirst
– Polyuria
– Dehydration
– Ketosis
– Hypotension
– Hyperventilation
– Vomiting
– Pain abdomen
– Altered sensorium
– Drowsiness
– Coma

## 2. LIPID METABOLISM

## (i) Digestion and Absorption of Lipid

### Digestion and absorption of lipid

**Problems/challenges with lipid absorption:**
• Lipids are not water soluble
• TAG are too large to be absorbed

### Major lipid in diet
• TAG (triacylglycerol)

• Phospholipids
• Fat-soluble vitamins (A, D, E and K) and a variety of lipids (including cholesterol) are absorbed dissolved in lipid micelle.

### Digestion: Fact file

Adult human digests 60-150 g lipid/day and TAG constitute > 90% of intake.

| Rest: | Phospholipid |
|---|---|
| | Cholesterol |
| | Cholesterol ester |
| | Free fatty acids |

• 90% of dietary fat: TAG
• Remaining: cholesterol, CE, PL, NEFA.
• Hydrophobic nature of fat excludes water-soluble digestive enzymes. Fat globules are needed to be emulsified before digestion can take place.

### Lipids secreted each day by liver
• 1-2 g cholesterol
• 7-22 g phospatidylcholine

### Dietary FA
• Comprise 30-60% of caloric intake in average diet
• Contain TAG, PL, sterol esters
• Principal sources: dairy products, meat

### Enzymes for lipid digestion
• Lingual lipase
• Gastric lipase
• Pancreatic lipase
• Intestine lipase
• Co-lipase
• Lipid esterase
• Phospholipase

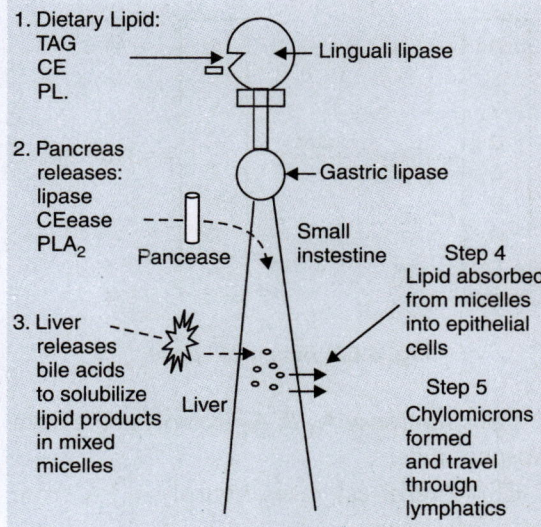

1. Dietary Lipid:
   TAG
   CE
   PL.
   — Linguali lipase

2. Pancreas
   releases:
   lipase
   CEease
   PLA$_2$
   Pancease
   — Gastric lipase
   Small
   instestine

3. Liver
   releases
   bile acids
   to solubilize
   lipid products
   in mixed
   micelles
   Liver

Step 4
Lipid absorbed
from micelles
into epithelial
cells

Step 5
Chylomicrons
formed
and travel
through
lymphatics

**Fig. 4.60.** Digestion of lipids.

## Stomach

- Heat helps in liquefying fat
- Peristalsis aid in emulsification
- Water insoluble TAG degraded to FA

## Gastric lipase

Hydrolyze TAG containing short, medium and unsaturated FFA to form FFA and 1, 2 DAG.

## Milk fat: Fate

Milk fat contains SCFA, MCFA:

- Good substrate for gastric lipase, tend to be esterified at *sn*-3 position
  - SCFA, MCFA absorbed via portal vein
  - LCFA dissolve in fat droplets and pass on to duodenum

Human milk contains bile salt activated lipase which ensures complete digestion of milk especially in premature infants where pancreatic secretions are not operational.

## Small intestine

- TAG enters small intestine as emulsion of lipid droplets.
- Specific lipases hydrolyze TAG to FA, MAG, and glycerol. They get packaged into micelles, get smaller in size.

## Pancreas

Secrete digestive enzymes and bicarbonate, which neutralizes acid from stomach.

### Pancreatic lipase

- Serine esterase
- Act on TAG; *sn* 1, 3 ester bonds
- TAG $\rightarrow$ sn-2 MAG + 2FA

### Pancreatic colipase

- 12 K Da protein
- Activated by trypsin
- Interacts with TAG and pancreatic lipase

## Lipase, colipase and PLA$_2$ are synthesized in proform

Lipase is activated by releasing a pentapeptide from amino terminal end.

Pancreatic lipase with the aid of colipase digests TAG to 2MAG & FFA which are packaged into micelle.

### Colipase

- Secreted from pancreas as procolipase
- Activated by trypsin
- Anchors lipase to micelle one colipase to one lipase (1:1 ratio)
- Lid region of lipase covers the active site and in presence of lipids is retracted towards colipase.
- Colipase deficiency causes steatorrhoea

- Pancreatic lipase inhibitors are used in treatment and prevention of:
  - Hyperlipidemia
  - Obesity
  - Cardiovascular diseases
  - CNS disorders
  - Diabetes
  - GI disorders

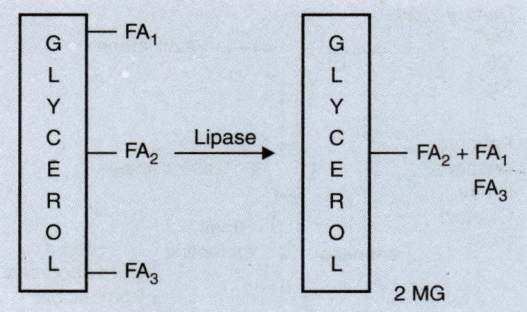

Fig. 4.62. Action of lipase.

**Phospholipase** $A_1$ & $A_2$ hydrolyze FA from phospholipids.

Cholesterol esterases hydrolyze FA from cholesterol esters.

**Micelles** are microdroplets emulsified by bile salts and also contain cholesterol and fat soluble vitamins.

### Micelle formation

- Complex of lipid material soluble in water
- Contains bile salts, phospholipids and cholesterol
- Combines with 2MAG, FFA and fat soluble vitamins to form mixed micelle

### Function

Allow digestion of products of lipid digestion to be transported through the environment of intestinal lumen and uptake into epithelium.

### Fate of lipid emulsion

As lipid emulsion enters duodenum, dietary lipid undergoes digestion.

Pancreatic lipase, colipase are secreted into lumen causing:

- Activation of lipase by colipase
- TAG hydrolyzed by lipase to form 2MAG

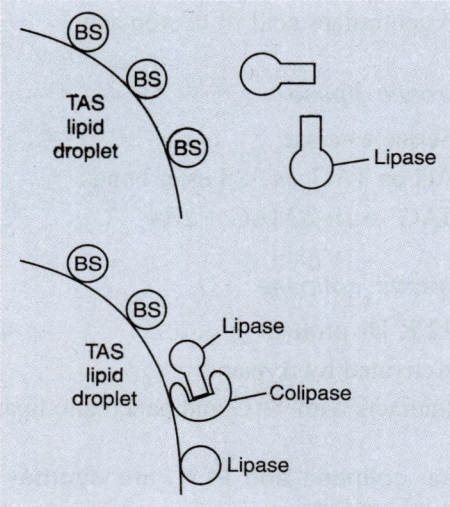

Fig. 4.61. Mechanism of action of colipase (BS = bile salts).

### Applied drugs:

- Panclicins
- Anti obesity drug: Orlistat inhibits pancreatic and gastric lipase

**Bile salts:** Synthesized in liver from cholesterol and secreted into bile that is stored in gall bladder. In response to hormones, bile passes into intestine where it emulsifies dietary lipids.

### Emulsification:

- Produces small lipid spheres giving greater surface area
- Lipases attack TG at 1 and 3 positions

**Table 4.13.** Lipid digestion

| | Step | Location | Enzyme |
|---|---|---|---|
| 1 | Minor digestion<br>TAG → DAG+FFA | Mouth, stomach | Lingual/gastric lipase |
| 2. | Major digestion<br>TAG → MAG + FFA<br>CE → Chols + ester<br>PL → FA + LysoPL | Small intestine | Pancreatic lipase<br>Cholesterol esterase<br>$PLA_2$ |
| 3. | Formation of mixed micelle | Lumen of small intestine | n/a |
| 4. | Passive absorption of lipolytic products | Intestinal epithelial cells | n/a |
| 5. | Assembly and export of chylomicrons | From intestinal cells to lymphatics | n/a |

n/a = not available

## Most of FA, 2MAG get absorbed into epithelial cells

- Water soluble lipids such as cholesterol are poorly absorbed (30-40%)
- Bile salts get absorbed from ileum and pass back to liver by EHC (enterohepatic circulation)

## Lipid absorption

### In lumen

- Micelle move to intestinal mucosal cells and release contents near cells
- Bile salts are reabsorbed further down the GIT (in ileum), transported to liver, finally recycled and secreted back into GIT.
- By passive diffusion; FA, 2MAG, cholesterol, cholesterol esters move down the concentration gradient.
- Repackaged in intestinal cells for transport to liver as chylomicrons, triglycerides.

### In enterocytel

- Glycerol and short chain FA (SCFA) directly enter mesenteric blood
- 2MAG and LCFA reformed into TAG

which then get packaged with proteins forming chylomicrons.
- Phospholipids get hydrolyzed to FFA
- FFA can enter circulation directly:
  - FFA (NEFA), short (12C) and medium chain FA enters liver via portal vein.
  - MCFA, SCFA (<10 C) – pass directly through cells to hepatic portal circulation
- FA >12C – bind to FA binding protein and get transferred to RER for resynthesis to TAG

## FA uptake

### SC FA, MCFA

- Enter portal circulation from enterocytes
- Form albumin – FFA complex in blood
- Oxidized in liver
- May get elongated and used for TG formation.

### LCFA

- Form chylomicrons
- Enter lymphatics via lacteal, then enter blood stream at thoracic duct.

## Digestion and absorption of TAG

- Hydrolysis:

  1 MAG → FA + glycerol

- Acetylation:

  2 MAG → TAG: MAG pathway

Glycerol thus released: In epithelium: passes into portal vein

In lumen: reutilized for TAG synthesis via normal phosphatidic acid pathway.

## Chylomicron formation

- Newly formed TAG accumulates as lipid droplets in ER, get coated with a protein layer to form chylomicrons.
- In golgi apparatus, carbohydrates are attached to the protein coat.

## Chylomicron absorption

Chylomicrons get absorbed from enterocytes into lacteals, enter blood via thoracic duct.

## Lipid malabsorption

They can be due to defective intestinal lipolysis or defective mucosal cell metabolism.

### Features

- Steatorrhoea
- Loss of fat soluble vitamins in stools

### Causes

- Tropical sprue
- Non-tropical sprue
- Celiac sprue
- Intestinal lipodystrophy (Whipple's disease)

## Comparison

|  | Fat synthesis | Fat oxidation |
|---|---|---|
| Carrier | Acyl Carrier protein | CoA |
| Activation by citrate | Yes | No |
| Inhibited by palmitate | Yes | No |
| Acyl/acetyl group carrier | Citrate (into cytosol) | Carnitine (cytosol to mitochondria) |
| Product | Palmitate | Acetyl CoA |
| Highest activity | Fed state | Fasting, starvation |
| Insulin/glucagon | High | Low |

## Comparison

|  | FA synthesis | FA degradation (oxidation) |
|---|---|---|
| Intermediates | Linked to –SH in proteins (acyl carrier proteins) | Linked to CoASH |
| Site | Cytosol | Mitochondria |
| Enzymes | Components of a single peptide | Separate polypeptides |
| Reducing equivalents | $NADP^+$ / $NADPH$ | $NAD^+$/$NADH$ |

# (ii) FA Biosynthesis

**Synthesis: Fact file**

- Occurs in cytosol, ER
- Starts with acetyl CoA:
  - Most acetyl CoA produced in mitochondria
  - Acetyl CoA can't traverse mitochondrial membrane
  - Moves out via its conversion to citrate
- Occurs when:
  - Energy needs are met (ATP>ADP)
  - Glycogen stores are full
  - Excess nutrients present

- Begins with acetyl CoA from:
  - Carbohydrates
  - Amino acids
  - Degraded lipids

## Where and when FA are synthesized?

FA synthesis occurs in:

- Liver (mainly)
- Lactating mammary gland
- Adipose tissue

**FA synthesized** from acetyl CoA derived from:

- Carbohydrates
- Protein

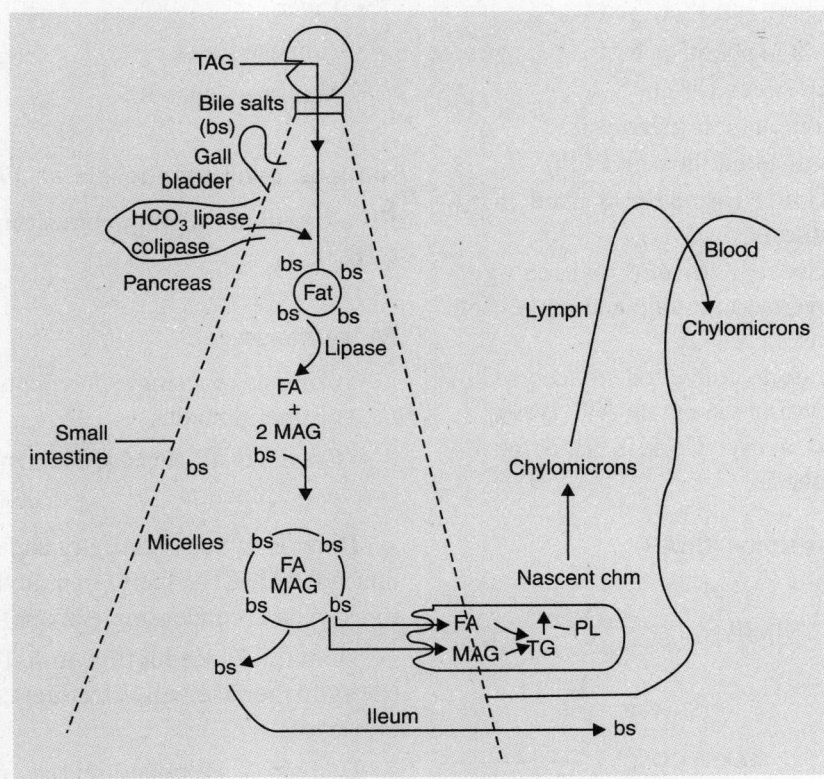

**Fig. 4.63.** Digestion and absorption of lipids (bs = bile salts).

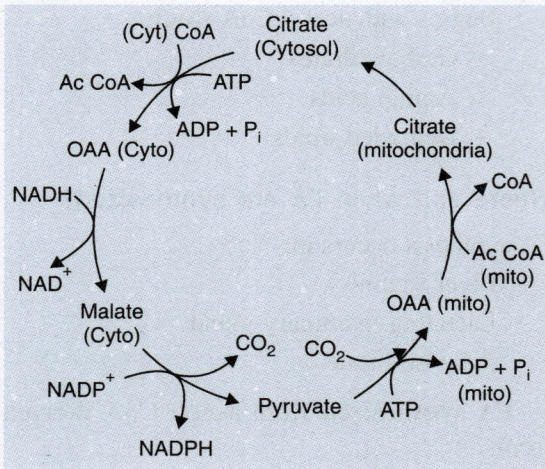

**Fig. 4.64.** Acetyl CoA in and out of mitochondria.

**FA synthesis uses:** ATP, NADPH

In fed state:

- Glucose is in abundance
- Glycogen stores fill-up
- ATP, citrate inhibit glycolysis
- Glucose diverted through PPP:
  - NADPH formed and used in FA synthesis
  - Pyruvate formed which gets converted to citrate and moves into cytosol.
  - Citrate is converted to acetyl CoA in cytosol via citrate ATP lyase.
  - This acetyl CoA is used for FA synthesis.

## Synthesis of malonyl CoA

$$\underset{\text{Acetyl CoA}}{CH_3COSCoA} + ATP + HCO_3^- \xrightarrow[\substack{\text{Carboxylase (ACC)} \\ ATP \quad ADP}]{\text{Acetyl CoA}} \underset{\text{Malonyl CoA}}{COCH_3COSCoA}$$

## Facts: ACC step

- Committed step
- Irreversible
- Regulated by:
  - Palmitoyl CoA
    (+) citrate
  - Malonyl CoA inhibits CPT I, thus blocks β-oxidation

## Advantage of storing excess feed or energy as fat:

Fat has high energy, low water content.

## Major producers of FA

- Liver
- Adipose tissue
- Mammary gland

## Humans can't synthesize all FA

EFA (essential FA) must come from diet (C18:2, C18:3).

## FA synthase

- Consists of a single polypeptide with three distinct domains
- Conducts all steps of FA synthesis except ACC function.

Domain 1: Substrate entry and condensation unit AT, MT, CE (Acetyl transacylase, malonyl transacylase, condensing enzyme)

Domain 2: Reduction unit DH, ER, KR (dehydrogenase, enoylreductase, ketoacyl reductase)

Domain 3: Palmitate release unit TE (thioesterase)

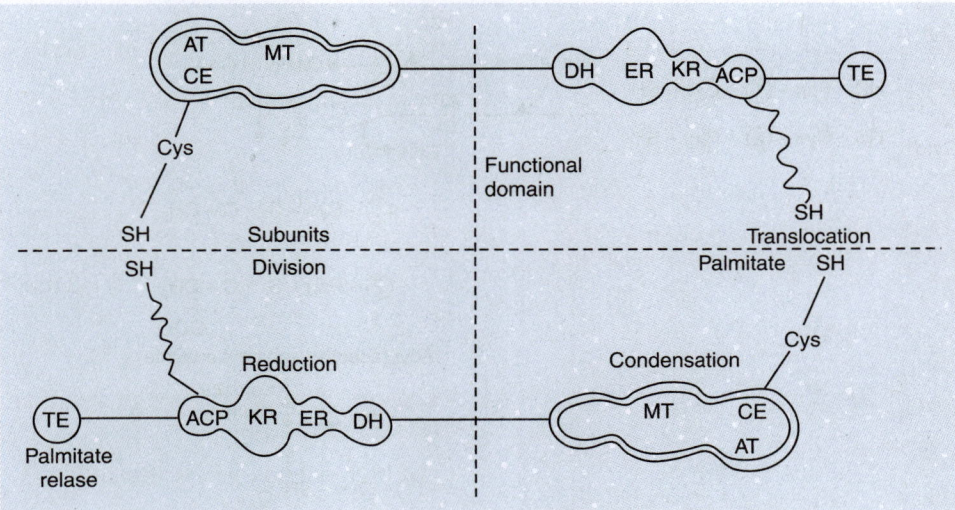

**Fig. 4.65.** Fatty acid synthase.

## SOURCES OF NADPH IN FA BIOSYNTHESIS

### HMP shunt

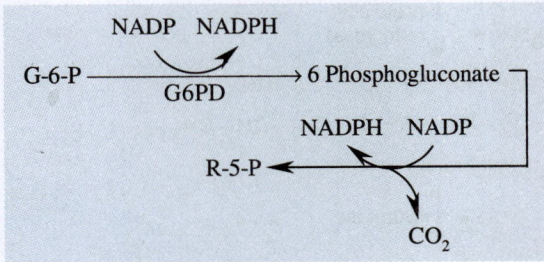

### Malic enzyme

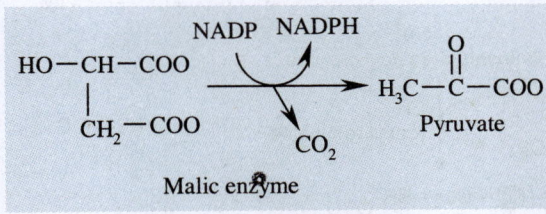

After seven cycles, palmitoyl-S-ACP is produced and palmitate released by thioesterase.

$$8 \text{ acetyl CoA} + 14 \text{ NADPH} + 14H^+ + 7 \text{ ATP} \rightarrow \text{Palmitate} + 8 \text{ CoA} + 14 \text{ NADP} + 7ADP + 7 \text{ Pi} + 7 \text{ H}_2\text{O}$$

### Elongation and desaturation

- Further elongation and desaturation of palmitate and dietary FA (if required) occurs in mitochondria and ER by diverse enzymes.
- Elongated by 2 carbon atoms at a time
- Cis double bond can be introduced not farther than C-9 from carboxylate end.

### FA modifications

Palmitate can be elongated:

- Addition of two carbon units at-COOH end of FA

### Desaturation

16:0 and 18:0 can be converted to 16:1 and 18:1 respectively.

$$CH_3(CH_2)_7 C = C^9 (CH_2)_7 COOH$$
$$\quad\quad\quad\quad | \quad |$$
$$\quad\quad\quad\quad H \quad H$$

Plants
Further unsaturation occurs primarily in this region

Animals
Further unsaturation occurs primarily in this region

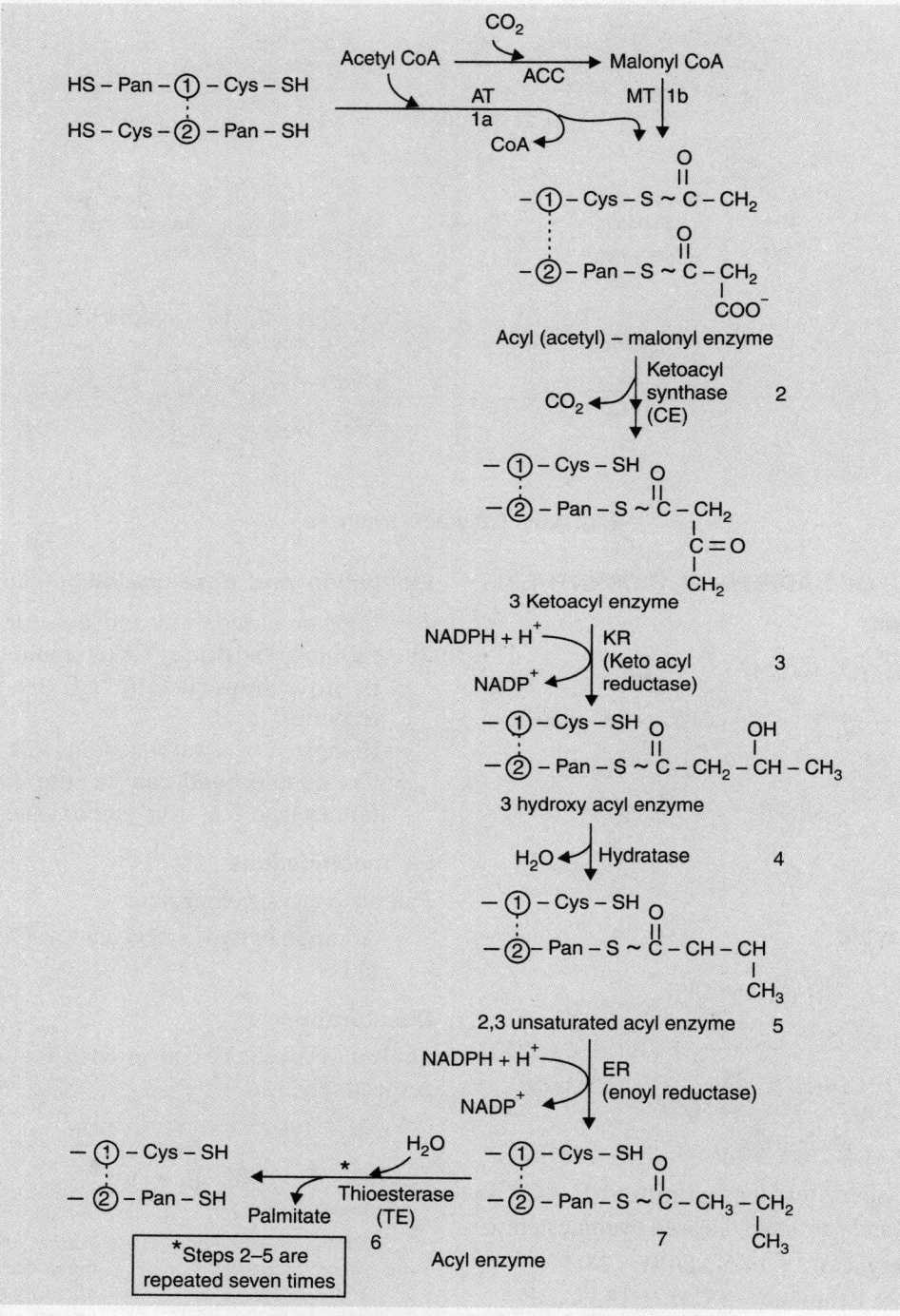

**Fig. 4.66.** Steps of FA synthesis.

## Regulation

### Primary signals
- Turned on by insulin
- Turned off by: glucagon, epinephrine

### Secondary signals
- Citrate: activates ACC
- **ACC:**
  Control point of FA synthesis:
  Inactivated by phosphorylation
  Activated by high concentration of citrate

### Allosteric regulation
- Citrate stimulates
- Inhibited by palmitoyl CoA

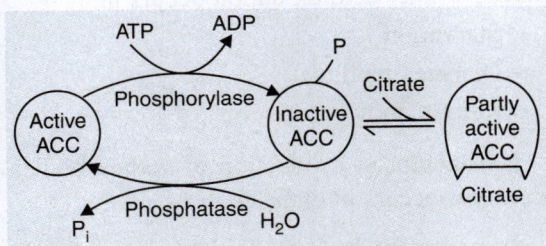

**Fig. 4.67.** Regulation of ACC.

(+) Insulin
(–) glucagon, epinephrine
(+) citrate
(–) palmitoyl CoA
(–) AMP

### Comparison of regulation

| **FA oxidation** | **FA synthesis** |
|---|---|
| *Stimulated by:* | *Stimulated by:* |
| Epinephrine | Insulin: (+) ACC |
| Glucagon | |

*Inhibited by:*

- Malonyl CoA CPTI inhibited
- NADH
- β hydroxyl acyl CoA DH

*ACC:*
*(+) by:*
Citrate:
(–) by
epinephrine
glucagon

## Lipid metabolism in fat cells

| *Fed state* | *Starved or exercising state* |
|---|---|
| Insulin | Glucagon, epinephrine |
| Stimulates LPL<br>  Increased uptake of FA | Stimulates adenyl cyclase |
| Stimulates glycolysis<br>  Increased glycerol phosphate synthesis | ↑ cAMP<br>Activate protein kinase |
| Induces HSL phosphatase | Activates HSL |
| Inactivates HSL<br>→ Net effect: TG storage | →net effect: TG mobilization and increased FFA |

## Essential FA

Body can synthesize all the FA it needs from carbohydrate, fat or protein except:

  Linoleic acid

  Linolenic acid

  Essential FA: ω-3, ω-6 FA

- Mammals lack enzyme to add double bond beyond C9
- Chains elongation and double bond addition yield arachidonic acid ($C_{20}$: 4) from linoleic acid ($C_8$: 2; ω-6)

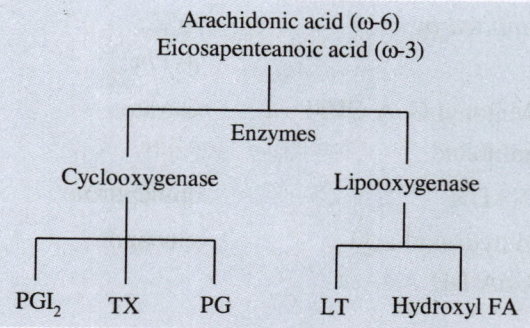

- ω6-linoleic acid
- ω3-linolenic acid
- Found in cold water fish
- Help to dissolve blood clots
- Lower blood pressure
- Dilates blood vessels.

## Trans-fatty acid

- Formed when margarine is processed
- Hydrogen molecules on opposite sides of point of unsaturation.

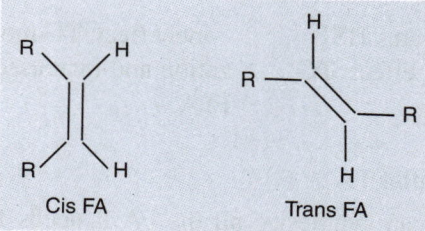

**Fig. 4.68.** Cis- and trans-FA.

## (iii) Fat Oxidation

### Major oxidation pathways of cell

- Glycolysis
- Fatty acid oxidation
- Citric acid cycle
- ETC coupled to oxidative phosphorylation

## FA oxidation

Fats provide a more condensed form of energy for storage than carbohydrates.

### Importance

- Fatty acids are both oxidized to acetyl CoA and synthesized from acetyl CoA.
- Synthesis and oxidation are entirely two different processes occurring in separate compartments of cell:
  - Oxidation in mitochondria
  - Synthesis in cytosol
- Oxidation is aerobic and involves acyl CoA derivatives, utilizes NAD and FAD; generates ATP.

### Clinical aspects

Increased fatty acid oxidation occurs in:

- Starvation
- Diabetes mellitus
- Ketone body production

**Ketoacidosis:** Production of ketone bodies in excess, occurs in diabetes

**Impairment in fatty acid oxidation leads to hypoglycemia:** Since GNG is dependent on fatty acid oxidation.

**Hypoglycemia occurs in:**

- Carnitine deficiency
- Deficiency of enzymes in fatty acid oxidation : CPT
- Inhibition of fatty acid oxidation occurs by poisons: hypoglycin

**MCAD deficiency:**

- Medium chain fatty acyl dehydrogenase deficiency:
- MCAD oxidizes FA between 8-10 carbon long resulting in hypoglycemia.

- **Zellweger syndrome:** Accumulation of VLCFA because peroxisomes are not properly formed.
- **Adrenoleukodystrophy:** VLCFA accumulate in brain and adrenal cortex due to inability to transport VLCFA into peroxisomes.

## Fat metabolism

- Controlled primarily by rate of TG hydrolysis in adipose tissue
- Regulated by hormonal mechanism:
  - Insulin
  - Glucagon
  - Epinephrine
  - Cortisol

### Fat acids are synthesized

- Primarily in:
  - Liver
  - Lactating mammary gland
  - Less so in adipose tissue
- From acetyl CoA, derived from excess proteins and carbohydrates
- Uses ATP and NADPH as energy source.

### Why should medical students be interested in lipid metabolism

1. Obesity epidemic
2. Lipids contribute to major diseases:
   a) Atherosclerosis, cardiovascular disease
   b) Cancer asthma
   c) NIDDM
   d) Fatty liver of alcoholism
3. Aberrant lipid metabolism causes diseases
4. Serum lipids serve as diagnostic agents

### Fact file: Lipids

- Relative small molecules: <500 Da MW (molecular weight)

- Soluble in organic solvents: chloroform/acetone, insoluble in water
- Transported by various carrier proteins
- Serve as source of energy
- Stored as TAG: very efficient fuel store.

### Principal organs involved in lipid metabolism

- Adipose tissue
- Liver
- Brain
- Skeletal muscle
- Intestine

### Adipose tissue: Fact file

- One of the largest organ
- White fat stores energy
- Brown fat dissipates energy
- Adipose cells:
  - Require glucose for synthesis of TAG
  - Glucose levels inside adipose cells determine whether FA are released into blood or not.

### Liver

Liver has a commanding role in lipid metabolism. Specific functions of liver in lipid metabolism:

- Conversion of carbohydrates and proteins to FA
- Synthesis of large quantities of cholesterol and phospholipids
- Formation of lipoproteins
- Oxidation of FA

### Brain

- Brain does not directly use FA as fuel
- Lipids are used in myelin formations, EPA deficiency causes hypomyelination.

## Organelles involved in lipid metabolism

| | |
|---|---|
| ER | Peroxisome |
| Mitochondria | Lysosomes |

## Organelles involved in lipid metabolism and their features

| ER | Features |
|---|---|
| ER, RER, SER | Contain enzymes involved in lipid metabolism |
| Mitochondria | Principal site of FA oxidation, source of acetyl CoA for FA synthesis |
| Peroxisomes | Degrade FA via β-, α-oxidation. Oxidation of side chain of cholesterol. Synthesis of other glycerolipids, cholesterol, dolichol. |
| Lysosomes | Principal site for degradation of macromolecules and complex lipids |

## Physiological role of FA in cell

- Building block of PL, GL
- Added into proteins to form lipoproteins
- Fuel molecule – source of ATP
- FA derivatives serve as hormones and intracellular messengers

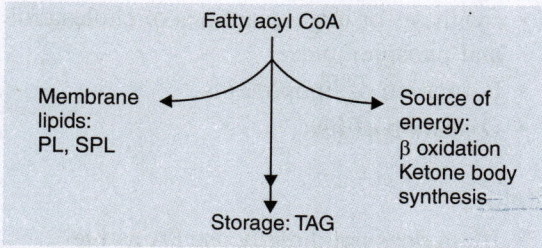

**Fig. 4.69.** Metabolic roles of long chain fatty acyl CoA.

## FATTY ACID OXIDATION

### Activation of fatty acids

- In cytosol, LCFA (long chain FA) are activated by ATP and CoA to form fatty acyl CoA.
- SCFA (short chain FA) are activated in mitochondria.

### β-oxidation

- Cleavage of FA to acetate in tissues occurs in mitochondria
- FA become esterified to carnitine and then transported into mitochondria

### β-Oxidation: Fact file

- Occurs in mitochondria of specialized tissue: skeletal, cardiac muscle, liver, adipose tissue.
- 4 repeated reactions for every two carbons
- Reactions mirror that of TCA
- One $FADH_2$ and one NADH produced per round
- Acetyl CoA produced in each round.
- Cleaves two carbons at a time from carboxyl end
- Acetyl CoA enters TCA
- NADH and $FADH_2$ enters ETC to yield ATP.

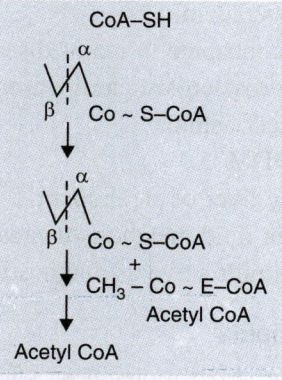

**Fig. 4.70.** β-Oxidation of FA.

## Carnitine shuttle

- Transfers FA from cytoplasm to mitochondria for oxidation
- Malonyl CoA (a precursor for FA synthesis) inhibits carnitine shuttle and slows down oxidation.

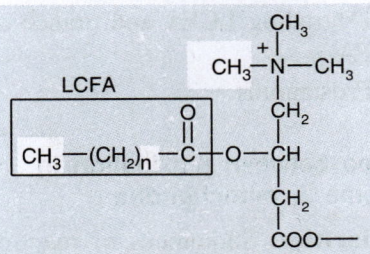

**Fig. 4.71.** Carnitine.

## Carnitine

- β-hydroxy trimethyl ammonium butyrate $(CH_3)_3 N^+ - CH_2 - CH(OH) - CH_2 - COO^-$

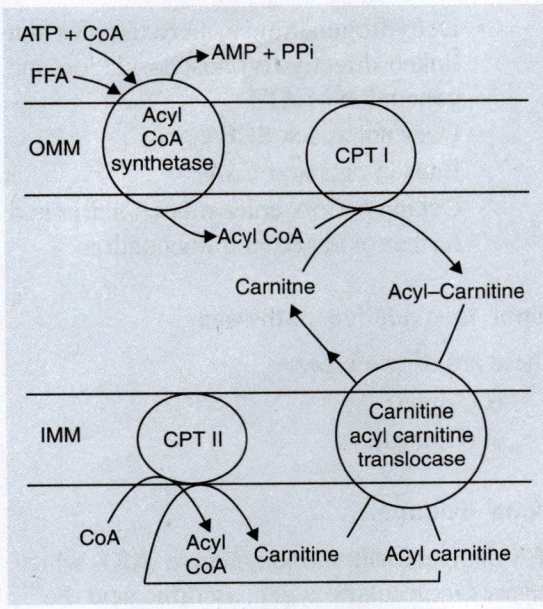

**Fig. 4.72.** Carnitine shuttle.

- Widely distributed, particularly abundant in muscle
CPT I: Carnitine acyl transferase I
   Membrane bound enzyme
   Resides on outer surface of IMM

### Steps in β-oxidation

- FA activation by esterification with CoA
- Membrane transport of fatty acyl CoA esters

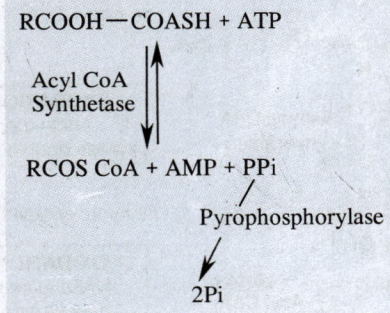

- Carbon back bone reaction sequence
- Dehydrogenation
- Hydration
- Dehydrogenation
- Carbon-carbon cleavage (thiolase reaction)

### Palmitate (C16:0) energetics

**C-C Cleavage:**

$1 FADH_2 + 1 NADH \rightarrow 5$ ATP

7 cleavage point × 5 ATP = 35 ATP

**Oxidation of acetyl CoA:**

8 acetyl CoA enter TCA = 8 × 12 ATP = 96 ATP

Total ATP = 35 + 96 = 131

131 – 2 ATP = 129 ATP

2 ATP are used for FA activation.

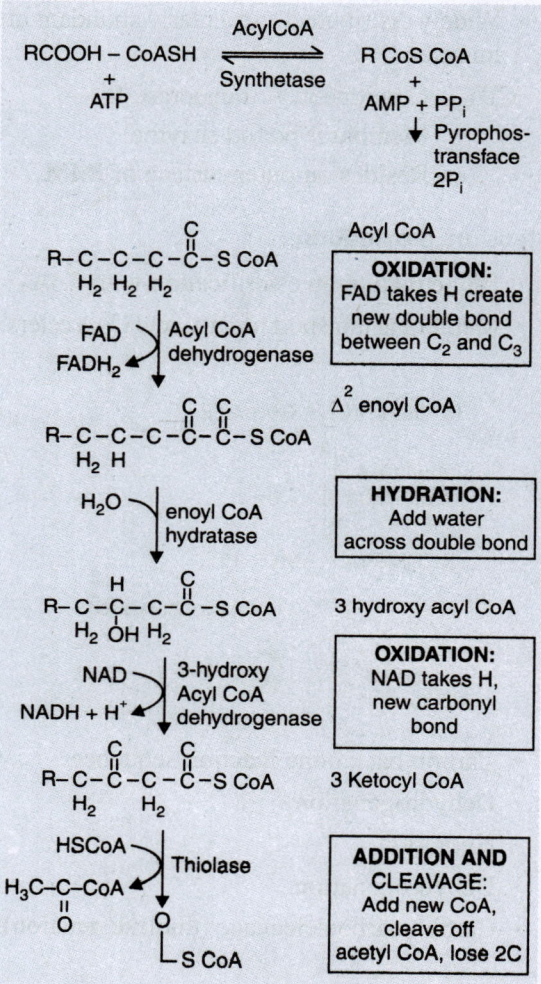

**Fig. 4.73.** β-Oxidation of FA.

## β-Oxidation: Regulation

- **Primary signals:**
  Hormone sensitive lipase:
  - Turned off by insulin
  - Turn on by glucagon, epinephrine, phosphorylation.

- **Secondary signals:**
  Malonyl CoA inhibits carnitine acyl transferase.

## Peroxisomal fatty acid β-oxidation

β-oxidation confined to FA up to 20C long, to generate energy.

In peroxisomes, β-oxidation has special functions:

- Retailoring of: VLCFA, C-27 bile acid intermediates
- Degrading LCFA and branch chained FA
- Prostanoids

## Difference between β-oxidation in peroxisome & mitochondria

**Similarities:** Sequences of reactions are same except:

- Acyl CoA oxidases which form $H_2O_2$ in peroxisosomes
- Multi-functional enzymes carrying out hydration and dehydrogenation
- Thiolase

**Differences:**

- Dehydrogenation in peroxisomes not linked directly to phosphorylation and generation of ATP.
- Does not attack SCFA
- Ends at octanoyl CoA
- Octanoyl CoA enter mitochondria and further oxidized in mitochondria.

## Minor fa oxidative pathways

These are of two types:

- α (Alpha)
- ω (Omega)

## Alpha oxidation

FFA interacts with monoxygenase (MO) which requires molecular oxygen, ascorbic acid, $Fe^{+2}$, producing corresponding α-hydroxy acid.

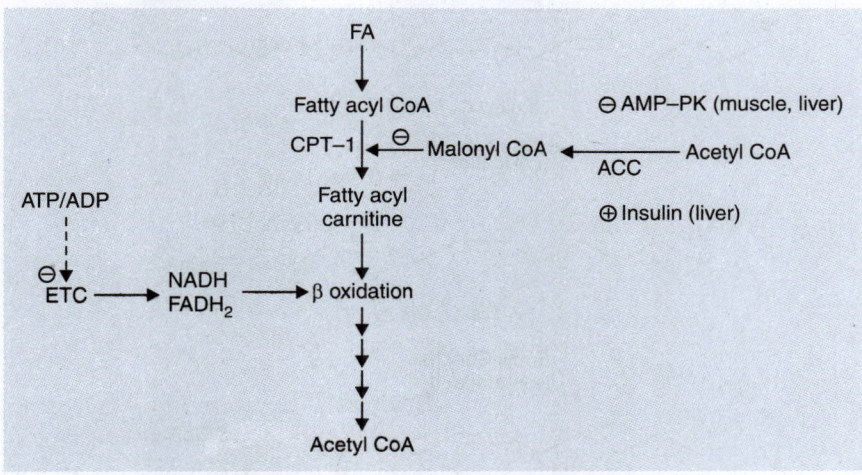

**Fig. 4.74.** Regulation of β-oxidation.

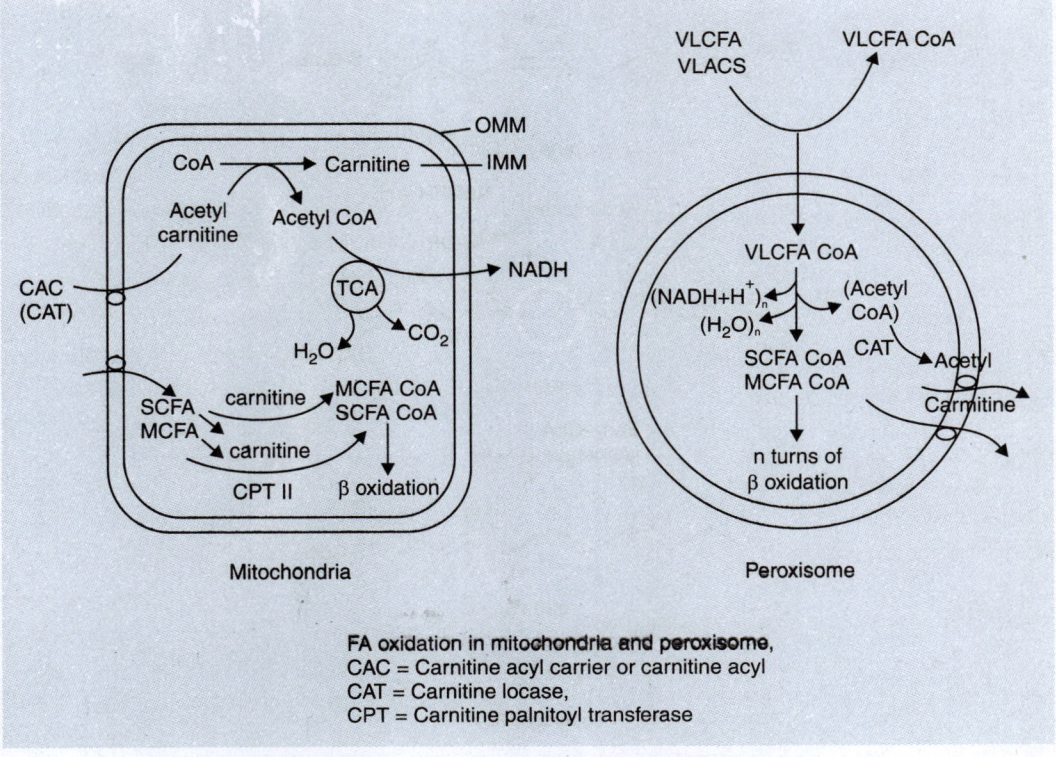

FA oxidation in mitochondria and peroxisome,
CAC = Carnitine acyl carrier or carnitine acyl
CAT = Carnitine locase,
CPT = Carnitine palnitoyl transferase

**Fig. 4.75.** FA oxidation in mitochondria and peroxisome.

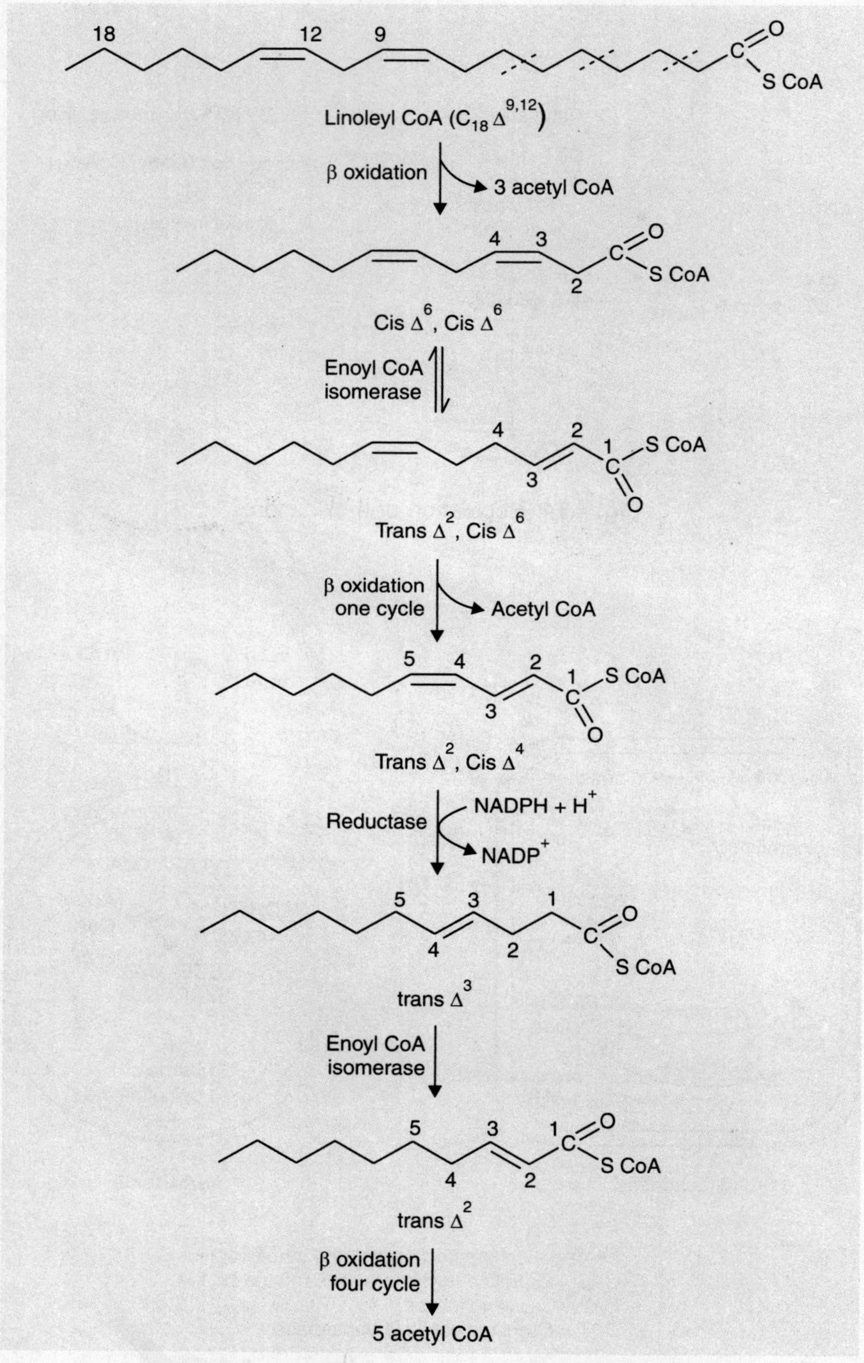

**Fig. 4.76.** ω-oxidation of FA to dicarboxylic acids.

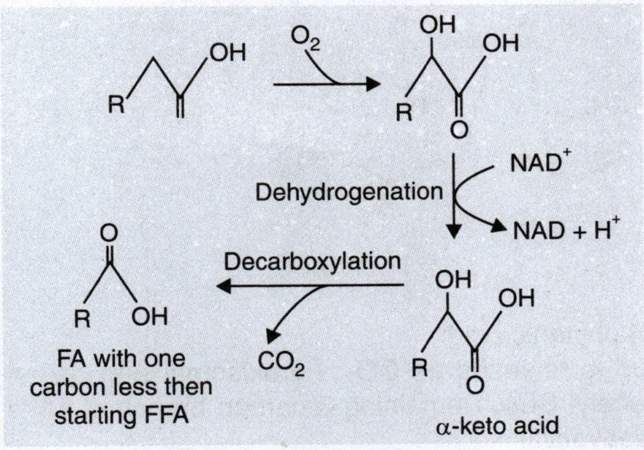

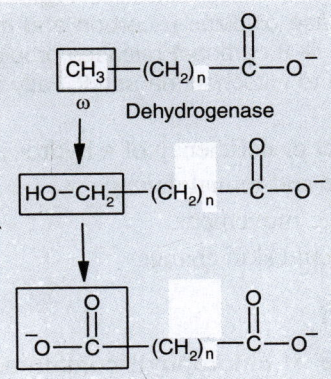

Fig. 4.77. α-Oxidation of fatty acid.

**FA with one carbon less then starting FFA**

**α-keto acid**

## Omega oxidation

Omega (last) carbon with respect to carboxylate group is oxidized to corresponding alcohol

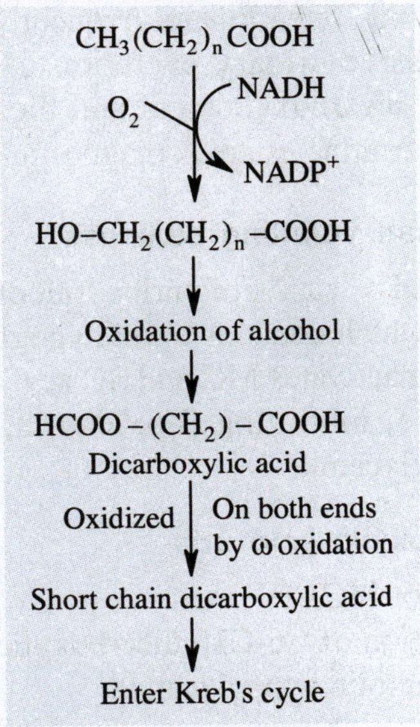

$$CH_3(CH_2)_n COOH$$

$O_2$ — NADH

NADP$^+$

$$HO-CH_2(CH_2)_n-COOH$$

Oxidation of alcohol

$$HCOO-(CH_2)-COOH$$
Dicarboxylic acid

Oxidized | On both ends by ω oxidation

Short chain dicarboxylic acid

Enter Kreb's cycle

## Importance of omega oxidation

Metabolism of drug molecules which contain alkyl chains get converted to dicarboxylic acid and become polar, so their excretion is facilitated.

## Unsaturated fatty acids

Unsaturated fatty acids must be saturated before β-oxidation.

- Isomerase converts cis to trans and moves double bond to 2 position.
- In poly unsaturated FA: reductase is required to add H to double bond.

$$CH_3-(CH_2)_n-\overset{O}{\underset{}{C}}-O^-$$
ω   Dehydrogenase

$$HO-CH_2-(CH_2)_n-\overset{O}{\underset{}{C}}-O^-$$

$$^-O-\overset{O}{\underset{}{C}}-(CH_2)_n-\overset{O}{\underset{}{C}}-O^-$$

Fig. 4.78. ω-Oxidation of FA to dicarboxylic acid.

## β-oxidation of odd chain FA

Odd chain FA degraded to form acetyl CoA and propionyl CoA.

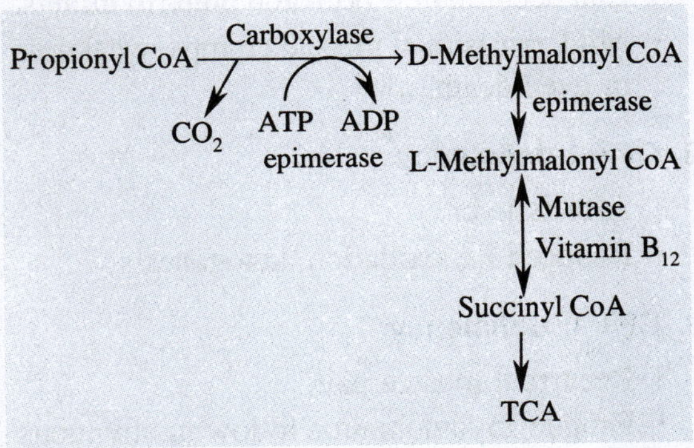

Propionyl CoA —Carboxylase→ D-Methylmalonyl CoA

$CO_2$   ATP   ADP   epimerase

epimerase   L-Methylmalonyl CoA

Mutase
Vitamin B$_{12}$

Succinyl CoA

TCA

## Refsum disease

Inherited disorders where phytanic acid accumulates in tissues:

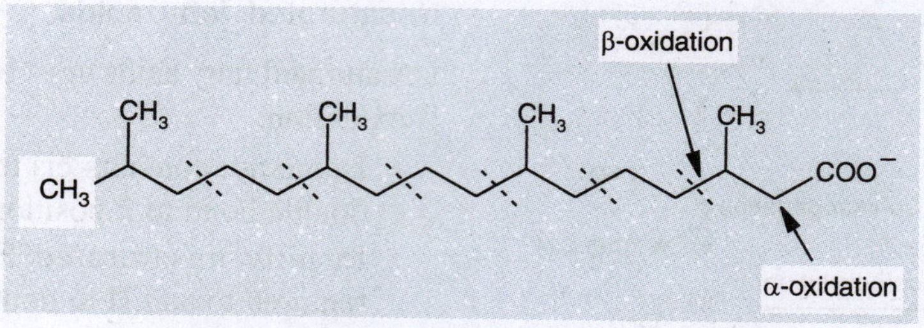

**Fig. 4.79.** Oxidation of phytanic acid:
$\alpha$-hydroxylase oxidizes $\alpha$-carbon and carboxylae group is releases as $CO_2$. Peroxisomal $\beta$-oxidation (continues till 8 carbons) releases propionyl CoA and acetyl CoA. Remaining 8 carbon branched FA is transferred to mitochondria as MCFatty acyl carnitine derivative.

- Defect or deficiency of a hydroxylase
- Nerve and retinal damage
- Spastic movement.
- Bone and skin changes

### Treatment

Avoidance of chlorophyll-containing foods, including meat from plant-eating animals.

## CLINICAL SIGNIFICANCE: BETA OXIDATION

### 1. Carnitine deficiency

- Inability to transport FA in mitochondria
- Can occur in new born and preterm infants.
- Mild, occasional muscle cramps, weakness or even death.

### 2. CPT I deficiency

- Affects liver
- Reduced FA oxidation, ketogenesis

### 3. CPT II deficiency

- Recurrent muscle pain
- Fatigue, myoglobinuria following strenuous exercise.

Carnitine acyl transferase can be inhibited by drugs:

Sulfonyl urea – tolbutamide and glyburide.

### 4. Acyl CoA dehydrogenase deficiency

Can affect VLCFA, LCFA, MCFA, SCFA.

### MCAD deficiency

- Medium chain acyl dehydrogenase (MCAD) deficiency
- Vomiting, lethargy and frequently coma
- Excessive urinary excretion of medium chain dicarboxylic acid and their glycine and carnitine esters is diagnostic.

### 5. Jamaican vomiting sickness

- Caused by eating of unripe fruit of the akee tree, which contains toxin hypoglycin.
- This inactivates MC and SC acyl dehydrogenase, inhibiting $\beta$-oxidation, causing hypoglycemia

### 6. Dicarboxylic acid uria

- Lack of MCAD
- Excretion of C6-C10 dicarboxylic acid
- Non ketotic hypoglycemia.

### 7. Zellweger syndrome

- Rare, inherited deficiency of peroxisomes
- C26-C68 polyenoic acids accumulate in brain
- Severe neurological symptom and fatal by 1st year of life.

# (iv) Cholesterol

## Cholesterol – fact file

- 386 Da, 27 carbon
- 17 carbon incorporated into 4 fused rings
- Perhydrocylopentane phenanthrene ring
- Planar
- Amphipathic lipid
- Important structural component of cell membrane and outer layer of PL.
- Major constituent of gall stones
- Chief role in genesis of atherosclerosis.
- All 27 carbons are derived from a single precursor: acetyl CoA.
- Acetyl CoA can be derived from β-oxidation of FA oxidation of ketogenic amino acids (leucine, lysine) PDH reaction.
- Carbons 1, 2, 5, 7, 9, 13, 15, 18, 19, 20, 22, 24, 26, 27 derived from methyl group of acetyl CoA.
- Remaining 12 carbons are derived from carboxylate atom of acetyl CoA.
- Requires reducing power, that is supplied by NADPH provided by G6PD and 6 phosphogluconate dehydrogenase of HMP shunt.

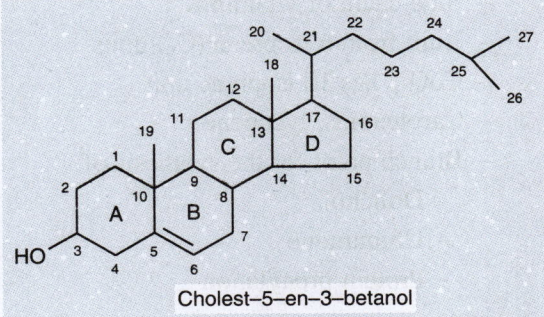

Cholest–5–en–3–betanol

**Fig. 4.80.** Cholest-5-en-3-betanol.

- Almost all mammalian cells can produce cholesterol. Most of cholesterol synthesis occurs in liver. Gut, adrenal cortex, gonads, placenta in pregnant women also produce magnificent amount of cholesterol.
- Entirely composed of C and H atoms with –OH group at C-3.
- Almost completely saturated with just one double bond between $C_5$ & $C_6$.

## Sources of cholesterol

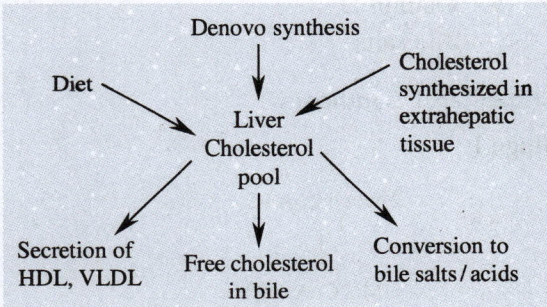

## Dietary cholesterol

### Source

- Animal products: eggs, meat, dairy products.
- 50% is absorbed, 1 g/day excreted as bile acids
- Increased intake decreases absorption.
- If intake is 400 mg/day: 200 mg absorbed, 100 mg excreted.
- 800 mg comes from denovo synthesis.
- Lowering cholesterol in diet has very little effect on blood cholesterol levels.

### Synthesis

- All tissues containing nucleated cells are capable of synthesizing cholesterol.
- Cholesterol synthesis occurs in cytosol, liver, also in adrenal cortex, gonads.

- Similar to ketogenic pathway
- Requires NADPH and ATP.
- Highly regulated
- 80% in liver, 10% intestine, ~5% skin
- Dietary cholesterol is brought to liver mostly in the form of free cholesterol. In VLDL, it is enesterified form (storage form)

### Cholesterol is precursor of:
- Steroid hormone
- Vitamin D
- Bile salts

## Cholesterol synthesis

### Stage 1

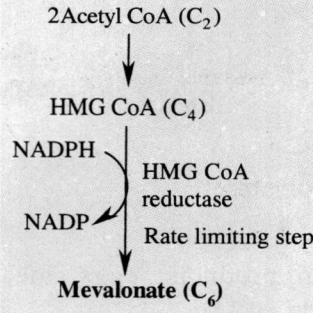

2 Acetyl CoA (C$_2$)

↓

HMG CoA (C$_4$)

NADPH ↘
        HMG CoA reductase
NADP ↙
        Rate limiting step

↓

**Mevalonate (C$_6$)**

### Stage 2:

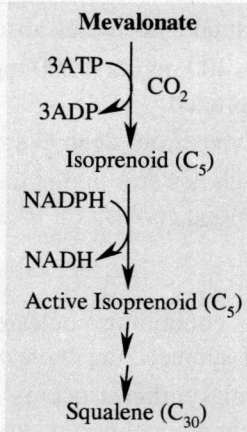

**Mevalonate**

3 ATP ↘
       CO$_2$
3 ADP ↙

Isoprenoid (C$_5$)

NADPH ↘

NADH ↙

Active Isoprenoid (C$_5$)

↓

Squalene (C$_{30}$)

## Stage 3

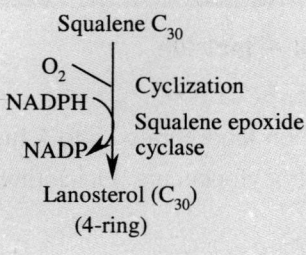

Squalene C$_{30}$

O$_2$ ↘
      Cyclization
NADPH ↘
      Squalene epoxide
NADP ↙ cyclase

Lanosterol (C$_{30}$)
(4-ring)

## Stage 4

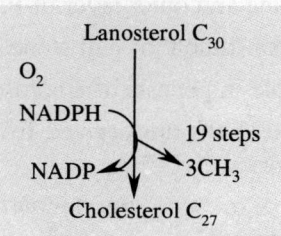

Lanosterol C$_{30}$

O$_2$ ↘
NADPH ↘
      19 steps
NADP ↙ 3 CH$_3$

Cholesterol C$_{27}$

## Isoprenoids

- Isopentanyl pyrophosphate (isoprene)
- Precursor for a variety of biomolecules:
  - Terpenes – Responsible for fragrances of many plants:
    Limonene (lemon oil C$_{110}$ H$_{15}$)
    Zingiberene (ginger oil C$_{15}$ H$_{24}$)
    Menthol from peppermint
- C$_{30}$ hydrocarbons:
  - Side-chain of vitamin K$_2$:
  - Built from 6 isoprene (C$_5$) units
  - CoQ$_{10}$ has 10 isoprene unit
  - Carotenoids, lycopene
  - Branch point for the synthesis of:
    - Dolichol
    - Ubiquinone
    - Protein prenylation
- Heme:
  - has farnesyl side chain

## Details

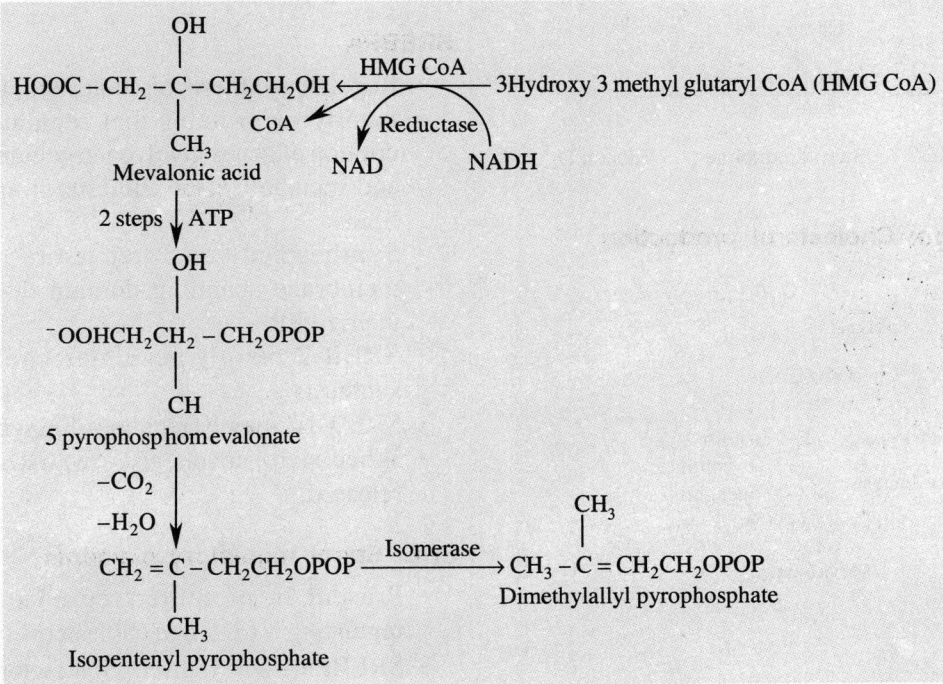

2CH$_3$COSCoA $\xrightarrow{\text{Thiolase}}$ CH$_3$COCH$_2$COSCoA    CH$_3$COSCoA
Acetyl CoA                     Acetoacetyl CoA

HMG CoA synthase

OH
|
HOOC – CH$_2$ – C – CH$_2$ COS CoA
|
CH$_3$

OH
|
HOOC – CH$_2$ – C – CH$_2$CH$_2$OH $\leftarrow$ $\overset{\text{HMG CoA}}{\underset{\text{CoA}}{\longleftarrow}}$ 3Hydroxy 3 methyl glutaryl CoA (HMG CoA)
|
CH$_3$                    Reductase
Mevalonic acid         NAD    NADH

2 steps ↓ ATP

OH
|
$^-$OOHCH$_2$CH$_2$ – CH$_2$OPOP
|
CH
5 pyrophosphomevalonate

–CO$_2$
–H$_2$O

CH$_2$ = C – CH$_2$CH$_2$OPOP $\xrightarrow{\text{Isomerase}}$ CH$_3$ – C = CH$_2$CH$_2$OPOP
|                                            |
CH$_3$                                      CH$_3$
Isopentenyl pyrophosphate              Dimethylallyl pyrophosphate

## Isoprenoid condensation

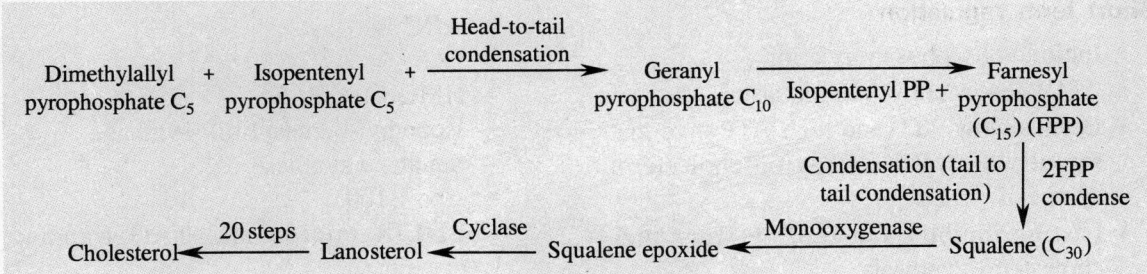

Dimethylallyl + Isopentenyl + $\xrightarrow[\text{condensation}]{\text{Head-to-tail}}$ Geranyl $\xrightarrow{\text{Isopentenyl PP +}}$ Farnesyl
pyrophosphate C$_5$   pyrophosphate C$_5$          pyrophosphate C$_{10}$          pyrophosphate
                                                                         (C$_{15}$) (FPP)

Condensation (tail to  | 2FPP
tail condensation)     | condense

Cholesterol $\xleftarrow{\text{20 steps}}$ Lanosterol $\xleftarrow{\text{Cyclase}}$ Squalene epoxide $\xleftarrow{\text{Monooxygenase}}$ Squalene (C$_{30}$)

## Natural products derived from isoprene

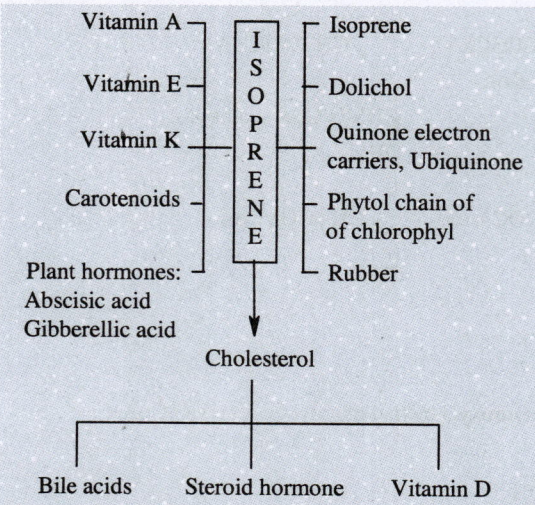

## Regulation: Cholesterol production

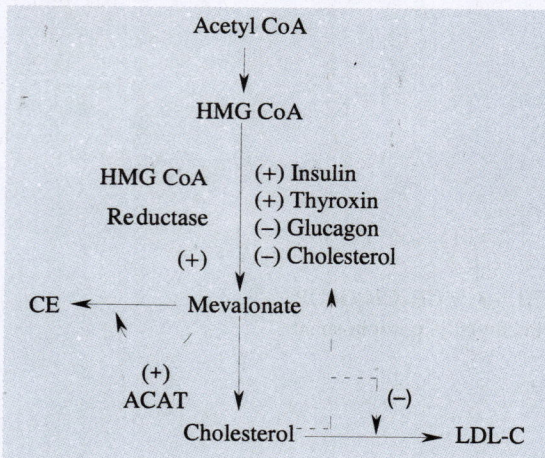

## Short term regulation

- Inhibited by phosphorylation
- AMP-dependent protein kinase
- Because low ATP and high ATP give that signal why waste energy on cholesterol synthesis
- Fasting inhibits and feeding stimulates cholesterol synthesis

## Long term regulation

- Proteolysis
- Degradation stimulated by cholesterol
- Sterol sensing domain

## Mechanism

Cholesterol and metabolites repress transcription of HMG CoA-R via:

Activation of sterol regulatory element binding protein (SREBP) transcription factor

## SREBPs

- Regulate synthesis of cholesterol and FA
- Family of proteins that regulate transcription of genes involved in cellular uptake and metabolism of cholesterol and other lipids
- Synthesized as precursors having membrane spanning domain that locate them in ER
- SREB-2 mainly regulates cholesterol synthesis
- SREB-1C mainly regulates FA synthesis
- When sterol levels are low, SREBP-2 is released.

## SRE: Sterol regulatory elements

- Present in promoter region of genes regulating VLDL and cholesterol synthesis
- SREBP: Act as transcription factor

Proteins encoded by genes responsive to SREBP:

- ACC
- FAS
- HMG CoA-R/-S
- Isopentyl/Farnesyl diP-synthase
- Squalene synthase
- Apo B100
- LDL-R microsomal TAG transfer protein

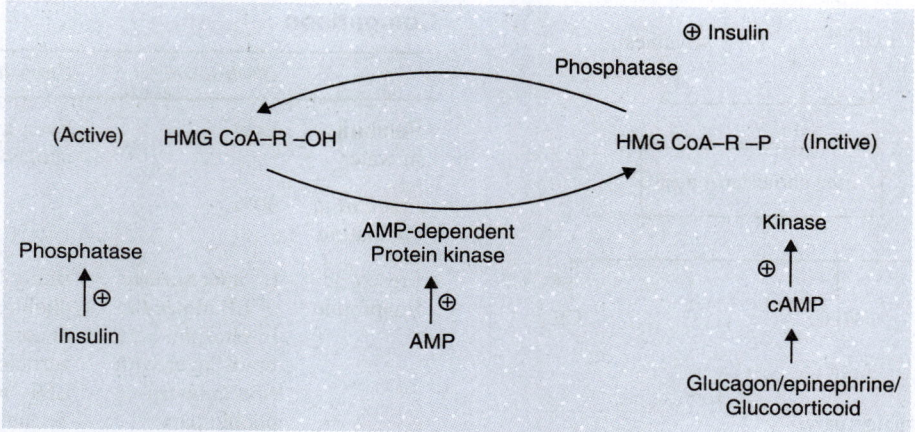

**Fig. 4.81.** Regulation by phosphorylation.

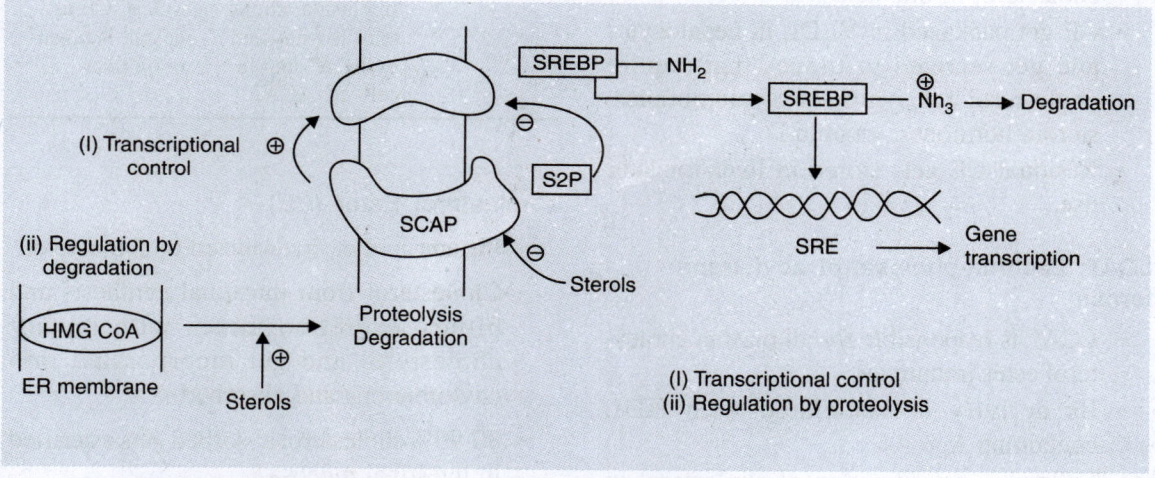

**Fig. 4.82.** Reguation of HMG CoA reductase. SCAP (SREBP cleavage activation reaction.

When mammalian cell is starved of cholesterol, SREBP is released from ER by proteolysis, enters nucleus, and activates transcription of genes having SRE.

Cellular cholesterol content exerts transcriptional control on:

– HMG CoA-R
– LDL-R synthesis

**Once synthesized in liver, cholesterol is exported out**

- Cholesterol is secreted via bile into small intestine
- Conversion to bile acids is followed by secretion into small intestine
- Conversion into cholesterol ester packaging into lipoproteins and export into the blood.

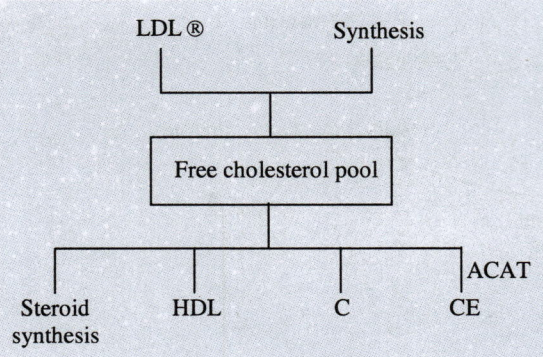

## Fate of cholesterol

- Used for: Synthesis of hepatic membrane
- Most cholesterol is secreted as CE, biliary cholesterol or bile acids.
- CE get packaged in VLDL in hepatocytes and get secreted to tissues that require cholesterol for synthesis of membranes, steroid hormones, vitamin D
- Residual CE gets stored in liver for later use.

## LCAT: Lecithin-cholesterol acyl transferase

- LCAT is responsible for all plasma cholesterol ester in humans
- Its activity is associated with HDL containing Apo A1
- Following esterification of cholesterol in HDL, a concentration gradient is created which draws cholesterol from tissues and other lipoproteins, enabling reverse cholesterol transport.

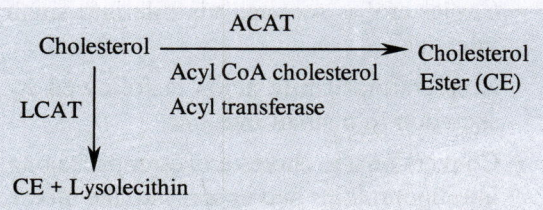

## Comparison

|  | *Cholesterol* | *Cholesterol ester* |
|---|---|---|
| Solubility in water | Low | Even less than cholesterol |
| Fraction in circulation | 30% | – |
| Present in lipoprotein | In outer surface of LP molecule In phospholipids layer with ring in hydrophobic part and –OH group at hydrophilic tail | Being hydrophobic, present in core of LP particle VLDL, LDL mainly Tissue storage form of cholesterol |
|  | In plasma, cholesterol is esterified by LCAT and in cells by ACAT | 80% of CE in plasma is taken up by liver |

## Cholesterol Ester (CE)

- Present in diet, hydrolyzed to cholesterol
- Cholesterol from intestinal synthesis and biliary excretion mixes with dietary cholesterol and get incorporated into chylomicrons and absorbed
- 80-90% cholesterol absorbed gets esterified in intestinal mucosa

## Dietary cholesterol: Fact file

- Dietery cholesterol takes several days to equilibrate with cholesterol in plasma; several weeks to equilibrate with cholesterol in tissues.
- Cholesterol turnover in liver is faster than total body cholesterol.
- Unesterified cholesterol in plasma and liver equilibrate within hours, exchanges and

transfers readily between cell membrane, plasma lipoproteins and RBC membrane.

## CE: Fact file

- Storage form of cholesterol in most tissues
- Transported in hydrophobic core of lipoprotein
- LDL mediates cholesterol and CE uptake in many tissues
- Free cholesterol removed from tissues by HDL and transported to liver.

### Energetics of cholesterol biosynthesis

1 mole of cholesterol requires:

18 moles of acetyl CoA

36 moles of ATP

16 moles of NADPH

18 acetyl CoA $\rightarrow$ 6 Mevalonate $(C_6)$

$\quad$ 2ATP $\rightarrow \downarrow \rightarrow$ 2ADP $\rightarrow$ 27C

$\quad$ 6 isoprene (CS) $\rightarrow$ 30 C Squalene

$\quad \rightarrow$ cholesterol

3 acetyl CoA $\rightarrow$ 1 Mevalonate

Each HMG CoA-R require 2 NADPH i.e., 6x2 = 12 NADPH

Squalene $(C_{30})$ to cholesterol $(C_{27})$ involves three decarboxylation reactions, an isomerization, reduction and NADPH is involved in four of these reactions: 12 + 6 = 16 NADPH

2ATP $\rightarrow$ Mevalonate $\rightarrow$ farnesyl

6 Mevalonate i.e., 6 × 2 ATP = 12 ATP

3 acetyl CoA $\rightarrow$ 1 Mevalonate, so 12 × 3 = 36 ATP

| Reaction | | ATP/NADPH consumed |
|---|---|---|
| HMG CoA – R | 6 reactions | 2 x 6 = 12 NADPH |
| Squalene $\rightarrow$ cholesterol | | 1 × 4 = 4 NADPH |
| $(C_{30})$ $\quad\quad$ $(C_{27})$ | | Total = 16 NADPH |
| 3 acetyl $\rightarrow$ 1 mevalonate | | |
| 6 mevalonate $\rightarrow$ 6 isoprene $\rightarrow$ | 30 C Squalene $\downarrow$ 27 C Cholesterol | 3 × 6 = 18 acetyl CoA |
| Mevalonate $\rightarrow$ isoprene | | 3 ATP |
| 6 isoprene required | | 6 × 3 = 18 ATP |
| Mevalonate $\rightarrow$ mevalonate -5-P $\downarrow$ 3 mevalonate -5-P $\downarrow$ Isopentenyl pyrophosphate | | |
| Isopentenyl PP $\rightarrow$ 2, 3 dimethylallyl PP $\quad \sqsubset\!\top\!\sqsupset$ $\quad\quad$ Geranyl | | 18 × 2 = 36 ATP |

## Excretion of cholesterol

Cholesterol is excreted from body in the bile as cholesterol or bile acids.

## Bile acids from cholesterol

- Formed from cholesterol in liver
- Stored in gall bladder in bile as bile salts (sodium and potassium)

## Bile

- Formed in liver, secreted down to bile duct to gall bladder
- Complex solution of salts and proteins
- Contain micelle composed to cholesterol, phospholipids and bile acids.
- Bile passes into intestine from gall bladder to facilitate degradation of ingested fats.

## Bile acids

- Cholyl CoA
- Chenodeoxy cholyl CoA
  - Get conjugated in peroxisomes as glycine or taurine conjugate in 3:1 ratio.
  - Deconjugation and $7\alpha$-hydroxylase in intestine form secondary bile acids
- Deoxycholic acid from cholic acid
- Lithocholic acid from chenodeoxy cholate.

## Cholic acid

- Cholic acid in bile acid is found in the largest amount in bile
- Primary bile acids: cholic acid 31%, chenodeoxy cholic acid 45%
- Converted to glycine or taurine conjugates
- In human glycine to taurine conjugates is 3:1

## Detergent character of bile salts

- Bile acids have a hydrophobic and hydrophilic face

- Detergent character of bile salts is due to hydrophobic-hydrophilic nature of molecules
- Presence of hydroxyl or sulfate and terminal carboxyl group on the tail gives molecule its hydrophilic face.
- Steroid ring with its puckered plane provides hydrophobic face.

## Functions of bile salts

- Emulsification of fats due to detergent activity
- Aid in absorption of fat soluble vitamins
- Accelerate action of pancreatic lipase
- Have choleretic action: stimulate liver to secrete bile
- Stimulate intestinal motility
- Keep cholesterol in solution (as micelles)

## Bile acid biosynthesis

- Two distinct series of bile acids are synthesized:
  - Cholic acid
  - Chenodroxycholic acid
- In cholic acid: all 3 hydroxyl groups project from the same surface of molecule.
- Bile acids are excreted in conjugated form: taurocholic or glycocholic acid (conjugated with taurine or glycine).

## Clinical aspects: Bile acids

Bile acids perform following physiological functions:

- Eliminate excess cholesterol
- Bile acids and phospholipids solubilize cholesterol in bile: preventing precipitation of cholesterol in gall bladder
- Facilitate digestion of dietary TAG by emulsification action.

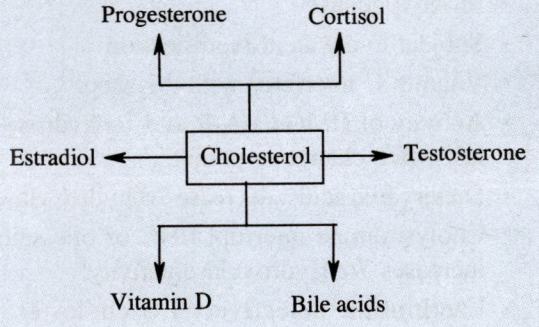

**Cholesterol**

NADP+ H$^+$ → Cyt P$_{450}$ ← Fe$^{+2}$ → O$_2$+H$^+$

NADP$^+$ ← Cyt P$_{450}$ ← Fe$^{3+}$ → H$_2$O

7α–hydroxylase

7α–hydroxy cholesterol

↓ Reduction, hydroxylation

3α, 7α diol

Chenocholic acid

↓ Oxidation

3α, 7α, 18α Triol

Cholic acid

**Fig. 4.83.** Synthesis of bile salts.

- Facilitate intestinal absorption of fat soluble vitamins

### Cholesterol breakdown: Fact file

- Cholesterol cannot be metabolized by mammalian cell
- Sterol ring of cholesterol cannot be degraded
- Cholesterol cannot be digested in gut
- Either excreted in free form or in form of bile acid
- 1 g cholesterol is eliminated from body per day through feces
- Approximately 50% is excreted after conversion to bile acids
- Rest excreted as coprosterol and cholesterol (by bacterial reduction)
- Most of bile acids (98-99%) return to liver after reabsorption in terminal ileum: EHC (enterohepatic circulation)
- Bile salts which are not absorbed are excreted.

### Transformation of cholesterol

Progesterone    Cortisol

Estradiol ← Cholesterol → Testosterone

Vitamin D    Bile acids

### Essential steps in conversion of cholesterol to bile acids

- Inversion of 3 –OH from β to α at C-3
- Removal of double bond between C-5 and C-6
- Insertion of three –OH groups at C-24.

## EHC (entero hepatic circulation of bile salts) -Fact file

- Bile acids non-covalently bind albumin and resecreted into bile.
- Total bile acid pool: 3 g
- Bile acids have to be recirculated 5-10 times a day.
- Pool of bile acids is kept constant via cholesterol synthesis by liver.

## Conversion of cholesterol to bile acids

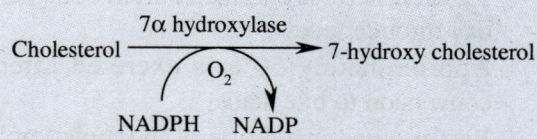

## 7 α-hydroxylase: Facts

- 1st committed step
- Rate-limiting step
- Microsomal enzyme
- Repressed by bile salts
- Induced by cholesterol
- Monoxygenase
- Subject to covalent modification
- Vitamin C interferes with this step.
- Activity of HMG CoA-R and 7α hydroxylase often change in parallel.
- Dietary bile acids: decrease 7α hydroxylase
- Cholystramine interrupt EHC of bile salts increases 7α Hydroxylase activity.
- Ezetimibine selectively (–) cholesterol absorption in small intestine by inhibiting cholesterol transporters in brush border

## Cholesterol transport between tissues

- Cholesterol is transported between tissues in plasma proteins
- Total plasma cholesterol is 5.2 mmol/L

- Greater part is in esterified form
- Transported in lipoproteins in plasma
- Highest proportion found in LDL

## Overview of whole body cholesterol metabolism

- Control of cholesterol level depends on rate of its excretion in bile as cholesterol or as bile salts
- Rate of synthesis of cholesterol regulated by HMG CoA-R by excess cholesterol
- Bile excreted in intestine is very efficiently reabsorbed
- All cholesterol circulation in blood is obtained in LP.

**Vitamin D causes:**

Intestinal absorption of Ca, $PO_4$.

Renal reabsorption of Ca, $PO_4$.

**Specific receptors of Vitamin D:**

Present in:

Intestine, bone, kidney.

## Serum cholesterol correlates with the incidence of atherosclerosis and coronary heart disease

- Changes in diet: reduce serum cholesterol
- PUFA and MUFA:
  (+) cholesterol excretion into intestine
  (–) oxidation of cholesterol to bile acids
  Up regulates LDL-R
- Changes in life style:
  Regular exercise
  Stop smoking

## Life style affects serum cholesterol levels

- High BP
- Smoking
- Male gender
- Obesity

## Overview

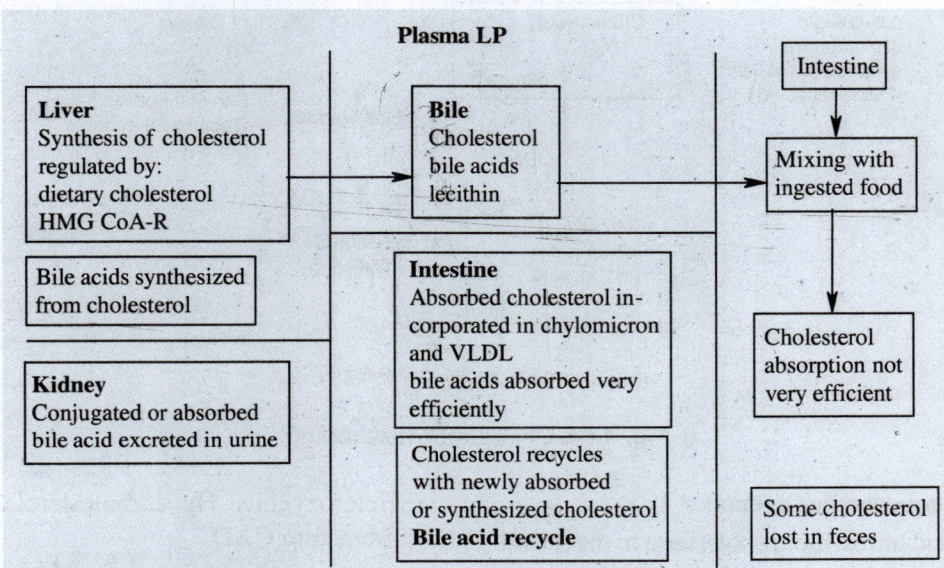

**Plasma LP**

| | | | |
|---|---|---|---|
| **Liver** Synthesis of cholesterol regulated by: dietary cholesterol HMG CoA-R | → | **Bile** Cholesterol bile acids lecithin | → |
| **Bile acids synthesized from cholesterol** | | **Intestine** Absorbed cholesterol incorporated in chylomicron and VLDL bile acids absorbed very efficiently | |
| **Kidney** Conjugated or absorbed bile acid excreted in urine | | Cholesterol recycles with newly absorbed or synthesized cholesterol **Bile acid recycle** | |

Intestine → Mixing with ingested food → Cholesterol absorption not very efficient → Some cholesterol lost in feces

## Photobiosynthesis of vitamin D₃:

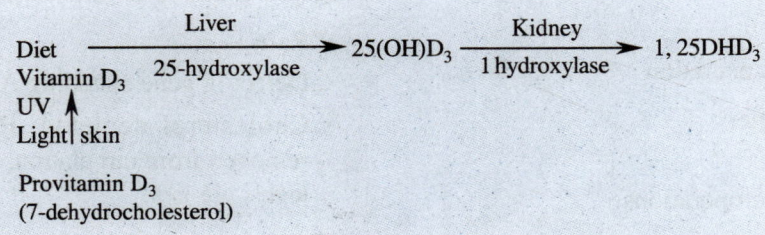

$$\text{Diet Vitamin D}_3 \xrightarrow[\text{25-hydroxylase}]{\text{Liver}} 25(OH)D_3 \xrightarrow[\text{1 hydroxylase}]{\text{Kidney}} 1, 25DHD_3$$

UV Light | skin

Provitamin D₃ (7-dehydrocholesterol)

---

- Lack of exercise
- Drinking soft water

### Non-dietary factors affecting cholesterol

- Stress, cigarette smoking, coffee increase LDL levels
- Aerobic exercise increase HDL levels
- Body shape correlated with cholesterol:
  - Fat in upper body correlated with high cholesterol level
  - Fat on hips and thighs correlated with low levels.

### Drugs lowering serum cholesterol & TG

**Statins:**

Lower serum cholesterol

Inhibit HMG CoA reductase

Up regulate LDL receptor activity

**Fibrates:**

(+) Secretion of VLDL

(+) LPL causing TAG hydrolysis in VLDL

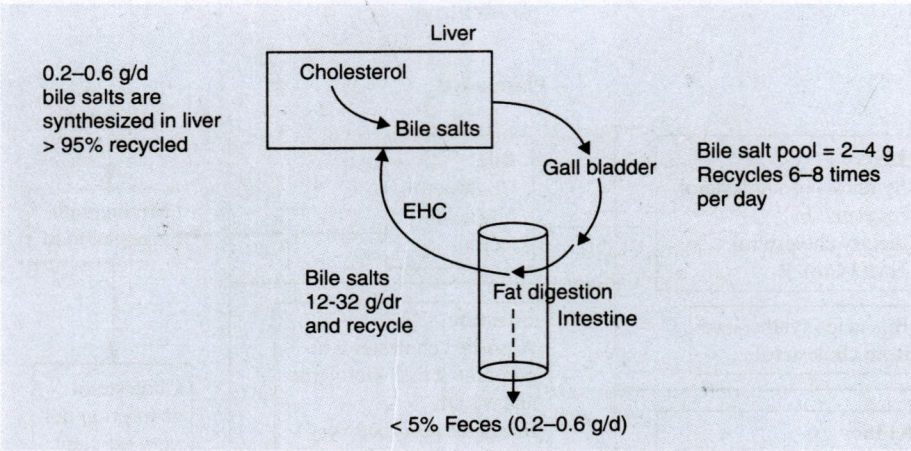

**Fig. 4.84.** Cholesterol metabolism.

**Bile sequestering agents**:
Bile acid utilize more cholesterol to make bile acids

**Oat bran**:
Soluble fiber, bond bile acids

**Niacin**:
Inhibit VLDL excretion

**Cholystramine**:
Interrupt EHC
Ileal exclusion operations

**Sitosterol**: Block absorption of cholesterol from GIT

**Probucol**: Increasing LDL catabolism

**Nicotinic acid**:
(–) Adipose tissue lipolysis
(–) VLDL production by liver

## Lipid Disorders

### Familial hyper cholesterolemia

- LDL receptor deficiency
  Gene for LDL-receptor on chromosome 19

- Heterozygous: Hypercholesterolemia and premature CAD
- Homozygous: Extremely high LDL-C, xanthoma, very early symptomatic CHD

### Tangier's disease & familial HDL deficiency

- Rare
- Defect in gene encoding ABC 1 protein
- Cholesterol depleted, HDL is rapidly removed from circulation, so plasma HDL levels are low.

Patients accumulate cholesterol in lymphoreticular system (hepatosplenomegaly).

### Xanthoma

- Raised, waxy appearing, often yellowish skin lesions associated with hyperlipidemia.
- Tendon xanthomas, common on Achilles and hand extensor tendons.
- Xanthoma of eyelids: generally associated with hypercholesterolemia
- Eruptive xanthomas associated with hypertriglyceridemia generally.

## LIPID DISORDERS

### Primary

**Table 4.14.** Lipid disorders

| Name | Defect | Features |
|---|---|---|
| Hypolipoproteinemia | No chm, VLDL or LDL formed defect in loading of apo B with lipid | Rare, blood acyl glycerol low Acylglycerols accumulate in intestine and liver – early death |
| Abetalipoproteinemia | No chm, VLDL or LDL formed defect in loading of apo B with lipid | Rare blood acyl glycerol low Acylglycerols accumulate in intestine and liver – early death |
| Familial $\alpha$-lipoprotein deficiency | All have low or near absence of HDL Absence of apo CII causing inactive LPL | Tendency towards hypertriacylglycerolemia Lower LDL levels, atherosclerosis |
| Familial LPL deficiency (Type I) | Hypertriglycerolemia apo CII, LPL deficiency | Slow clearance of chm, VLDL Low LDL, HDL No increased risk of CHD. |
| Familial hypercholesterolemia (Type IIa) | Defective LDL receptor or mutation in ligand region of apo B-100 | Elevated LDL levels, hypercholesterolemia, CHD, atherosclerosis |
| Familial type III hyperlipoproteinemia (broad beta disease) | Deficiency in remnant clearance by liver due to abnormality in apo E | Increase in Chm, VLDL remnant hypercholesterolemia, xanthoma, atherosclerosis |
| Familial hypertriacyl glycerolemia (type IV) | Over production of VLDL glucose intolerance hyperinsulinemia | Cholesterol levels rise with VLDL concentration LDL, HDL subnormal CHD, type II DM, obesity |
| Familial hyper alpha lipoproteinemia | Increased concentration of HDL | Rare, beneficial |
| Hepatic lipase deficiency | Deficiency of enzyme LPL leads to accumulation of large TAG rich HDL & VLDL remnants | Xanthoma, CHD |
| Familial LCAT deficiency | Absence of LCAT leads to block in reverse cholesterol transport HDL remains discoidal incapable of taking up and esterifying cholesterol | Low plasma LCAT, CE, Lysolecithin. Abnormal LDL fraction: LPLX VLDL abnormal |
| Familial Lp(a) excess | Lp (a) consists of 1mol of LDL attached to 1mol of apo(a) | Premature CHD, thrombosis |

## (v) Ketone Body Metabolism

### Ketone bodies

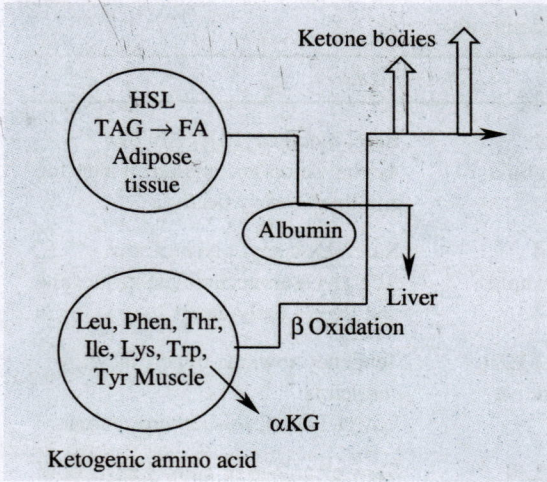

Ketogenic amino acid

Ketone bodies (KB) are important source of energy, especially in starvation

### Ketogenesis: Ketone body production

**Ketone bodies:**

Acetoacetate

$$CH_3CCH_2COO^-$$
$$\parallel$$
$$O$$

β-hydroxybutyrate

$$CH_3CHCH_2COO$$
$$|$$
$$OH$$

Acetone

$$CH_3C-CH_3$$
$$\parallel$$
$$O$$

Ketones bodies are:

- Formed in liver to free up CoA for oxidation.
- Metabolized in other tissues including brain as an energy source.

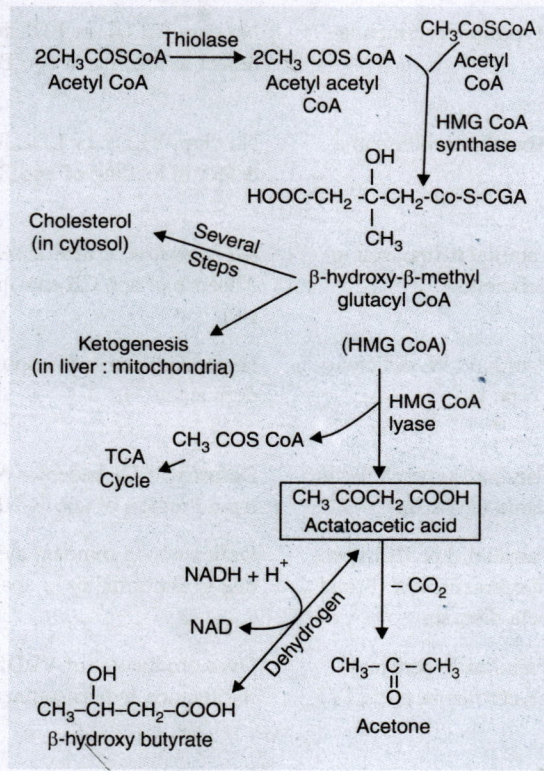

**Fig. 4.85.** Formation of KB.

### Formation of ketone bodies

- Occurs when there is a high rate of FA oxidation in liver.
- Under high rate of FA oxidation, liver produces considerable amount of acetoacetate and β-hydroxybutyrate
- Acetoacetate and β-hydroxybutyrate are spontaneously decarboxylated to acetone.
- Ketone bodies produced in liver flow to

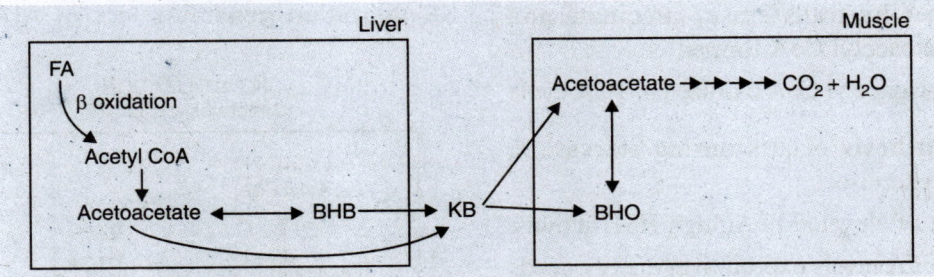

**Fig. 4.86.** Ketone body synthesis and utilization.

extrahepatic tissues where their rate of utilization is very low.

## Ketone bodies as energy source

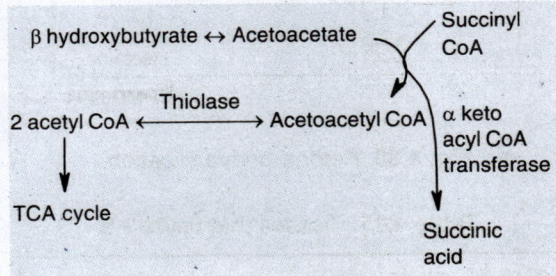

**Fig. 4.87.** Ketone body as energy source.

Formation, utilization and excretion of KB.

### Use of KB

KB serve as a fuel for extrahepatic tissues, preferential fuel in heart muscle

- In liver, acetoacetate is produced from acetoacetyl CoA:
  - Once formed can't be reactivated directly except in cytosol
  - In cytosol, acetoacetate is used as a precursor for cholesterol synthesis
- In extrahepatic tissues:
  - Acetoacetate is activated to acetoacetyl

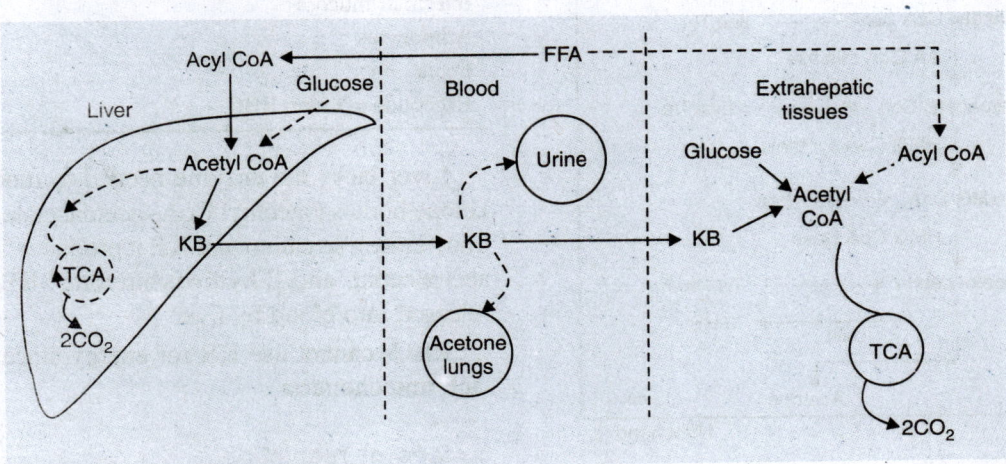

**Fig. 4.88.** Ketone body metabolism.

CoA by transferase, succinate and acetoacetyl CoA formed

– Acetoacetyl CoA oxidized in TCA cycle

**KB synthesis** occurs during starvation, prolonged exercise:

- Result of elevated FFA, high HSL activity
- High FFA levels exceed liver energy needs
- KB are partially oxidized FA

### Utilization of KB by extrahepatic tissues

- KB oxidation starts when its concentration is 1-3 mM.
- In brain, succinyl CoA- acetoacetyl CoA transferase is induced, allowing brain to utilize KB as energy source.
- Also, it reduces glucose needs and protein catabolism for GNG.

### Ketogenesis in liver mitochondria

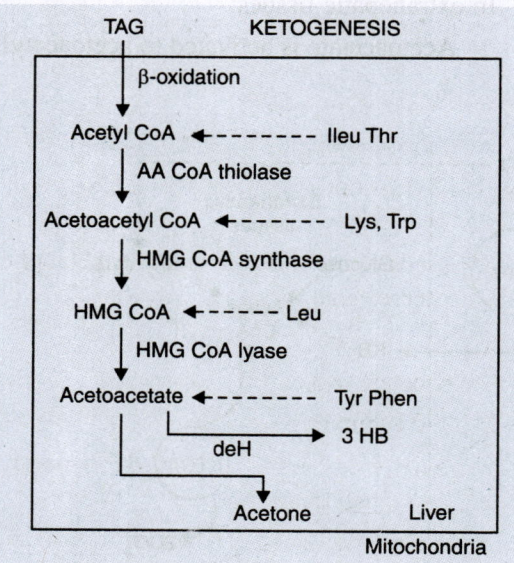

**Fig. 4.89.** Ketogenesis.

### KB utilization generates lots of ATP

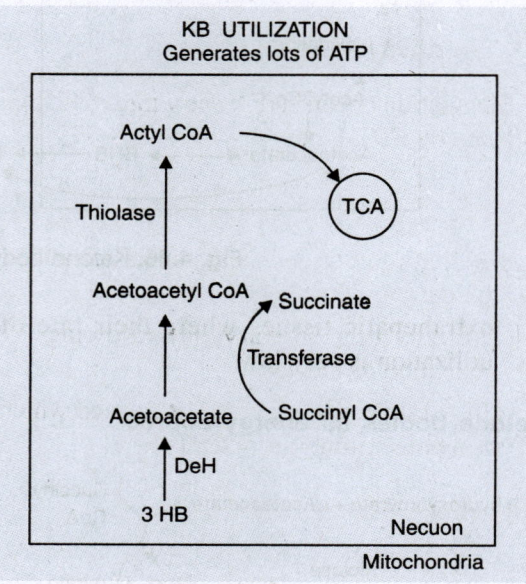

**Fig. 4.90.** Ketone body utilization.

**Table 4.15.** Tissues that utilize KB

| |
| --- |
| Skeletal muscle |
| Heart |
| Brain |
| Intestinal mucosa |
| Adipocytes |
| Fetus |
| Exception = Liver, RBC |

Liver lacks the enzyme needed to mobilize ketone bodies (succinyl CoA- acetoacetate CoA transferase), so cannot use KB it produces. Thus, acetoacetate and β-hydroxybutyrate (HB) are released into blood by liver.

RBCs cannot use KB for energy since they lack mitochondria.

### 3 steps of regulation

After uptake by liver, FFA are oxidized to:

- $CO_2$
- KB
- Esterified to TAG & PL

Regulation occurs at FA entry into oxidative pathway by CPT-I.

## CPT-I

- Activity low in fed state depression of FA oxidation
- Activity high in starvation allowing FA oxidation to increase
- In fed state, malonyl CoA is formed which is a potent inhibitor of CPT-1.

## Regulation: Ketogenesis

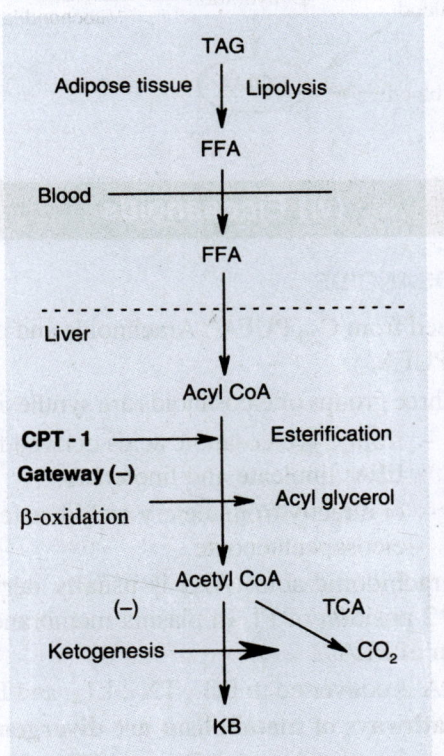

**Fig. 4.91.** Regulation ketogenesis.

## Clinical aspects

Impaired FA oxidation gives rise to diseases often associated with hypoglycemia:

- Carnitine deficiency
- CPT-1 deficiency
- Defects in enzymes of oxidation and ketogenesis
- Jamaican vomiting sickness
- Refsum's disease
- Zellweger syndrome

## Carnitine deficiency

- Occurs in newborn, more so in preterm infants due to inadequate biosynthesis or renal leakage
- Occurs in hemodialysis.

### Symptoms

- Hypoglycemia (impaired FA oxidation)
- Muscle weakness

### Treatment

- Oral carnitine supplementation

## KB in diabetes mellitus

$\downarrow$ Glucose in cells $\rightarrow$ $\uparrow$ GNG $\rightarrow$ $\downarrow$ OAA

$\uparrow$ FA oxidation $\rightarrow$ $\uparrow$ Acetoacetyl CoA $\rightarrow$ $\uparrow$ KB

Increased acetoacetate can result in metabolic acidosis, decreasing affinity of Hb for $O_2$.

$pK_a$ of:

Acetoacetate = 3.6

$\beta$ Hydroxybutyrate = 4.7

In healthy subjects, KB are normally produced in small quantities.

In diabetic patients, cells have a reduced capacity to take up glucose and these cells must depend on FA metabolism.

## KB in diabetes mellitus

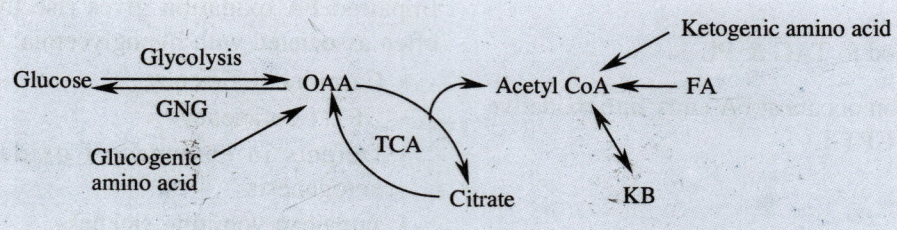

## Mechanism

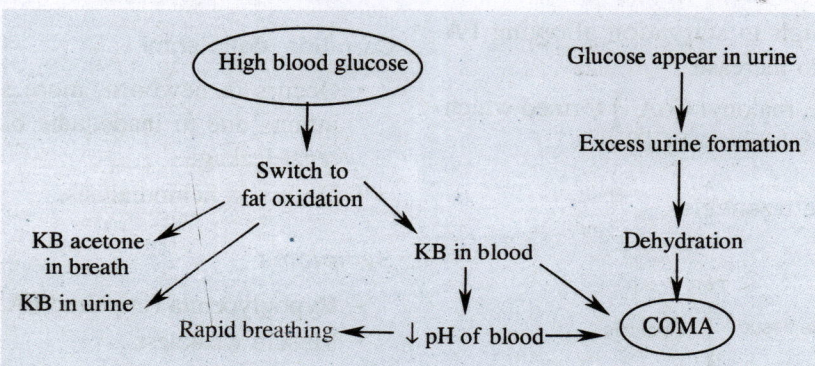

Thus, KB production can be drastically elevated under these conditions and can result in ketoacidosis, ketogenic coma.

### Energy production from oxidation of KB

One acetoacetate produces two acetyl CoA, each can generate about 12ATP via TCA of i.e., total 24 ATPs.

However, activation of acetoacetate results in generation of one less ATP because GTP is not produced when succinyl CoA is used to activate acetoacetate. Therefore, oxidation of acetoacetate yields net 23 ATP.

When β-hydroxybutyrate is oxidized, additional 3 ATP are formed oxidation of β-hydroxybutyrate to acetoacetate produces NADH (One NADH → 3ATP).

## (vi) Eicosanoids

### EICOSANOIDS

Formed from $C_{20}$ PUFA : Arachnoids and other $C_{20}$ PUFA.

Three groups of eicosanoids are synthesized:
- from $C_{20}$ eicosanoic acids derived from EFA: linoleate and linolenate.
- or directly from dietary archidonate and eicosapentaenoate.

Arachidonic acid (AA) is usually derived from 2 position of PL in plasma membrane by action of $PLA_2$.

AA is converted to $PG_2$, $TX_2$, $LT_4$, and $LX_4$.

**Pathways of metabolism are divergent:**
- Synthesis of PG and $TX_2$ series: Cyclooxygenase pathway (C.O.)

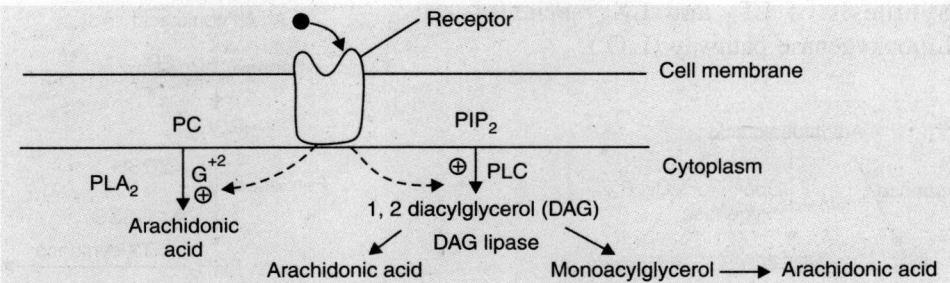

**Fig. 4.92.** Release of arachidonic acid from membrane lipids.

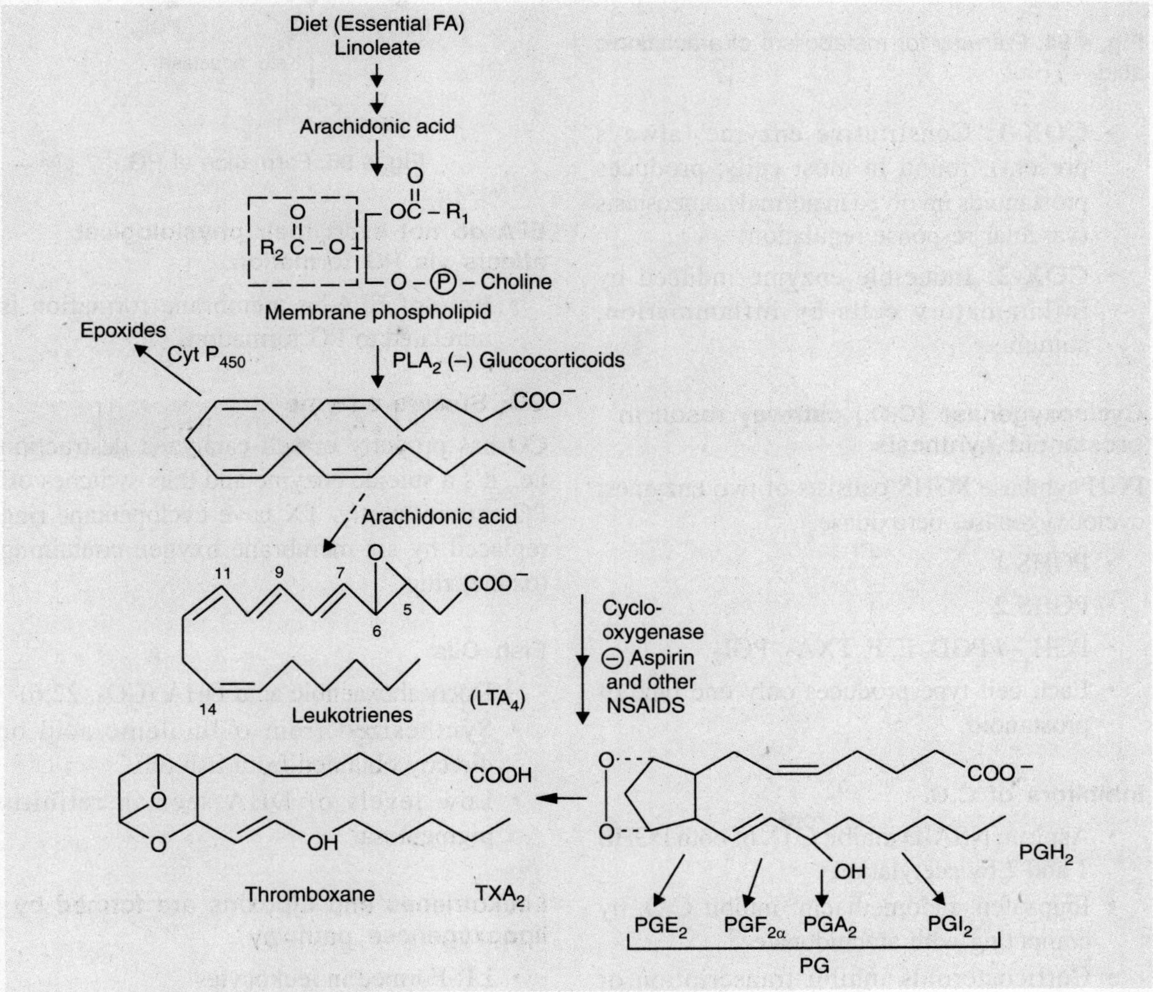

Diet (Essential FA)
Linoleate
↓↓
Arachidonic acid
↓↓

O
‖
OC — R₁
O
R₂ C — O
‖
O
O — Ⓟ — Choline

Membrane phospholipid

Epoxides ← Cyt P₄₅₀

PLA₂ (–) Glucocorticoids

COO⁻

Arachidonic acid

11    9    7    O
6    5    COO⁻

14    Leukotrienes    (LTA₄)

Cyclo-oxygenase ⊖ Aspirin and other NSAIDS

COOH

O
O
OH

Thromboxane    TXA₂

O
O
COO⁻

OH

PGH₂

PGE₂    PGF₂α    PGA₂    PGI₂

PG

**Fig. 4.93.** Overview of eicosanoid metabolism.

– Synthesis of $LT_4$ and $LX_4$ series: Lipooxygenase pathway (L.O.)

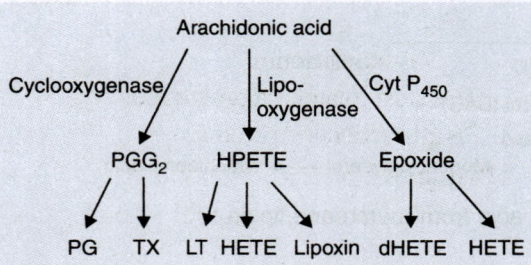

**Fig. 4.94.** Pathway for metabolism of arachidonic acid.

- **COX-1:** Constitutive enzyme (always present), found in most cells, produces prostanoids involved in normal homeostasis (vascular response regulation)
- **COX-2:** Inducible enzyme induced by inflammatory cells by inflammation, stimulus.

## Cyclooxygenase (C.O.) pathway result in prostanoid synthesis

PGH synthase PGHS consists of two enzymes: cyclooxygenase, peroxidase

- PGHS 1
- PGHS 2
- PGH → PGD, E, F, $TXA_2$, $PGI_2$
- Each cell type produces only one type of prostanoid.

## Inhibitors of C.O.

- Aspirin: NSAID inhibit C.O. of both PGHS 1 and 2 by acetylation
- Ibuprofen, indomethacin: inhibit C.O. by competing with arachidonate
- Corticosteroids inhibit transcription of PGHS-2.

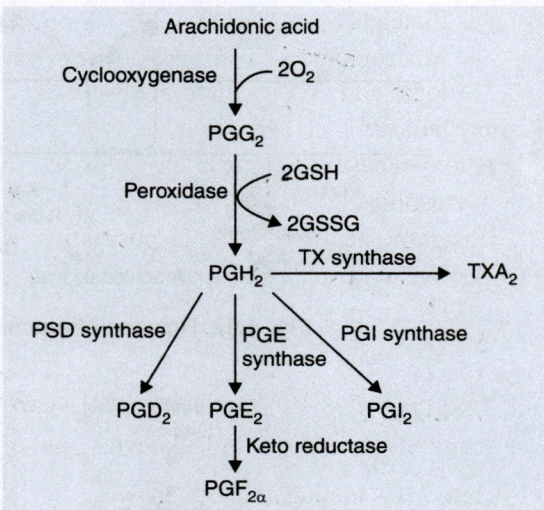

**Fig. 4.95.** Formation of PG.

## EFA do not exert their physiological effects via PG formation

- Role of EFA in membrane formation is unrelated to PG formation

## CO: Suicide enzyme

CO has property of self-catalyzed destruction i.e., it's a suicide enzyme and thus switches off PG activity partly. TX have cyclopentane ring replaced by six-membrane oxygen containing (oxane) ring.

## Fish Oils

- Docosahexaenoic acid DHA ($CO_3$, 22:6)
- Synthesized from α-linolenic acid or directly obtained from fish oils.
- Low levels of DHA seen in retinitis pigmentosa

## Leukotrienes and Lipoxins are formed by lipooxygenase pathway

- LT: Formed in leukocytes
  - Mastocytoma cells

- Platelets
- Macrophage in response to immunologic and non-immunologic stimuli

**Lipoxygenase:**
- Dioxygenase:
- Cytosolic:
  Insert oxygen into 5, 12, 15 position
- Various types of LO:
  3 LO
  5 LO
  12 LO
  15 LO
- Only 5LO forms LT in leukocytes

  **Lipoxins** – conjugated tetraenes.

## 15 HPETE

Basophil, PMN, (polymorphonuclear cells) macrophage, mast cells, organs undergoing inflammatory response.

**Prostanoid:**

PGs

TXs

Vasoconstriction: $TXA_2$, $LTC_4$, $D_4$, $E_4$

Vasodilation: $PGI_2$, $P_4$, $E_1$, $E_2$, $D_2$

Increase permeability:  LT $C_4$, $D_4$, $E_4$

Chemotaxis, leukocyte adhesion: $LTB_4$, HETE, LX

**$PGD_2$:**
- Vasodilation
- Inhibit platelet aggregation
- Relaxation of GI muscle
- Uterine relaxation

**$PGF_{2\alpha}$:**
- Myometrial contraction
- Luteolysis (cattle)
- Bronchoconstriction (dog)

**$PGI_2$:**
- Vasodilation

- Inhibit platelet aggregation
- Rennin release and natriuresis: via effects on tubular reabsorption of $Na^+$

**$TXA_2$:**
- Vasoconstriction
- Cause platelet aggregation
- Bronchoconstriction

**$PGE_2$:**
- $EP_1$: Bronchial and GI smooth muscle contraction
- $EP_2$: Bronchodilation, vasodilation, (GI) smooth muscle relaxation (+) intestinal fluid secretion
- $EP_3$:
  - smooth muscle contraction
  - inhibit gastric acid secretion
  - increase gastric mucus secretion
  - stimulate uterus contraction

**PGE** is implicated production of fever; antipyretic action of NSAID is partly by inhibition of $PGE_2$ synthesis in hypothalamus. Compounds of 2-series derived from arachidonic acid are principal PG in humans and are of greatest significance biologically.

## PROSTANOIDS ARE POTENT BIOLOGICALLY ACTIVE SUBSTANCES

### TX
- Synthesized by platelets
- 6-member O-containing ring
- Upon release cause vasoconstriction, platelet aggregation (action opposite to $PGI_2$)
- Inhibited by low dose aspirin

### $PGI_2$
- Produced by blood vessel walls – vasodilation
- Potent inhibitor of platelet aggregation

**TXA$_2$ and PGI$_2$ are antagonists**

- PGI$_2$ as potent antiaggregator of platelet
- TXA$_3$ weak aggregator

**PG$_3$, TX$_3$**

- Formed from eicopantaenoic acid (EPA) in fish oils
- Inhibit release of arachidonate from PL.

**Use**

**PG$_2$, TX$_2$**

- Prevention of conception
- Induction of labor at term PGE$_2$, F$_{2\alpha}$
- Termination of pregnancy
- Prevention of alleviation of gastric ulcers
- Control of inflammation

**PGE**

- Hypotension
- Relief of asthma, nasal congestion

**TXA$_2$**

- Constriction of vasculature, glomerular mesangium, smooth muscle

**PGI$_2$**

- Inhibit platelet aggregation – epopustenol is used – if heparin is contraindicated.

**LEUKOTRIENES AND LIPOXINS**

- **SRS A** is mixture of LTC$_4$, D$_4$ and E$_4$.

- **LT:** Potent constrictor of bronchial airway musculature, vasoactive.
- **LTB$_4$-E$_4$:** Cause vascular permeability and attraction and activation of leukocytes and important regulators of inflammation or immediate hypersensitivity reaction, 1000 times more potent than histamine in constricting pulmonary airways.
- **Lipoxins** – Vasoactive, immunoregulatory – counteregulatory compounds of immune regulation
- **L.O.:** Cytosolic, lung, platelet, mast cells, WBC.
- **LTB$_4$:** Chemotactic agent in neutrophil and macrophages
- **LtD$_4$:** Bronchoconstriction, increase mucus reaction, decrease blood pressure (vaso-constriction)
- **LX:** Oppose action of LTB$_4$
  A$_4$, B$_4$ generated by platelets by 12 L.O. (Fig. 4.96).

**LTB$_4$**

- Mediate chemotaxis
- Stimulate adenyl cyclase
- Induce PMN to degranulate and release lysosomal hydrolytic enzyme

**LTC$_4$ and D$_4$**

- Humoral agents
- Promote smooth muscle contraction
- Constriction of pulmonary airways, trachea, intestine
- Increase capillary permeability (edema)

| | Arachidonate | Eicosapentaenoate | Site of synthesis | Action |
|---|---|---|---|---|
| PGI$_2$ | PGI$_2$ | PGI$_3$ | Vascular Endothelium | Vasodilation, antiaggregator |
| TX | TXA$_2$ | TXA$_3$ | Platelets | Vasoconstriction |
| LT | LTB$_4$ | LTB$_5$ | Leukocytes | Chemotaxis |

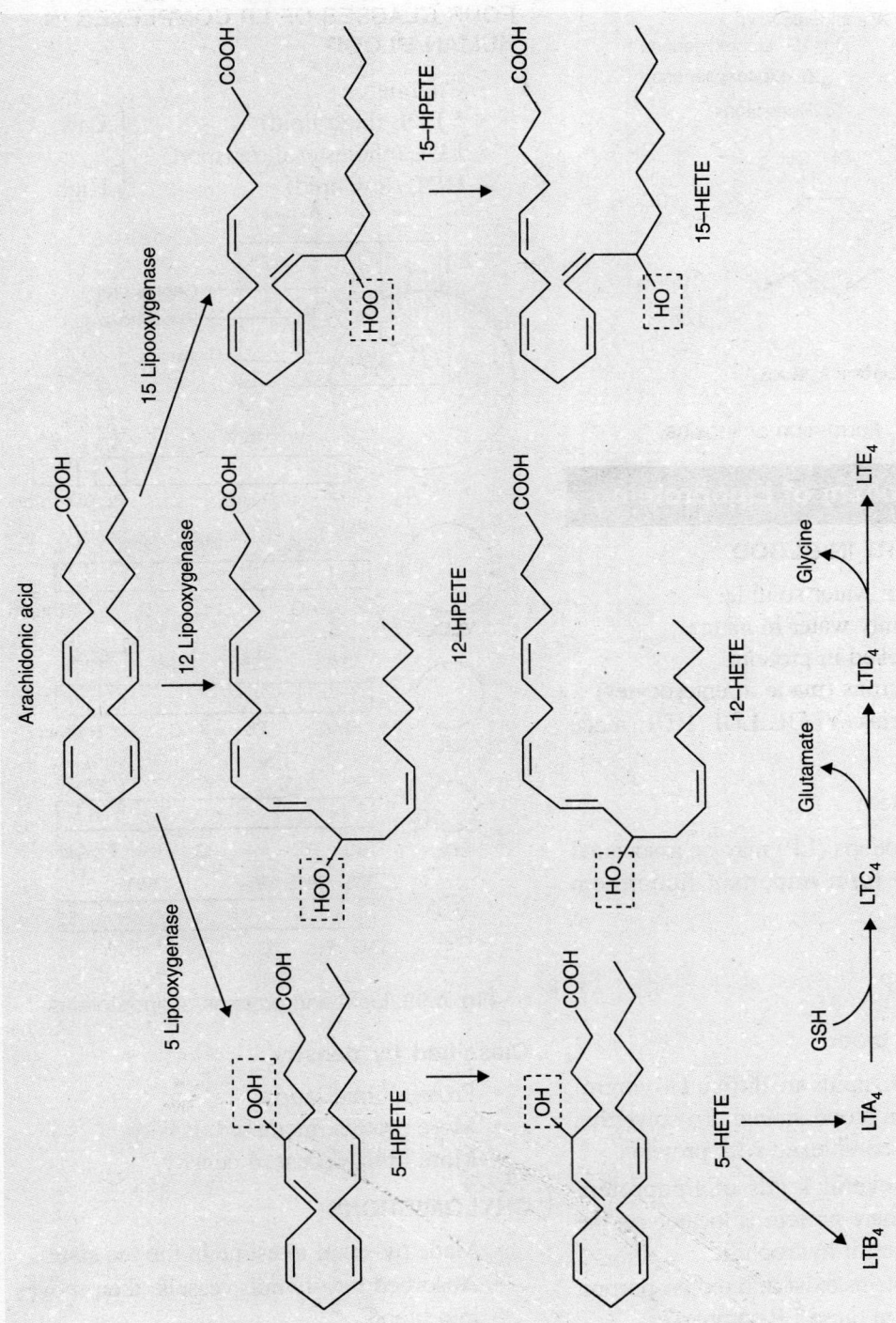

**Fig. 4.96.** Action of lipooxygenases on arachidonic acid.

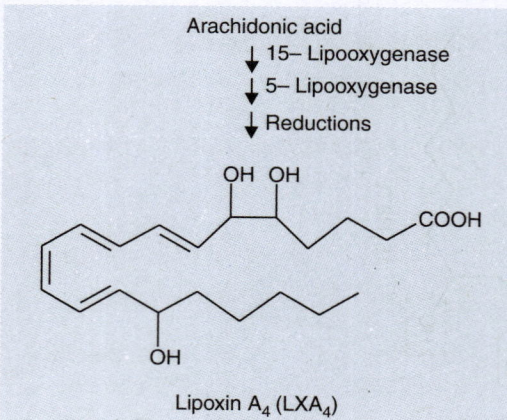

**Fig. 4.97.** Formation of lipoxins.

## (vi) Metabolism of Lipoprotein

### LIPID TRANSPORT IN BLOOD

- Lipids are not water soluble:
  Blood is mainly water in nature
- Lipid are packed in protein:
  - Chylomicrons (made in enterocytes)
  - Lipoproteins (VLDL, LDL, HDL, made in liver).

### Lipoprotein system

Lipids and lipoproteins (LP) may be associated noncovalently to form important lipoprotein system:

1. Transport LP
2. Membrane LP

### Transport LP of blood

Being hydrophobic, lipids are difficult to control and move about in blood stream. To solve this problem, they are complexed with proteins.

- They form several kinds of lipoprotein complexes where protein is located on the outside, making it hydrophilic
- Lipid and proteins exist in fixed proportion to each other in these LP complexes.

## FOUR CLASSES OF LP COMPLEXES IN HUMAN BLOOD

- Chymicron
- VLDL (high lipid)
- LDL (cholesterol transport)
- HDL (low lipid)

Low

High

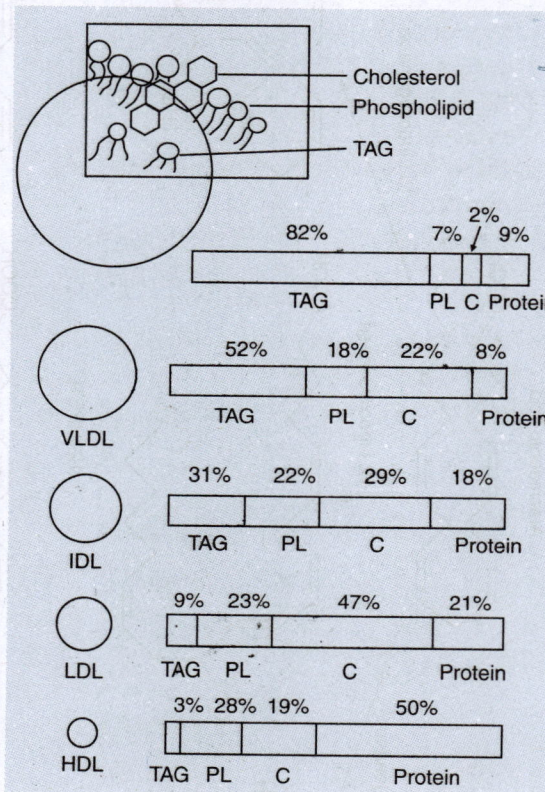

**Fig. 4.98.** Lipid and proteins of lipoproteins.

### Classified by density

- Protein: lipid ratio
- More protein, increased density
- More lipid, deceased density

### CHYLOMICRONS

- Made by small intestine in the fed state
- Absorbed into lymph vessels, then moves into blood

- Rich in TAG (TG)
- Function: to deliver TG to body cells for their use as fuel

## VLDL

- Made in liver from excess dietary carbohydrate and protein along with chylomicron remnant.
- Secreted into blood stream
- Rich in TG
- Contain apo $B_{100}$
- Similar to chylomicrons, but made by different tissues.

  **Function**: They deliver TG to body cells

## LDL

- Once VLDL loses much to its TG, it becomes LDL
- Made in liver as VLDL
- Secreted into blood stream

- Rich in cholesterol
- Function: to deliver cholesterol to all body cell
- **Bad cholesterol,** associated with plaque formation in blood vessels.

## HDL

- Made in liver and small intestine
- Secreted into blood stream
- Removes cholesterol from cells and LP
- Deliver cholesterol to liver for excretion: Converted into bile salts and excreted in feces
- **'Good cholesterol'**
- **Function:** picks up cholesterol from body cells and takes its back to the liver: **reverse cholesterol transport**
- Potential to help reverse heart disease.

## Lipoprotein processing (Fig. 4.99)

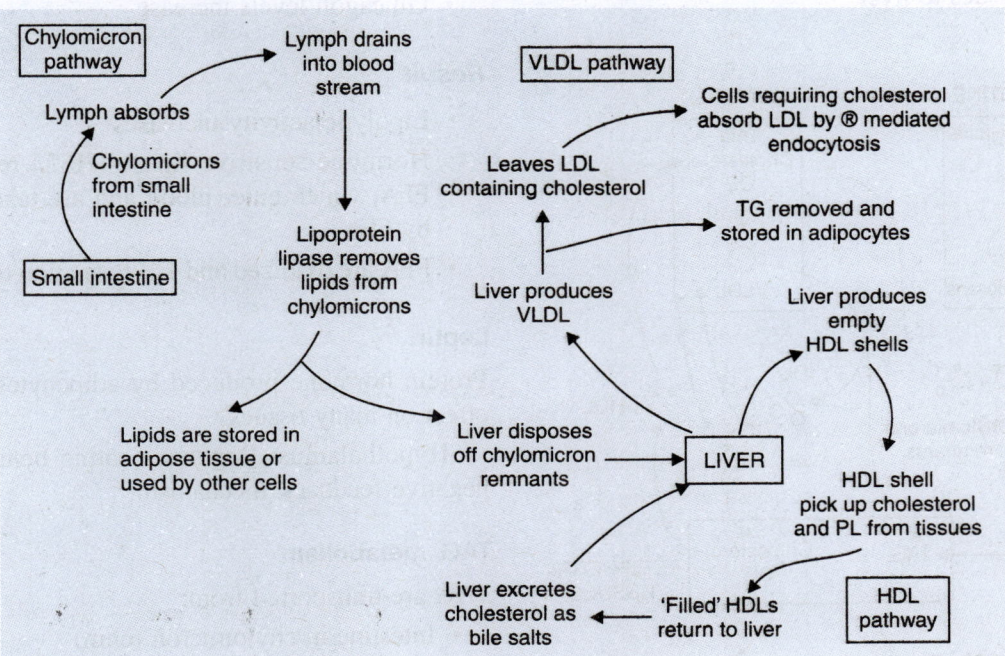

**Fig. 4.99.** Lipoprotein processing.

### Is cholesterol 'bad' for you?

No.

Cholesterol is required for synthesis of steroid hormones, bile salts and present in cell membrane.

### SUMMARY: LIPOPROTEIN METABOLISM

- Chymicrons, largest of lipoproteins, are formed in intestinal cells; carry dietary TAG to peripheral tissues including muscle and adipose tissue.
- Chylomicron remnants deliver CE to liver
- VLDL assemble in liver and carry endogenous lipids to peripheral tissues
- VLDL when degraded, pick up cholesterol and CE from HDL and become LDL which carry cholesterol to nonhepatic tissues.
- HDL deliver cholesterol from peripheral tissues to liver

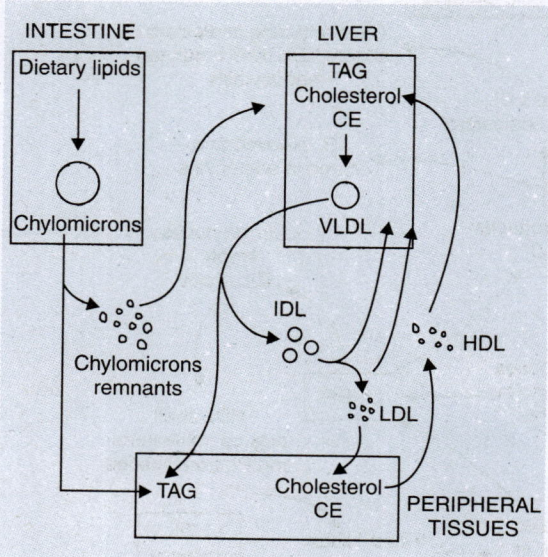

**Fig. 4.100.** Summary: Lipoprotein metabolism.

### LIPID TRANSPORT

- Apart from mammary gland, intestine and liver are the only tissue which secrete particulate lipid.
- FFA are transported as complex with albumin in blood
- Lipids are rapidly removed from blood to enter:
  - Liver
  - Fat depot
  - Other tissue

### ADIPOSE TISSUE

- Major storage site for TG
- Contains up to 85% lipid

#### In fasting

- Blood glucose level and insulin levels decrease
- Glucagon levels increase

#### *Result*

- Lipolytic activity increases

  Hormone-sensitive lipase (HSL) release FFA, which enter blood and are taken up by FFA
- FFA are oxidized and KB formation occurs

### Leptin

Protein hormone produced by adipocytes, has effect on many tissues.

Hypothalamus: Regulates eating behavior, negative-feedback mechanism.

### TAG metabolism

TAG are transported from:

- Intestine in chylomicron (chm)
- Liver in VLDL

## TG catabolism

- Hydrolysis of TG yields one glycerol and 3 FFA
- Glycerol is used for energy, GNG
- Glycerol enters glycolysis
- FFA are oxidized to $CO_2$ and water via β-oxidation in mitochondria

**Remember:**
FA as such cannot be used for GNG

## Mechanism of formation of CHM & VLDL

- Apo B synthesized by ribosomes in RER and incorporated into lipoprotein (LP) in SER
- LP pass to golgi apparatus where carbohydrate residues are attached to LP
- Chm pass into spaces between intestinal cells, and finally making way into lacteals draining intestine
- VLDL secreted by hepatic cells enter into space of Disse, then into hepatic sinusoids.

## CHM & VLDL formation are similar

Nascent chm and VLDL contain little Apo C and E and take up apoproteins once they enter circulation.

## Hydrolysis of TAG & VLDL occurs by LPL

## LPL-lipoprotein lipase

- Anchored on the cell membranes in blood vessels
- Releases glycerol and FFA from chylomicron and lipoproteins
- Located on wall of blood capillaries
- Anchored to endothelium by heparin sulfate
- Require PL, apo C-II a cofactors
- Found in: Heart, adipose tissue, spleen, lung, renal medulla, aorta, diaphragm, lactating mammary gland, neonatal liver.

Chylomicrons form chylomicron remnants:

- Cholesterol rich
- Taken up by liver and FFA are metabolized there.

Lipid is repackaged in liver to VLDL

## Key enzymes in LP metabolism

- LPL: Hydrolysis of TG-rich particles
- LCAT: Participates in removal of excess cholesterol from peripheral tissues/cells

## Key receptors in LP metabolism

- LDL receptor:
  Catabolism of LDL, apo B ligand
  ABCA 1 transporter: Transports excess cholesterol from cells, apo A-1 ligand
- Scavenger receptor A1 (SR-A1): Uptake of oxidized and modified LDL by macrophages.
- SR-B1 receptors: Selective uptake of excess cholesterol from HDL apo A-1 ligand.

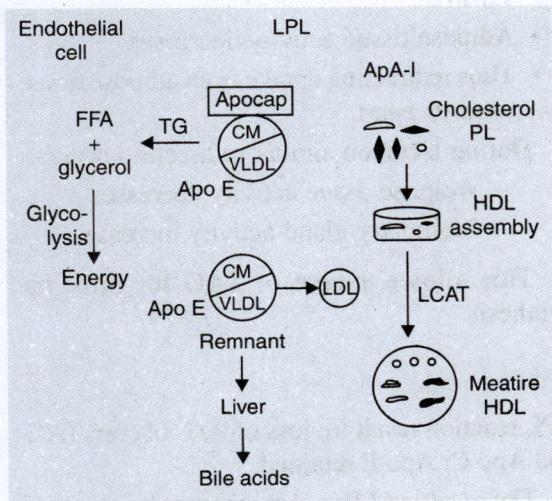

**Fig. 4.101.** LPL and LCAT.

## Other lipases

1. Hormone-sensitive lipase (HSL): Hydro-lyze TAG before uptake into extrahepatic tissues, inhibited by insulin.
2. Hepatic lipase: Found on endothelial cells of liver
   - Released from liver by heparin
   - Does not react readily with chm
   - Concerned with chm and HDL meta-bolism
   - Act as ligand to LP and hydrolyze TAG and PL

## Lipase hydrolyze TAG

TAG → DAG →→ MAG → FFA + glycerol
FFA enter circulation and bind to albumin

## Redirection of TAG

- Heart LPL: Low km of TAG
- Adipose LPL: 10 times km for TAG

As concentration of TAG decrease in transition from fed to starved condition:

- Heart enzyme remains saturated with substrate
- Adipose tissue activity decreases
- Thus redirecting uptake from adipose tissue towards heart.

During lactation similar redirection occurs:

- Adipose tissue activity decreases
- Mammary gland activity increases

This allows uptake of TAG for milk fat synthesis

## CHM remnant

LPL reaction result in: loss of 90% of chm TAG and Apo C; Apo E retained.

The resulting LP is chm remnant having half

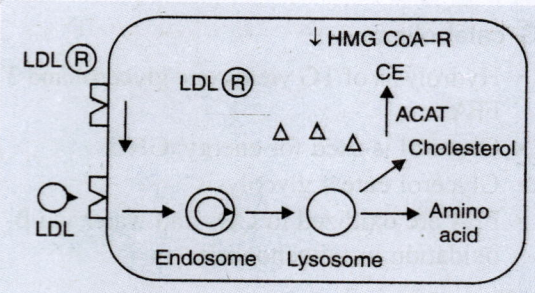

**Fig. 4.102.** LDL receptor.

LDL- ® (Apo - E ®) regulates cholesterol synthe-sis and plasma cholesterol level

diameter of parent chm, relatively enriched with C & CE.

## ELECTROPHORETIC MOBILITY OF LP

- α LP (HDL) migrate farthest towards an anode followed by
  pre-β (VLDL)
  β-LDL
- Chylomicrons remain at cathodic end (origin of electrophoretic strip)

## Cholesterol homeostasis in cell

LDL is taken by various cells by endocytosis and cholesterol in LDL is released:

- Cholesterol released from CE can be used for synthesis of cell membranes, bile salts in liver, steroid hormones in endocrine tissues.
- Cholesterol inhibits HMG CoA reductase thus decreasing rate of cholesterol synthesis by cell
- Cholesterol inhibits synthesis of LDL-R, thus reduces the amount of cholesterol taken up by cells
- Cholesterol activates ACAT which converts cholesterol to cholesterol ester for storage in cells

### Sources of intracellular cholesterol

- Newly synthesized cholesterol within the cell
- Derived from chylomicron remnants that carry cholesterol
- VLDL-LDL pathway

Intracellular cholesterol concentration is a key factor in regulating cellular cholesterol synthesis.

## LIPOPROTEIN METABOLISM

### Action of LPL on TG in CHM

- It forms chm remnants
- Chm loses 90% of TG and apo C
- Apo E retained.
- Chm remnant has half diameter of parent chm and relatively enriched with cholesterol & CE.
- In VLDL, similar changes occur with formation of VLDL remnant or IDL.

Two fates await IDL:
- Taken up by liver directly via LDL-®
- Converted to LDL

### LDL

- Derived from VLDL
- 70% degraded in liver
- 30% degraded in liver extrahepatic tissues

### LPL-metabolic gate keeper?

LPL deficiency (chylomicronaemia)

- Massive accumulation of chm-TG in plasma
- Cannot clear TG normally

LPL over expression causes:
- Decrease in plasma TG
- Increase in FA uptake in skeletal muscle, protect against obesity when fed high-fat diet

## HORMONES & ADIPOSE TISSUE

- Adipose tissue is an endocrine organ!
- Adipose tissue is not just a big fat depot; it produces a number of hormones that regulate fat storage.

**Hormones produced:** Leptin, adiponectin, resistin, ASP

**Growth factors produced:** VEGF, TNFα, 1L-6.

### 1. Leptin

Decrease food intake/increase energy utilization, intake.

### 2. Acylating stimulating protein (ASP)

- Chm stimulate production of ASP
- Anabolic effects similar to insulin
- Promote adipocyte glucose uptake and FA reesterfication.

| Hormone | Action |
|---|---|
| Leptin | Regulate food intake<br>    Energy expenditure<br>Neuroendocrine function:<br>    Decrease appetite<br>    Increase thermogenesis |
| Adiponectin | Has insulin-sensitizing effect: decreases blood glucose |

### Summary of lipoprotein functions

| Lipoprotein | Function |
|---|---|
| Chylomicron | Deliver FA as part of TAG from dietary fat to muscle, adipose tissue |
| Chylomicron remnant | Deliver dietary cholesterol to liver |
| VLDL | Deliver FA attached to TAG, derived from liver synthesis |
| LDL | Formed from VLDL delivers cholesterol, derived from liver synthesis to various tissues |
| HDL | Collects (scavenges) cholesterol from non-hepatic tissues and deli-vers to liver |

## Summary of apoproteins

| LP | Apo | Function |
|---|---|---|
| Chm | B48 | Chm formation |
| | CII | Activates LPL |
| | CIII | Transferred to remnants |
| Chm remnants | E | Binds liver receptor for remnants to enter cell |
| VLDL | B-100 | Assembly of VLDL |
| | CII | Activates LPL |
| | E | Binds LDL receptor, for VLDL to enter cell |
| LDL | B-100 | Binds LDL-R for LDL to enter cell |
| HDL | AI | Facilitates cholesterol efflux from cells |
| | CII | HDL stores it, transfer to chm/VLDL |
| | E | Binds liver ® for HDL to enter cell |

## Reverse Cholesterol Transport (RCT)

Process by which excess cholesterol in peripheral cells, especially foam cells is returned to liver for degradation and excretion.

Involves apo A-1, ABCA1 and LCAT as well as receptors on the liver for the uptake of the excess cholesterol.

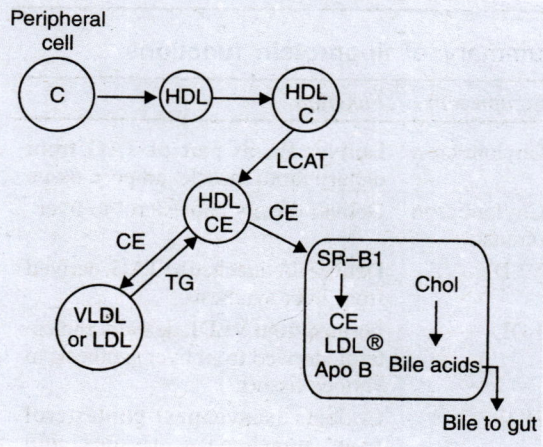

**Fig. 4.103.** Reverse cholesterol transport.

## Scavenger receptor (SR-A1)

### How macrophages deal with oxidized or modified LDL?

- The scavenger receptor recognizes modified and/or oxidized LDL and internalizes it.
- Accumulation of these modified LDL in the cell leads to accumulation of cholesterol droplets in macrophage and formation of foam cells.

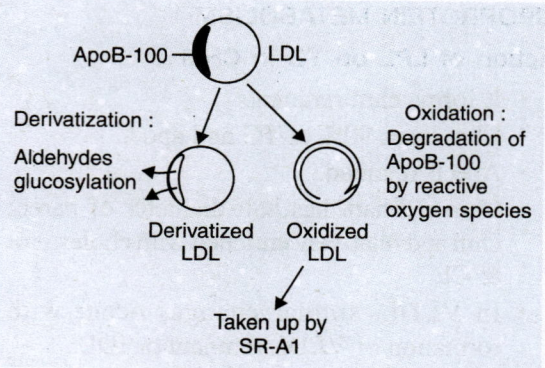

**Fig. 4.104.** Modification of LDL.

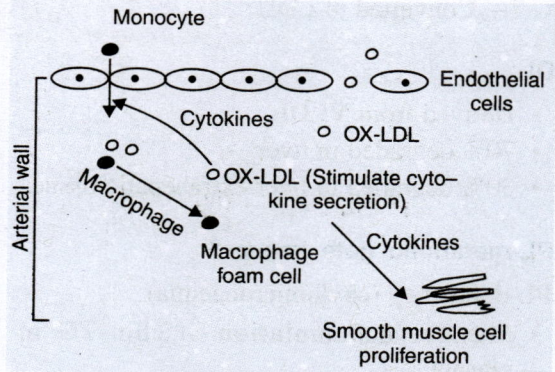

**Fig. 4.105.** LDL and atherosclerosis.

## Drugs for treatment of hyperlipoproteinemia

Statins: Target liver

Inhibit cholesterol biosynthesis

Increase LDL receptors

*Examples*: Lovastatin
Simvastatin
Atorvastatin (lipitor)

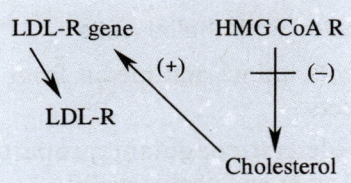

## Bile acid sequestrants

- Cholystramine
- Colestipol
- Bind and remove bile in intestine
- Increases conversion of cholesterol to bile
- Increases LDL clearance
- Lowers plasma cholesterol

## TG reducers

Fibric acid: Gemofibrozil, fenofibrate

### Mechanism

- Reduces synthesis of VLDL in liver
- Increases catabolism of VLDL
- Lowers plasma TG
- Increases HDL

## Ezetimibe

- Blocks uptake of dietary cholesterol in small intestine.
- Inhibit ABC transporter receptor on surface of intestinal absorptive cells
- Lowers plasma cholesterol
- Used with statin (lipilator): extremely powerful in reducing plasma cholesterol.

## New drugs beyond statin

- Synthetic HDL
- CETP inhibitor: Torcetrapib

## Principal enzymes in LP metabolism

| Enzyme | Substrate | Site of action |
| --- | --- | --- |
| LCAT (+apo B II) | Phosphatidylcholine, cholesterol | LP, especially nascent LDL |
| LPL (+apo CII) | TAG in VLDL and Chm | Capillary surface |
| Hepatic lipase | TAG and PL in IDL and HDL | Liver sinusoids |
| Acid lipase | TAG and CE | Lysosomes |

## LP in human disease

### LDL/HDL

LDL is enriched in cholesterol and delivers it to peripheral tissues through circulatory system:

- Cholesterol deposits in vessel wall: atherosclerosis
- HDL removes cholesterol from plasma and non hepatic cells, returning it to liver.

## Abetalipoproteinemia

- Due to lack of Apo B-100
- Patients can't synthesize chm, VLDL and LDL

### Features

- Fat malabsorption
- Accumulation of lipid droplets in enterocytes
- Spiny shaped RBCs
- Neurological disease (ataxia and retardation)

## Apo E and type III hyperlipidemia

- Defect in gene encoding Apo E
- Reduced uptake of chm and VLDL remnants
- Increased risk of atherosclerosis

## Apo E and Alzheimer's disease

Apo E gene has three common alleles:

- Apo E3 (78%), Apo E4 (15%), Apo E2 (7% population)
- Individuals with Apo E4 have 16-fold increased risk of Alzheimer's disease.

## LCAT deficiency

- Results in inability to convert cholesterol associated with HDL to CE
- Ordinarily these CE are transferred to other LP which would then be taken up by receptors in liver.
- Thus, for continued removal of cholesterol from periphery, LDL is required.

- Results in defects in kidney, RBC and cornea of eye.

## ATHEROSCLEROSIS

### Functions of endothelial cells

- Protects intima and media from foreign invaders
- Provide anticoagulant properties for platelets or endothelial wall
- Prevent adhesion of leukocytes or platelets to the wall of artery
- Control of tissue permeability, allowing specific molecules to pass through endothelium (i.e., LDL)

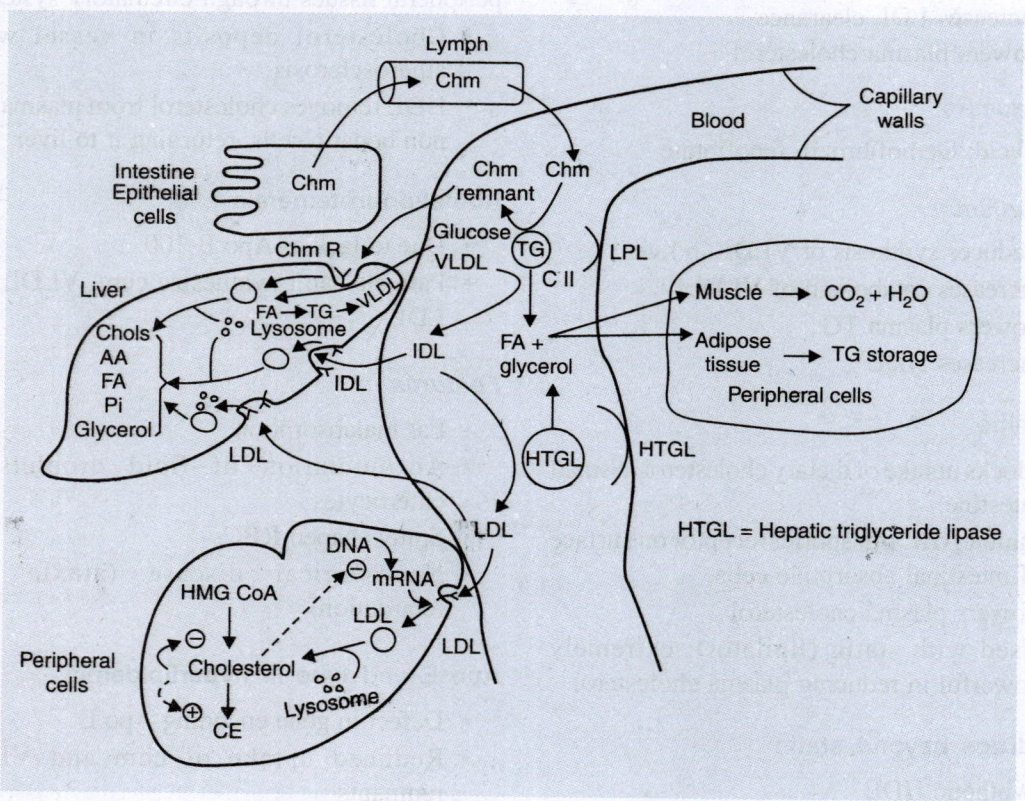

**Fig. 4.106.** Lipoprotein metabolism.

- Production of vasodilating molecules such as nitric oxide to keep the artery patent

### Factors that can cause endothelial dysfunction

- Modified LDL
- Homocysteine
- Free radicals
- Infection
- Hypertension
- Once the endothelium is irritated, an inflammatory response follows.
- Ist phase of inflammatory response is increased permeability to lipoproteins and other plasma constituents.

  Permeability of endothelium is controlled by:
  - Nitric oxide
  - $PGI_2$
  - Platelet derived growth factor (PDGF)
  - Angiotensin II
  - Endothelin

### Lipoporteins are primary intruders via increased endothelial permeability

- Primary lipoprotein passing through endothelial barrier is LDL
- Oxidized LDL too becomes irritant for endothelium
- At the same time, leukocyte adherence to endothelium increase.
- Once leukocytes adhere to endothelial wall, they migrate into artery wall.
- Along with increased leukocytes adhesion, platelets adhesion is increased.
- Monocytes engulf the oxidized LDL molecules to foam cells
- Foam cells occlude the artery

### Platelet aggregation releases several factors

- Serotonin
- Clotting factors
- PG
- Enzymes
- Myogenic factors
- PDGF

### Atherosclerotic lesion formation

- Growth factors from platelet and other inflammatory players cause smooth muscle fibers to proliferate and migrate from intima to media
- Excess smooth muscle proliferation protrudes into lumen of artery
- Increased smooth muscle, foam cells and other debris protrude into lumen of artery, creating atherosclerotic lesion.
- Advanced lesion contains a fibrous cap which can wall off the lesion from the lumen.
- Fibrous cap becomes calcified.
- Inflammatory process continues as long as endothelial irritation persist
- Partial occlusion of artery lumen produces ischemia and total occlusion produces tissue infarction.

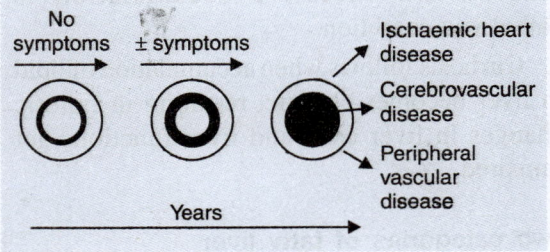

**Fig. 4.107.** Time course of atherogenesis: chronic to acute atheroma

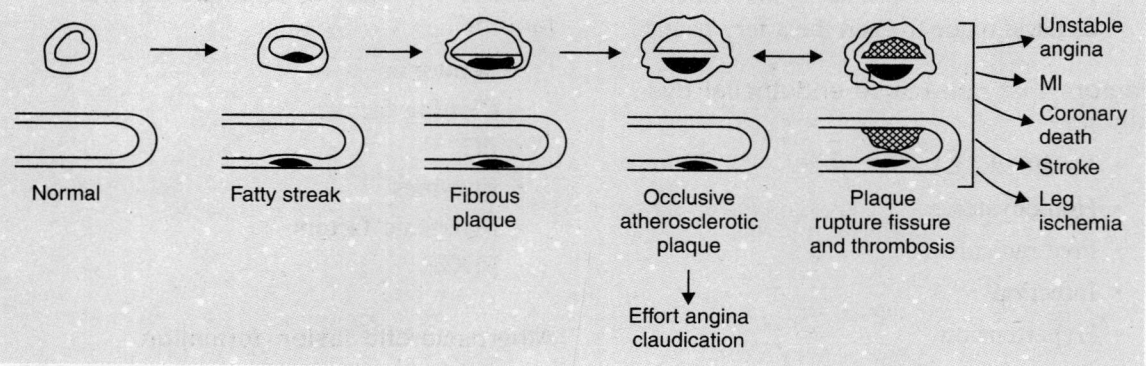

**Fig. 4.108.** Atherosclerosis process.

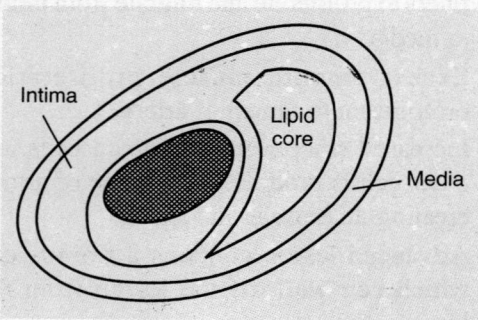

**Fig. 4.109.** Anatomy of plaque

- Artery health is key to control and prevent hypertension, heart disease and stroke.

## FATTY LIVER

TG can accumulate in liver for a variety of reasons and excessive accumulation is pathologic condition.

Cirrhosis follows when accumulation of lipid in liver becomes chronic, resulting in fibrotic changes in liver cells and liver functions get impaired.

## Two categories of fatty liver

1. Associated with raised plasma FFA:
   Results from fat mobilization from adipose tissue or TG hydrolysis by LPL in extrahepatic tissues.

   When production of VLDL does not keep pace with increasing influx and esterification of FFA: this allows TG to accumulate causing fatty liver, seen in starvation and high fat diet.

2. Due to metabolic block in production of plasma lipoprotein causing TG to accumulate.

**Theoretically fatty liver can be due to :**

- Block in apolipoprotein synthesis
- Block in synthesis of LP from lipid and apolipoprotein
- Failure in provision of PL for LP synthesis.
- Failure in secretory mechanism
- In rats: deficiency of choline (lipotropic factor)
- Puromycin
- Ethionine
- Carbon tetrachloride
- Chloroform
- Phosphorus
- Lead
- Arsenic

## Carbon tetrachloride

- Causes lipid peroxidation
- Vitamin E supplementation protects against this.

## Pathogenesis: Causes of fat accumulation

- Hepatic steatosis: It is TG accumulation in liver
- Excessive import of FFA from tissues to liver:
- Diminished fat export by VLDL
- Increased delivery (obesity)
- Excessive conversion of carbohydrate and protein to fat.
- Impaired VLDL synthesis
- Impaired beta oxidation

## Liver is highly susceptible to toxicity

- 60% of liver failure is due to toxicity
- 2-4% of jaundice are associated with drugs.

## Main problems

- Loss of functional liver cells by cell death
- Impaired bile flow
- Faulty fat processing
- Liver toxicity can be predicted by blood parameters namely bilirubin, AST, ALT, GGT

## Functional asymmetry in liver

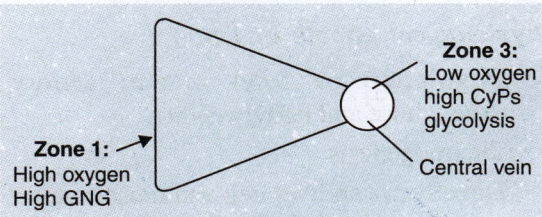

**Fig. 4.110.** Functional asymmetry in liver.

## Essential fatty acid

- Omega 3 – linolenic acid
- Omega 6 – linoleic acid

### Functions

- Formation of healthy cell membrane
- Proper development and functioning of brain and nervous system.
- Production of hormone like substances: eicosanoids:

  Thromboxane, prostaglandin, leukotriene which are responsible for regulating blood pressure, blood viscosity, vasoconstriction, immune and inflammatory response.

### Sources

- Eicospentaenoic acid (EPA)
  Fish liver oil, fish, egg
- ω-3:
  Source: Walnut wheat germ oil, flax seed/canola oil, fish liver oil, fish, egg, human milk

  *Benefits:*
  - Lower $PG_2$
  - Anti inflammatory
  - Low TG and cholesterol
  - Prevent cancer
  - Maintain kidney
  - Increase insulin sensitivity
  - Enhance thrombogenesis and lipid metabolism
  - Inhibit platelet adhesion
  - PGE for placental development
  - PGF causes leuteolysis
- ω-6:
  *Source*: Corn oil, peanut oil, cotton seed oil, soybean oil

*Benefit*: Reduce inflammation in rheumatoid arthritis:
- Relieve discomfort of premenstrual tension, endometriosis and fibrocystic breasts
- Reduce symptoms of eczema, psoriasis
- Clear up acne and rosacea
- Prevent and improve diabetic neuropathy

**EFA deficiency causes:**
- Hemorrhagic dermatitis
- Skin atrophy
- Scaly dermatitis
- Dry skin
- Weakness
- Impaired vision
- Tingling sensation
- High blood pressure
- High TG
- Immune deficiency
- Hematological disturbances
- Impaired growth.

## Who are at risk for deficiency?
- Patients on long term total parenteral nutrition (TPN)
- Cystic fibrosis
- Low birth weight infant
- Premature infants
- Severally malnourished patients
- Patients with fat malabsorption

## Disease where EFA deficiency can occur
- Acrodermatitis Enteropathica
- Hepatorenal syndrome
- Sjogren syndrome
- Crohn's disease
- Cirrhosis and alcoholism

- Reye's syndrome
- Short bowel syndrome

## Triene: Tetraene (T/T) Ratio

T/T ratio is marker used to diagnose EFA deficiency.

*Characterized by*:
- A decrease of arachidonic acid (C20:4)
- An increase of Mead's acid (C20:3: produced in excess during EFA deficiency)
- T/T > 0.4 is EFA deficiency

*Recommendations*:
- EFA requirement is 1 to 2% of dietary calories for adults.
- 0.2 to 1% of total calories should be provided by ω-3 fatty acids.

## Leptin
- 16KDa protein encoded by ob gene
- Expressed and secreted by adipocyte, placenta, gastric epithelium.
- Directly proportional to total amount of fat in the body.
- Member of helical cytokine family, composed of four antiparallel helices, each about 5-6 turn long.
- Leptin receptor is homologous to cytokine receptor and activates JAK/STAT
- Acts via P1-3 kinase signaling pathway

## Physiological effects of leptin
- Regulation of food intake, energy expenditure and body weight.
- Thermogenesis
- Directly act on liver cell and muscle cells
- Related to inflammatory response
- Contribute to early hematopoiesis

## Role of leptin in regulation of food intake & body weight

- Decrease hunger and food consumption inhibits neuropeptide Y synthesis
- Food intake linked to its ability to regulate neuroendocrine system.

### Effect on lipid metabolism

- Activate AMP
- Activate protein kinase
- Inhibit acetyl CoA carboxylase (ACC)
- Increase FA oxidation
- Reduce fat tissue in muscle and liver
- Increase insulin sensitivity

## Regulation of leptin expression

Two transcription factors:

- PPAR γ-promote leptin expression
- C/EBP- decrease leptin expression
- Environmental and hormonal factors regulate leptin expression.
- Intake of food trigger output of gluco-corticoids and insulin that favors fat accumulation and increase leptin
- Leptin travels to hypothalamus and regulate body mass, body energy intake and energy expenditure.
- Hypothalamic insensitivity to leptin is fundamental mechanism of obesity.

## Leptin resistance

- Mutation of gene for leptin receptors in brain occurs
- Post receptor abnormalities in leptin signal transduction
- Impaired leptin transport across blood-brain barrier.

## PPAR

- Peroxisome proliferator-activated receptors.
- Nuclear hormone receptor super family α, β, γ, δ
- Unique tissue distribution

| PPAR | Activators |
|------|------------|
| α | FA (derivatives), Hypolipidemic drugs (fibrates), Industrial solvents |
| β | PGI$_2$, Thiozoladinediones (TDZ) (Troglitazone) |
| δ | FA, FA derivative |

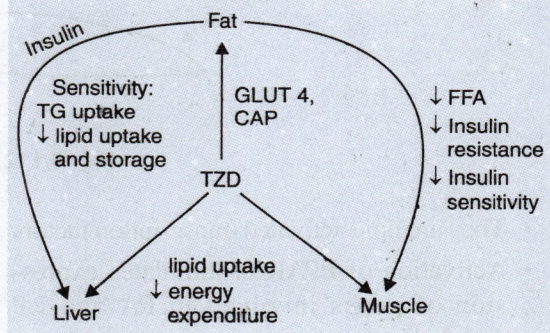

**Fig. 4.111.** PPAR actions.

| PPAR | Organ | Function |
|------|-------|----------|
| PPAR α | Liver, kidney, heart, muscle | Liver FA catabolism target of lipid lowering fibrate |
| PPAR β | Adipose tissue | Adipose FA catabolism Potential lipid lowering target, participates in brain lipid metabolism and affects proliferation and differentiation of adipocyte |
| PPAR γ | Brown and white adipose tissue | Adipose tissue differentiation , Target of TZD, Affects cells differentiation, insulin action and FA synthesis (+) TG synthesis and storage. |

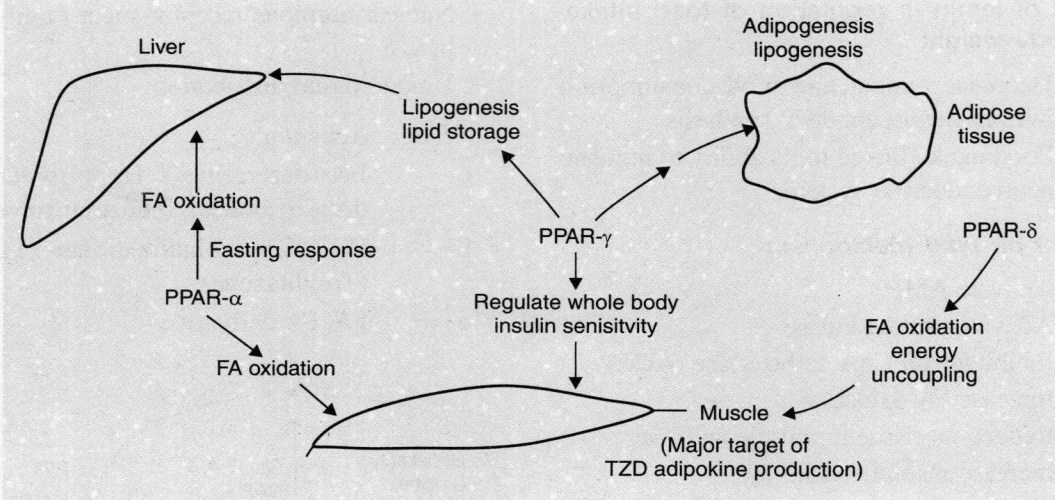

**Fig. 4.112.** TZD action.

- They are lipid activated transcription factors
- Activation of PPAR α-stimulates expression of genes involved in FA and LP metabolism.
- PPAR-α activators such as fibrates decrease TAG by increasing expression of Apo A-I and A-II.
- PPAR-α activation by fibrates improves insulin sensitivity and decrease thrombosis and vascular inflammation.

## LXR

Liver X-receptors

- Regulate genes involved in cholesterol metabolism, FA metabolism
- Has nuclear receptors like PPAR
- Act as transcription factor
- Possesses DNA – binding domain and ligand binding domain.
- PPAR and LXR form heterodimers: PPAR/RXR, LXR/RXR with retinoid receptors RXR.

## TAG biosynthesis

- In the final stage of lipogenesis, TAG are synthesized by addition of two fatty acyl CoA to glycerol-3-phosphate to form phosphatidic acid. This is the hydrolyzed to diacylglycerol which gets acylated to TAG.
- In post absorptive state, TAG is synthesized in liver. This TAG is then exported in

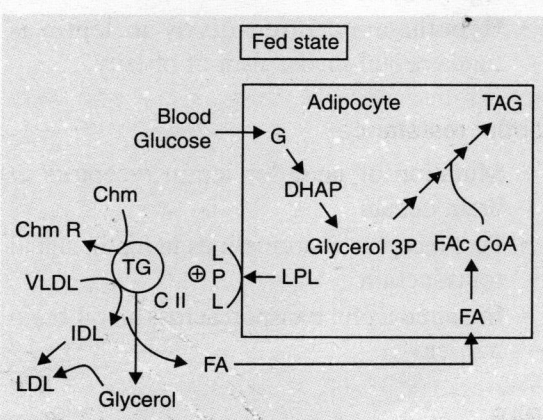

**Fig. 113.** Formation of TAG in adipocyte.

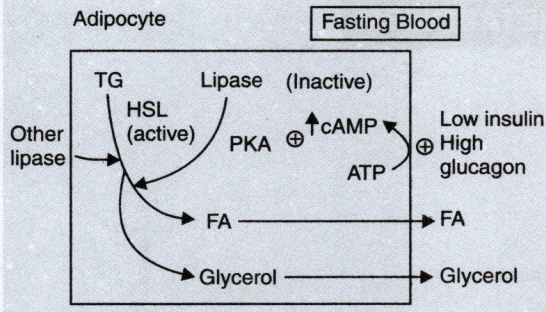

**Fig. 114.** Mobilization of adipocyte TAG.

lipoproteins (VLDL) and finally stored in adipose tissue.

### Storage of fats

- Fatty acids in diet or produced by *denovo* synthesis are stored and transported as triacylglycerol (triglycerides, TG)

- In liver, TG are produced from glycerol-3-phosphate and phosphatidic acid. This glycerol-3-P is formed by glycerol by action of glycerol kinase.

- In adipose tissue, glucose (via DHAP) is source of glycerol-3-phosphate, since adipocytes lack a glycerol kinase enzyme.

- Thus, storage of TG in adipocyte occurs only when glycolysis is active in fed state.

### Mobilization of lipid during GNG and work

Direction and rate of glucose and glycogen metabolism in liver is controlled by following hormones:

- Insulin
- Glucagon
- Epinephrine
- Cortisol

During fasting and starvation, there is:

a. Activation of hepatic GNG by glucagon: precursors for this GNG come from:

(i) Muscle: protein degradation which releases amino acids.

(ii) Adipose tissue: TG lipolysis releases FFA and glycerol.
HSL in adipocytes is activated by glucagon
Remember: Insulin inhibits both GNG and lipolysis.

b. Lipolysis is stimulated by glucagon which provides inputs to GNG. Also, there is increased concentration of FFA, glycerol and ketone bodies.

### Lipid metabolism in alcoholism

- Alcohol metabolism produces increased amount of NADH which inhibits FA oxidation.

- Since oxidation of fats is inhibited, FA reaching liver (dietary or mobilized from adipocytes) get reesterified with glycerol to form TG.

*Result*:

- Raised VLDL and TG in serum
- Later stage, liver damage starts and there is failure to produce lipoproteins and TG accumulate in liver causing fatty liver.

### Regulation of total body fat stores:

Adiposity signals regulate total body stores.

Excess dietary proteins results in:

- Oxidation for energy
- Conversion into fat for storage
- Amino acids must be deaminated prior to oxidation for energy.

### Dynamic state of body

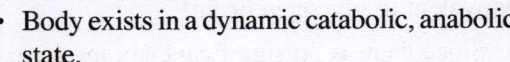

- Body exists in a dynamic catabolic, anabolic state.

- Organic molecules are continuously broken down and rebuilt.

- The body's total supply of nutrients constitutes its nutrient pool.

# 3. AMINO ACID METABOLISM

## INTRODUCTION

### Sources and fate of amino acids

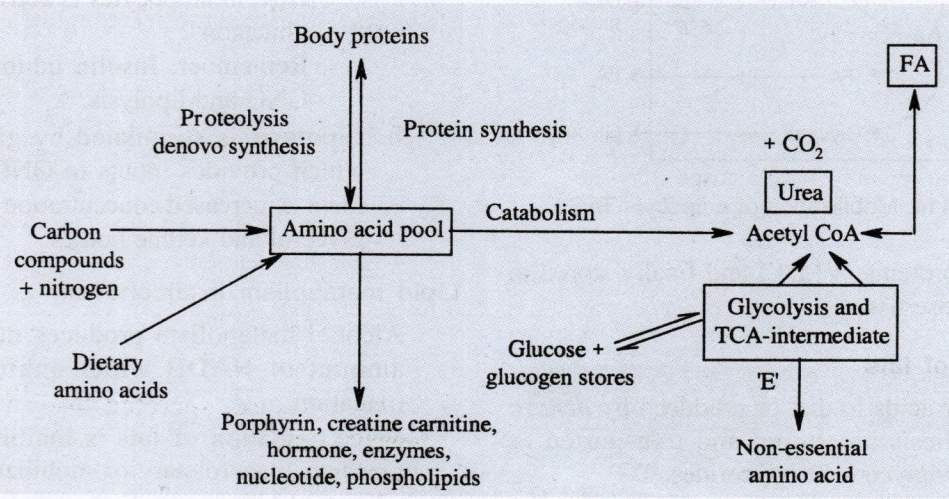

## Amino acids

Amino acids are building blocks for peptides and proteins.

They are precursors of:
- Neurotransmitter
- Hormones

They are source of energy:
- Under normal conditions, not used for 'E' production.
- Glucogenic amino acids form glucose via GNG: occurs under extended fast.

**Remember:** Unlike carbohydrate and lipids, amino acids do not have a dedicated storage form equivalent to glycogen or fat!

Since there is no significant storage form of nitrogen or amino compounds in humans, nitrogen metabolism is dynamic and balance between nitrogen ingestion and secretion is normally maintained.

Amino acids when metabolized, release nitrogen and carbon skeletons.

Excess nitrogen is removed in form of ammonia which is converted to urea. Urea is neutral, less toxic and very soluble to be excreted in urine.

>80% nitrogen is excreted in form of urea. About 25-30 g/d is excreted as urea in urine.

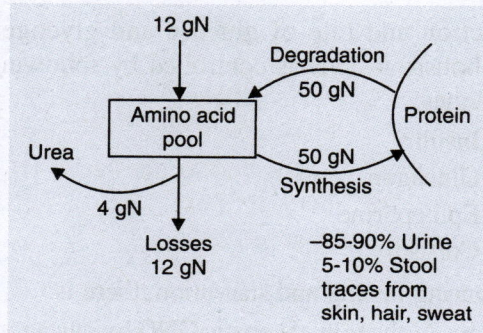

**Fig. 4.115.** Nitrogen excretion.

Small amount is excreted as: uric acid, creatinine, ammonium ion.

## Essential amino acids

Must be supplied in diet and cannot be synthesized in body.

### *METTVILPHLY!*

Methionine, Threonine, Tryptophan, Valine, Isoleucine, Leucine Phenylalanine, Lysine.

## Non essential amino acids

Not required in diet and can be synthesized in the body.

## (i) Digestion and Absorption

### Sources of amino acids

- Exogenous: Dietary proteins.
- Endogenous: breakdown of defective and unneeded cellular proteins.

### *Digestion*

- Digestion of protein begins in stomach with the action of pepsin.
- In small intestine, pancreatic secretions act on contents emptied by stomach, releasing free amino acids that are being transported to portal vein.

### Pepsin

- Produced as inactive zymogen pepsinogen by chief cells in stomach
- Pepsinogen is activated to pepsin by $H^+$, pepsin itself (autocatalysis)
- Pepsin is active at pH 2.0

In intestine, protein digestion begins by enzymes:
- Serine protease

- Trypsin
- Chymotrypsin
- Elastase
- Carboxy peptidase

Enzymes in pancreatic secretion are:
*Endopeptidase*:
- Trypsin
- Chymotrypsin
- Elastase

*Exopeptidase*:
- Carboxy peptidase

### Activation of trypsinogen

- Enterokinase
- Endopeptidase, secreted by intestinal mucosa
- Hydrolyzes a lysine peptide bond in zymogen, releases a small peptide from trypsinogen, allowing the molecule to unfold as active trypsin.
- Once trypsin is formed, it will attack additional molecules of trypsinogen and other zymogens namely, chymotrypsinogen, proelastase, procarboxy peptidase.

### Characteristics of proteolytic enzymes:
- Synthesized as zymogen
- Activated by enterokinase.

### Activation of zymogen

| Zymogen | Active form | Bond specificity |
|---|---|---|
| Trypsinogen | Trypsin | Basic amino acid |
| Chymo-trypsinogen | Chymotrypsin | Aromatic amino acid |
| Proelastase | Elastase | Broad specificity |
| Pro carboxy peptidase | Carboxy peptidase | Carboxy Terminal (exopeptidase) |

## Site of action of proteolytic enzymes

| Enzyme | Site |
|---|---|
| Trypsin | Peptide bond of basic amino acid (lys, arg) |
| Chymotrypsin | Peptide bond of aromatic amino acid |
| Elastase | Broad specificity: attack bonds next to small amino acid residues such as alanine, glycine, serine |

## Intestinal secretions complete the digestive process

Enzymes of small intestine are:

- Endopeptidase
- Exopeptidase
- Amino peptidase
- Dipeptidase

These enzymes complete the digestion of peptides and dipeptides to free amino acids which are then absorbed.

| Enzyme | Mechanism of action |
|---|---|
| Carboxy peptidase | Exopeptidase, attack carboxy terminal peptide releases single amino acid |
| Amino peptidase | Exopeptidase attack peptide bond next to amino terminal |
| Dipeptidase | Digest dipeptides to free amino acids |

Also, proteins are broken down to amino acids and oligopeptides in intestinal lumen. Free amino acids and dipeptides enter enterocyte, and finally enter blood stream (Fig. 4.116).

## ABSORPTION

### Fact file: digestion of proteins

- Dietary proteins are almost completely digested (by endo – and exo peptidase)

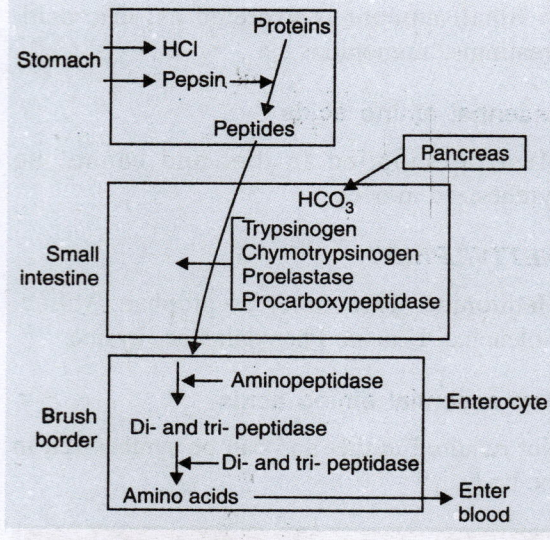

Fig. 4.116. Digestion of proteins.

- End products of digestion are absorbed across enterocyte membrane by carrier-mediated membrane transport.
- 50-100g proteins are lost in feces

## Absorption of amino acids

- Natural L-isomer of amino acids are actively absorbed
- At brush – border transporter are present:
  - Na – dependent symporters
  - H dependent symporters

This transport is 'E' dependent and may require pyridoxal phosphate.

| Symporter | Amino acids |
|---|---|
| Neutral amino acid | Ser, Thr, Ala |
| Neutral amino acid with aromatic amino acid side chain | Phen, Tyr, Met, Val, Leu, Ile |
| Imino acid | Proline, Hydroxyproline |
| Basic amino acid | Lys, Arg, Cys |
| Acid amino acid | Asp, Glu |
| β amino acid | β-alanine, taurine |

## Gamma glutamyl cycle

Located in cell membrane:

- Group transfer transport system for amino acid
- Utilizes 3 ATP to transport a single amino acid
- Functions in kidney mainly.
- Operative for transport of cysteine and glutamine.
- Important for metabolism of GSH

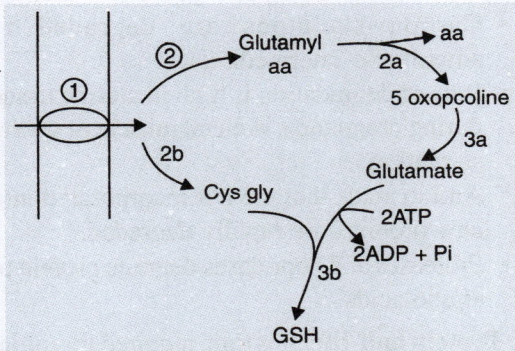

**Fig. 4.117.** Gamma glutanyl cycle.

### Steps

1. Enzyme glutamyl transpeptidase is located in membrane and shuttles GSH to cell surface to interact with amino acid.
2. a. γ-Glutamyl amino acid is transported into cell and hydrolyzes to liberate amino acid (aa) and oxyproline
   b. Cysteinyl is cleaved to its component amino acid.
3. To regenerate GSH, glutamate is reformed from 5 oxoproline and 2 ATP are required in this reaction.

### Clinical implications: Absorption

Absorption of undigested polypeptides may cause antigenic reactions.

| Disease | Defect |
|---|---|
| Nontropical sprue | Gluten absorption |
| Celiac disease | Protein and amino acid absorption |
| Hartnup disease | Neutral amino acid carrier defect |

### Hartnup disease

Defect in transport of neutral amino acid.

*Features*: **Pellagra:**
- Due to deficiency of niacin (which may be synthesized from tryptophan)

**Cystinuria:** Defect in transport of basic amino acid cysteine

*Features*: Cystine crystal deposition

**Glycinuria:** Defect in transport of glycine and imino acid proline and hydroxy proline.

*Features*: increased excretion of these amino acid, no clinical abnormalities.

## (ii) Removal and Addition of Amino Acid 'N'

### Catabolism of proteins and amino acid nitrogen (Fig. 4.118)

### Protein balance

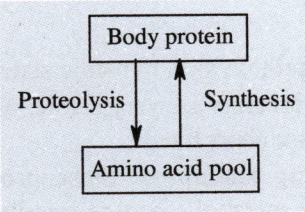

### Positive balance

Protein synthesis > degradation e.g., growth, body building

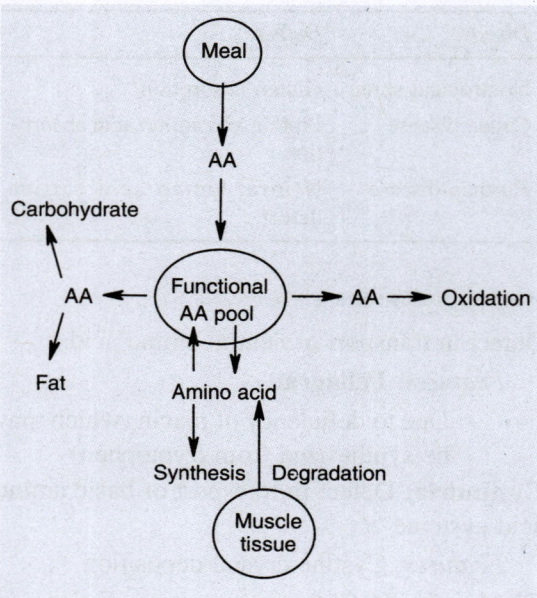

**Fig. 4.118.** Protein metabolism.

## Negative balance

Protein synthesis < degradation e.g. Starvation, trauma, cancer cachexia

## PROTEIN TURNOVER

- Protein turnover involves both synthesis and degradation of proteins
- Key physiologic process in all live forms
- Takes place in all life forms, all cell types constantly.

## Fact-file

- Body protein is in dynamic state
- Some proteins are very stable, while many other are short lived.
- Altering amount of these proteins can change metabolic pattern rapidly
- Cells have mechanism for detecting and removing damaged cells
- Even a significant proportion of newly synthesized proteins are defective

- Proteins that are first synthesized as normal protein may undergo oxidative damage.
- Removal of senescent, damaged, abnormal and oxidatively damaged protein is part of protein turnover.
- Adults degrade 1-2% of their total body protein, principally muscle protein.
- About 1-2% of total body proteins degraded daily
- 75-80% of amino acids liberated are reutilized for protein synthesis
- 20-25% remaining nitrogen forms urea
- Carbon skeletons are degraded to amphibolic intermediates.
- Rate of degradation is high in uterine tissue during pregnancy, skeletal muscle in severe starvation
- Amino acids that are not incorporated into new proteins are rapidly degraded.
- Proteases and peptidases degrade protein to amino acids.

**Protein half-life**: It is time required for initial amount of protein to be reduced to half.

Susceptibility to degradation is expressed as half life (t½).

| Protein /enzyme | t ½ |
|---|---|
| Liver proteins | 30 min–150 hr |
| Tryptophan oxygenase, Tyrosine transaminase, HMG CoA-R | 0.5–2 hr |
| LDH, Cyt, aldolase | >100 hr |

## Tissue protein half life

| Type of tissue | t ½ |
|---|---|
| Muscle proteins | 160 d |
| Body proteins | 80 d |
| Liver proteins | 6 d |
| LDH, cytochrome | >100h |
| HMG CoA-R | <2h |
| Oncogene product | <2h |

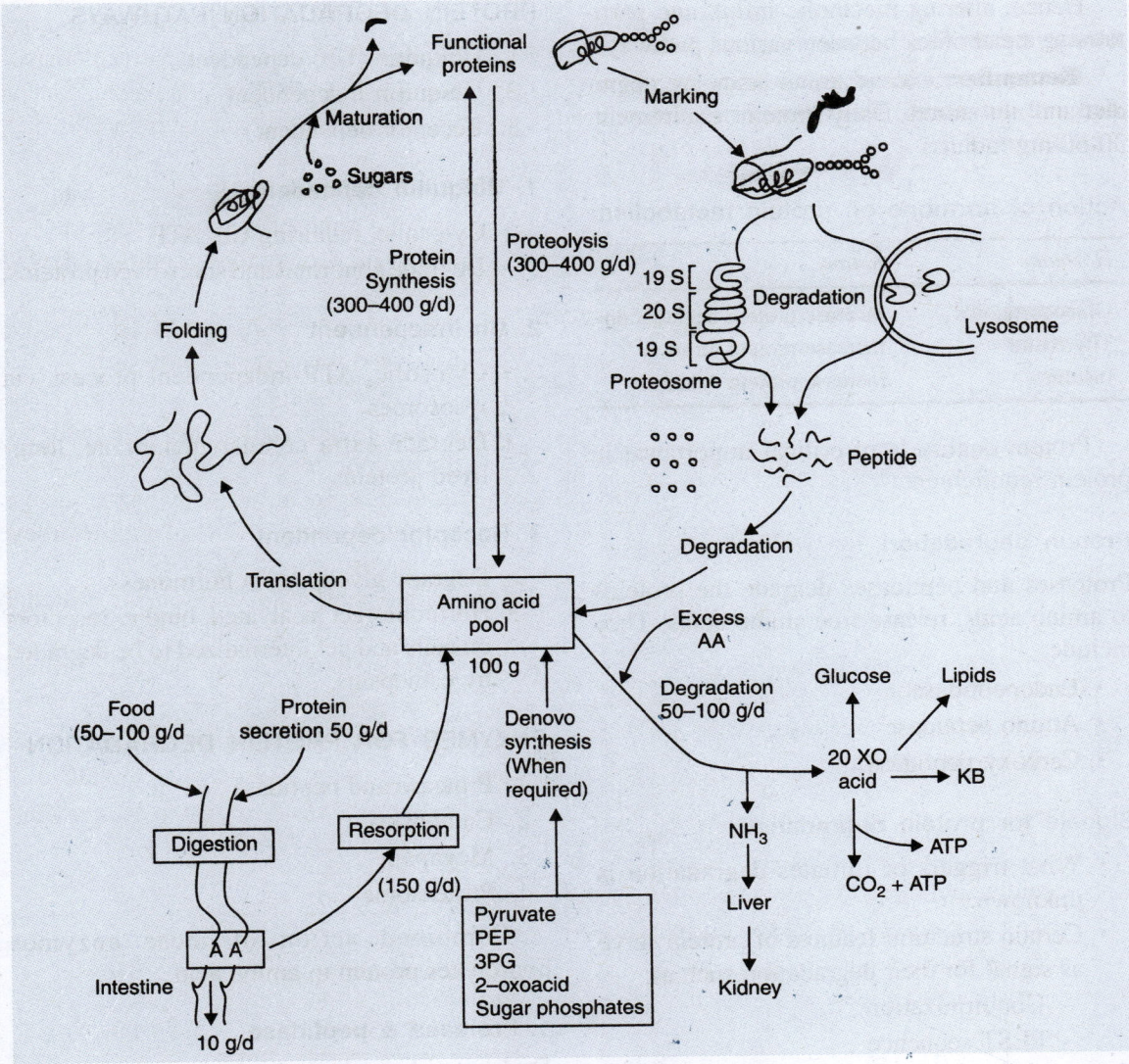

**Fig. 4.119.** Overview of protein metabolism.

## PEST sequence

Proteins with short half lives have PEST sequence regions rich in amino acids:

- Proline (P)
- Glutamine (E)
- Serine (S)
- Threonine (T)

These sequences target them for rapid degradation.

According to physiologic demand, degradation of key regulated enzyme may be:

- Accelerated
- Retained
- Altering enzyme level

Hence, altering metabolic influx and partitioning metabolites between various pathways.

**Remember:** excess amino acids are degraded and not stored. Daily protein requirement: 30-60 mg (adults)

## Action of hormone on protein metabolism

| Hormone | Action |
|---|---|
| Glucocorticoids | Increase protein degradation |
| Thyroxine | Increase protein turnover |
| Insulin | Increase protein synthesis |

Protein quality is of critical importance in protein requirement.

## Protein degradation

Proteases and peptidases degrade the proteins to amino acids, release free amino acids. They include:

- Endopeptidase
- Amino peptidase
- Carboxy peptidase

## Signals for protein degradation

- What triggers or initiates degradation is unknown.
- Certain structural features of protein serve as signal for their degradation such as:
  - Ubiquitinization
  - PEST sequence
  - N-terminal amino acids e.g. arginine, lysine, phenylalanine, aspartate oxidized amino acids

## What is the purpose of protein degradation

- Removal of abnormal, defective, damaged protein
- Removal of inducible enzyme after its action.

## PROTEIN DEGRADATION PATHWAYS

1. Ubiquitin (Ub) dependent
2. Ubiquitin independent
3. Receptor dependent

### 1. Ubiquitin dependent

- Cytosolic, requiring Ub, ATP
- Degrade abnormal and short-lived proteins.

### 2. Ub independent

- Cytosolic, ATP-independent process via lysosomes
- Degrade extra cellular membrane, long-lived proteins

### 3. Receptor dependent

- Degrade glycoprotein hormones
- Hormones get asialyated, bind to receptors on cells and get internalized to be degraded by cathepsins.

## ENZYMES FOR PROTEIN DEGRADATION

1. Protease and peptidase
2. Cathepsins
3. Megapain
4. Proteasome

Combined action of these enzymes hydrolyzes protein to amino acid.

### 1. Protease & peptidase

**Endopeptidases include:**

- Trypsin
- Chymotrypsin
- Elastase
- Calpain
- Collagenase

**Exopeptidases include:**

- Carboxy peptidase
- Amino peptidase

## 2. Cathepsins

They degrade intracellular proteins and glycoprotein hormone

## 3. Megapain

- HMM protease found in liver, muscle, retics.
- Degrade protein in presence of Ub.

## 4. Proteasome

- Cytosolic, has multicatalytic function.
- Eukaryotic system for protein modification had evolved from pre-existing prokaryotic pathway for coenzyme biosynthesis (proteasome).

## UBIQUITIN (Ub)

- Ub targets intracellular proteins for degradation
- 8.5 kDa protein, present in all eukaryotic cells.

Ub conjugation involves three enzymes:

- E1: Ub activating enzyme
- E2: Ub conjugating enzyme
- E3: Ub protein ligase

## 1. E1

- $Ub\ COOH + E1 - SH + ATP \rightarrow AMP + PPi + UbCO\text{-}S\text{-}E1$

Terminal carboxyl group of Ub forms thioester bond with $\varepsilon$ group of lysyl residue in protein $\varepsilon1$.

## 2. E2

- $Ub\ CO\text{-}S\text{-}E1 + E2 - SH \rightarrow E1\text{-}SH + UbCO\text{-}S\text{-}E2$
- $Ub\text{-}CO\text{-}S\text{-}E2 + 2HN - \varepsilon\ Protein \rightarrow E2 - SH + Ub\text{-}CO\text{-}NH\text{-}\ \varepsilon\ protein$

Thioester exchange reaction transfer Ub to E2.

## 3. E3

Catalyzes transfer of Ub to $\varepsilon$ lysyl group of target protein.

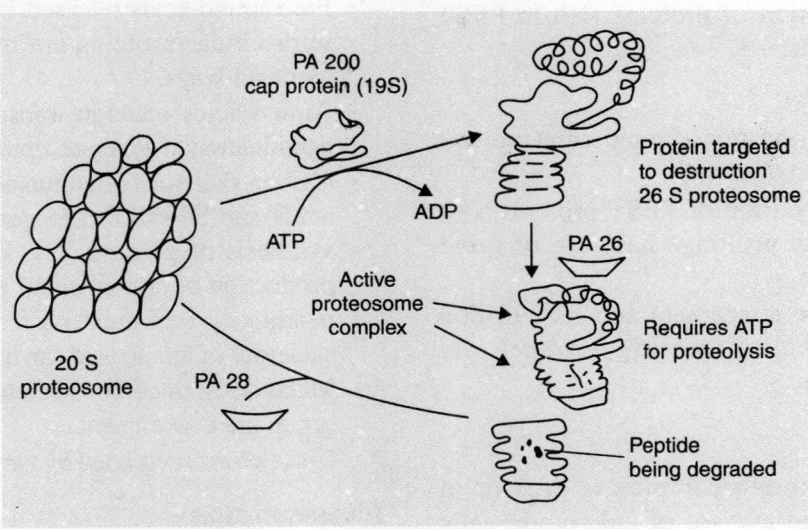

**Fig. 4.120.** Proteosome and proton degradation.

## Many biological functions are regulated by protein degradation

Protein degradation exert control by altering stability and abundance of regulatory proteins e.g. NF-κB.

## Process regulated by protein degradation

- Gene transcription
- Cell cycle progression
- Organ formation
- Circadian rhythm
- Inflammatory response
- Tumor suppression
- Cholesterol metabolism
- Antigen processing

Some disease – causing viruses target host cell proteins for degradation in proteasome by either activating Ub ligase to ubiquitinate host protein or encoding their own Ub ligase.

## Regulation of ubiquitination

- Some proteins regulate or facilitate Ub conjugation.
- Phosphorylation of PEST domains activates ubiquitination of proteins rich in PEST amino acids:

Regulation by:

- Phosphorylation of some target proteins has been observed
- Glycosylation of PEST proteins with GlcNAc prolongs half-life of these proteins
- GlcNAc attachment acts as nutrition sensor by increasing extracellular glucose

## Proteasome

- A large protein complex is present in nucleus and cytosol of eukaryotic cells which encloses a cavity with three compartment joined by narrow passage ways.
- Proteasome core complex has 20S sedimentation coefficient, contains two each of different polypeptides:
  - 7A type proteins: form each of two A rings at the cylindrical structure
  - 7B type proteins: form each of two central B rings

Protease activity is associated with 3 of the β subunits, each having different substrate specificity.

## Protein catabolism

Protein catabolism occurs when:

- Dietary protein intake exceeds requirement
- Composition of absorbed amino acids is unbalanced.
- GNG is increased

General rule is that there is loss of amino group followed by catabolism of C-skeletons in central pathway (TCA, glycolysis, ketone body).

## Metabolism of amino acids

- Free amino acids released from dietary or intracellular proteins are metabolized in identical ways.
- Amino acids undergo transamination and deamination to generate ammonia and urea.
- Carbon skeletons of amino acids from keto acids can be utilized to generate energy, synthesis of glucose, FA, ketone bodies, production of non essential amino acids.
- α-amino group must be removed before skeletons of amino acid can be metabolized.
- Metabolism of carbon skeletons and amino group are coordinated.
- C-skeleton is degraded by various pathways

## Transamination

Removal of amino group from amino acid to a

suitable keto acceptor, common keto acid are: αKG, OAA.

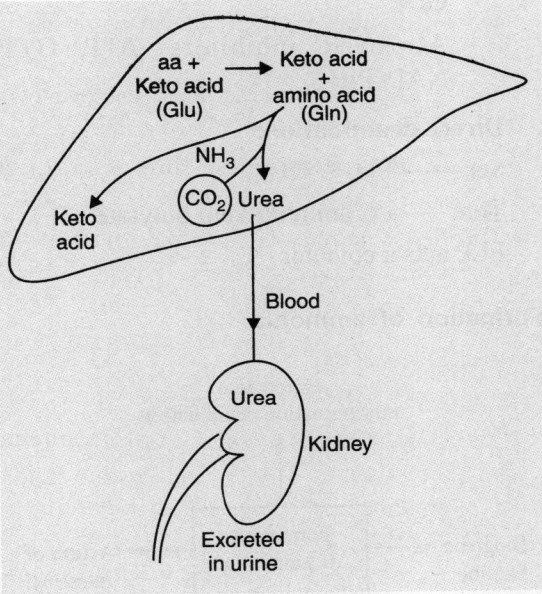

**Fig. 4.121. Transamination.**

- It interconverts a pair of α amino acid and a pair of α keto acids.
- Most amino acids undergo transamination
  *Except*:
  - Lysine
  - Threonine
  - Proline, Hydroxyproline

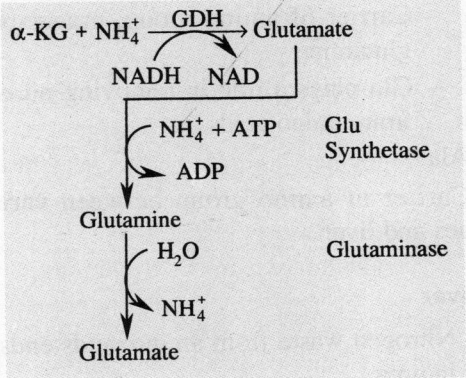

**Glutamine synthetase:** fixes $NH_3$ as glutamine and $NH_3$ is rapidly removed from circulation by liver

### Metabolic flow of amino 'N'

Amino acid derived 'N' is metabolized by sequential action of:
- Amino transferase
- GDH (glutamate dehydrogenase)
- Urea Cycle

Nitrogen atoms are incorporated in urea from two sources:
- Glutamate (GDH reaction)
- Aspartate

$$\text{Aspartate + Citrulline}$$
$$\downarrow$$
$$\text{Arginino – succinate}$$
$$\downarrow$$
$$\text{Fumarate + arginine}$$

### GDH

Glutamate dehydrogenase:
- Ubiquitous enzyme
- Uses either NAD or NADP
- Occupies a central position in 'N' metabolism
- Catabolically channels 'N' from glutamate to urea
- Anabolically, channels amination of αKG by free amino acid.

$$NAD(P) \longleftarrow \qquad \longrightarrow NADPH + H^+$$
$$\text{L-Glu} \qquad \alpha KG \qquad NH_3$$

### Transamination

- Freely reversible
- Can function in both amino acid catabolism and synthesis

- Pyridoxal $PO_4$ residues at catalytic site of all transaminases.

## Common transaminases

- Transaminases are specific for one pair of substrate:
  - Ala-pyr transaminase
  - Glu-aKG transaminase
- Transamination not restricted to a-amino group.
- δ Amino group of ornithine is readily transaminated to form glu γ-semialdehyde.

### Significance of transamination

- Synthesis of non essential amino acid
- Interconversion of different amino acid
- Catabolism of amino acid and transfer of amino group of various amino acid, finally to glutamate
- Since amino acid cannot be stored, transamination channelizes excess amino acid for energy production.
- Important for malate aspartate shuttle (transport of OAA from mitochondria to cytosol).

## Oxidative deamination

- Occurs in mitochondrial Enzyme is GDH (glutamate dehydrogenase)

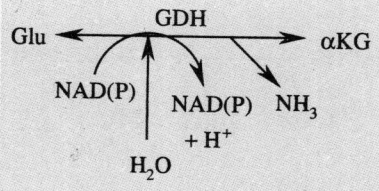

- Glutamate can recycle as a 'N' acceptor, enter TCA or serve as precursor in GNG.
- GDH can use both NAD and NADP as cofactor:

- Requires pyridine nucleotide coenzyme
- Allosteric activators of GDH: ADP, GDP
- Allosteric inhibitors: ATP, GTP, NAD(P)H

## Direct deamination:

$$Ser \longrightarrow Pyr + NH_3$$

$$Thre \longrightarrow \alpha \text{ amino } \beta \text{ keto butyrate}$$

PLP acts a cofactor

## Formation of ammonia

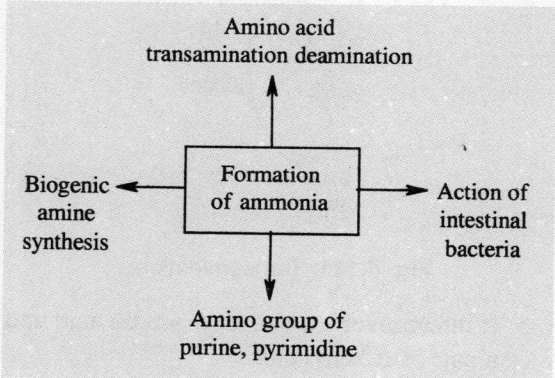

## Amino group transporters

Glutamate and alanine are key transporters of amino group between muscle and liver:

Glutamate:

- Carrier of amino group, precursor of glutamine
- Glu plays a role in removing nitrogen from amino acids.

Ala:

Carrier of amino group between various tissues and liver

## In liver

- Nitrogen waste from amino acids ends up in urea

- Amino acids are derived from:
  - Proteins break down in various tissues
  - Protein synthesized in these tissues

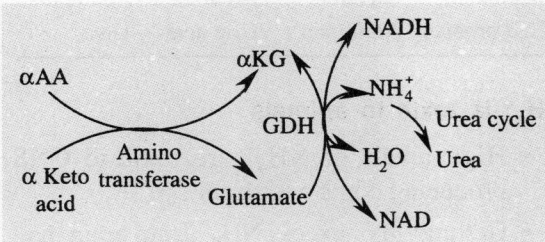

### In non hepatic tissues

GDH and glutamine synthetase remove two ammonia molecules from tissues as a way of getting rid of tissue of nitrogen waste.

$$\alpha KG + NH_4^+ \xrightarrow[\text{GDH}]{\text{NADH} \quad \text{NAD}} \text{Glutamate}$$

Glutamate → (ATP, $NH_4^+$ → ADP) → Glutamine (Glutamate synthetase)

### Glutaminase

Most urea is synthesized from ammonia that has been reduced by glutamine by glutaminase.

This enzyme is located in perivenous area of hepatic lobule (surrounding central vein) (Fig. 4.111).

Enzymes of urea synthesis are periportal in location in 90% of lobules (peripheral region of lobule). Thus, any ammonia that escapes urea cycle is scavenged by glutamine synthetase which is present in remaining 10% of hepatocyte lobules. This glutamine is secreted into blood and can be hydrolyzed in kidney with release of ammonia into urine.

### Brain

- Brain tissue can form urea, but does not appear to play a significant role for $NH_3$ removal.
- Major mechanism for detoxification of $NH_3$ is glutamine formation.
- If blood $NH_3$ levels are elevated, supply of blood glutamine available to brain becomes limiting.
- Brain, therefore must synthesize glutamate from $\alpha KG$ which would deplete TCA intermediates.

### Glutaminase, Asparaginase

- Deaminate glutamine and asparagine
- Glucose catalyze interconversion of free ammonium ions
- Analogous reaction catalyzed by asparaginase.

### *Clinical correlation*

- Certain tumors exhibit abnormally high requirement for glutamine and asparagine.
- Asparagine and glutamine are anticancer agents!

### Glu, Gln, aKG

- 'C' skeletons are same!
- Interconvertible via:
  - Amino transferase
  - Gln synthetase
  - Glutaminase

### Functions of ammonia

- $NH_3$ is not just a waste product
- It synthesizes:
  - Non essential amino acids
  - Purine
  - Pyrimidine
  - Amino sugars
  - Asparagine

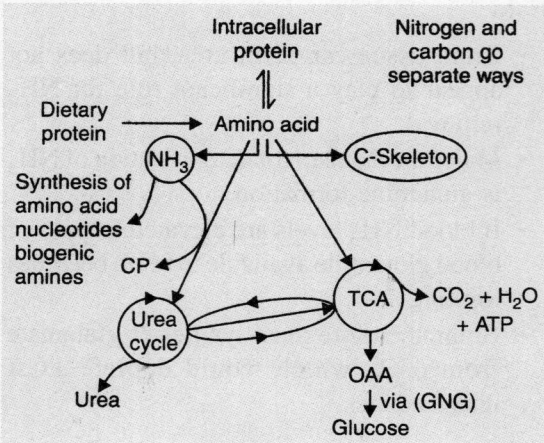

**Fig. 4.122.** Amino acid catabolism.

- Maintains acid-base balance
- Interorgan exchange maintains circulating levels of amino acid

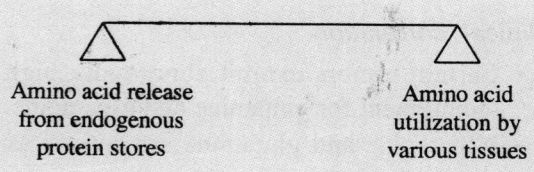

| Amino acid release from endogenous protein stores | Amino acid utilization by various tissues |
|---|---|
| Transamination, serine dehydratase amine oxidase (mitochondria), Glutaminase, glycine cleavage to $NH_4^+$ and $CO_2$, purine, pyrimidine deamination | Synthesis of glutamate, glutamine, urea, excretion as $NH_4^+$ in urine |

Maintenance of steady stage concentration of amino acid between meals depends on net balance between release and utilization.

### Ammonia: fact file

- Ammonia is in equilibrium with ammonium ion with pka of 9.3
- Freely diffusible across membrane.

## Ammonia disposal

| Type | Aminotelic | Uricotelic | Ureatelic |
|---|---|---|---|
| Animal | Aquatic | Birds | Mammals |
| End product | Ammonia | Uric acid | Urea |

### $NH_4^+$ is toxic to animals

- High levels of $NH_4^+$ are toxic to CNS producing coma and death
- Getting rid of excess $NH_4^+$ from brain may reduce $\alpha KG$ levels and inhibit TCA cycle
- Moreover, glutamine and $\gamma$-amino butyric acid (GABA) are neurotransmitter
- Brain needs to maintain [ATP] at very high levels.

### Important nitrogen carriers

- Most amino acid metabolism occurs in the liver
- In cytosol, $\alpha KG$ receives amino groups transferred from other amino acids to form Glutamate
- Glutamate and glutamine then pass to liver mitochondria for further metabolism
- Glutamine is most important ammonia carrier from other tissues by transamination of glutamine, except muscle, where alanine is used.

Ammonia is also produced by bacteria in gut and travels to liver via portal vein.

### Ammonia transport

In adult, ~ 70-90g/d protein is catabolized to form 15-20g $NH_3$/day:

Plasma ammonia : 10-20 µg/dL

Blood glutamine : 10 µg/dL

i.e., ammonia level is 100 times less as compared to glutamine

## Free ammonia is toxic even in traces

Ammonia is transported in the form of glutamine, alanine. Under normal conditions, liver maintain blood $NH_3$ levels with in normal limits by converting it into urea.

## Transport of nh₃ as glutamine

From brain and peripheral tissues except muscle, $NH_3$ released from amino acids is transported to liver and kidney.

Ammonia travels to liver from other tissues in the form of alanine and glutamine.

## Transport of NH₃ as alanine

Glutamine activity is low in muscle and $NH_3$ formed is released by deamination. $NH_3$ is transported in form of alanine to liver where it is converted to pyruvate which returns to muscle.

## Where does nitrogen go and how does it get there?

### Glucose alanine cycle

* Muscle contraction releases pyruvate and amino groups.

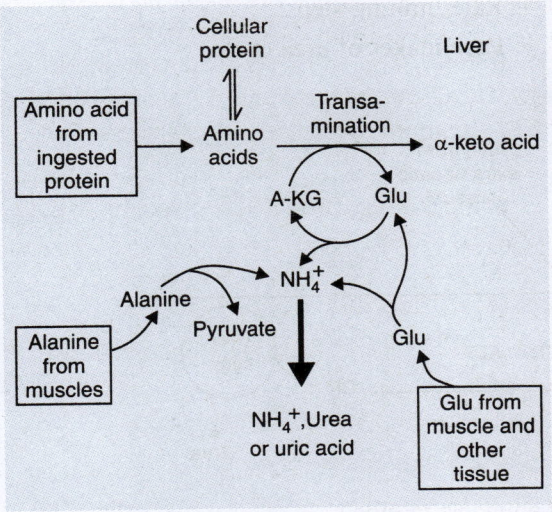

**Fig. 4.123.** Sources and fate of ammonia.

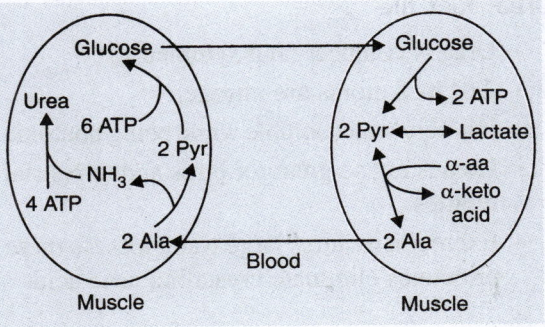

**Fig. 4.124.** Glucose alanine cycle.

* ALT (alanine amino transferase) makes alanine which goes to liver and get reconverted to pyruvate, then to glucose (via GNG) to be exported back to muscle).

## How to get rid of toxic ammonia?

| Amino acids (ingested protein) | Glutamine (muscle and other tissues) | Alanine (muscle) |
|---|---|---|
| 0.7 g/d | 0.8 g/d | 1.5 g/d |
| ↓ | ↓ | Uricotelic, |
| $NH_3$ | Uricotelic | excrete it |
| Aminotelic | | as creatinine |

Ammonia above 50 mm is toxic to CNS

## (iii) Urea Cycle

### Urea: What's so great about it?

Urea synthesis is essential to humans, because:

* Proteins are required in diet to provide amino acids.
* Proteins can't be stored, unlike fats and carbohydrates
* The resultant excess nitrogen after conversion to ammonia must be excreted as urea.
* It will circulate in the blood stream and be toxic if it rises above certain levels.

## Urea: fact file

- Urea is compact (and symmetric)
- 2 of its 8 atoms are nitrogen
- It is very water soluble while being nontoxic
- Urea is not so great for birds and terrestrial reptiles
- Excretion requires large water loss, so these uricoteles eliminate crystalline uric acid.

## How ammonia is converted to urea for excretion?

## Sources of nitrogen for urea cycle

**2N:**
- One from glutamine
- 2nd from aspartate
- 1C: from $HCO_3$

## Biosynthesis of urea

**4 Stages:**
- Transamination
- Oxidation deamination
- Ammonia transport
- Reactions of urea cycle

A human subject consumes 100 g protein/d

and excretes 16.5 g/d nitrogen: 95% in urine, 5% feces.

## Urea synthesis

- Urea is formed from $NH_3$ $CO_2$ and aspartate
- Synthesis of 1 mol urea requires:
- 3 mol ATP
- 1 mol $NH_4^+$
- 1 mol a- amino nitrogen of aspartate
- 5 enzymes: CPS I, OTC, AS synthase, ASase, Arginase

## Urea cycle

$1^{st}$ two reactions (CPS I, OTC) occurs in mitochondria, rest occur in cytosol

## CPS I

- Carbamoyl phosphate synthase I
- Mitochondrial enzyme
- Location: Hepatic
- Uses $CO_2$, $NH_3$, ATP
- Requires NAc glutamate as cofactor (allosteric)
- Rate limiting step
- Pace maker of urea cycle.

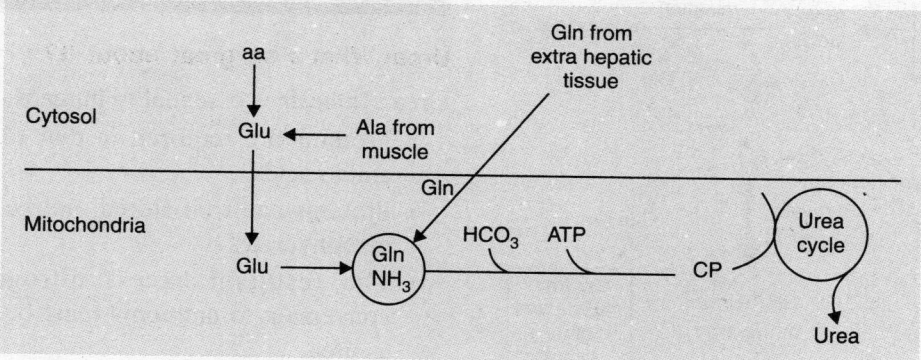

**Fig. 4.125.** Conversion of ammonia to urea
(Glu = glutamate, Gln = glutamine)

$$HCO_3 + NH_2 + 2\ ATP \longrightarrow$$

$$\underset{\underset{\parallel}{O}}{H_2N - C - OPO_3^{2-}} + 2\ ADP + P_i$$

**Fig. 4.126.** CPSI.

### NAcGlu

N-acetyl glutamate (NAcGlu) is allosteric activator of CPS I.

NAcGlu synthesized from acetyl CoA and glutamate, when cellular glutamate concentration is high, signaling an excess of free amino acids due to dietary intake or protein breakdown. Rate of synthesis of acetyl CoA and glutamate determine concentration of NAc Glu.

Starvation elevates CPS I enzyme levels to cope up with increased production of $NH_3$ due to protein degradation i.e., urea cycle enzymes are up regulated during increased demands to excrete nitrogen.

|  | *CPS I* | *CPS II* |
|---|---|---|
| Site | Mitochondria | Cytosol |
| Synthesis | Urea | Pyrimidine |
| Amino group donor | Asp | Gln |
| Regulation | Allosterically: NAc Glu | Does not require NAc Glu activated by PRPP and inhibited by CTP |
| Location | $CO_2 + NH_3 \rightarrow CP$ | $CO_2 + Gln \rightarrow CP + Glu$ |

- CPS I and II work independently under normal conditions and in different cellular compartment
- In ODC deficiency, a block in urea cycle occurs causing spilling of accumulated mitochondrial CP into cytosolic compartment.

- This CP in cytosolic compartment may stimulate pyrimidine synthesis and there is built up of orotic acid in blood and urine.

$$Acetyl\ CoA \underset{+}{\overset{AGA}{\underset{Synthase}{\xrightarrow{\hspace{1.5cm}}}}} N\text{-acetyl glutamate (AGA}$$
$$Glutamate$$

- AG synthase in activated by arginine.

### 5 enzymes of urea cycle:

- CPS I (carbamoyl phosphate synthase I)
- OTC (ornithine transcarbamoylase)
- ASS (arginino succinate synthetase)
- ASase (arginino succinase)
- Arginase

### 5 amino acids in urea cycle

- Arginine
- Aspartate
- Glutamate
- Ornithine
- Citrulline

**Function of glutamate:**
To regenerate asparatate from OAA.

**ATP required in urea cycle:** Three
 – Two: To make CP
 – Third: To provide energy for aspartate condensation with citrulline

| *Energetics* | | *ATP* |
|---|---|---|
| CPS | $CO_2 + NH_3 + 2ATP \rightarrow$ $CP + 2ADP + Pi$ | – 2 ATP |
| ASS | Citrulline + Asp + $ATP \rightarrow AS + AMP + PPi$ | –1 ATP |

- ATP consumption: 3 moles of ATP consumed for synthesis of 1 mole of urea

- 3 participating amino acid:
  - Glutamate
  - Aspartate
  - Arginine
  - $NH_4^+$ and aspartate provide nitrogen to produce urea and carbon dioxide provides the carbon.

For each cycle, citrulline must leave mitochondria and ornithine must enter mitochondrial matrix. Ornithine/citrulline transporter in IMM facilitates this flux.

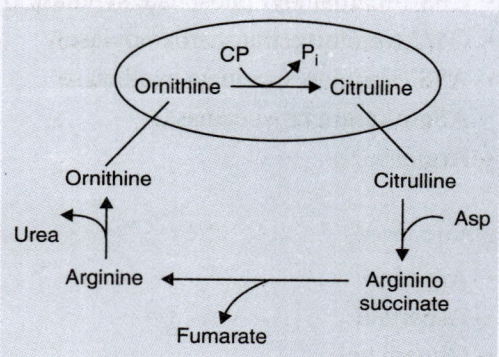

**Fig. 4.127.** Urea cycle outline.

## Ornithine

Required for:

- Urea cycle
- Putrescine, spermine, polyamine synthesis.

To regenerate aspartate from fumarate, cytosolic isoenzymes of some Kreb's cycle enzymes are involved.

## Arginase

- Catalyzes cleavage of guanido group to release urea
- Present in liver, renal tissue, brain, mammary gland, testes, skin
- Ornithine and lysine are potent competitive inhibitors of arginase.

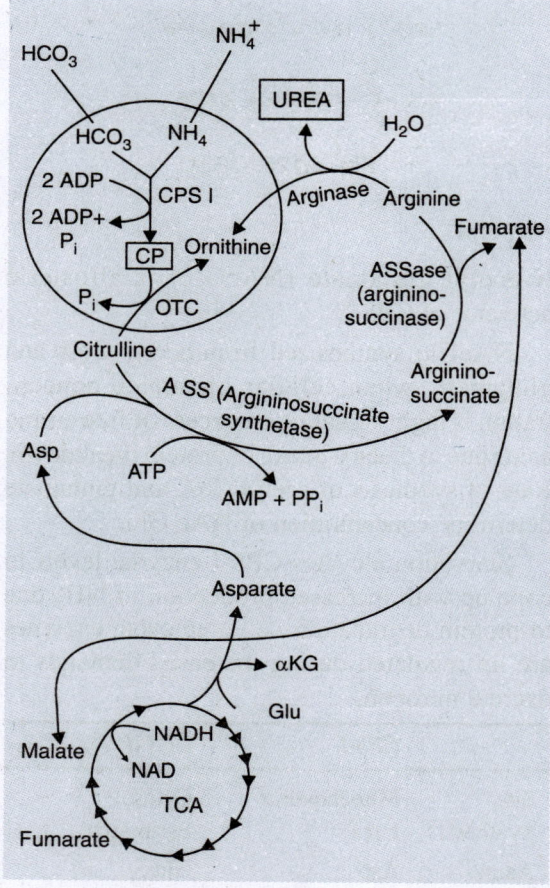

**Fig. 4.128.** Urea bicycle.

## Urea bicycle

- Aspartate – argininosuccinate shunt.
- 2 cycles are going on:
  - One takes ornithine to arginine and returns arginine to ornithine
  - 2nd takes fumarate from argininosuccinate and returns to aspartate.

### Regulation

- NAcGlu: Activator of CPS I
- Arginine: Stimulates synthesis of NAcGlu

Urea cycle is activated by glucocorticoids and

glucagon, both activate the gene encoding CPS I.

## Hereditary deficiency of urea cycle enzymes

- Hereditary deficiency of any of the urea cycle enzymes leads to: hyperammonemia – elevated ammonia in blood
- Total lack of any of the enzyme of urea cycle is lethal
- Elevated ammonia is toxic, especially to brain.
- If elevated ammonia is not treated immediately after birth, severe mental retardation results.

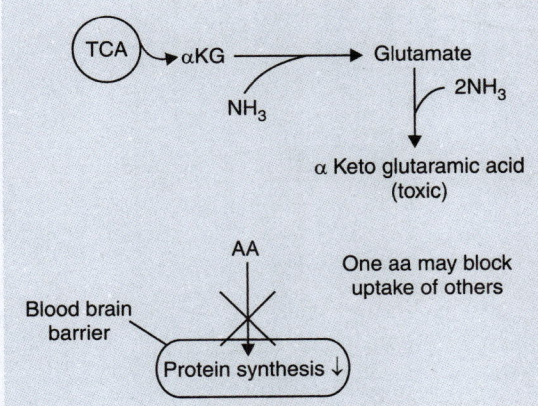

**Fig. 4.129.** Possible mechanism of $NH_3$ toxicity in brain.

## Postulated mechanism for toxicity of high ammonia

1. High ammonia drive glutamine synthase
   $$Glu + ATP + NH_3 \rightarrow Gln + ADP + Pi$$
   This depletes glutamate, (excitatory) neurotransmitter and precursor for synthesis of (inhibitory), neurotransmitter GABA.
2. Depletion of glutamate and high $NH_3$ level drive GDH to reverse:

$$Glu + NAD (P) \rightarrow \alpha KG + NAD(P) H + NH_4^+$$

This depletes aKG, an essential TCA cycle intermediate, thus impairing energy metabolism in brain.

**CPS I deficiency** results in inability for nitrogenous wastes (ammonia) to be metabolized via urea cycle. Ammonia levels rise, leading to brain damage, coma or death.

## Treatment of deficiency of urea cycle enzyme

- Limit protein intake and add α-keto acid analogs of essential amino acids
- Liver transplant
- Gene therapy

## Treatment hyperammonemia with benzoic acid or phenylacetic acid

$$Benzoic\ acid \xrightarrow{Glycine} Hippuric\ acid$$

$$Phenylacetic\ acid \xrightarrow{Gln} Phenylacetyl\ glutamine$$

## Metabolic disorders of urea cycle

| Disease | Enzyme defect | Features |
|---------|---------------|----------|
| Hyperammonemia I | CPS I | Rare |
| Hyperammonemia II | OTC | X-linked aversion to high protein diet |
| Citrullinemia | ASS | Lethargy, seizures |
| AS aciduria | ASase | Friable, tufted hair, fatal in early life |
| Hyperargininemia* | Arginase | Raised arginine |

*Arginase deficiency does not result in severe hyperammonemia

## Krebs' cycle (Fig. 4.129)

Connecting TCA cycle via aspartate – arginino succinate shunt

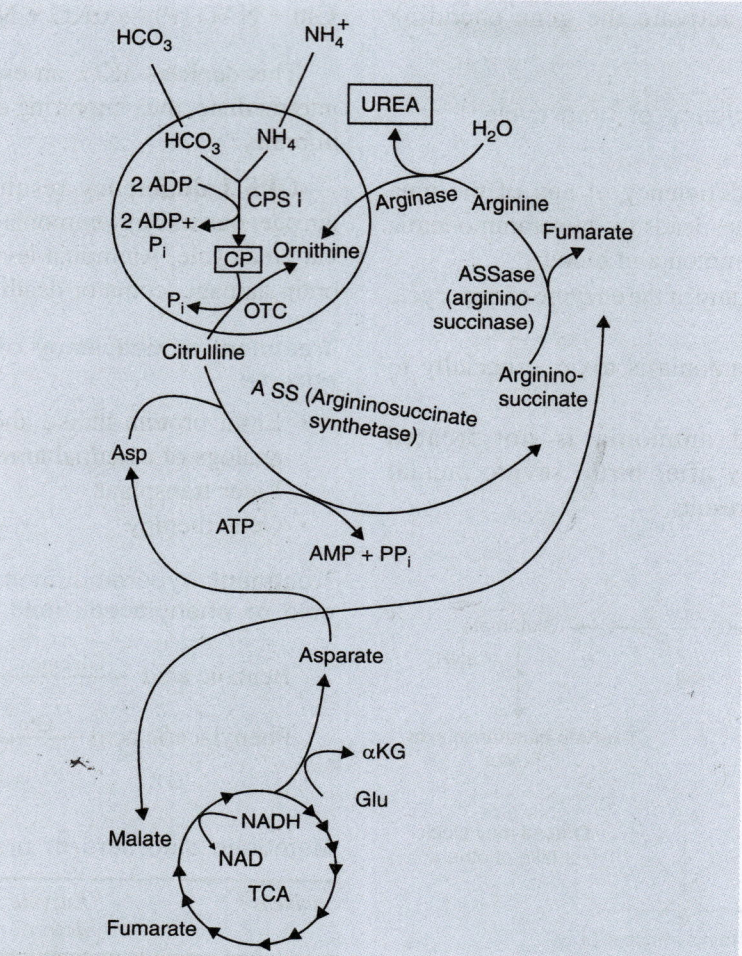

**Fig. 4.130.** Urea bicycle (Kreb bicycle).

## Biochemical screening tests

| Test | Compound | Interpretation |
|---|---|---|
| Ferric chloride Phenistix | Phenyl pyruvate | Green, PKU |
| Dinitrophenyl hydrazine | α keto acids | Yellow, MSUP, Keto acidosis |
| Cyanide nitroprusside | Disulfide bonds | Red purple, cystinuria, homocystinuria, |
| Nitrosanaphthol | OH-phenolic acids | Orange red, Tyrosinemia, liver dysfunction |
| Merckoquant sulfite | Sulfite | Pink, Sulfide oxidase, molybdenum decrease |
| Benedict's (clinitest) | Reducing substance | Green → orange, glycinuria |
| Acetest | Acetone acetoacetate | Purple, acetoacetate |
| P nitroaniline | Methylmalonic acid | Emerald green, MMA (methyl malonyluria) |

\* Antibiotics can interfere

# (iv) Synthesis and Degradation of Amino Acid

## Degradation of amino acid

When carbon skeletons of amino acids are degraded, major products are:
- Pyruvate
- Intermediates of TCA cycle
- Acetoacetate, i.e. Amino acid can be:
  - Glucogenic from pyruvate or intermediates of TCA
  - Ketogenic (from acetyl CoA or acetoacetate)

Amino acids that can be converted to pyruvate are glycine, serine, cystine, and alanine).

## AMINO ACID CATABOLISM: CARBON SKELETONS

### Fact file

Virtually all carbon skeletons can be converted into intermediates of:
- Glycolytic pathway
- TCA cycle
- Lipid metabolism

### 1st step

- Transfer of a amino group by transamination to αKG or OAA.
- This provides glutamate and aspartate: source for 'N' in urea cycle.

*Exception*:
Lysine, proline, hydroxyproline, threonine
Do not undergo transamination

## Amino acid carbon skeletons

Amino acids are deaminated to α-keto acids that are fed into major metabolic pathways (e.g. TCA)

Amino acids can be grouped as:

- Glucogenic
- Ketogenic

Based on whether or not their carbon skeletons can be converted to glucose.

## Glucogenic Amino acid

- Carbon skeletons of glucogenic amino acid are degraded to:
  - Pyruvate
  - 4C, 5C-intermediates of TCA cycle
- These carbon skeletons serve as precursor for glucose via GNG

## Ketogenic Amino acid

- Carbon skeletons of ketogenic amino acids are degraded to:
  - Acetyl CoA
  - Acetoacetate
- They cannot be converted to glucose

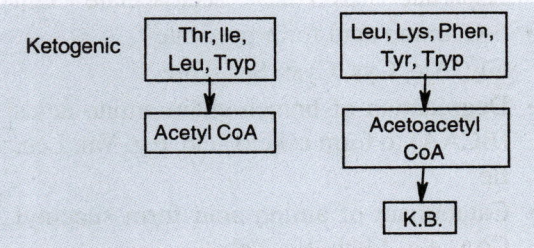

**Fig. 4.131.** Metabolic fate of carbon skeletons

## Glucogenic

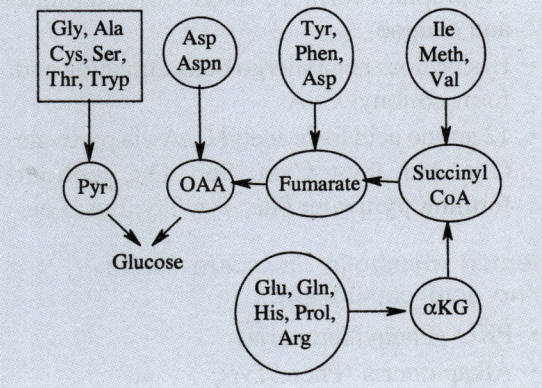

## Fate on 'N' released

- Either reutilized for anabolic process: protein synthesis or converted to urea and excreted.
- Partially oxidized hydrocarbon skeletons may be degraded to amphibolic intermediates.

## Fate of 'C' – skeletons

- 3-C amino acids form pyruvate e.g. alanine, serine, cysteine, threonine. Glycine also forms pyruvate

$$\text{Alanine} + \alpha KG \rightleftharpoons \text{Pyruvate} + \text{glutamate}$$
Amino
Transferase

- 4-C amino acids for OAA, e.g. Aspartate, asparagine.
- 5-C amino acids form Glutamate (precursor of Gln) e.g. Glu, his, arg, prol.

$$\text{Aspartate} + \alpha KG \rightleftharpoons \text{acetoacetate} + \text{Glu}$$

- 6-C amino acid form pyruvate
Gly, Ala, Cys, Cyst, Ser, Thre
- Degradation of branch chain amino acids (BCAA) to form α keto acid, e.g. Val, Leu, Ile
- Catabolism of amino acid form succinyl CoA, e.g. Meth, Ile, Val
- Aromatic amino acid form fumarate, acetoacetate, e.g. Phe, Tyr
- Tryptophan form crotonyl CoA, formate and alanine
- Lysine does not undergo transamination and form crotonyl CoA.
- 12 amino acid form acetyl CoA via pyruvate Gly, Ala, Cys, Cyst, Ser, Thr, without forming pyruvate: Phe, Tyr, Try, Lys, Leu

## Inherited metabolic disorders (IMD): amino acid catabolism

- PKU (Phenylketonuria)
- Alkaptonuria (Phen, Tyr)

- Tyrosinemia (Phen, Tyr)
- Methylmalonyluria (Met, Val, Ile)
- Isovalterate academia (Ile, Leu, Val)
- Histidinemia (His)
- Hyperprolinemia (Pro)

**IMD of amino acid results in:**

- Accumulation of intermediate in blood or urine.
- Severity of disease depends on toxicity of accumulated metabolites
- Treatment: low protein diet

## Biosynthesis of amino acids

- Evolution has left human beings without ability to synthesize almost half the amino acid.
- 20 amino acid are used to build peptides and proteins
- Amino acid biosynthesis involves:
  - Synthesis of 'C' skeletons for corresponding α keto acids
  - Addition of amino group via transamination

Nutritionally amino acid can be:

- Essential
- Non essential
- Biologically all amino acid are essential in nature
- Nutritionally non-essential amino acids are most important to cell than essential ones!

## Essential Amino acid

- Met, His, Phen, Trys
- Ile, Leu, Lys, Val
- Thre, Arg

## Non essential amino acids

- Ala, Glu, Gly
- Asp, Aspn

- Cys, Ser
- Gln, Tyr, Proline

All amino acids (except tyrosine) are synthesized from common metabolic intermediates in cell:

- Pyruvate
- OAA
- αKG
- 3PG

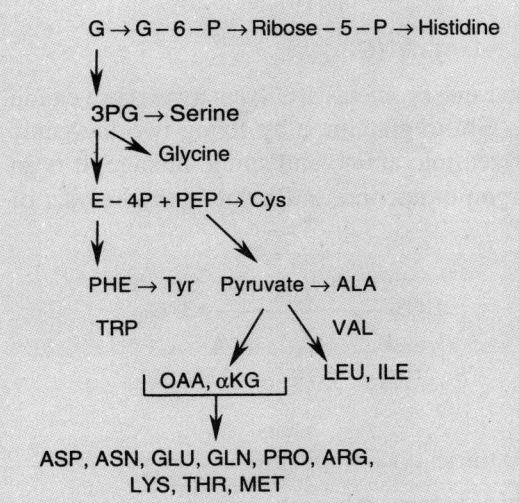

$$G \rightarrow G-6-P \rightarrow Ribose-5-P \rightarrow Histidine$$

$$3PG \rightarrow Serine$$

Glycine

$$E-4P+PEP \rightarrow Cys$$

PHE → Tyr    Pyruvate → ALA

TRP                              VAL

OAA, αKG         LEU, ILE

ASP, ASN, GLU, GLN, PRO, ARG, LYS, THR, MET

**Fig. 4.132.** Biosynthesis of amino acids from metabolic intermediates

Nine essential amino acid must be derived from diet: Met, Thr, Val, Iso, Leu, Lys, Phen, Trp, His.

Eleven non essential amino acid are synthesized in body: Ala, Asp/Aspn, Glu/Gln, Arg, Prol, Ser, Gly, Cys, Cyst.

The eleven amino acids we can make [Ala, Asp/Aspn, Glu/Gln, Arg, Prol, Ser, Gly, Cys, and Cyst]

The rest we must ingest (Met, Thr, Val, Ile, Lys, Phen, Trp, His).

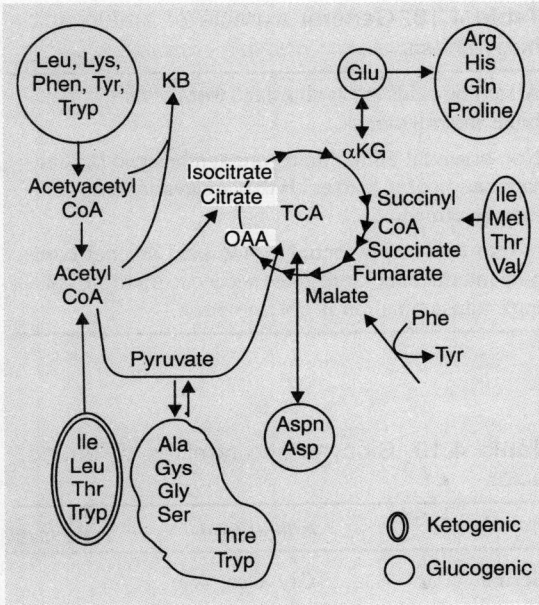

**Fig. 4.133.** Fate of amino acids.

### Table 4.16. Essential amino acids

| | |
|---|---|
| Arginine* | Methionine |
| Histidine | Phenylalanine |
| Isoleucine | Threonine |
| Leucine | Tryptophan |
| Lysine | Valine |

\* Arginine is essential in infants and children and most of synthesized arginine is converted to ornithine and urea via urea cycle

### Table 4.17. Non-essential amino acids

| | |
|---|---|
| Alanine | Glutamine |
| Asparagine | Glycine |
| Aspartate | Proline |
| Cysteine* | Serine |
| Glutamate | Tyrosine+ |

\* Cysteine gets its sulfur atom from methionine
+ Tyrosine is hydroxylated phenylalanine, it is not essential.

## Table 4.18. General aspects of amino acid biosynthesis

All amino acids are synthesized from common metabolic intermediates

Non-essential amino acids are synthesized by transamination of α-keto acids that are available as common intermediates.

α-keto acids of essential amino acid are not common intermediates (enzymes needed to them are lacking), transamination is not an option.

### Biosynthesis

## Table 4.19. Biosynthetic families of amino acids

| Family | Amino acids |
|--------|-------------|
| Serine | Gly, Cys, Ser |
| Aromatic | Phen, Tyr, Trp |
| Gln | Glu, Gln, Pro, Arg, HO-Pro |
| Asp | Asp, Aspn |
| Pyr | Ala, HO-Lys |

### Amino acid biosynthesis

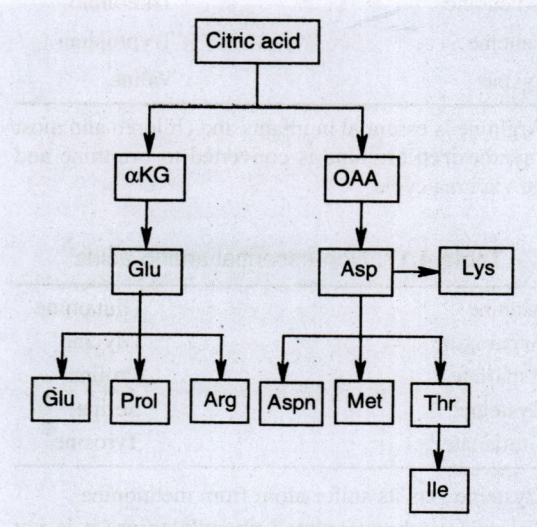

**Fig. 4.134.** Amino acid biosynthesis.

## 1. Glutamate (Glu)

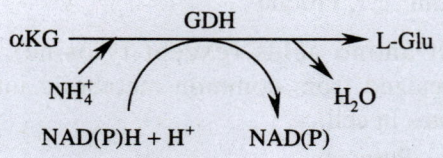

Glutamate dehydrogenase (GD) catalyzes reductive amination of αKG to L-glutamate and this reaction is key regulatory step in biosynthesis of many amino acids.

## 2. Glutamine (Gln)

Glutamine synthetase (GS) catalyzes conversion of L-Glu to glutamine by fixing two inorganic nitrogen into amino and amide linkage. It is an exergonic reaction and involves hydrolysis of ATP.

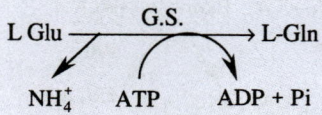

## 3. Alanine and Aspartate

Alanine is formed by transamination of pyruvate and aspartate by transamination of oxaloacetate.

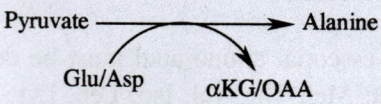

## 4. Asparagine (Aspn)

Asparagine synthetase catalyzes formation of Aspn from Asp (resembles Gln synthesis)

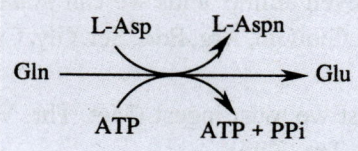

## Metabolic fate of amino acid carbon skeletons

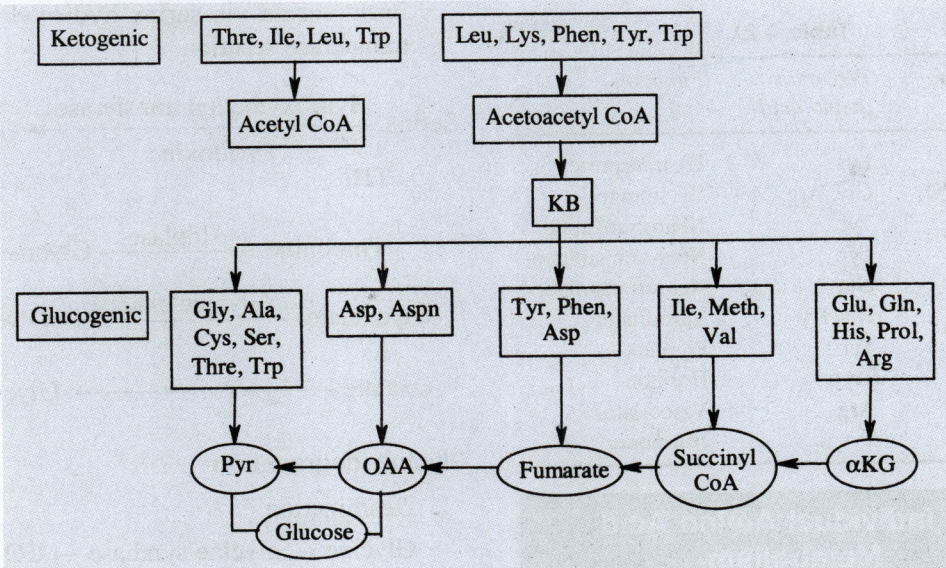

## 5. Serine

Serine is formed from glycolytic intermediate 3-phosphoglycerate (3PG)

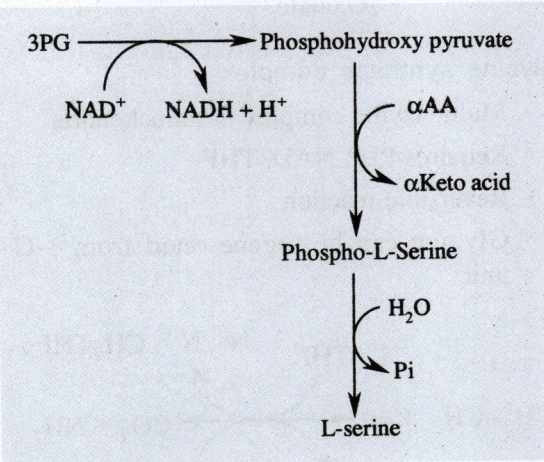

Rest will be discussed under individual amino acid metabolism.

## Biosynthetic families of amino acids

| Table 4.20 | | |
|---|---|---|
| *Glucogenic* | *Ketogenic* | *Both* |
| Gly, Ser, Cys | Leu | Ile |
| Ala | | Lys |
| Phen, Tyr, Trp | | Phen |
| Glu/Gln, Asp/Aspn | | Trp |
| Prol, Arg, His, Meth, Thre | | Tyr |
| BCAA (Val, Leu, Ile) | | |

## Amino acids form pyruvate

- Serine family (gly, cys, ser)
- Pyruvate family (ala)
- Aspartate family (thre)

## Serine family

It includes glycine, cysteine and serine.

## Amino acid derivatives of importance

### Table 4.21.

| Compound | Precursor amino acid | Function |
|---|---|---|
| Carnitine | Lys | FA transporter |
| Creatine $PO_4$ | Gly, Arg, Met | 'E' storage |
| Dopamine | Tyr | Neurotransmitter |
| Epi/NE | Tyr | Neurotransmitter |
| GABA | Glu | Neurotransmitter |
| Histamine | His/Try | Vasodilator |
| Melanin | Tyr | Pigment |
| Melatonin | Tryp | Hormone |
| NO | Arg | Vasodilator |
| Thyroxine | Tyr | Hormone |

# (v) Individual Amino Acid Metabolism

## Serine family

Gly, Ser, Cys (synthesized from pyruvate)

**Glycine:**

$$H_3N^+ - \overset{\displaystyle COO^-}{\underset{\displaystyle H}{C}} - H$$

- Most abundant amino acid
- Non essential
- Optically inactive
- Glucogenic
- Synthesized by living cells
- Act as inhibitory neurotransmitter
- Involved in synthesis of many specialized products: ser, gly 1-C metabolism

### Synthesis

- Transmination of glycine from glyoxalate and glutamine or alanine via glycine transaminase

- From choline
- From serine via serine hydroxyl methyl transferase reaction

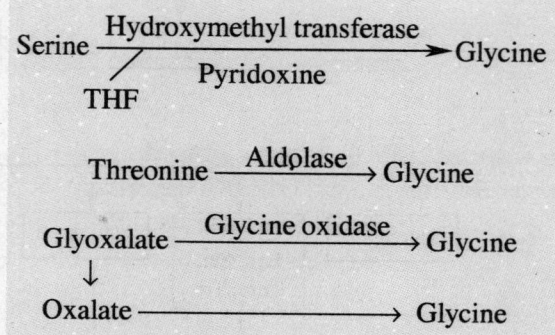

$$Serine \xrightarrow[\text{THF}]{\text{Hydroxymethyl transferase} \atop \text{Pyridoxine}} Glycine$$

$$Threonine \xrightarrow{\text{Aldolase}} Glycine$$

$$Glyoxalate \xrightarrow{\text{Glycine oxidase}} Glycine$$
$$\downarrow$$
$$Oxalate \longrightarrow Glycine$$

## Glycine degradation

1. Deamination

   Glycine ← glycine synthase → $CO_2$ + $NH_4$ + IC

2. Glycine ↔ serine $\xrightarrow{\text{Dehydratase}}$ pyruvate

3. Glycine → glyoxalate $\xrightarrow{\frac{1}{2}O_2}$ formate
   $$\downarrow \qquad\qquad\qquad \downarrow$$
   $$Oxalate \qquad\qquad I\text{-}C$$

## Glycine synthase complex

- Multienzyme complex in mitochondria
- Requires PLP, NAD, THF
- Reversible reaction:

  Glycine can be regene-rated from 1-C unit

$$NH_3 - CH_2 - C = 0 \longleftrightarrow CO_2 + NH_3$$

THF, $N^5, N^{10}, CH_2THF$, NAD, NADH + $H^+$

Glycine synthase

Specialized products synthesized from glycine:

| | |
|---|---|
| Glucose | Creatine |
| Protein | Porphyrin |
| Serine | GSH |
| Oxalate | Conjugates |
| Formate | Purine |

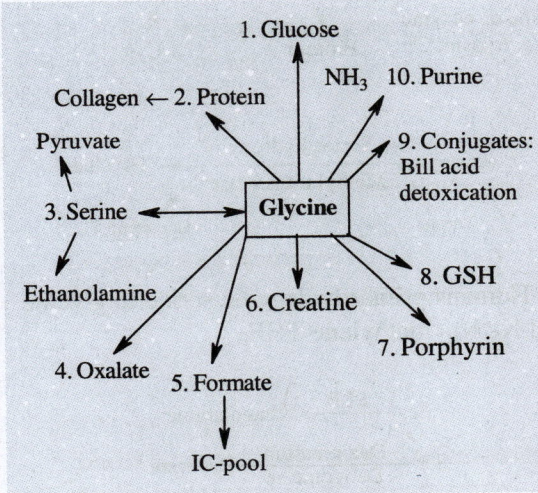

## Creatine synthesis

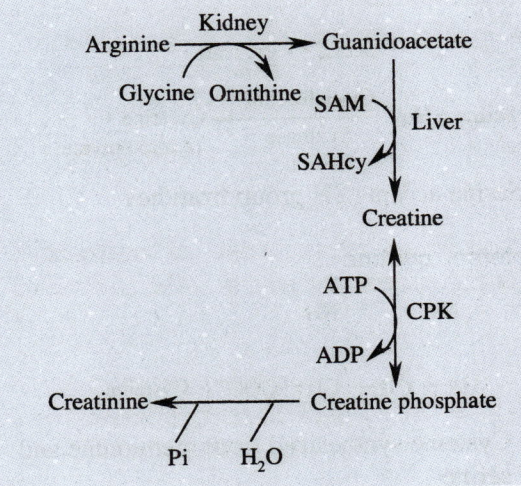

## GSH (glutathione)

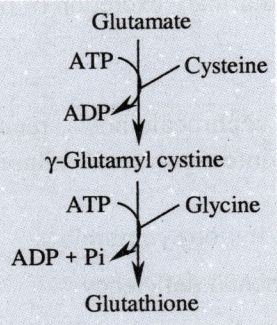

## Porphyrin

$$\text{Succinyl CoA} + \text{glycine} \xrightarrow[\text{Synthase}]{\text{Ala}} \text{Ala} \ (\delta\text{-amino leuvinic acid})$$

## Conjugation reaction

Cholic acid + glycine → glycocholic acid

*Detoxification reaction*:

Benzoic acid + glycine → hippuric acid

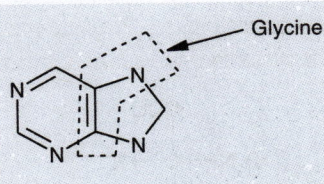

**Fig. 4.135.** Contribution of glycine in purine ring.

## Metabolic disorders of glycine

- Glycinuria
- Primary hyperoxaluria

## Glycinuria

Defect in renal tubular reabsorption.

## Primary hyperoxaluria

- Defect in failure to catabolize glycoxalate arising from deamination of glycine.

- Glyoxalate get oxidized to oxalate causing increased urinary excretion of oxalate

## Features

Urolithiasis, nephrocalcinosis, recurrent UTI (urinary tract infection), renal failure, HT.

## Non-Ketotic hyperglycinemia

- Severe mental deficiency
- Should be distinguished from ketoacidosis of BCAA metabolism abnormality
- Deficiency of glycine cleavage complex in 3 of 4 components of complex is known!
- Glycine being major inhibitory neurotransmitter may be responsible for neurological complications.

$$\text{Glycine} \xrightarrow{\text{THF, NAD, NADH}^+\text{H, CO}_2} N^5N^{10} \text{ methylene FH}_4$$

## Serine

$$
\begin{array}{c}
\text{COO} \\
| \\
\text{H}_3\text{N} - \text{C} - \text{H} \\
| \\
\text{CH}_2\text{OH}
\end{array}
$$

- Non essential amino acid
- Glucogenic
- Interconvertible with glycine
- Synthesized from 3PG
- αOH group oxidized by dehydrogenase to oxo group via NAD$^+$

Then, transaminated → phosphoserine, then dephosphorylated to serine.

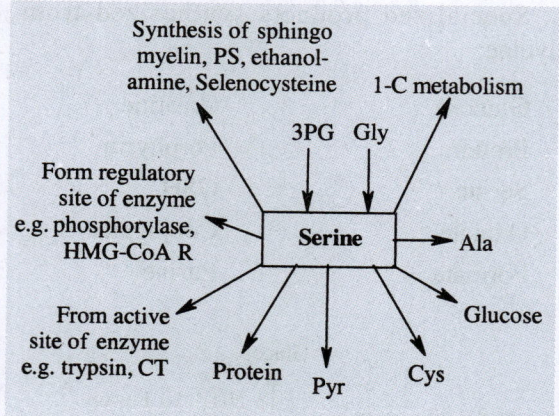

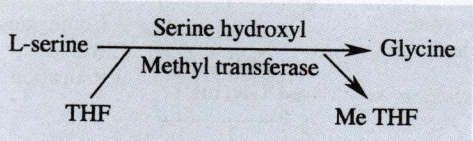

Humans primarily degrade serine to glycine and $N_5 N_{10}$ methylene THF.

$$\text{Ser} \xrightarrow{\text{PLP}} \text{Ethanolamine}$$

$$\text{Ser} \xrightarrow[\text{Dehydratase}]{\text{Deamination}} \text{Pyruvate}$$

Serine deaminated by dehydratase to pyruvate

$$\text{Serine} \rightarrow \text{Pyruvate}$$

$$\text{Serine + Hcy} \xrightarrow[\text{Synthase}]{\text{Cystathionine}} \text{Cysteine +}\ \alpha \text{ keto butyrate}$$

Serine accepts SH group from hcy

## Cysteine, cystine

$$
\begin{array}{c}
\text{NH}_3 \\
| \\
\text{HS} - \text{CH} - \text{CH} - \text{COO}^-
\end{array}
\quad \text{Cysteine}
$$

- Cysteine synthesized from methionine and serine

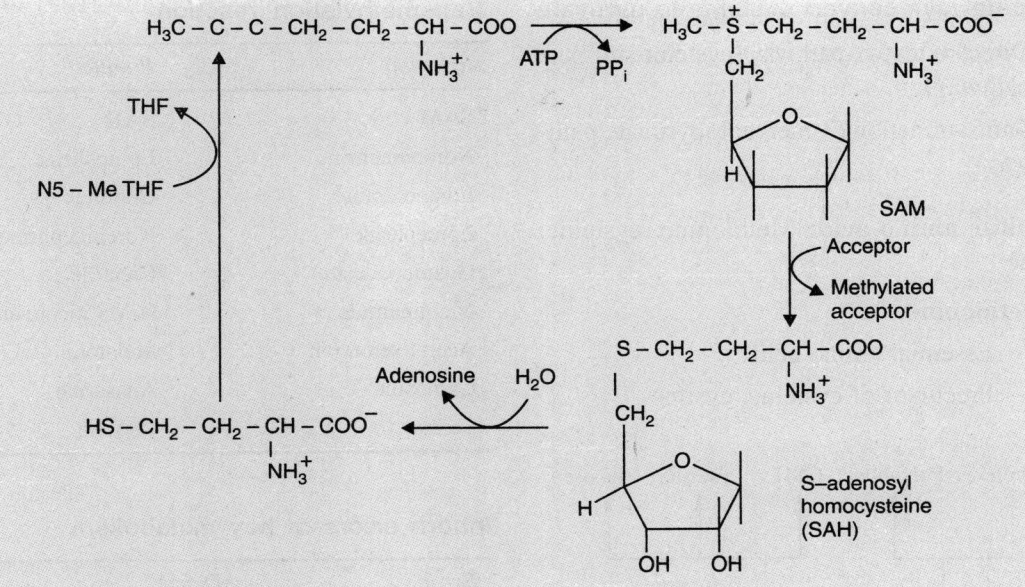

**Fig. 4.136.** Cysteine and cystine interconversion.

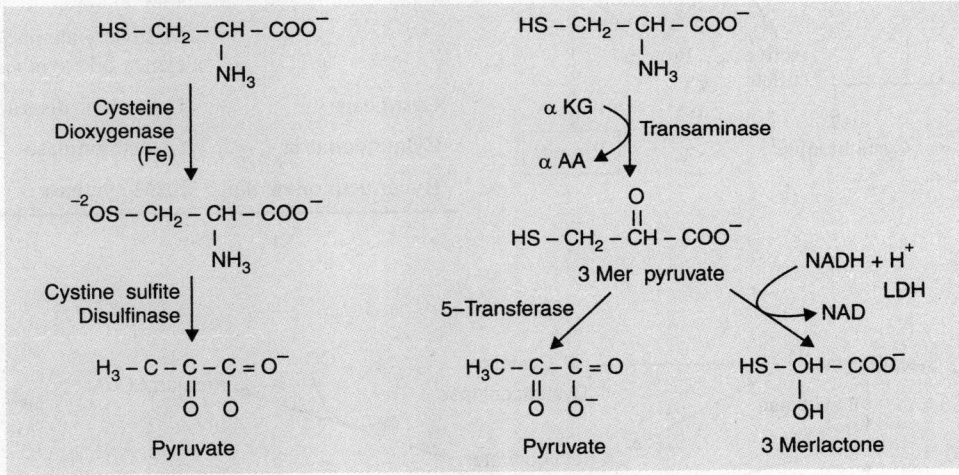

**Fig. 4.137.** Cysteine metabolism.

- Methionine first converted to hcy via SAM and SAH

  Meth + Ser → Hcy → cystathionine → homoserine + cysteine

  Cystine reductase reduces cystine to cysteine

and catabolism of cystine then merges with that of cysteine

$$L\text{-cystine} \xrightarrow[\text{NADH + H} \quad \text{NAD}]{\text{Reductase}} 2L\text{-cysteine}$$

## Two pathways convert cysteine to pyruvate

1. Direct oxidative pathway (cysteine sulfinate pathway)
2. Transamination (3-mercaptopyruvate pathway)

**Sulfur amino acid:** Methionine, cysteine, cystine

### Methionine:

- Essential amino acid
- Precursor of cysteine, cystine

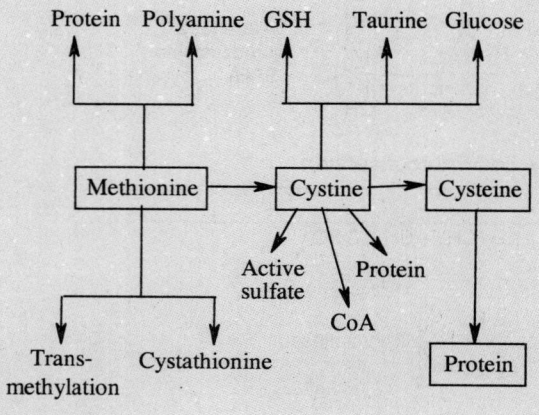

## Transmethylation reaction

| Reactant | Product |
|---|---|
| SAM | SAH |
| Norepinephrine | Epinephrine |
| Ethanolamine | Choline |
| Epinephrine | Norepinephrine |
| Guanidoacetate | Creatine |
| Nicotinamide | N-Me nicotinamide |
| Acetyl serotonin | Melatonin |
| Carnosine | Anaserine |
| Serine | Choline |

## Inborn errors of hcy metabolism

| Error | Defect |
|---|---|
| Homocystinuria | Cystathione synthase, Me THF-R |
| | Methylcobalamin deficiency and synthesis |
| Cystinosis | Lysosomal disorder |
| Cytathioninuria | Cystathioninase |
| Hypermethioninemia | SAM synthase |

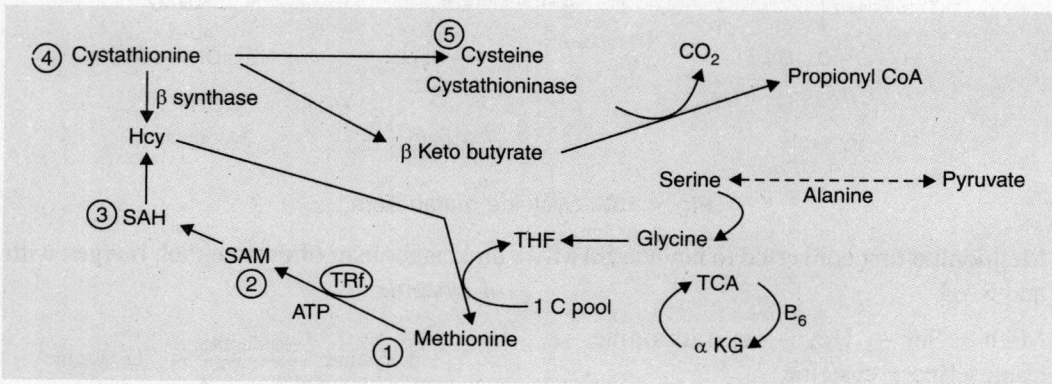

**Fig. 4.138.** Synthesis of sulfur containing amino acid.

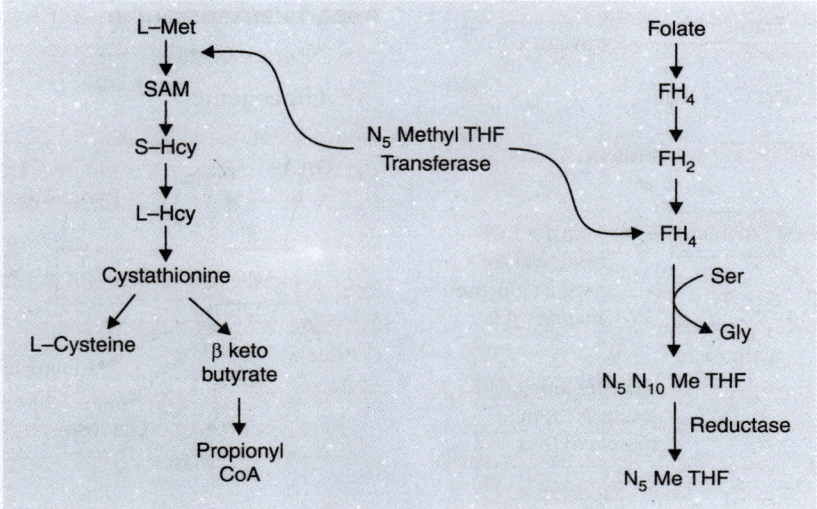

**Fig. 4.139.** Metabolism of sulfur amino acids

## IMD-Sulfur amino acid

Disease Defect

Hcyturia

I    Cystathionine synthase

II   N5 N10 Me THF

III  Low N5 Me THF

IV   Low N5 Me THF, defective intestinal absorption

V    Hypermethioninemia

VI   Cystathioninuria    Cystathioninase deficiency

Sulfituria    Sulfate oxidase deficiency

Disulfiduria    3 Mer S transferase deficiency (3 Mer → Pyr)

Methionine MAS (malabsorption):

Cystinuria

Cystinosis

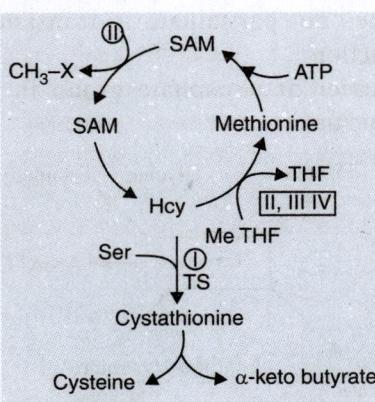

**Fig. 4.140.** IMD sulfur amino acids.

## Alanine

- Non essential amino acid
- Major plasma amino acid
- Glucogenic
- No known metabolic defects
- Synthesized from pyruvate

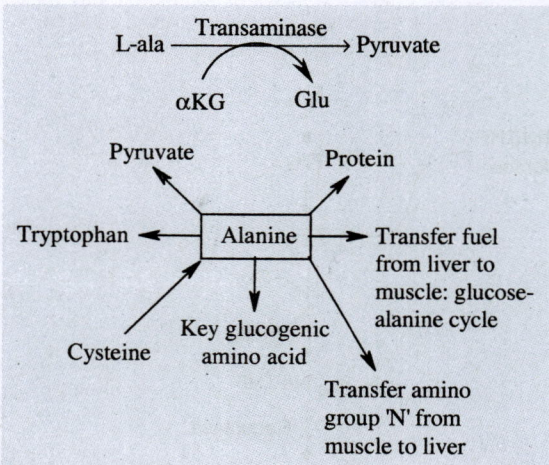

## Aspartate/Asparagine

- Non essential
- Glucogenic

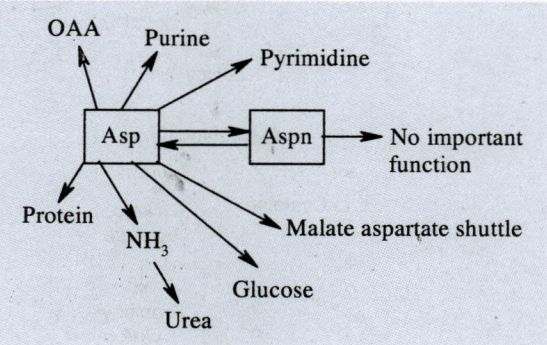

## Threonine

- Essential amino acid
- Glucogenic
- Does not participate in transamination reaction
- Carrier of phosphate group in protein structure.

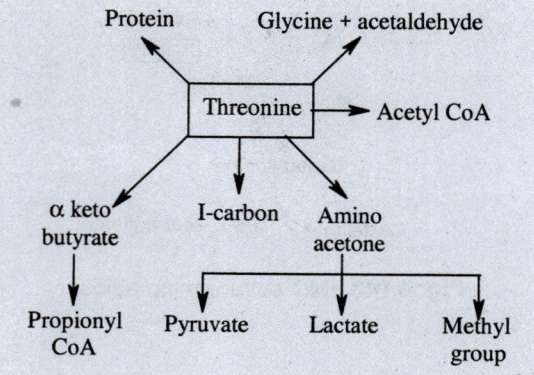

- Threonine undergoes deamination by threonine dehydratase
- Threonine is cleaved to glycine and acet-aldehyde by hydroxyl methyl transferase
- Dehydrogenation followed by decarboxy-lation of threonine results in amino acetone which may be converted by pyruvate or lactate.

## Aspartate transaminase

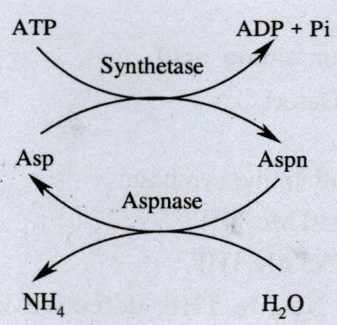

## Synthesis

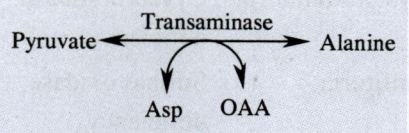

## Transamination of OAA yields aspartate

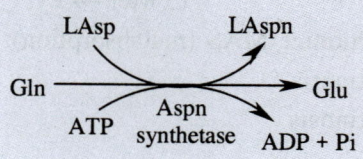

## Catabolism

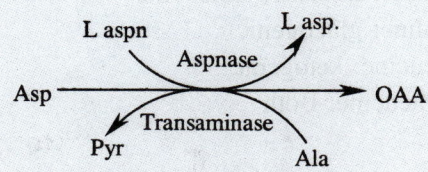

There is no known metabolic defect of this pathway

## Glutamate

- Glu/Gln

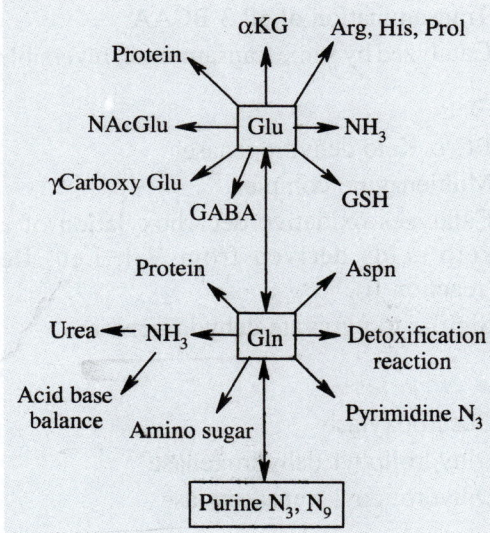

- Non essential amino acid
- Glucogenic
- Directly involved in final transfer of amino acid for urea synthesis

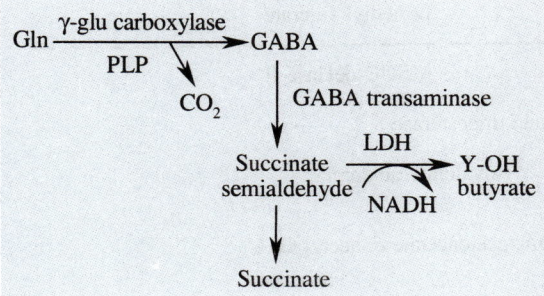

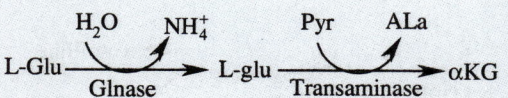

**Glutamine:** Storage form of $NH_3$
Freely diffusible
'N' donor
Source of $NH_3$ in kidney for maintaining acid-base balance

**Histidine, Proline, Arginine:**
- Semi essential amino acid
- Generate 1-carbon unit
- Converted to glutamate by a series of reaction that transfer its forimino group to THF

**Figlu** accumulates in $B_{12}$ deficiency:

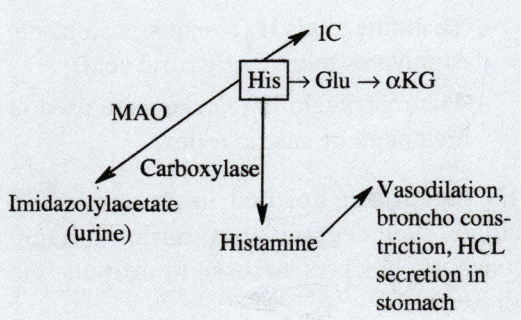

**Histidinemia:**
- Rare
- Histidase deficiency
- Histidine ———|→ urocanate
- Mental retardation

**Argininine:** NO nitric oxide:

**Synthesized** and liberated during conversion of arginine to citrulline by NOS (nitric oxide synthase).
- NOS: 3 isoforms:
- Neuronal NOS (nNOS, NOS-1)
- Macrophage or inducible NO (iNOS, NOS-2)
- Endothelial NOS (eNOS, NOS-3)

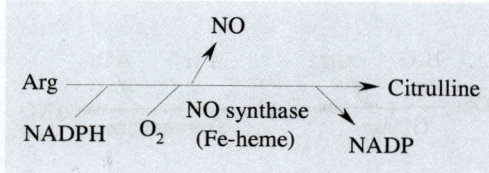

## Functions

- iNOS: Bactericidal in macrophages for creating NO for generation of free radical.
- NO: Activate cGMP which causes vascular dilatation

  Also known as EDRF (endothelium-derived relaxation factor)

  Nitrates (nitroglycerine, nitroprusside) release NO that control blood pressure.

### $H_1$ receptors:

- Histidine binds $H_1$ reactors in stomach, stimulates release of gastric acid.
- Pharmacologic $H_1$ blockers are used in treatment of gastric reflex.

**$H_2$ receptors:** Located in basophils and stimulate their degranulation during allergic response. $H_2$ blockers are used to treat allergic conditions.

## BCAA Branch chain amino acid

- Valine, Leucine, Isoleucine
- Valine: glucogenic
- Leucine: ketogenic
- Isoleucine: Both

## BCAA

- All are essential amino acid
- BCAA transaminase loosely bound to IMM which is a common enzyme for all 3 BCAA.
- $1^{st}$ two catabolic reactions of 3 BCAA are common:
- Transamination of all 3 BCAA: Catalyzed by same transaminase, reversible

## BCKD

- BC α Keto dehydrogenase
- Multienzyme complex
- Catalyzes oxidative decarboxylation of a keto acids derived from Val, Leu, Ile (reaction II).
- Similar to pyruvate dehydrogenase

## Three enzymes

- Decarboxylase
- Dihydrolipoyl dehydrogenase
- Dihydrolipoyl transacetylase

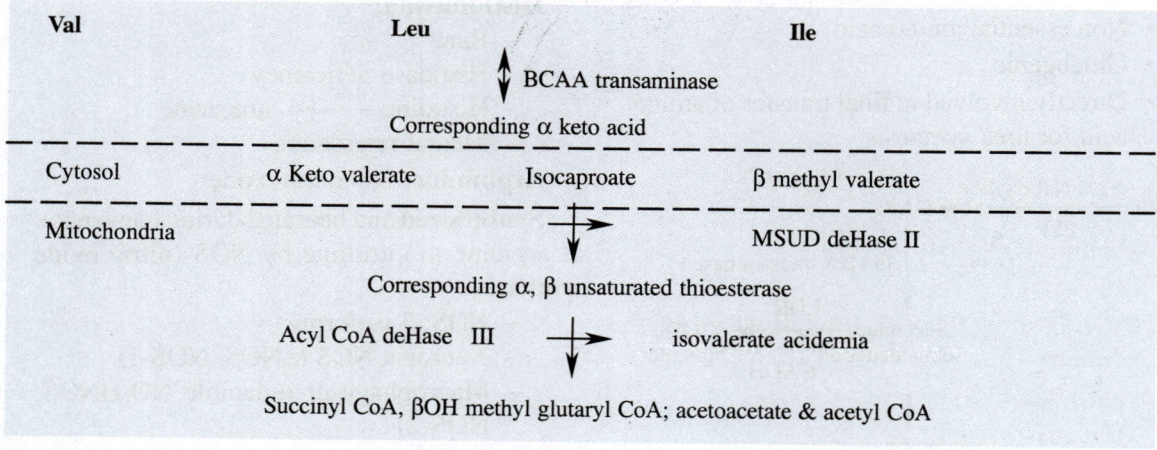

## Four vitamins

- Thiamin (TDP)
- Riboflavin (FAD)
- Pantothenic acid (CoA)
- Niacin (NAD)

### Regulation: BCKD

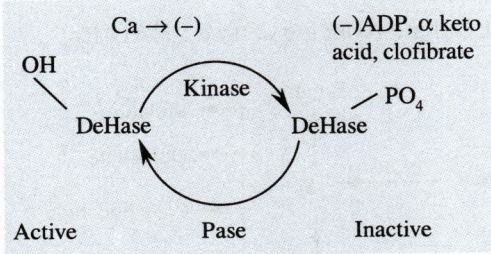

**Catabolism of BCAA** occurs in

- Liver
- Kidney
- Muscle
- Heart
- Adipose tissue

**IMD: BCAA**

**MSUD: Maple syrup urine disease**

Branch chain amino aciduria

Defect: BCKD (dehydrogenase), AR

Urine: Maple syrup / burnt sugar odor

↑ Plasma and urine levels of Leu Ile, Val and their keto acids

### Features

- Evident by end of first week of life
- Difficulty to take feed
- Vomiting
- Lethargy
- Extensive brain damage: mental retardation.
- Death by $1^{st}$ year of life
- Poor myelination
- Mechanism: not known

## Treatment

- BCAA free – diet

### Intermittent BC Ketonuria

- Variant of MSUD
- α Keto decarboxylase defect
- Symptoms appear later in life, only intermittently
- Prognosis by diet therapy favorable.

### Isovalerate academia

- Isovaleryl CoA dehydrogenase defect
- Isovaleryl accumulation – cheesy odor of breath and body fluids.

### Features

- Vomiting
- Acidosis
- Coma precipitated by ingestion of excessive proteins
- Distinct 'Sweaty Odor'
- NM irritability
- Mental retardation

### Methylmalonic aciduria

- Occurs in hereditary deficiency of methyl malonyl CoA mutase, acquired vitamin $B_{12}$ deficiency.
- Valine metabolism: $B_{12}$ dependent reaction: methyl malonyl CoA mutase defective.
- Responsive to pharmacologic doses of $B_{12}$

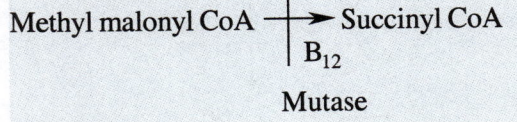

### Features

Vomiting, dehydration, seizures, failure to thrive, developmental delay, Propionyl acidemia. Propionyl CoA accumulates which condenses with OAA to form methyl citrate.

**Propionyl CoA carboxylase deficiency** in isoleucine metabolism.

High serum propionyl levels

Propionyl CoA $\xrightarrow[\text{Carboxylase}]{}$ d-methyl malonyl CoA

## (vi) Aromatic Amino Acid Metabolism

### Aromatic amino acids

- Phenylalanine
- Tyrosine
- Tryptophan
- Phen: essential amino acid
- Tyr: non essential amino acid

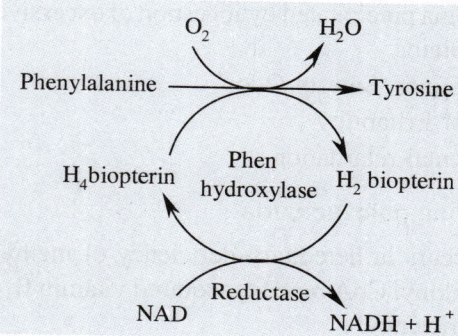

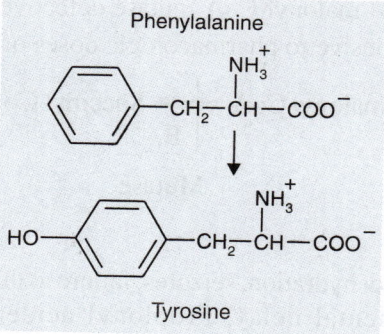

**Fig. 4.141.**

### Phenylalanine hydroxylase

- Mixed function oxygenase
- Present in mammalian liver
- One atom of molecular oxygen incorporated into para position of phenylalanine.
- $2^{nd}$ atom of oxygen reduced to form water
- Immediate source of reducing power: $H_4$ biopterin
- Ultimate reducing source : NAD(P)

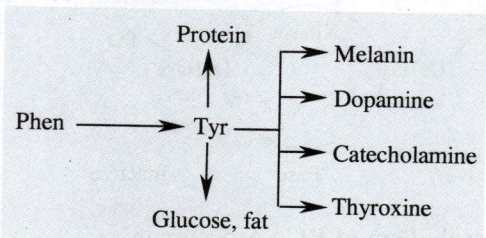

| Table 4.22. | | |
|---|---|---|
| *Adrenal medulla* | *Thyroid* | *Melanocyte* |
| Tyrosine | ↓ | Tyrosine |
| BH$_2$ ← | hydrolase | ↓ | Tyrosinase Albinism |
| L-dopa | ↓ | L-dopa |
| CO$_2$ ← | decarboxylase | ↓ | ↓ |
| Dopamine | | |
| ↓ | β hydroxylase | ↓ | ↓ |
| Norepinephrine | T3, T4 | Melanin |
| SAM ⟍ | Methyl-transferase | |
| SAH ⟋ | | |
| Epinephrine | | |

### Ultimate fate of phenylalanine

- L-Phen → fumarate + acetoacetate + $CO_2$
- Catabolism: Phenylalanine

## AKU (alkaptonuria)

- Alkaptonuria
- Homogentisate oxidase deficiency.
  - Alkapton, a product of Phen and tyrosine metabolism accumulates.
  - Homogentisate autoxidizes to form dark color pigment that accumulates in various tissues, especially cartilages namely nose, ear.
  - Urine darkens on standing.

## IMD: Phen

| Table 4.23. PKU Phenylketonuria | |
| --- | --- |
| *Type* | *Defect* |
| I-III | Phenylalanine hydroxylase defect (absent/immature, decreased) |
| IV | Dihydrobiopterine reductase defect |
| V | Dihydropiopterine biosynthesis defect |

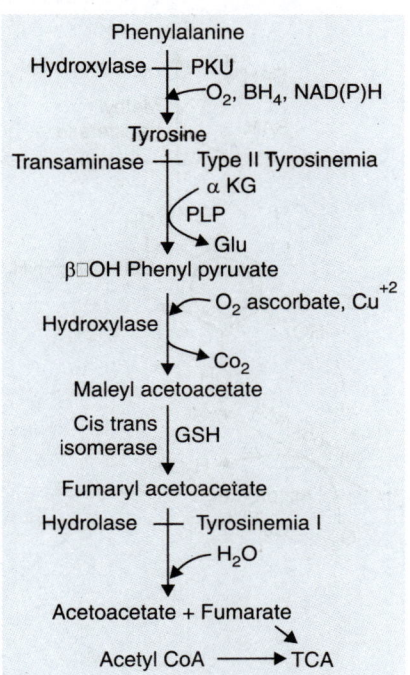

**Fig. 4.142.** Catabolism: Phenylalanine.

## Tyrosinemia

| *Type* | *Defect* |
| --- | --- |
| I | Fumaryl acetoacetate hydroxylase defect: neonatal tyrosinemia |
| II | Tyrosine transaminase |
| Neonatal tyrosinemia | p-OH phenyl pyruvate hydroxylase deficiency |
| AKU (alkaptonuria) | Homogentisate oxidase deficiency |

## PKU (Phenylketonuria)

Genetic deficiency of phen hydroxylase (PH) phenylalanine and products of phenylalanine deamination (phenyl pyruvate) via transaminase accumulate in blood and urine.

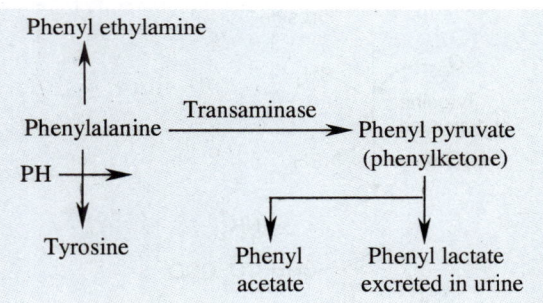

Altered brain functions: blocks other amino acid transport, myelin formation, and neurotransmitters.

## PKU: Features

- Incidence 1 : 10,000 live births
- Screening of new born in mandatory in USA
- Increased urine phenyl pyruvate detected by $FeCl_3$ (ferric chloride test)
- Mental retardation results unless treatment begins immediately after birth

## Treatment

- Limit phenylalanine intake till 6 years of age (because brain development occurs till that age)
- Supply tyrosine in diet

## Catecholamine synthesis

- Epinephrine and norepinephrine are secreted by adrenal medulla, sympathetic and central nervous system. Cells of neural crest origin convert epinephrine to norepinephrine.
- DOPA is intermediate in formation of melanin and norepinephrine.

- Different hydroxylases act on tyrosine via melanocytes and other cell types.

Parkinson's disease:

- Decreased production of dopamine
- Common feature are tremors, difficulty in initiating voluntary movement, mask-like face, shuffling gait.
- Dopamine is important in substantia nigra to mediate motor activity of brain.

## Treatment

Dopa, which crosses blood brain barrier and get converted to dopamine.

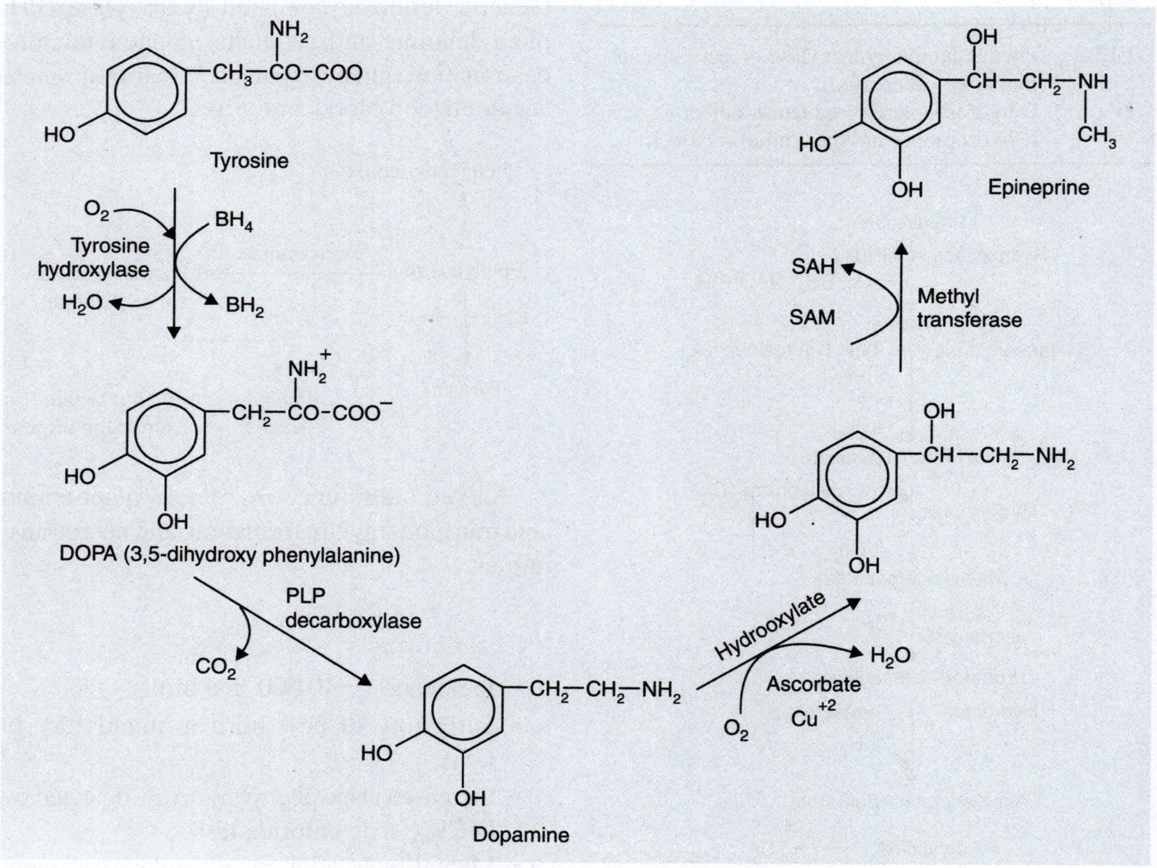

**Fig. 4.143.** Catecholamine synthesis

## Inactivation of catecholamines

- Inactivated by MAO (monoamine oxidase)
- Producing $NH_4^+$ and $H_2O_2$ and catecholamine is converted to an aldehyde. COMT (catecholamine-O-methyl transferase) methylates 3-hydroxy group. Inhibition of MAO and COMT are used in treatment of neuropsychiatric disorders such as depression, Parkinson's disease.

**VMA:** Vinyl mandelic acid is major urinary excreted product of deaminated, methylated catecholamines. In pheochromocytoma, over-production of catecholamines from adrenal tyrosine result in increased excretion of VMA.

## THYROID HORMONE SYNTHESIS

### Melanins

- Pigments in skin and hair
- Polymers of tyrosine catabolites (quinine) of dopa

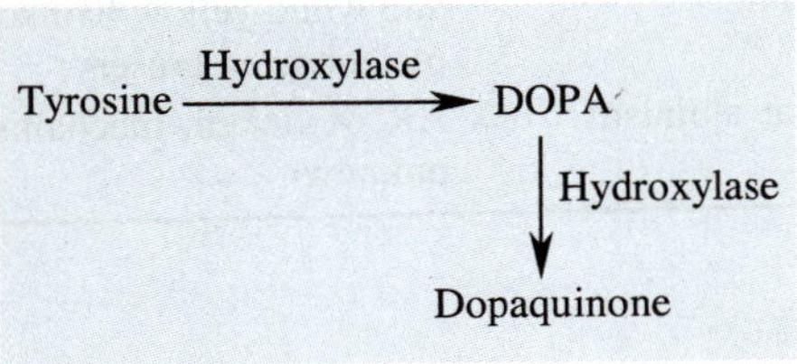

Tyrosine $\xrightarrow{\text{Hydroxylase}}$ DOPA $\xrightarrow{\text{Hydroxylase}}$ Dopaquinone

### Albinism

Defect in conversion of tyrosine to melanin. Hypomelanosis is due to inheritable defects in eyes, skin, melanocytes, and hair.

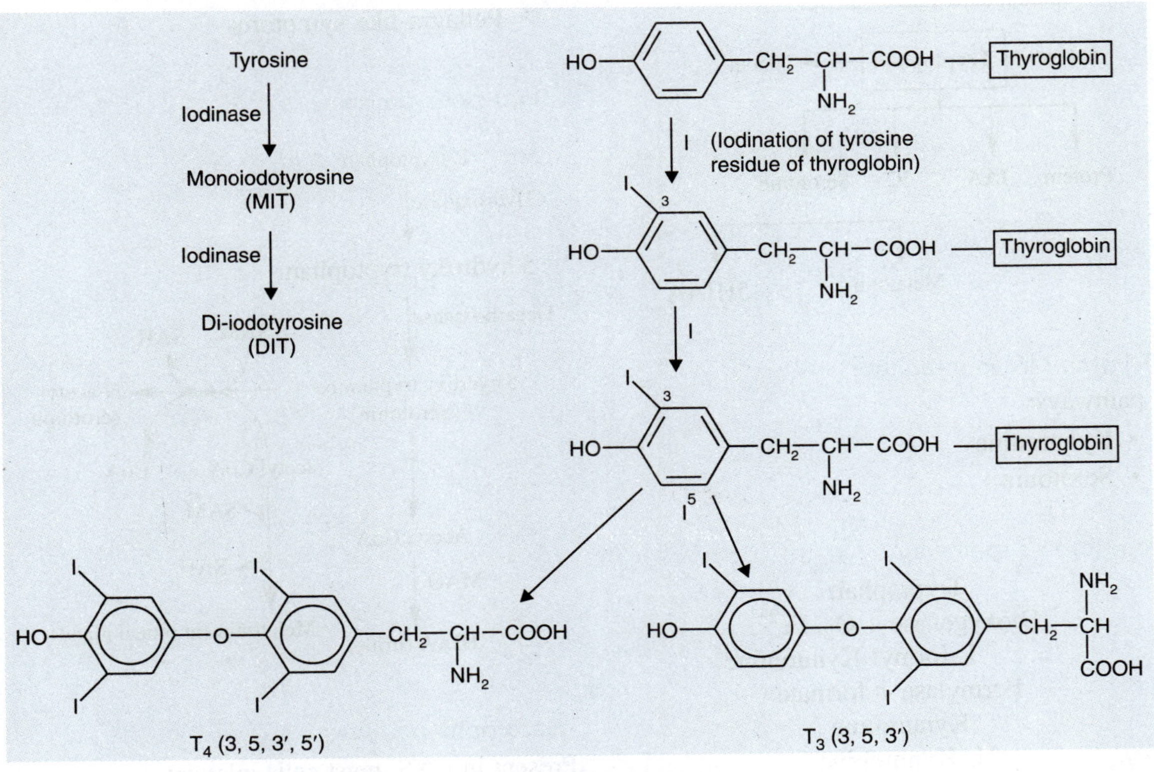

Fig. 4.144. Thyroid hormone synthesis.

| Table 4.24. | |
|---|---|
| *Defect* | *Features* |
| Tyrosine hydroxylase negative | Lacks all visual pigments, hair bulb fail to convert tyrosine to pigment |
| Tyrosine hydroxylase positive | Have some visible pigment and white-yellow hair some melanocytes present |
| Ocular albinism | AR, X-linked, mechanism: unknown |

## Tryptophan

- Essential amino acid
- Contain indole ring
- Both glucogenic and ketogenic

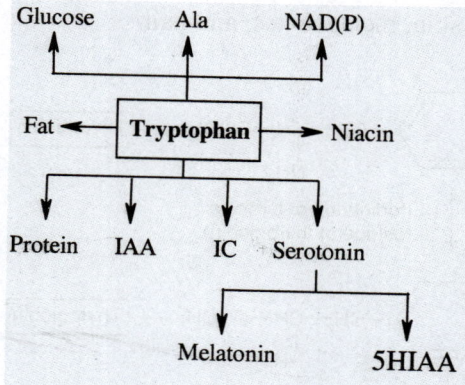

## Tryptophan metabolism

2 pathways:

- Kynurenine
- Serotonin

### Kynurenine pathway

Tryptophan
Dioxygenase $\downarrow O_2, Fe^{2+}$
L-formyl Kynurenine
Formylase $\downarrow$ formate
Kynurenine
L-Kynurenine

Hydroxylase $\downarrow O_2$, NADPH
3-hydroxy Kynurenine
Kynureninase
$\searrow$
alanine
3-hydroxy
Anthranilate
Oxidase $\downarrow$ PLP
2acroleyl-3-amino fumarate
$\downarrow$
$\alpha$ Keto adipate

**In $B_6$ deficiency:** Kynurenine $\rightarrow$ xanthurinate which accumulate in urine

### Hartnup disease

- AR, Defect in intestinal and renal transport of neutral amino acids including tryptophan.
- Increased excretion of indole derivative
- Pellagra-like symptoms

### Serotonin pathway

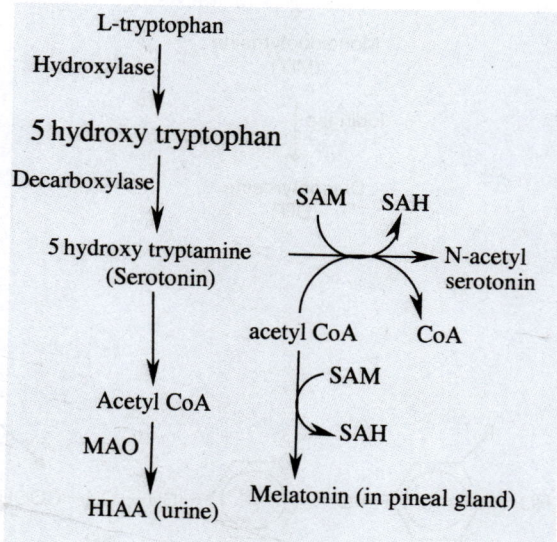

### Serotonin pathway

Present in CNS, mast cells, platelet.

## Actions

- Potent vasodilator
- Muscle contraction
- Neurotransmitter, stimulatory neurotransmitter

## Carcinoid syndrome

Argentiffinoma, overproduction of serotonin.

## Features

- Hypertension, flushes, respiratory distress, diarrhea, wheezing, increased HIAA in urine.
- Decreased nicotinic acid causing pellagra, since tryptophan is not available for synthesis of vitamin niacin.

## Biosynthesis of niacin

60 mg tryptophan forms 1mg equivalent of niacin.

## Catabolism

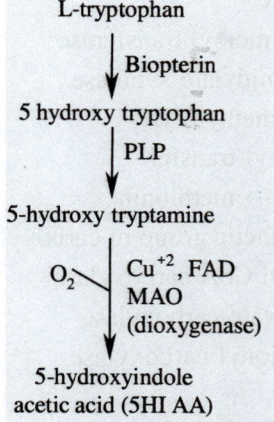

L-tryptophan
↓ Biopterin
5 hydroxy tryptophan
↓ PLP
5-hydroxy tryptamine
↓ $O_2$ | $Cu^{+2}$, FAD MAO (dioxygenase)
5-hydroxyindole acetic acid (5HI AA)

## Polyamine

- Ornithine and arginine form polyamines
- Polyamines are important for:
- Cell proliferation and growth
- Protein synthesis

**Include:** Putrescine, spermine, spermidine.

## ODC

- Ornithine decarboxylase
- Shortest half life
- t1/2 of 10 minute

Stimulated by:
- GH
- Corticosteroids
- Testosterone
- EDGF (epidermoid derived growth factor)

Target for cancer chemotherapy

ODC enzyme directed chemotherapy is given in malignancy.

## Synthesis

Monoamines: biogenic amino: dopamine, norepinephrine, epinephrine, serotonin, histamine.

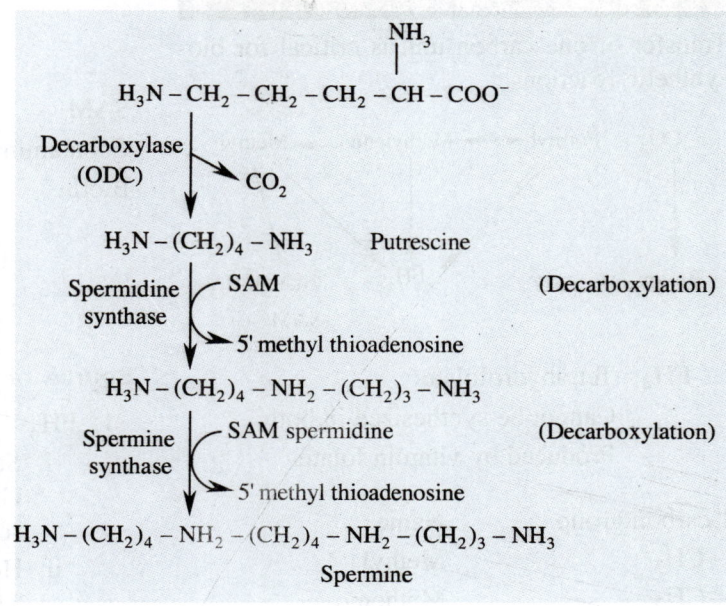

$$H_3N - CH_2 - CH_2 - CH_2 - CH - COO^-$$
with $NH_3$ on the $CH$

Decarboxylase (ODC) → $CO_2$

$H_3N - (CH_2)_4 - NH_3$    Putrescine

Spermidine synthase ↙ SAM    (Decarboxylation)
↘ 5' methyl thioadenosine

$H_3N - (CH_2)_4 - NH_2 - (CH_2)_3 - NH_3$

Spermine synthase ↙ SAM spermidine    (Decarboxylation)
↘ 5' methyl thioadenosine

$H_3N - (CH_2)_4 - NH_2 - (CH_2)_4 - NH_2 - (CH_2)_3 - NH_3$
Spermine

## Amino acids as precursors of signaling molecules

### Neurotransmitters

Amino acid acting directly as neurotransmitters:
- Glycine
- Aspartate
- Glutamate, Glutamine

### Amino acids converted to neurotransmitter

- GABA
- Serotonin
- Histamine
- Melatonin
- NO (from arginine)

### Hormones synthesized from amino acids

- Thyroxine
- Catecholamines:
- Dopamine, epinephrine
- Norepinephrine

## (vii) One-Carbon Metabolism

Transfer of one carbon unit is critical for biosynthetic reactions.

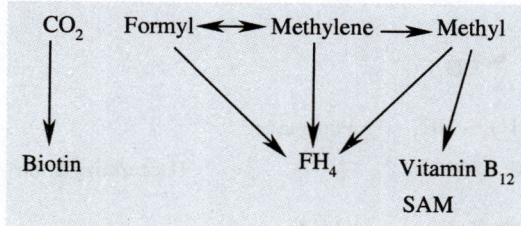

**FH$_4$:** Tetrahydrofolate
Cannot be synthesized in body
Produced by vitamin folate.

| 1 carbon group | Name |
|---|---|
| —CH$_3$ | Methyl |
| —CH$_2$— | Methenyl |

| | |
|---|---|
| —CH— | Formyl |
| —CHNH— | Formimino |
| —COOH | Formate |
| $CO_2$, $HCO_3$ | – |

### I-C carriers

| I-C carrier | I-C carried |
|---|---|
| Folic acid | —CH$_3$, —CH$_2$, —CH<br>—CHNH$_2$ —CHO |
| SAM | —CH$_3$ |
| Biotin | $HCO_3$ or $CO_2$ |

**1C attachment sites:** C, N, S atoms mainly

| | |
|---|---|
| THF | N$_5$, N$_{10}$ carbon |
| SAM | S atom |
| Cobalamin | Co attaches methyl group |
| Biotin | $CO_2$ attaches to 'N' of imidazole |

### Utilization of 1-C

| | |
|---|---|
| FH$_4$ | Serine hydroxyl methyl transferase |
| | Hcy methyl transferase |
| | Thymidylate synthase |
| | N$_{10}$ methyl THF |
| SAM | Methyl transfer |
| Cobalamin | Hcy → methionine |
| Biotin | Prosthetic group of carboxylase:<br>acetyl CoA carboxylase<br>pyruvate carboxylase<br>propionyl carboxylase |

### Source of 1-carbon

1. FH$_4$
   i. Serine hydroxyl methyl transferase: Glycine + N$^5$ N$^{10}$ methylene THF ↔ serine + THF
   ii. Hcy methyl transferase: Hcy + N5 Me THF ↔ Methionine + THF

iii. Thymidylate synthase: $2'$ deoxyuridylate + $N^5 N^{10}$ methylene THF $\leftrightarrow 2'$ deoxy thymidylate

iv. $N^{10}$ Methyl THF

$N^{10}$ MeTHF $\rightarrow$ C2 purine

2. SAM:
   - Methyl transfer from SAM to acceptor: when SAM transfers its methyl group, 5-adenosyl homocysteine (SAH) is produced, hcy gets methylated by vitamin $B_{12}$ to form SAM
   - Synthesized from methionine and ADP
   - Supplies methyl group and used in following conversions:

   Guanido acetate $\rightarrow$ creatine

   Phosphatidylethanolamine $\rightarrow$ phosphatidyl choline

   Norepinephrine $\rightarrow$ epinephrine

   Polynucleotide $\rightarrow$ methylated polynucleotides

   Acetyl serotonin $\rightarrow$ melatonin

## Transmethylation reaction

| Reactant | Product |
|---|---|
| SAM | SAH |
| Norepinephrine | Epinephrine |
| Ethanolamine | Choline |
| Epinephrine | Norepinephrine |
| Guanidoacetate | Creatine |
| Nicotinamide | N-methyl nicotinamide |
| Acetyl serotonin | Melatonin |
| Carnosine | Anaserine |
| Serine | Choline |

3. Cobalamin: Hey $\rightarrow$ methionine requires $N^5$ methyl THF

4. Biotin: Prosthetic group of carboxylase, e.g.
   - Acetyl CoA carboxylase
   - Pyruvate carboxylase
   - Propionyl carboxylase

## Source of 1-carbon

### Serine, glycine:
- Predominant source
- Serine degradation $\rightarrow N^5 N^{10}$ Methyl THF
- Glycine breakdown:
  - $N^5 N^{10}$ methylene THF

### Histidine catabolism: formate:
- Tryptophan $\rightarrow$ formate $\rightarrow N^{10}$ formyl THF
- Glycine $\rightarrow$ formate

**Table 4.25.** Summary 1C-metabolism

| Source | Carriers | Products |
|---|---|---|
| Gly, Try $\rightarrow$ formate | $N^{10}$ formyl THF | C2 purine |
| His $\xrightarrow{\text{Folate}}$ FIGLU | $N^5$ formimino THF | Formyl |
| Ser + THF $\leftrightarrow$ Gly | $N^5 N^{10}$ methylene THF | Gly $\rightarrow$ Ser $\rightarrow B_{12}$ thymidylate (TMP) deficiency |
| Choline + THF $\rightarrow$ betaine Transmethylation synthesis of creatinine, epinephrine, choline, melatonin | $N^5$ methyl THF $\rightarrow$ Hcy $\downarrow B_{12}$ $CH_3 \leftarrow$ SAM | |

## 1-C carried by $FH_4$

Serine, glycine, formaldehyde, histidine, formate transfer 1C to $FH_4$ which are then transferred to other compounds.

Dihydrofolate reductase        Dihydrofolate reductase

NADPH   NADP          NADPH   NAD

Folate $\leftrightarrows FH_2$ (dihydrofolate) $\leftrightarrows FH_4$

**1-C groups carried by FH$_4$:**

Formyl, methyl, methenyl, methylene

**Recipients of 1-C groups:**

- Purine:
  C2 and C8 from FH$_4$
  Deoxyuridine monophosphate (dUMP) forms dTMP
- Methotrexate:
  Inhibits dihydrofolate reductase, thus inhibits purine synthesis, used in cancer, rheumatoid arthritis
- Trimethoprim:
  Folate analog, binds bacterial dihydrofolate reductase: anti bacterial compound used with sulfonamides
- Spina bifida and anencephaly: Neural tube defects are reduced by preconception supplementation with folic acid.

# 4. NUCLEOTIDE & PORPHYRIN METABOLISM

## (i) Purine Metabolism

**Synthesis**

Two types: Salvage, Denovo

**Table 4.26.**

| Salvage | Denovo |
|---|---|
| Activated ribose (PRPP) | Activated ribose (PRPP) |
| Base → nucleotide | A.A. + ATP + CO$_2$ → nucleotide |
| Base is attached | Base is synthesized (require ATP) |
| Preformed bases recovered and reconnected to ribose unit | Nucleotide base assembled first then attached to ribose: pyrimidine in purine: base synthesized piece by piece over ribose-based structure |

Purine ring built up using:
Amino acids:
    Glycine, aspartate, glutamine
THF
CO$_2$

**Fact file: Purines**

- Purines are not metabolized to central metabolites
- Ring structure is retained in birds reptiles and primates
- Other organisms can further breakdown ring before excretion
- Pyrimidine base catabolized to form intermediates of central metabolism piece by piece on ribose-based structure

**Purine synthesis**

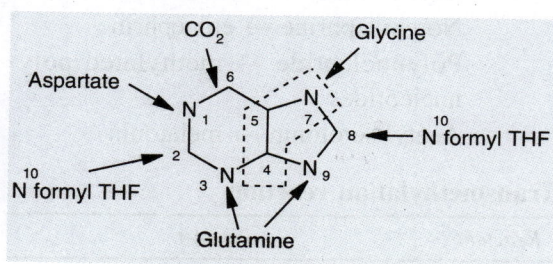

**Fig. 4.145.** Purine synthesis.

1st step: PRPP (phosphoribosyl pyrophosphate) synthesis

$$\text{Ribose-5-P} + \text{ATP} \xrightarrow[\text{synthase}]{\text{PRPP}} \text{PRPP} + \text{AMP}$$

PRPP provides ribose moiety to glutamine to form PRA (phosphoribosylamine)

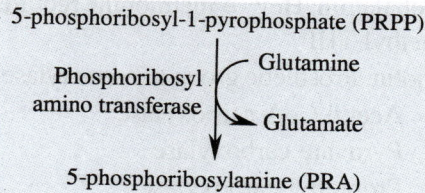

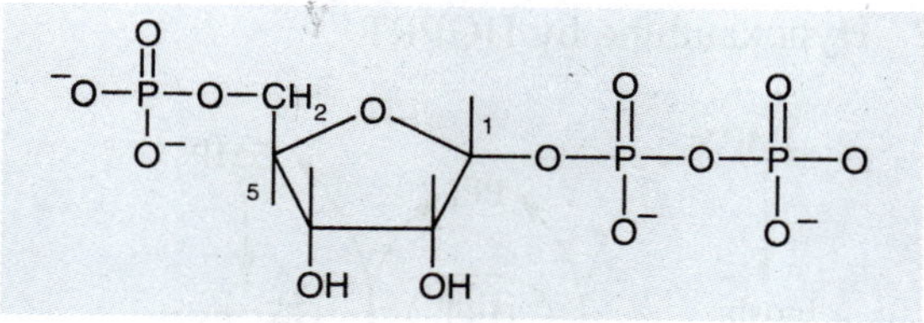

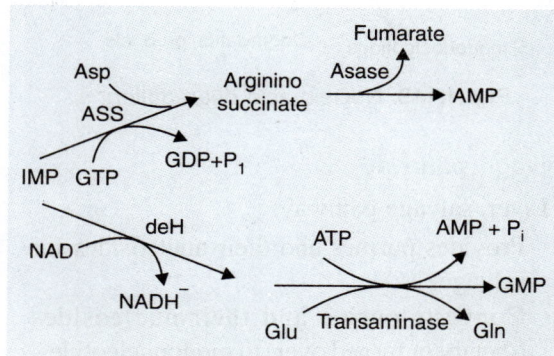

**Fig. 4.146.** PRPP.

## Aminotransferase

- Committed step
- Important regulated step
- Inhibit by IMP, GMP, AMP

## APPLIED ASPECTS

### Over activity of PRPPS

- X-linked disorder
- Resulting in overproduction of nucleotides leading to increased degradation, hyperuricemia, gout and kidney stones.

### Next steps

- Then, glycine molecule is added to growing purine precursor
- $C_8$ by formyl THF
- $N_4$ by glutamine
- $C_6$ by $CO_2$
- $N_1$ by aspartate
- $C_2$ by formyl THF
- Inosine monophosphate, IMP which contains base hypoxanthine is generated.
- IMP can be converted to free base in liver or to nucleotide (by dephosphorylation).
- IMP is precursor for both AMP and GMP and IMP is converted to XMP by IMP dehydrogenase and finally to GMP by GMP synthetase.

### AMP is formed from IMP

IMP is first converted to adenyl succinate by enzyme adenyl succinate synthetase and finally to AMP by adenyl succinase.

Each product (AMP, GMP) regulates its own synthesis by feedback inhibition of first two steps of synthesis.

- AMP and GMP can be phosphorylated to triphosphate level (ATP and GTP).
- Ribose moiety is reduced to deoxyribose at diphosphate level by ribonucleotide reductase and requires thioredoxin.

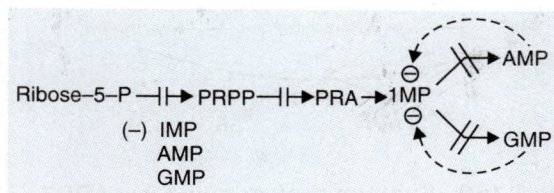

**Fig. 4.147.** AMP and GMP synthesis.

### Regulation

Key regulatory steps:

- PRPP synthase (PRPPS)
- PRPP amidotransferase (ART): committed step

Hydroxyurea is an inhibitor of ribonucleotide reductase, used in treatment of myelogenous leukemia, polycythemia.

**Fig. 4.148.** Regulation of purine synthesis.

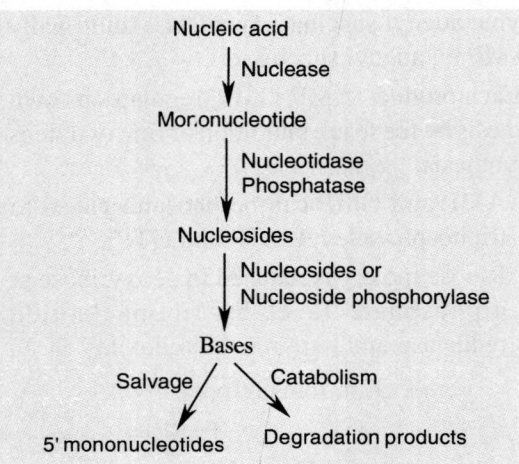

**Fig. 4.149.** Nucleic acid degradation.

## Salvage pathway

In Liver, salvage pathway:

- Provides purines and their nucleosides for salvage
- Converts purine and their nucleosides (dietary or turned over) to mononucleotides.

### Salvage pathway:

- Requires less energy than denovo
- Involves ribosylation of free purine
- Occurs in brain, RBC, polymorphs:
- lack APRT: cannot synthesize PRA and polymorp utilize exogenous purines to form nucleotides.

### Ribosylation of free purine by PRPP

1. Adenine

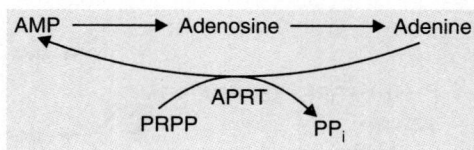

**Fig. 4.150.** Synthesis of adenine by APRT (Adeninophosphoribosyl transferase)

2. Hypoxanthine by HGPRT

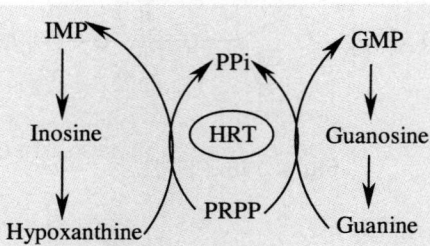

3. Direct ribosylation of purine ribonucleotide

$$
\text{Adenine} \xrightarrow[\text{Kinase}]{\text{Adenine}} \text{AMP}
$$
$$
\text{Deoxy adenine} \xrightarrow{\text{AK}} \text{dAMP}
$$
$$
\text{Deoxycytidine} \xrightarrow{\text{dCK}} \text{dCMP}
$$
$$
\text{Adenine} \xrightarrow{\text{dCK}} \text{AMP}
$$

## Purine degradation

- During degradation of purine nucleotides, phosphate and ribose are removed first, and then the nitrogenous base is oxidized.
- GMP is degraded to guanine by 5' NTDase which is further degraded to guanine and ribose-1-P by PNP.
- Guanine is then converted to xanthine.

## Breakdown of nucleic acid

## Catabolism

Intracellular purine catabolism

- Nucleotides are broken into nucleosides by action of 5'nucleotidase (5'NTDase)
- Purine nucleoside phosphorylase (PNP) converts:

  Inosine → hypoxanthine

  Xanthosine → xanthine

  Guanosine → Guanine
- Ribose-1-P splits off and can be isomerized to ribose-5-P.

- Adenosine is deaminated to inosine by adenosine deaminase (ADA).
- Adenosine $\xrightarrow{\text{ADA}}$ Inosine

## Xanthine

- It is point of convergence of metabolism of purine bases
- Converted to uric acid by xanthine oxidase.

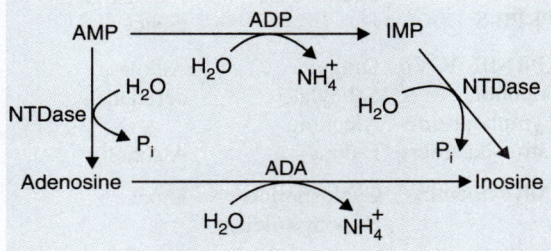

**Fig. 4.151.** Synthesis of inosine.

## Applied

### Deficiency of PNP

Leads to SCID (severe combined immunodeficiency)

- dATP and dGTP accumulate
- T-, B- and natural killer cell deficiency.

AMP is degraded to adenosine, by RNTDase,

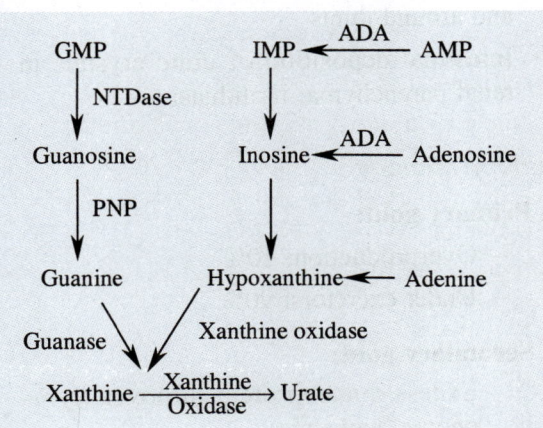

then to inosine finally by adenosine deaminase enzyme.

Then, xanthine is converted to uric acid by xanthine oxidase.

Inosine is degraded by PNP to hypoxanthine and R-1-P. Hypoxanthine is oxidized to xanthine by xanthine oxidase.

### Xanthine Oxidase

- Homodimeric protein
- Contain electron transfer proteins:
  - FAD
  - Mo-pterin complex
  - Two Fe-S clusters
- Transfer electrons to $O_2$ forming $H_2O_2$
- $H_2O_2$ is toxic converted to $H_2O$ and $O_2$ by catalase

### Catabolism of uric acid

- Humans excrete uric acid.
- Uric acid is very insoluble at high levels it precipitates out and causes gout

### Uric acid

- $pK_1 = 5.8$
- $pK_2 = 10.3$
- Only monosodium urate salt is present in body fluids.
- Urate: More water-soluble than uric acid
- Total body urate pool:
  - 1200 mg in males
  - 60 mg in females

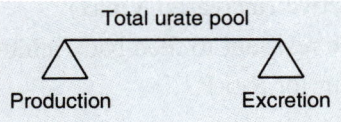

**Fig. 1.152.**

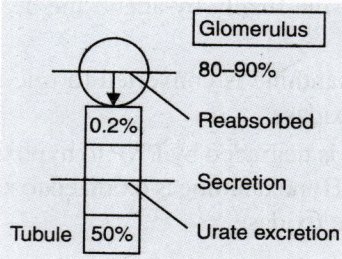

**Fig. 1.153.**

## METABOLIC DISORDERS OF PURINE CATABOLISM

### Hyper/hypouricemia

### Hyperuricemia

Serum uric acid levels > 7 mg/dL

### *Causes*

### Gout

Peripheral arthritis resulting from deposition of sodium urate crystals in one or more joints.

### What happens in gout?

R-5-P —||→ PRPP ||→ PRA → IMP

AMP    GMP

PRPPS not inhibited by IMP, AMP, GMP

### *Defect*

1. PRPPS enzyme defect:
   Superactive (increased Vmax)
   Enzyme resistant to feed back inhibition
   Low Km for R-5-P.
2. HGPRT deficiency
   PRPP levels increased.

| Table 4.27. | | |
|---|---|---|
| *Increased production* | *Decreased urate excretion* | *Combined* |
| Primary idio-pathic | Primary idio-pathic | G-6-Pase deficiency (GSDI) |
| HGPRT deficiency | DKA | |
| Increased PRPP-S | Lactacidosis | F1-Pase deficiency |
| GSD-III, V, VII Alcohol Lymphoprolife-rative disorders | Drugs: Salicylate Alcohol L-dopa | Aldolase deficiency Alcohol |
| Polycythemia | Cyclosporine Hypothyroidism | Shock |
| Aldolase deficiency | Alcohol Shock | |
| Secondary | Sarcoidosis Renal insuffi-ciency | |

## Gout

Hyperuricemia

- Attacks of actuate, monoarticular, inflammatory arthritis.
- Tophaceous deposition of urate crystals in and around joints
- Intestinal deposition of urate crystals in renal parenchyma: urolithiasis.

### *Pathophysiology*

**Primary gout:**

- Overproduction: 10%
- Under excretors: 90%

**Secondary gout:**

- Excess nucleoprotein turnover (lymphoma, leukemia)

– Increased cell proliferation cell death (psoriasis)

**Rare genetic disorder:** Lesch-Nyhan syndrome

### Treatment

- NSAID (non-steroidal antiinflammatory drugs)
- Colchicine
- Intrarticular corticosteroid
- Prednisone
- ACTH
- Opiates

### Adenosine deaminase (ADA) deficiency

$$Adenosine \xrightarrow{ADA} Indosine$$

- Autosomal recessive disorder, infant prone to bacterial, candida, viral, protozoal infections
- Both T and B-cells significantly reduced

### Lesch Nyhan Syndrome

- Defect in production or activity of HGPRT
- Increased level of hypoxanthine and guanine
- Increased degradation to uric acid
  – PRPP accumulates
- Causes gout like symptoms
- Neurological symptoms: Spasticity, aggressiveness, Self mutilation.

## (ii) Pyrimidine Metabolism

### PYRIMIDINE

Uridine monophosphate (UMP) is synthesized first: CTP is synthesized from UMP. Pyrimidine ring synthesis is first completed, and then attached to ribose-5-P.

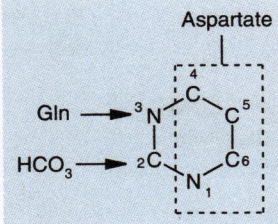

**Fig. 4.154.** Pyrimidine synthesis.

Pyrimidine ring is assembled as free base orotic acid which is then converted to nucleotide orotidine monophosphate (OMP).

Glutamine reacts with $CO_2$ and two ATP molecules to form carbamoyl phosphate in the presence of carbamoyl phosphate synthase II (CSP).

Starts with carbamoyl phosphate. (This reaction is similar to $1^{st}$ step of urea synthesis: CPS I)

CPS II is inhibited by UTP.

Aspartate adds to carbamoyl phosphate and molecule closes to yield a ring which is oxidized to form orotate. Orotate reacts with PRPP forming OMP (orotate monophosphate).

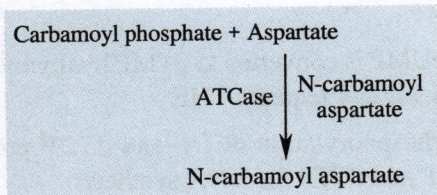

OMP is decarboxylated to form UMP by UMP synthase enzyme complex.

Most of the pathway takes place in cytoplasm.

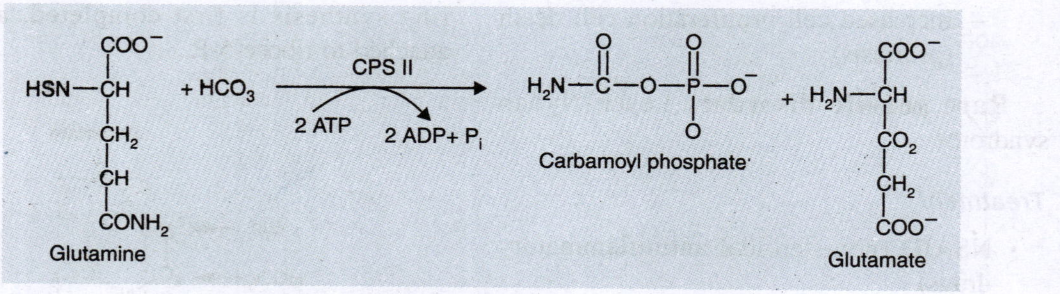

**Fig. 4.155.**

Have two multifunctional enzymes:

- CAD (CPS II, ATCase, DHOase)
- UMP synthase (OPRT, OMP-DC)

Only one reaction takes place in mitochondria (ODH).

## OMP decarboxylase

- Most catalytically proficient enzyme
- Final reaction of pyrimidine pathway
- Does not require cofactor
- Does not involve high energy carbanion intermediate.

UMP is phosphorylated to UTP which is then aminated to CTP (glutamine is amino group donor). CDP is reduced to dCDP by ribonucleotide reductase (RNR) which is deaminated to dUMP.

dUMP is converted to dTMP by thymidylate synthase and requires THF.

Phosphorylation dCDP and dTDP produce dCTP and dTTP for DNA synthesis.

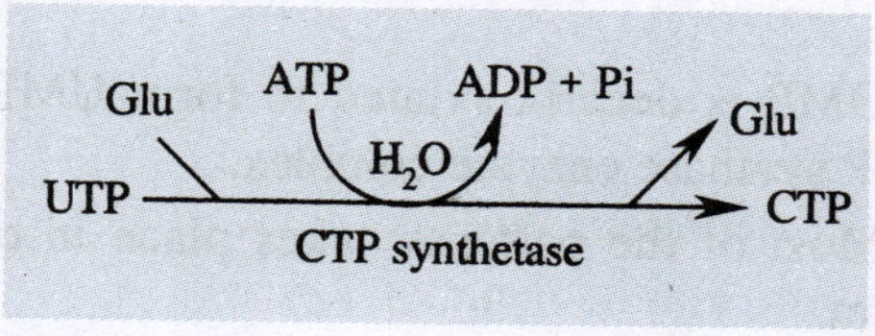

## Synthesis of deoxynucleotides

- Ribonucleotide must be reduced to deoxy nucleotides to serve as substrate for DNA synthesis.
- Ribonucleotide diphosphate is reduced by reductase and requires NADPH.

## Applied

## Orotic aciduria

- Caused by defect in enzyme UMP synthase complex (OPRT, ODC). Pyrimidines cannot be synthesized: increased excretion of orotic acid occurs in urine.
- Retarded growth, severe megaloblastic anaemia.
- Oral administration of uridine bypasses the metabolic block and provides a source of pyrimidine.

## Degradation of pyrimidines

CMP, UMP degraded to bases by:

- Dephosphorylation
- Deamination
- Glycosidic bond cleavage
- Uracil reduced in liver to form β-alanine which gets converted to malonyl CoA and finally FA synthesis.
- In pyrimidine degradation, carbon skeleton produce $CO_2$, water-soluble products, β-

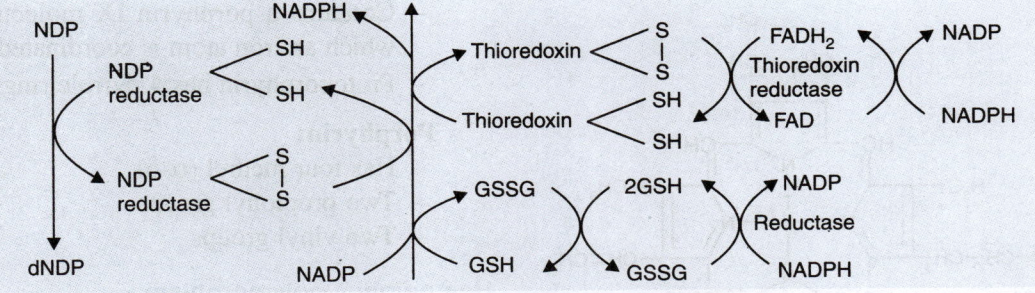

**Fig. 4.156.** Synthesis of deoxynucleotides.

alanine and some nitrogen is released as ammonium ion.

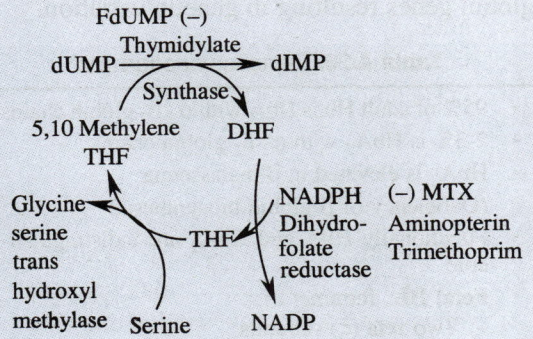

Fluorouracil is presence of enzyme thymidylate synthase converted to Flurodeoxy uridylate (FdUMP or FdU) (Suicide inhibitor of thymidylate synthase) FdUMP or FdU remains bound to enzyme as suicide inhibitor.

### Salvage pathway

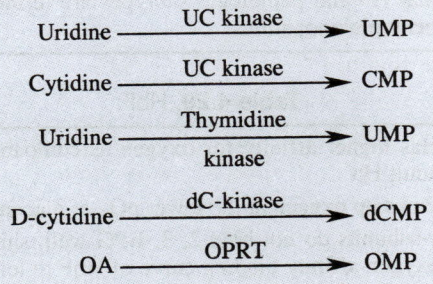

### Nucleotide analogs

- AZT (azidothymidine): AIDS,
- ddC dideoxy cytidine): antiviral, stop DNA or RNA synthesis directly

## (iii) Heme

### Hemoglobin

Hemoglobin, found in RBCs, carrier of oxygen from lungs to tissue and carbon dioxide from tissues to lungs.

### Hemoglobin (Hb): salient features

**Normal concentration:**
  – 14-16 g/dl (males)
  – 13-15 g/dl (females)

Each RBC contains 280 million Hb molecules

**Hemoglobin: Conjugated protein:**

Contains:
  – globin (apoprotein, prosthetic group)
  – Heme (non-protein, prosthetic group)
  – Tetrameric allosteric protein

### Structure: Hb

Dimer of heteromers: $(\alpha\text{-}\beta)_2$.

(a) **Globin:** soluble metabolic protein

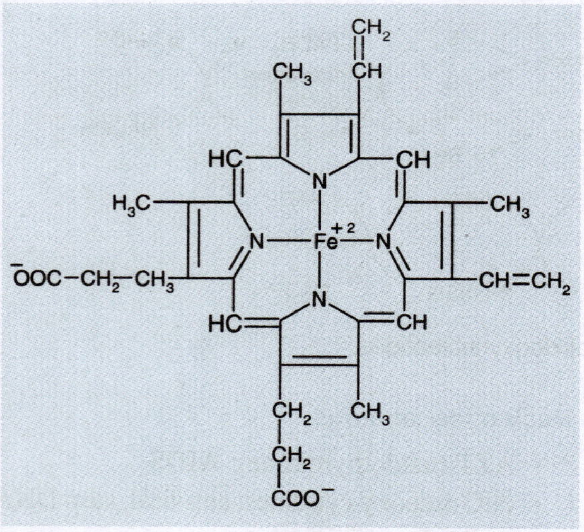

**Fig. 4.157.** Heme structure.

– Consists of four chains (two pairs of identical chains):
- $\alpha_1 \alpha_2$
- $\beta_1 \beta_2$

$\alpha$-Chain: 141 amino acids

$\beta$-Chain: 146 amino acids

**Bonds in globin chains:**
– Few bonds between two $\alpha$ or two $\beta$-chains
– Strong hydrophobic between $\alpha$, $\beta$ chains (responsible for determining oxygen, binding and release)
– Bonds between $\alpha$- and $\beta$-monomer stronger than $\alpha$-$\alpha$ or $\beta$-$\beta$ bonds or between $\alpha$-$\beta$ dimer
– Urea treatment of hemoglobin always results in $\alpha$-$\beta$ dimer.

(b) **Heme:**
– Responsible for red color of hemoglobin.
– Synthesized from porphyrin and iron
– Contains type III porphyrins

– Contains a porphyrin IX molecule to which an iron atom is coordinated
– Protoporphyrin has 4 pyrrole rings

**Porphyrin:**
– Has four methyl ($\alpha$-$\delta$)
– Two propionyl groups
– Two vinyl groups

### Hemoglobin polymorphism

Several different types of hemoglobin can be found in adult humans and during human development. In addition, different subunits of various hemoglobin are product of different globin genes resulting in genetic variation.

**Table 4.28.** Genetic variation: Hb

- 95% of adult Hb is HbA with $\alpha_2 \beta_2$ globin chains
- 2-3% is HbA$_2$ with $\alpha_2 \delta_2$ globin chains
- HbA$_2$ is elevated in $\beta$-thalassemia (Deficiency of $\beta$-globin biosynthesis)
- Functionally HbA and HbA$_2$ are indistinguishable.
- **Fetal Hb**: Tetramer of:
  – Two zeta ($\xi$) subunits
  – Two epsilon ($\in$) subunits i.e., $\xi_2 \in_2$ units evolutionarily similar to $\alpha$-subunits.
  – After 6 months of development, $\xi$ subunit replaced by $\alpha$ subunit i.e., $\in$ fetal Hb: HbF is $\alpha_2\gamma_2$
- Later embryonic life and just after birth, $\gamma$-subunits replaced by $\beta$-subunits.
- More than 600 mutations in gene encoding $\alpha$ and $\beta$-globin have been documented
- Several hundred mutations giving rise to abnormal Hb and pathologic subtypes are termed as hemoglobinopathies.

**Table 4.29.** HbF

- Has higher affinity for oxygen as compared to adult Hb
- Picks up oxygen at the lower pO$_2$ of placenta
- $\gamma$-subunits do not bind 2, 3, BPG well, shifting oxygen-affinity binding curve of HbF to left.

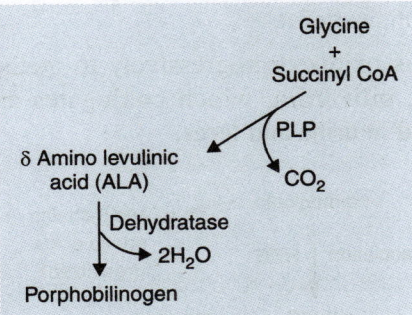

Glycine
+
Succinyl CoA

δ Amino levulinic acid (ALA)

PLP

$CO_2$

Dehydratase

$2H_2O$

Porphobilinogen

**Fig. 4.158.**

## Table 4.30. HbA

- More efficient transfer of $O_2$ from maternal HbA to fetal Hb
- Decreases shortly after birth due to gene switching on chromosome 11
- HbF variant increases up to 15-20% in adults with mutant adult Hb e.g. sickle cell disease.

## Table 4.31. Function: Hb

- Oxygen transport from lungs to tissues
- Carbon dioxide transport from tissues to lungs.
- Maintain acid-base balance: erythrocyte Hb functions as buffer:
  Buffers the hydrogen generated from carbonic anhydrase i.e., carbonic acid.

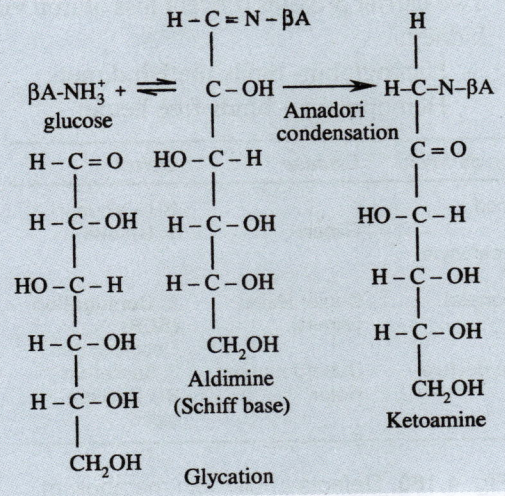

# Heme metabolism

## Table 4.32. Salient feature- heme metabolism

- 85% heme synthesized in erythroid cells to provide heme for Hb
- Heme produced in liver to provide cyt $P_{450}$ enzymes.
- Under physiological conditions in human adults: $1-2 \times 10^8$ RBCs destroyed per hour.
- 70 kg human turns around 6 g of Hb daily
- 1 g Hb yields 35 mg bilirubin.

## NO

- NO binds reversibly with Hb in two ways:
  - Binds to heme $Fe^{+2}$
  - Forms an adduct with surface exposed $Cys^{93}$ β side chains to form nitrosyl-Hb or S-nitroso-Hb.

Thus, NO has a role in transport and delivery of a third gas (NO).

## Glycated Hb

Glucose reacts with N-terminal amino acid residues (valine) of β chains of (HbA) to form $HbA_{1c}$ via formation of Schiff's base via ketoamine formation (glucose-$CH_2$-NH-βA)

This reaction is a continuous process occurring slowly over the life span of RBC. This phenomenon is not confined to Hb and a number of other glycated proteins have been reported. The concentration of $HbA_{1c}$ correlates with degree of diabetic control and reflects patient average blood glucose concentration over a long period (i.e., 2-3 months).

Normal $HbA_1c$ is 4-6% of total HbA and levels below 7% indicate acceptable control of diabetes.

## Heme containing protein:

- Hb
- Myoglobin

- Cytochrome
- Cytochrome $P_{450}$
- Catalase
- Tryptophan pyrrolase

## Heme biosynthesis

Heme is a constituent of hemoglobin, myoglobin and cytochromes is synthesized in most cells of the body.

Heme is synthesized from glycine and succinyl coenzyme A which condense to form δ-amino leuvulinate (δ-ALA) catalyzed by δ-ALA synthase in mitochondria.

### Table 4.33. ALA synthesis- Fact file

- Synthesized from glycine and succinyl CoA in mitochondria
- Catalyzed by ALA synthase
- PLP acts as a cofactor
- Rate-limiting step
- Committed step
- Regulated by level of heme:
  Inhibited by: Heme
  Transcription of ALA synthase repressed by heme.
- ALA synthase is inducible enzyme:
  Drugs metabolizing through cyt $P_{450}$ increase utilization of heme, causing depression of enzyme

Subsequently, in cytosol, two molecules of ALA condense in cytosol to form a pyrrole ring porphobilinogen (PBG). Four PBG molecules combine to form a linear tetrapyrrole: compound hydroxymethylbilane (HMB).

HMB cyclizes to uroporphyrinogen III which gets decarboxylated to coproporphyrinogen III. Finally, coproporphyrinogen decarboxylated in mitochondria to yield protoporphyrinogen III and finally protoporphyrin IX. Iron ($Fe^{+2}$) is added to protoporphyrin IX to form heme.

## Catabolism-heme

Heme is oxidized progressively to methemoglobin, biliverdin, which conjugates and is excreted in urine and feces.

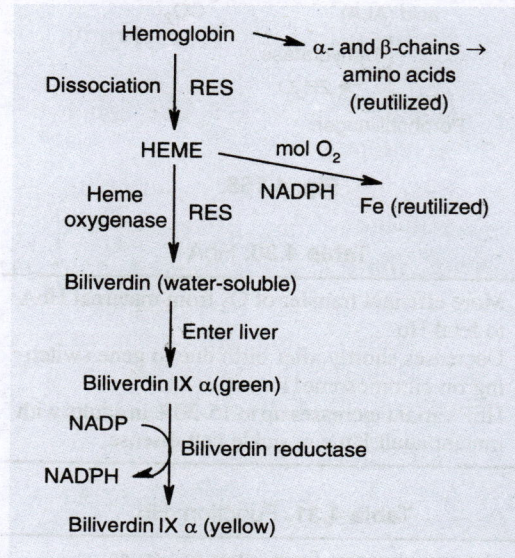

**Fig. 4.159.** Metabolic fate-Bilirubin

## RBC destruction

- Occurs in spleen, liver
- When occurs elsewhere: hemolytic anaemia
- Two carrier proteins prevent loss of iron via kidney:
  - Haptoglobin- binds metHb dimers
  - Hemoprexin – binds free heme.

| Compartment | Disease | Defect |
|---|---|---|
| Blood | | BR + albumin |
| | Gilbert | 1. Uptake |
| Hepatocyte BR | | |
| Neonatal | Crigler Najjar Gilbert | 2. Conjugation (SER) Deconjugated |
| Bile ductule | Dubin Johnson, Rotor | 3. Secretion BR Deconjugated |

**Fig. 4.160.** Defects in bilirubin metabolism.

When in excess, bilirubin imparts yellow colour to skin and is termed as **jaundice: Hyper bilirubinemia.**

## Causes of jaundice

- **Prehepatic** – increased production of bilirubin
- **Hepatic** – impaired uptake, conjugation or secretion of bilirubin
- **Post hepatic** – obstruction to biliary drainage.

   Note that:

   – Conjugated bilirubin glucuronide is water-soluble and excreted in both bile and urine.

   – Biliary obstruction leads to jaundice, pale, stools and dark urine.

## Neonatal jaundice

- Caused by production of insufficient amount of UDP-glucuronyl transferase by infant (pre-maturity)
- Free bilirubin accumulates causes serious brain damage (basal ganglia): **Kernicterus.**
- **Treatment:** phototherapy (photo isomerization of bilirubin to soluble forms), phenobarbitone (induces conjugation), exchange blood transfusion.

### Table 4.34. Causes of jaundice

| Prehepatic | Hepatic | Post hepatic |
|---|---|---|
| Hemolysis ineffective erythropoiesis | **Pre microsomal:** Drugs e.g., Rifampicin (interferes with uptake) **Microsomal:** Prematurity Hepatitis: Viral Drug Gilbert's Crigler Najjar | Gallstone Stricture CA pancreas CA biliary tree |
| | **Post microsomal:** **Impaired excretion:** Hepatitis Drugs (methyltestosterone) Dubin Johnson **Intrahepatic obstruction:** Hepatitis, cirrhosis, infiltration (lymphoma, amyloid), tumor | |

## Disorders of hemoproteins and porphyrins

The inherited disorders of hemoglobin fall into three categories:

   i. Structural Hb variants

### Table 4.35. Liver function tests

| Test → condition ↓ | S. Bilirubin | AST/ ALT | ALT | Urine urobilinogen | Urine bilirubin | Fecal urobilinogen |
|---|---|---|---|---|---|---|
| Prehepatic | ↑(Unconjugated) | N | N | ↑ | – | ↑ |
| Hepatic | ↑ (both) | ↑ | N | May be ↑ (Intrahepatic cholestasis) | May be + (Intrahepatic cholestasis) | ↓ |
| Post hepatic | ↑ (conjugated) | N | ↑ | – | + | –/traces |

ii. Thalassemia: characterized by a reduced rate of production of either $\alpha$ or $\beta$ globin chains

iii. Defects in normal switch from fetal to adult Hb.

## Hemoglobinopathies

Hemoglobinopathies are genetically determined abnormalities of Hb synthesis.

Constitute two groups:
- Qualitative known as substitutions
- Quantitative known as Thalassemia

### Qualitative hemoglobinopathies

This group include amino acid substitutions causing synthesis of abnormal Hb e.g., HbS, HbC.

Usually only one amino acid substitution occur in either of the $\alpha$- or $\beta$-chains of the hundreds of hemoglobinopathies so far described, some have no symptoms or impairment, while others may have severe impairment.

### SICKLE CELL ANAEMIA

#### Fact file

- One of the first hemoglobinopathy described
- Inherited structural abnormality in $\beta$ globin chain.
- Single point mutation where glutamic acid at sixth position in $\beta$ chain is replaced by valine [Glu$^6$ $\beta$ → Val]
- $\alpha$-chain normal
- Resulting hemoglobin HbS has:
  - Two normal $\alpha$-globin chains
  - Two abnormal (mutant) $\beta$-globin chains.
- Most common hemoglobinopathy in USA.

#### Defect in sickle cell disease:

HbA remains true solute at high concentrations and non-reactive with nearby Hb molecules. On deoxygenation, HbS is less soluble and forms rod-like filaments which precipitate and distorting erythrocyte morphology to sickle shape.

Polar glutamine is replaced by non-polar valine on mutant $\beta$-globulin and valine fits into a complementary pocket (sticky patch) formed on $\beta$-globin subunit of another Hb molecule after releasing $O_2$ in tissue capillaries.

**Table 4.36.** Sickled erythrocytes

- Formed in deoxygenated state
- Contain HbS which polymerizes within RBCs on deoxygenation
- Exhibit less deformability and no longer move freely through microvasculature, blocking blood flow especially in spleen and joints.
- Sickled erythrocytes lose water, become fragile and have shorter life span.
  (10-15 days) leading to :
  - Hemolysis
  - Anaemia
  - Sickle cell crisis and cumulative organ damage
  - Death

### Sickle cell trait

They are heterozygous for the gene and have both kind of Hb in equal amounts. Heterozygosity is symptom-free and associated with increased resistance to falciparum malaria. This is an example of a selective advantage, which HbA/HbS heterozygote exhibits over HbA/HbA normal or HbS/HbS homozygote. That is why HbS gene persists in gene pool.

Protection against falciparum malaria provided by two mutations:

1. Sickle cell trait (HbA/HbS)
2. Glucose-6-phosphate dehydrogenase

deficiency: Depleting parasite of reduced glutathione

## Techniques of detection of Hb variants and mutations

- Electrophoresis
- Iso electric focusing
- Ion exchange chromatography
- Complete blood count
- DNA analysis

## Hemoglobin C

- Second most common hemoglobinopathy
- $GLu^6\beta \rightarrow Lys$
  Glutamic acid in 6th position in $\beta$ chain mutated to lysine
- No sickling occurs, but crystals of HbC may form in RBCs.
- Anaemia occurs in these patients.

## Qualitative hemoglobinopathy

Hereditary hemolytic disorders caused by insufficient production of either:

- $\alpha$ or $\beta$ subunits of Hb.
- $\alpha$-Chain deficiency: $\alpha$-Thalassemia
- $\beta$-Chain deficiency: $\beta$-Thalassemia

## Defect

Defect in production of $\alpha$ or $\beta$-chain due to: gene duplication or substitution, mutation in promoter, gene regulatory region of globin chain, nonsense or frame shift mutation.

## Classes of thalassemia

1. $\alpha$-Thalassemia:
   - Caused by defect in synthesis of $\alpha$-globin chain (normally four copies of gene)

- Deficient expression of:
  - Single $\alpha$-globin – normal and carrier
  - Two $\alpha$-globin-thalassemia traits [mild anaemia]
  - Three $\alpha$-globin – HbH disease (hemoglobin H) [severe anaemia]
  - Four $\alpha$-globin – Homozygous thalassemia [lethal, still birth]

2. **$\beta$-Thalassemia:**
   Defect in $\beta$-globin chain (normally two copies of gene)

   **$\beta$-Thalassemia major:** Carry two mutated gene: severe anaemia and hemolysis, hepatosplenomegaly, cardiomegaly, early death.

   **$\beta$-Thalassemia minor:** Carry one mutated gene
   - Chance finding when evaluated for anaemia.

## Porphyria

Inherited or acquired disorders of specific enzymes of heme biosynthetic pathway resulting in accumulation of intermediates of heme biosynthesis which cannot be further metabolized in body

**Classified as:**
- Hepatic (neuropsychiatric)
- Erythropoietic (cutaneous or mixed)

## Biochemical cause: porphyria

Mutation in DNA $\rightarrow$ abnormal enzymes of heme synthesis $\rightarrow$ Accumulation of ALA and PBG and/or $\downarrow$ in heme in cell and body fluid $\rightarrow$ Neuropsychiartic signs.

Accumulation of PBG in skin and tissues: Phototo-sensitivity $\rightarrow$ Spontaneous $\rightarrow$ Porphyrins

**Table 4.37.** Types of porphyria

| Type | Defect | | Porphyrin excretion | |
|------|--------|---|---------------------|---|
| EPP (erythropoietic porphyria) | HEME ↑ **8. Ferrochelatase** Protoporphyrin IX | a | In urine | In stool Proto IX |
| VP (Variegate) | ↑ **7. proto-oxidase** protoporphyrinogen III | a, b, c | ALA, PBG, copro III | Copro III Proto IX |
| HCP (hereditary copro) | ↑ **6. copro oxidase** | a, b, c | ALA, PBG, Copro III | Copro III |
| PCT (porphyria cutanea tarda) | **5. Uroporphyrinogen decarboxylase**, Uroporphyrinogen III | ~ | Uro I, porphyrin | Uro, copro |
| CEP (congenital Cutaneous | ↑ **4.Uro III synthase** | - | Uro I | Copro I |
| **Hepatic:** | | | | |
| AIP (acute intermittent) | Hydroxymethylbilane, ↑**3. Uroporphyrinogen I synthase** | | ALA, PBG | - |
| Deficiency (rare) | Porphobilinogen, ↑ **2. ALA dehydratase** ALA | | ALA, copro III | - |
| ALA (no porphyria) | ↑ **1. ALA synthase**, Succinyl CoA + glycine | (X – linked sideroblastic anaemia) | | |

a. photosensitivity, b. Neuropsychiatric signs, c. Abdominal pain

**Table 4.38.** Porphyria

* Inherited as autosomal dominant except congenital erythropoietic porphyria (CEP) [autosomal recessive]

* Can be:

    Hepatic

    Erythropoietic

* Acquired:

    Due to drugs:

    Barbitone

    Steroid

    Alcohol

    Due to heavy metals:

    Lead

* Hepatic porphyrias present with abdominal pain, neuropathy, neurological symptoms, and mental disturbance.

* Erythropoietic or cutaneous porphyria present with photosensitivity.

**Oxidation of porphyrinogens**

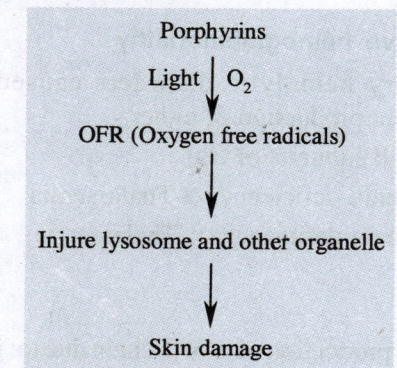

Porphyrins

Light ↓ $O_2$

OFR (Oxygen free radicals)

↓

Injure lysosome and other organelle

↓

Skin damage

# 5. INTEGRATION OF METABOLISM

## (i) Metabolic Fuel, Dietary Requirement

Major food stuffs are interconvertible, but few are not.

## Fact file: metabolic fuels:

- Metabolic fuels are substances used by body as source of carbon, free energy for anabolic processes and cellular functions.
- Metabolic fuels are: glucose, carbohydrates, triacylglycerol, and body protein.
- Energy produced by oxidizing fuels:
  - Carbohydrate (4 Kcal/g)
  - Protein (4 Kcal/g)
  - Fat (9Kcal/g)
- BMR of 24 Kcal/kg body weight/day (about 1680 Kcal) for 70 kg man

| Table 4.39 | |
|---|---|
| *Fuel* | *Recommended composition in diet (of daily calorie intake)* |
| Carbohydrate | 45-65% |
| Lipids | 30% |
| Protein | Rest (0.8g/kg body weight/day) |

- Metabolic fuels are used during:
  - **Fed state:** Fuels used by tissues may be derived from ingested, digested and absorbed food
  - **Fasting state:** Fuels used by tissues are derived from mobilized stores of fuel.
  - **Starvation:** occurs after extended fasting
- Other nutrients: vitamins, mineral.
- Metabolic fuels play structural and metabolic role.
- Regulation of fuel intake and its distribution to various tissues for utilization is important. The regulatory mechanisms of breakdown e.g. hormonal imbalance or metabolic imbalance result in pathological aberrations.

A number of central metabolic pathways are common in most cells and organisms. These pathways of synthesis, degradation and interconversion of important metabolites and referred to as **intermediary metabolism.**

## Major metabolic routes of intermediary metabolism

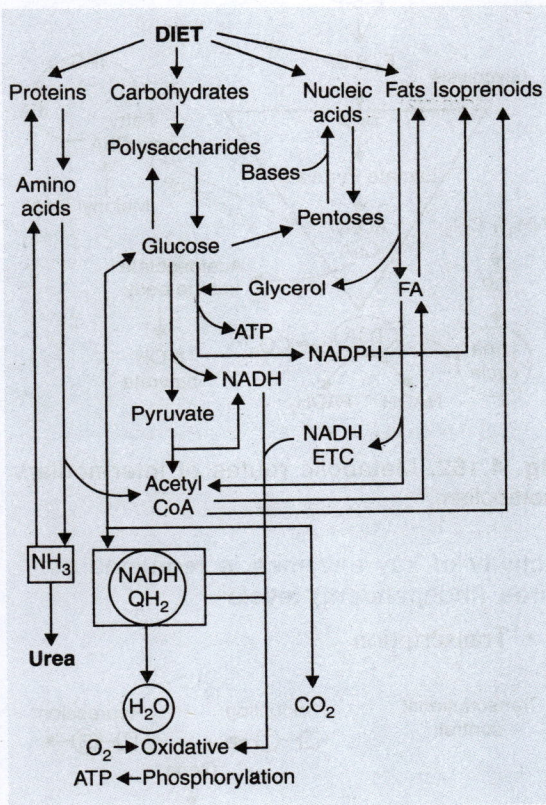

**Fig. 4.161.** Overview of intermediary metabolism

## REGULATORY MECHANISMS

### Fundamental mechanism of metabolic regulation

All metabolic pathways are under precise regulation to adjust synthesis and degradation of metabolites to physiological requirements. This is mainly determined by activity of key enzymes.

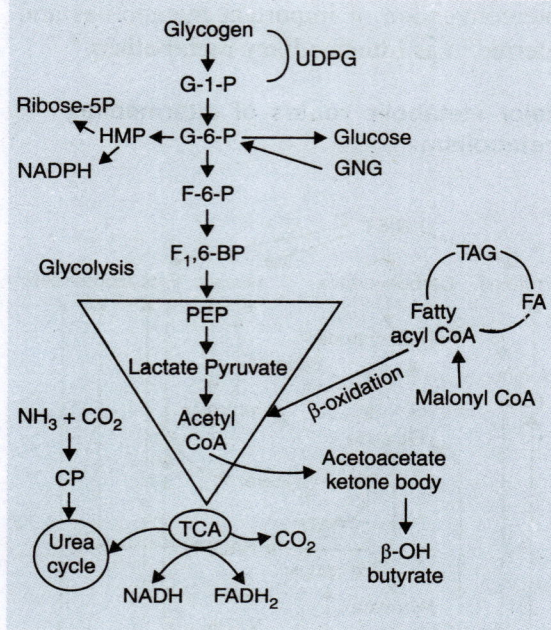

**Fig. 4.162.** Metabolic routes of intermediary metabolism.

## Activity of key enzymes is regulated at three (independent) levels

- Transcription

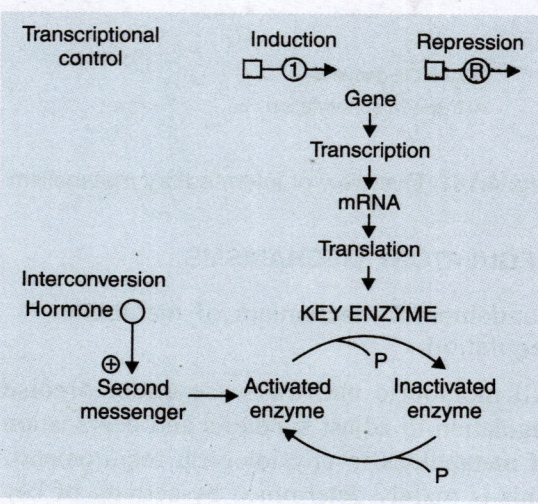

**Fig. 4.163.** Regulation of key enzymes.

- Interconversion
- Modulation by ligands

### 1. Transcription control

Biosynthesis of enzyme is influenced at genetic level by affecting synthesis of corresponding mRNA (i.e., transcription).

This can be mediated by:

- Regulatory proteins (transcription factors).
- The regulatory proteins act on promoter region causing induction (increased) or repression (reduced) of protein synthesis.

### 2. Interconversion of key enzymes

- Faster than transcriptional control.
- Requires second messengers to activate or inactivate enzyme, e.g. ATP dependent phosphorylation and dephosphorylation: covalent modification.

### Hormonal regulation of metabolic pathway

| Table 4.40 | | |
|---|---|---|
| *Metabolism* | *Action of insulin* | *Action of glucagon/ epinephrine* |
| **Carbohydrate** | | |
| Glycolysis | + | – |
| Glycogenesis | + | – |
| Glycogenolysis | – | + |
| Gluconeogenesis | – | + |
| PPP | + | – |
| **Lipid** | | |
| Fatty acid oxidation | – | + |
| Fatty acid synthesis | + | + |
| Cholesterol synthesis | + | – |
| **Protein** | | |
| Protein synthesis | + | – |
| Proteolysis | – | – |

## 3. Modulation by ligands: Allosteric effectors

- Ligands: substrate, products, coenzymes or other effectors.
- Precursor availability regulates flow through a metabolic pathway.
- Also, coenzyme availability has a limiting effect.
- Key enzymes are often inhibited by immediate reaction products, by end products of reaction (feedback inhibition), by metabolites from completely different metabolic pathways (Fig. 4.164).

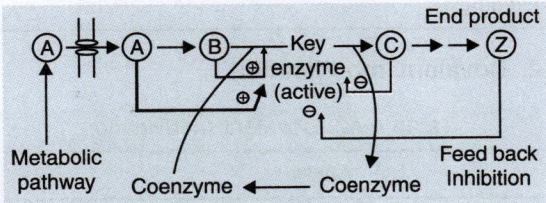

**Fig. 4.164.** Modulation by ligands.

## Allosteric regulation

- ATCase (aspartate transcarbamoyl transferase) (Fig. 4.165).

- Key enzyme of pyrimidine synthesis is classical example of allosteric regulation (Fig. 4.166)..

ATCase exihibits sigmoidal (S-shaped) substrate saturation curve.

## ATCase: Fact file

- Six catalytic sub units
- Six regulatory subunits binds effects or ATP, CTP.
- Has two conformations:
  - T (tense) state
  - R (relaxed) state
- Increase in asparate concentration shifts equilibrium towards R form and ATP stabilizes R form.
- CTP promotes transition to T state by binding to regulatory subunit.

## Action of insulin

### Insulin

- Signals fed state
- Stimulates synthesis of glycogen, fat, protein

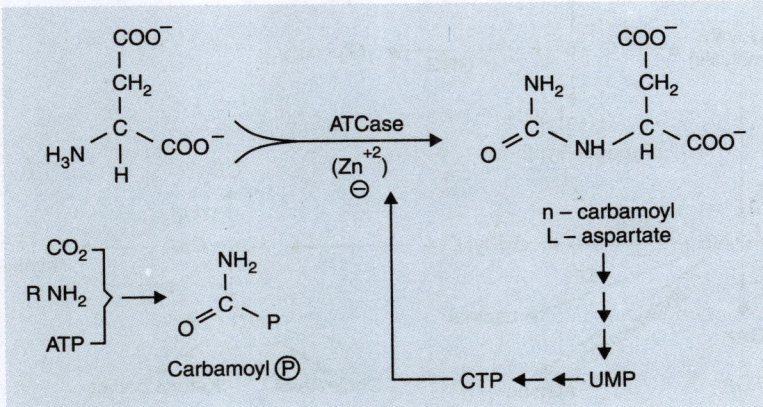

**Fig. 4.165.** AT case.

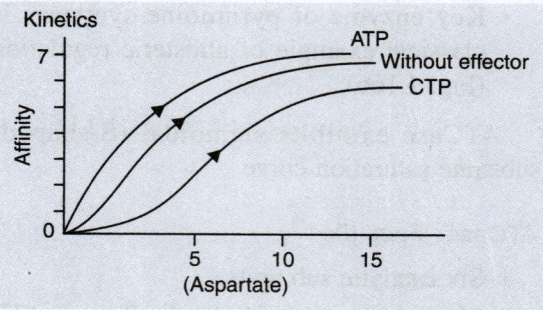

Fig. 4.166. Allosteric regulation.

- Inhibits degradation of glycogen, fat and protein
- Insulin release triggered by glucose.

### Glucagon

**Signals fasting state:**

- Stimulates degradation of glycogen, fat and protein.
- Inhibits synthesis of glycogen, fat and proteins.
- Muscle cell **lack** glucagon receptor and do not respond to it.

### Epinephrine

Epinephrine mobilizes fuel to meet the requirements of stressful state.

## NON-HORMONAL REGULATION OF METABOLIC PATHWAY

### 1. Allosteric control

**Table 4.41.** Allosteric control

| Pathway | Enzyme | Activator | Inhibitor |
|---|---|---|---|
| Glycolysis | PFK | F2, 6BP AMP | ATP |
| Gluconeo-genesis | F1, 6BPase | Citrate ATP | F2, 6BP, AMP |
| Fatty acid synthesis | ACC | Citrate | Palmitoyl CoA |

### 2. Covalent modification

**Table 4.42.** Covalent modification

| | Enzyme | |
|---|---|---|
| Glycogenesis | Glycogen synthase | Active in dephos-phorylated form |
| Glycogenolysis | Glycogen phosphorylase | Active in phos-phorylated form |

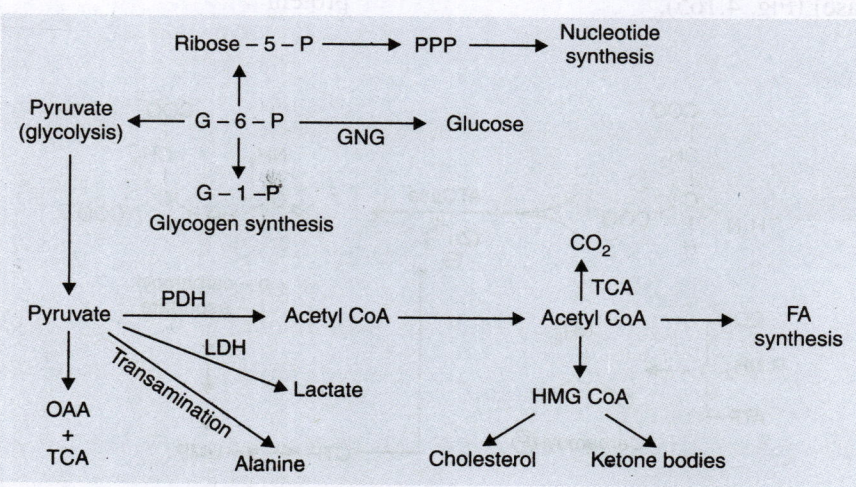

Fig. 4.167. Key intermediates of various pathways.

## 3. Respiratory control

To match the need of cell for ATP, respiratory control is exerted on following pathways:

- Citric acid cycle
- Fatty acid synthesis
- Oxidative phosphorylation

## 4. Substrate availability

It determines flux of metabolites through the following pathways:

- Pentose phosphate pathway
- Urea cycle

## Key intermediates of various pathways

- Glucose-6-Phosphate
- Pyruvate
- Acetyl CoA

## Interorgan metabolic pathways

Liver supplies glucose, ketone bodies to other tissues. Adipocytes make FA available to other tissues. Circulatory system transports metabolic fuels, intermediates and waste products among tissues. Also, certain metabolic pathways occur in multiple tissues namely,

- Cori cycle
- Glucose alanine cycle

### (ii) Metabolism of Specialized Tissues

## Liver

Central metabolic clearing house

- Play central role in regulation of blood glucose and other metabolic fuels
- Metabolic pathways in liver:
  - Glycogen storage: synthesis and break down
  - Gluconeogenesis
  - Fatty acid synthesis, ketone body synthesis
  - Ketone body synthesis
  - Synthesis of plasma lipoprotein: VLDL, HDL
  - Urea synthesis
  - Degradation of nucleic acid
  - Oxidation of alcohol
  - Creatine synthesis
  - Fructose metabolism

## Skeletal muscle

Greatest consumer of oxygen and metabolic fuel (glucose from glycogen)

- Glycogen storage
- Protein storage
- Fatty acid oxidation
- Gluconeogenesis
- Muscle carbohydrate metabolism serves only the muscle

## Cardiac muscle

- Aerobic tissue, richly endowed with mitochondria.
- No fuel reserve can metabolize FA, ketone bodies, glucose, pyruvate and lactate.

## Adipose tissue

Release FA and glycerol through HSL on TAG during metabolic need.

**Signals for release:**
- Low glucose
- Hormones

Derives most of its FA for storage from circulation.

70 Kg man contains ~15 kg fat i.e., 590,000 kcal of energy which can maintain life for 3 months!

**Functions of adipose tissue:**
- TAG storage
- Synthesis of TAG
- Oxidation of TAG

## Brain tissue

- Has no fuel reserve, high respiration rate.
- Uses glucose as fuel
- Adapts to ketone body as fuel under extreme starvation (3-5 days)
- Blood glucose levels if <30mg/dL, coma can develop.

## Kidney

- Excreted urea, uric acid, creatinine, $NH_4$, phosphoric acid
- Maintains blood pH by generating $HCO_3$, excreting excess $H^+$

## RBC

- Lack mitochondria
- No TCA, $\beta$-oxidation of FA, ETC.
- Glucose major fuel, converted to lactate
- Transport $O_2$ and $CO_2$

## ADAPTATION DURING STARVATION

### Protein

- After overnight fast, GNG provides glucose from amino acids.
- During first three days of starvation, GNG from amino acids increases.
- Then, body adjusts to metabolism to use ketone bodies as primary fuel source.

### Fats

GNG from amino acids declines, on prolonged starvation and FFA mobilized till reserves of TAG allow.

## Ketone bodies

High levels of acetyl CoA in liver drive the formation of ketone bodies by third day. Cardiac and skeletal muscles and brain use ketone bodies at high plasma levels of ketone bodies.

## Disorders of fuel metabolism

Fuel metabolism is regulated precisely and permits body to respond to changing energy demands and to accommodate changes in the availability of various fuels, maintaining reasonable metabolic homeostasis.

Disturbances in fuel metabolism occur in:
- Starvation
- Diabetes mellitus
- Obesity

# 6. BIOCHEMISTRY OF TISSUES

## MUSCLE CONTRACTION

### Morphology of muscle

- Skeletal muscles are striated
- Consists of parallel bundles of fibers known as myofibrils.
- Each myofibril is composed of repeating unit called sarcomere.
- **Sarcolemma:** plasma membrane of muscle fiber.
- Sarcoplasm: Cytoplasm of muscle fiber
- Sarcoplasmic reticulum: ER of muscle cell.

### Sarcomere

Consists of striated components between Z bands at the centre of I band.

EM shows band structure of sarcomere:
Dark (A) and light (I) bands:
- In A band lies a lighter zone: H zone.
- In middle of H zone is dark: M line

- I band separates adjacent sarcomere along a dark, dense, marrow Z line.
- Thus a sarcomere is Z line to Z line repeat
- A band contains thick filament
- I band contains thin filament
- These filaments are linked by cross bridges where they overlap.
- Thick filament contains mainly myosin.
- Thin filament contains mainly actin
- Both thick and thin filaments do not change length or width during muscle contraction, but, they overlap.
- Thin filaments are formed by end-to-end polymerization of globular actin subunit and referred to as F-actin, fibrous actin.
- Tropomyosin and troponin are associated with F-actin.

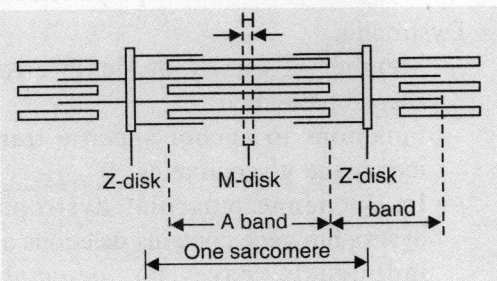

**Fig. 4.168.** Myofibril.

### Actin

- 43,000 MW size, globular protein (globular or G actin)
- One molecule of ATP bind to each actin
- Each G-actin has two binding sites, one for ATP and second to divalent metal $Mg^{+2}$.
- G-actin-ATP-$Mg^{+2}$ complex aggregates to form F-actin
- Exist as double stranded helix, their ends anchored to Z-disks of sarcomeres

- Helices grooves of actin filament are occupied by tropomyosin.

### Tropomyosin

- Rod shaped protein with two dissimilar subunits $\alpha$ and $\beta$.
- Forms aggregates in head to tail configuration
- Interact in flexible manner.
- One tropomyosin interacts with seven actin monomer
- One troponin complex binds to every tropomyosin

### Troponin ($T_n$)

- Complex of three polypeptides TnT, TnI, TnC.
- TnT binds to tromyosin
- TnI binds to actin, inhibits binding of actin to myosin
- TnC is calmodulin-like protein, binds $Ca^{+2}$.
- At high calcium concentrations found in contracting muscle ($10^{-5}M$), TnC undergoes a conformational change, releasing TnI from actin and causing tropomyosin to move deeper into its binding groove, exposing myosin-binding site of actin.
- There are 7 thin filaments surrounding each thick filament. Each thick filament interacts with multiple thin filaments.

### Myosin

- Thick filament contain myosin
- Myosin is long fibrous molecule with two globular heads on each end.
- 6 polypeptide: consists of 2 heavy chain and two pairs of different light chains.
- Light chains are calmodulin like proteins
  – Two types: I, II
    - Type I not found in muscle cells

- Type II required for muscle contraction
- N-terminal is globular structure to which L chains are bound
- Two H chains are attached through coiling of their α-helical tails in coiled tail structure.
- Tail sections are aligned in parallel manner on both sides of M line of H zone in sarcomere, with head group pointing towards Z line.
- N-terminal can bind to filamentous actin (F-actin)
- Each thick filament contains 400 myosin
- Cross bridges between thick and thin filament are seen in A band by binding of N terminal head group of myosin to actin.
- Myosin head contains ATPase activity to provide energy for contraction and actin binding.
- Under physiological conditions, several hundred myosin molecules aggregate to form a thick filament with globular heads projecting on sides of the both ends.

## Minor proteins in muscle

- α Actinin, desmin, vimentin present in 2 disks to which thin filaments are anchored.
- C protein, M protein present in M disk, where thick filaments are anchored.
- Titin - unusual protein:
  - Longest known polypeptide chain
  - 3-6 molecules of titin associate with each thick filament between M and Z-disks
  - Function as metabolic bunge cord to keep thick filaments centered on sarcomere
  - Compresses during muscle contraction, during relaxation resists sarcomere extension past the point where thin and thick filaments have started to slide past each other.
- Nebulin
  - a helical protein associated with thin filament
  - Act as template for actin polymerization
- Dystrophin
  - Member of family of flexible rod-shaped proteins
  - Functions to anchor specific trans-membrane glycoproteins.
  - In Duchenne muscular dystrophy, dystrophin gene contains deletions and individuals have no detectable dystrophin in their muscles.

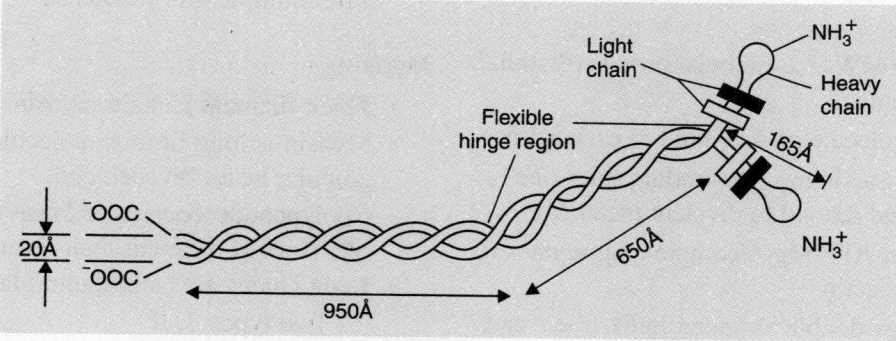

**Fig. 4.169.** Myosin molecule

## Mechanisms muscle contraction

### Sliding filament model

- Each myosin cross-bridges to actin, repeatedly detaches and reattaches itself and free energy for this is provided by ATP hydrolysis.
- Each sarcomere of a myofibril shortens and thin filaments slide across the thick filaments.
- Shortening of sarcomeres result in significant reduction in length of myofibrils.

## Basic contraction

### Four stages

1. Myosin along with ADP and Pi bound to it diffuses to make contact with actin and its binding with actin becomes tight following loss of Pi.
2. This binding induces conformational change in myosin.
   Actin pulled across thick filament, ADP released, conformation of myosin changes.
3. ATP binds to myosin, releasing it from actin.
4. Hydrolysis of ATP by myosin and conformation change in myosin occurs so that it is free to bind actin.
   This cycle continues till $Ca^{+2}$ and ATP are present.

## ENERGY RESERVOIRS FOR MUSCLE CONTRACTION

CPK, Adenylate kinase.

### 1. Creatine phosphokinase (CPK)

$$Phosphocreatine + ADP \rightleftharpoons ATP + creatine$$

If metabolic activity is insufficient to keep up with the need for ATP, CPK helps to maintain constant cellular levels.

### 2. Adenylate kinase

Provides additional ATP via:

$$2ADP \rightleftharpoons ATP + AMP$$

### Regulation

Key regulatory molecule: Calcium.

Calcium is sequestered in sarcoplasmic reticulum.

- **Presence of Ca:**
  - Ca binds to TnC, causes conformation change in Tn-Tropomyosin complex.
  - Tropomyosin moves away from myosin binding site on actin, allowing myosin to bind and carry out contraction.
- Absence of calcium: Tropomyosin lies in groove of actin helix and myosin ADP-P complex cannot bind
- On electrical excitation, depolarization of sarcolemma results in release of calcium from sarcoplasmic reticulum.
- Calcium is removed from sarcoplasm and tropomyosin-Tn complex conformation reversed
- Tropomyosin returns to groove on actin helix, inhibiting binding of myosin to it.

# CHAPTER 5

# Endocrinology

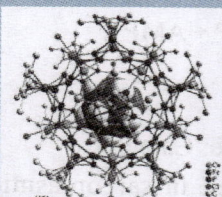

## ENDOCRINES

### Introduction

### Fact file

- Provide communication between cells, tissues and organs to regulate wide range of functions such as growth, development, reproduction, homeostasis and response to external stimuli and stress.
- Hormones can be endocrine, paracrine or autocrine in nature
- Tight homeostatic control exists to regulate hormone synthesis, secretion
- One hormone may control several processes and several hormones control one process
- Hormone can be chemically modified amino acids, polypeptides, glycoproteins, or derived from lipids.

**Endocrine hormones:** synthesized from endocrine glands and transported in blood to target cells.

| Table 5.1 | |
|---|---|
| *Chemical nature* | *Example* |
| Amino acids: | |
| Single amino acid derived | Catecholamine, Serotonin, Dopamine, Thyroxine |
| Tripeptide | TRH |
| Small peptide | ADH, Somatostatin |
| Peptides | Insulin, PTH, glucagon |
| Glycoproteins | TSH |
| Lipid derived: | |
| Fatty acid derivative | PG, LT |
| Cholesterol | Cortisol, estradiol, testosterone, Vitamin D |
| Phospholipids | Platelet activating factor |

**Paracrine hormones:** synthesized near target of action, and act locally.

**Autocrine hormones:** affects the cells that synthesize them.

## Table 5.2. Classification of hormone

| Hormone | Site of action |
|---|---|
| 1. Endocrine | Act on cells to which they are carried by blood |
| 2. Autocrine | Act on cells that synthesize them |
| 3. Paracrine | Act on neighbouring cells |
| 4. Neuroendocrine | (Can be paracrine or endocrine). Hormone synthesized in neuron and released either adjacent to target cell or carried to target cell via bloodstream |
| 5. Neural | Released by one neuron and act on adjacent neuron |
| 6. Pheromone | Release of volatile hormones into atmosphere and recognized as olfactory signal |

## (i) Mechanism of Hormone Action (Fig. 5.1)

## Table 5.3. Hormone: site of action

| Intracellular® | Membrane® | | |
|---|---|---|---|
| | cAMP | PI$_3$ | Unknown |
| Steroid Hormone | | | |
| Gonadotrophs | ACTH | TRH | GH |
| Estrogen | FSH | GnRH | PRL |
| Progesterone | LH | | Oxytocin |
| Androgens | hCG | | |
| GC (gluco-corticoids) | TSH | | Insulin |
| MC (mineralo-corticoids) | PTH | | IGF-1 & II |
| Vitamin D | ADH | | |
| T$_3$ T$_4$ | Epi/NE | | |

® = Receptor

## Mechanism of Hormone action

Hormones interact with target cells through a primary interaction with receptors that recognize hormones selectively.

Different Receptors (®) System:
1. Channel – linked (ionotropic) ®
2. G-protein coupled (metabotropic)
3. Kinase linked ®
4. Steroid ®

## Table 5.4

| Receptor | Example | Response (time scale) |
|---|---|---|
| 1. Ionotropic | Nicotinic AcH ® | Milliseconds |
| 2. G-protein-coupled | Muscarinic AcH ® | Seconds |
| 3. Kinase-linked | Insulin ® | Minutes |
| 4. Steroid ® | Estrogen ® | hours |

Receptors can be membrane-bound or intracellular ®

### Membrane receptors

Charged ions such as peptides, neurotransmitters bind to ® on cell membrane and cause a conformational change in other membrane proteins to activate enzymes that synthesize second messengers. Second messengers, in turn, activate phosphorylating enzymes.

### Structure: Membrane receptors (Fig. 5.2)

**Membrane receptors have 3 regions:**
- Extracellular domain
- Membrane-spanning domain
- Intracellular domain

**Second messengers:**
- G-protein
- Adenylate cyclase system
- Inositol triphosphate system.

### 1. G-Protein

- Have extracellular and intracellular domain
- Peptide chain span the membrane
- Following binding of hormone to extracellular domain, shape of ® changes

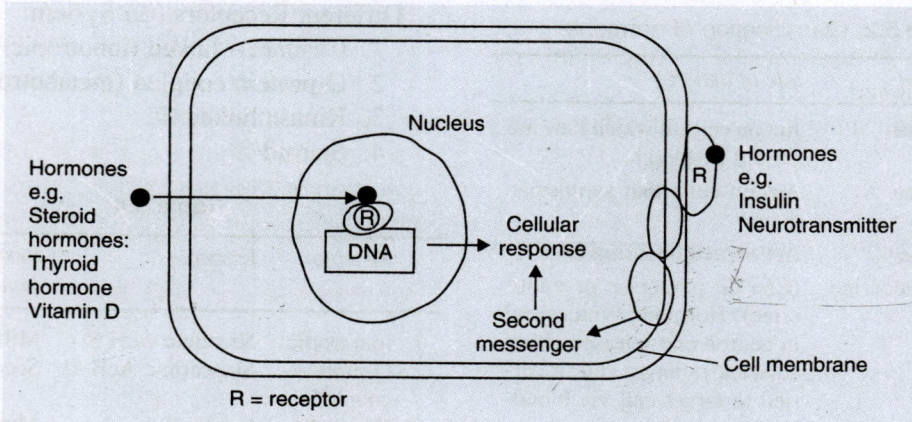

**Fig. 5.1.** Mechanism of hormone action.

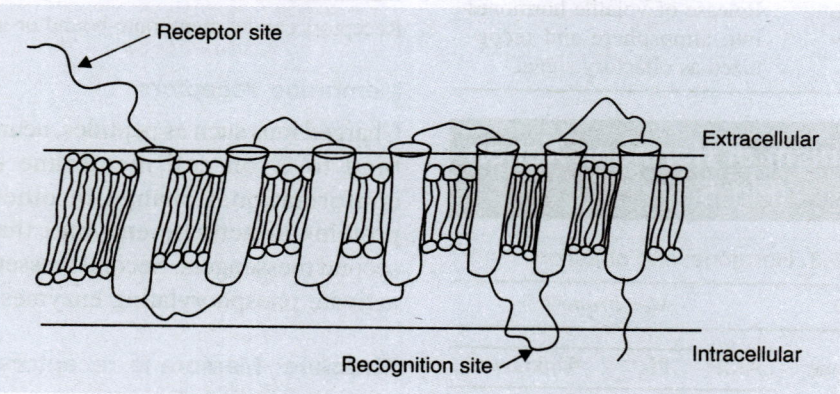

**Fig. 5.2.** Structure of membrane receptor.

**Table 5.5**

| Domain | Sites | Specific site for binding |
|---|---|---|
| 1. Extracellular domain | Hormone binding Glycosylation binding | Cysteine – rich |
| 2. Trans membrane | Helically arranged hydrophobic sites for hormone binding and anchoring ® in membrane | Hydrophobic charged amino acid |
| 3. Intracellular | Effector region linked to membrane protein system e.g., G-protein kinases | - |

causing intracellular domain to active G-protein.
• Has 3 parts:  α subunit
               β subunit
               γ subunit

• On activation α-subunit substitutes GDP molecule for a GTP molecule resulting in activation of G protein.

## 2. Adenylate cyclase

Hormones ® that activate G-protein and GDP gets exchanged for GTP.

G protein subunit activate adenylate cyclase

$$ATP \xrightarrow{AC} cAMP \xrightarrow{\text{Phospho-diesterase}} AMP$$

cAMP activate catalytic unit of protein kinase A (PKA)

## IP₃ system

- Hormone-®-G protein complex trigger enzyme phospholipase (PLC) to catalyze conversion of $PIP_2$ to $IP_3$ and DAG
- $IP_3$ generates $Ca^{+2}$ ions from ER (endoplasmic reticulum).
- Free $Ca^{+2}$ ions along with DAG activate protein kinase C (PKC) stimulating the transcription of effector proteins.

## Membrane ® agonists and antagonists

- **Agonist** – molecule binds to a ® and elicit a normal response

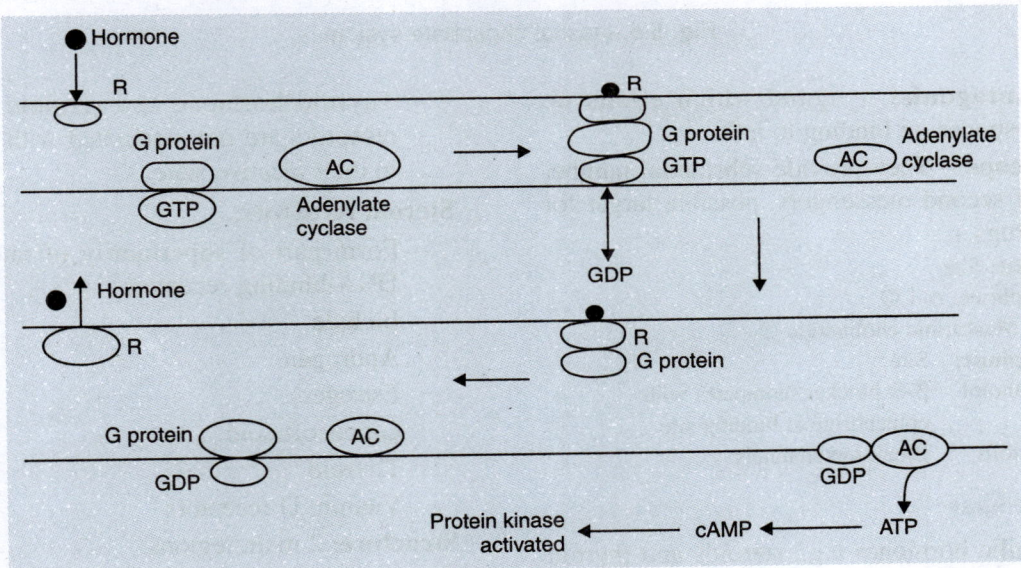

**Fig. 5.3.** Adenylate cyclase.

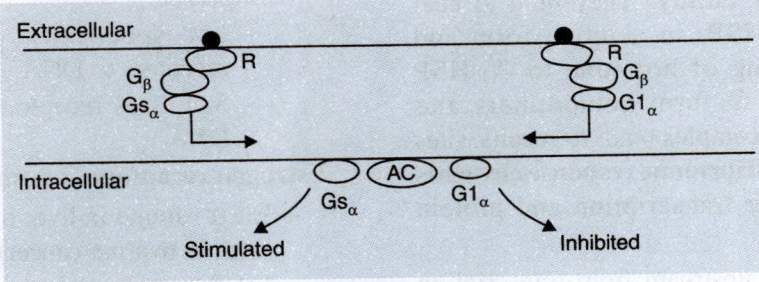

**Fig. 5.4.** G-proteins.

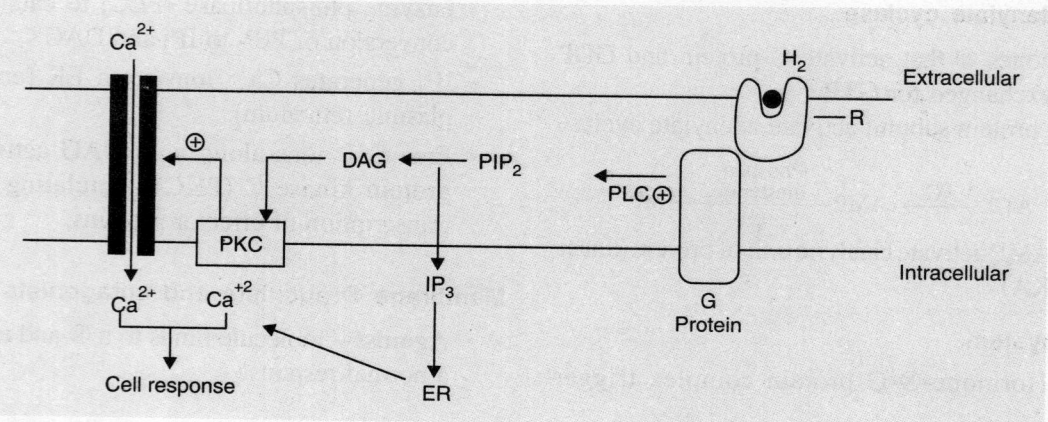

**Fig. 5.5.** Inositol phosphate system.

- **Antagonist** – ligand which elicits no response on binding to a ®.

   **Scope** – They provide substantial number of second messengers, possible target for drugs.

   **Agonist:** Site
   Epinephrine: $\alpha$-1 ®
   AcH: Muscarinic cholinergic ®
   **Antagonist:** Site
   Propranolol  $\beta$-® blocker (competes with epinephrine at binding site
   Phenytoin  Block ion channels

### Intracellular

Lipophilic hormones e.g., steroids and thyroid hormones, traverse plasma membrane to enter the cell to combine with specific ® proteins.

   **Steroid super family:** They bind to heat shock protein (HSP) in inactive form and following binding of hormone to ®, HSP dissociates and ® form homodimers and hormone receptor complex binds to specific sites in DNA termed as **Hormone response elements (HREs)** and alter transcription and protein synthesis.

   – HRE lies upstream from transcription initiation sites.

   – Thyroid hormone and retinoic acid receptors are not associated with HSP in their inactive state.

**Steroid receptors:**

   – Form part of superfamily of nuclear DNA-binding receptors
   – Include:
   Androgen
   Estrogen
   Glucocorticoid
   Thyroid
   Vitamin D receptors

**Structure:** 2 main regions:

   – Hormone-binding region (hydrophobic)
   – DNA-binding region (having two zinc fingers):
     - For specificity of binding of receptors to DNA
     - Stabilizes receptors to its HRE of DNA

**Estrogen receptors:** 2 forms :

   – ER $\alpha$ - found in liver but (predominant form in ovarian cancer)
   – ER $\beta$ - predominant form in prostate, ovary

They have different affinities for estradiol and different anatomic distribution.

**Antagonist:** used in prevention and treatment of breast cancer.

**SERM:** **S**elective **E**strogen **R**eceptors **M**odulators e.g., tamoxifen, raloxifen, toremifene, used in CA breast, osteoporosis, for lowering cholesterol.

## Thyroid hormone receptors

They also function as hormone- activated transcription factors.

## Anterior pituitary hormones

3 categories:
- GH-PRL-CS (chronic somatomammotrophs)
- Glycoprotein hormone
- POMC peptide family (pro-opiomelanocortin)

## GH-PRL-CS group

Constitute one group:
- Show considerable sequence homology, share common antigenic determinant.
- Size range from 190-199 amino acids
- Production: GH-PRL by anterior pituitary
- CS by syncytiotrophoblast cells of placenta.
- GH-CS gene – linkage group q22-24 long arm of chromosome 17
- PRL gene – chromosome 6

## GH

## Synthesis of GH

Synthesized in somatotrophs (a subclass of acidophilic cells) in anterior pituitary gland.

## Structure of GH

- Single polypeptide
- Molecular mass 22 kDa
- Composed of 191 aa
- Structural homology with PL, PRL.

## GH-Receptor

- Member of cytokine- hematopoietin receptor super family
- 70 kDa
- Single membrane- spanning domain
- GH binding causes dimerization of two GH receptors

## Mechanism of action of GH

GH receptor is associated with JAK2 tyrosine kinase

## Signaling pathways of GH interaction with GH receptor involve:

- STAT protein phosphorylation
- SHC/Grb2 – associated activation of MAP kinase
- IRS phosphorylation with a activation of $PI_3$ kinase
- PLC activation with formation of DAG and activation of protein kinase C.

## Hormone transport

In circulation, small or hydrophobic hormones are transported bound to carrier proteins.

| Table 5.6 | |
|---|---|
| *Hormone* | *Binding proteins* |
| Thyroxine | Thyroxine binding globulin (TBG) |
| Cortisol, Progesterone | Cortisol binding globulin (CBG) |
| Testosterone, estradiol | SHBG (steroid hormone binding globulin) |
| IGF-1 IGF-II | IGF binding proteins |
| Vitamin D | Vitamin D binding protein |

## Transport proteins

- Hormones bind to protein through non covalent interaction

- Bind most soluble circulating hormone and free hormone is a small portion of total
- Binding capacity of transport protein does not exceed normal concentration of hormone in plasma
- Modest decrease in transport protein level or modest increase in hormone concentration can lead to large increase in free hormone levels.
- Role: Facilitate even delivery of hormones across target tissue
- Transport protein increase half-life of hormone in circulation, increase concentration of smaller hormones that would be otherwise eliminated from circulation in liver or kidney.

## Transport of hormone across membrane

Nuclear receptor ligands being hydrophobic traverse phospholipids bilayer and this transport mechanism exists across membrane.

## Metabolism and elimination of hormones

Hormone inactivation occurs by metabolism e.g. hydroxylation, conjugation, proteolysis followed by excretion of metabolites.

## Peptide hormones

Degraded through binding to cell surface receptors and non receptor hormone-binding sites with subsequent uptake (internalization) and degradation by lysosomal enzymes.

## Steroid hormones

- Metabolic inactivation by reduction and conjugation to glucuronide and sulfate group results in water-soluble inactive forms that are effectively eliminated.
- Metabolism of prohormones to active forms occurs in case of testosterone (to dihydrotestosterone).

- $T_4$ is deiodinated to more active $T_3$ in peripheral tissues and hydroxylation reactions of liver and kidney result in more active form of vitamin D.
- Hormones produced locally in target tissues get metabolized to provide high local concentration of hormones and thus providing additional control of hormone response, e.g. testosterone produced from androstenedione and dehydroepiandrostrone; estradiol from testosterone.

## Catecholamines and eicosanoids

Catecholamines are degraded to catechol-O-methyltransferase (COMT) and monoamine oxidase (MAO). $PG_s$ are rapidly metabolized within seconds- by widely distributed enzymes via oxidation of 15-hyroxyl group.

## Histology anterior pituitary

Anterior pituitary cells are classified as based on H & E staining:

    Acidophils (Secrete GH)
    Basophils
    Chromopobe

## Based on immunocytochemical and election microscopy

| Cell | Hormone secreted |
| --- | --- |
| Somatotrophs | GH secreting |
| Lactotrophs | PRL – secreting |
| Thyrotrophs | TSH |
| Corticotrophs | ACTH |
| Gonadotrophs | CLH, FSH |
| Thyrotrophs | TSH |
| | Basophils secrete and PAS (periodic acid Schiff stain) |
| Lactotrophs | PRL secreting (10-20%), second in distribution basophil containing |

*(Contd.)*

| Cell | Hormone secreted |
|------|------------------|
| | 2 types: |
| | Sparsely granulated |
| | Densely granulated |
| Corticotrophs | ACTH and related peptides |
| | 15-30% of cells |
| | Basophilic |
| Gonadotrophs | Basophil staining |
| | Secretes LH, FSH |
| | 10-15% of cells. |
| Somatotrophs | Acidophilic |
| | Present in lateral portion |
| | Account for 5% of anterior pituitary |

## (ii) Pituitary Hormones

### Anterior pituitary hormones

Three groups:

- Corticotrophin related peptide (ACTH, LPH, MSH, endorphin)
- Somatotropin – related peptide (GH, PRL)
- Glycoproteins (LH, FSH, LH)

### ACTH and related peptides

### ACTH

39 amino acid peptide hormone, processed from large precursor molecule: proopiomelanocortin (POMC)

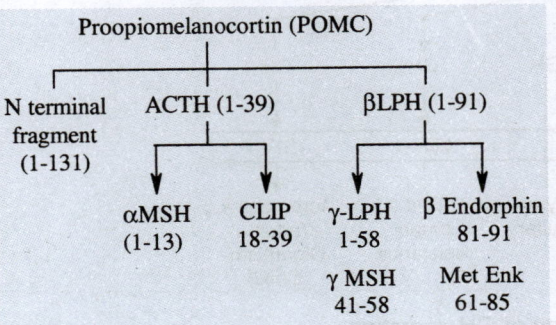

αMSH is identical to ACTH (1-13) represents ACTH 18-39.

### Function

- ACTH stimulates secretion of glucocorticoids, mineralocoides and androgen steroids from adrenal cortex.
- Hyperpigmentation in ACTH hypersecretion (Addison's disease) is primarily due to ACTH binding to MSH receptor.

### Secretion

CRH (corticotrophin – releasing hormone) stimulates ACTH release.

### Diurnal rhythm

- ACTH peak before awakening and decline as day progress.
- Stress, pain, trauma, hypoxia, cold, surgery, depression stimulate ACTH and cortisol secretion.

### GH

Secretion of GH is mediated by two hypothalamic hormones: growth hormone – releasing hormone (HRH) and somatostatin (growth hormone inhibiting hormone).

**Table 5.7.** Metabolic effects of GH

| | Decrease | Increase |
|------|----------|----------|
| Carbohydrate metabolism | Glucose uptake in extrahepatic tissues, insulin sensitivity | Hepatic glucose output, hepatic glycogen stores, plasma glucose |
| Lipid metabolism | - | Lipolysis, plasma FFA, plasma ketone bodies |
| Protein metabolism | Nitrogen excretion | Amino acid uptake, protein synthesis |

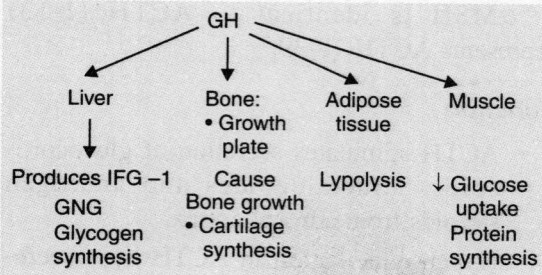

**Fig. 5.6.** Anabolic effects of GH.

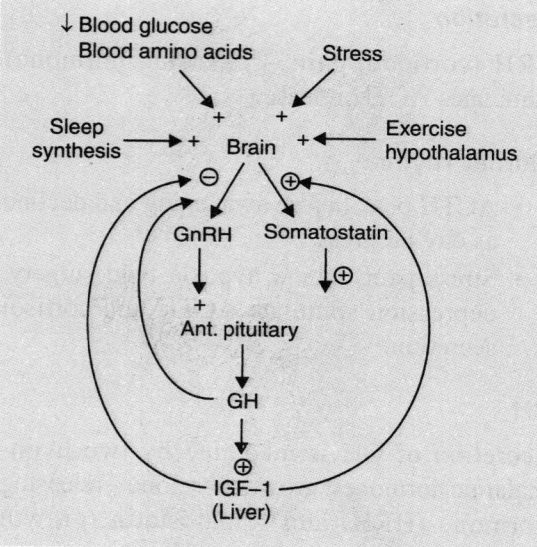

**Fig. 5.7.** Control of secretion of GH.

## PRL (Prolactin)

198 amino acid polypeptide hormone synthesized from lactrophs of anterior pituitary.

### Function

Stimulate lactation in postpartum.

### Secretion

- Hypothalamic control of PRL secretion is predominantly inhibitory, dopamine is most important inhibitory factor.
- TRH evokes release of PRL.

## Causes of hyperprolectinemia

- Physiological: Pregnancy.
- Drugs: Dopamine blockers, dopamine depleting drugs, $H_2$ agonist, MAO inhibitors.

### Diseases

Prolactinoma, pituitary tumor, CRF, primary hypothyroidism

### Thyrotropin

### TSH

- Glycoprotein, composed of two non covalently linked alpha and beta subunits
- Structure of alpha subunit of TSH is identical to that of FSH, LH and hCG and

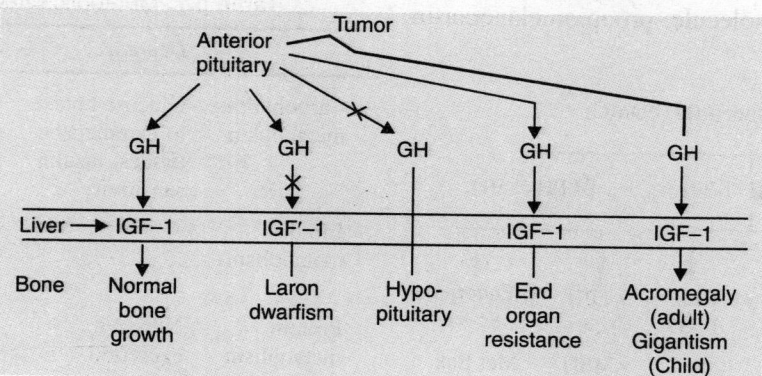

**Fig. 5.8.** Pathophysiology of GH secretion.

beta subunit differs, providing biologic and immunologic specificity.

## Function

Beta subunit of TSH attaches to receptors in thyroid, stimulating iodide uptake, hormone synthesis and release of $T_3$, $T_4$.

## Secretion

- Controlled by both stimulatory (TRH) and inhibitory (somatostatin) influence of hypothalamus.
- Modulated by feedback inhibition of thyroid hormone on hypothalamic – pituitary axis.

## Gonadotropins: LH, FSH

### LH and FSH

Glycoproteins, composed of $\alpha$- and $\beta$-subunits, synthesized by same cells.

## Function

LH and FSH bind to receptors in ovary and testis and regulate gonadal function by production of sex steroids and gametogenesis.

**In men:**
- LH stimulates testosterone production from Leydig cells of testes.
- Maturation of sperm requires both LH and FSH.
- FSH stimulates testicular growth and enhances production of androgen binding protein by Sertoli cells to promote high local concentration of testosterone.

**In women:**
- LH stimulates estrogen and progesterone production from ovary
- LH surge in mid menstrual cycle is responsible for ovulation.
- Continued secretion of LH results in stimulation of corpus luteum to produce more progesterone.

- Development of ovarian follicle in largely under FSH control.

## Secretion

- Secretion of LH and FSH is controlled by GnRH.
- Circulating sex steroids affect GnRH secretion.

## Clinical correlates: Hypothalamic, pituitary disorders

In adults, most common cause of hypothalamic, pituitary dysfunction is pituitary adenomas which are in great majority hypersecreting.

- Hypogonadism is most frequent presentation
- Sella enlargement and local manifestations such as headache and visual loss follow later.
- In children, pituitary adenomas are uncommon, craniopharyngioma and other hypothalamic tumors occur mainly.
- Manifest as endocrine disturbances: low GH level, delayed puberty, diabetes insipidus prior to development of headache and visual loss.

## Manifestations

### Pituitary hypersecretion

- Gonadal dysfunction, secondary gonadotropin deficiency, galactorrhea
- Enlargement of sella turcica
- Acromegaly (hypersecretion of GH)
- Cushing's (hypersecretion of ACTH)

## Causes of Hypothalamic pituitary dysfunction

**Invasion:**
- Craniopharyngioma
- Primary CNS tumor
- Pituitary adenoma

**Infraction, infiltration, injury:**
– Spontaneous, postpartum
– Sarcoidosis, Haemochromatosis, head trauma

**Immunologic:**
– Iatrogenic
– Isolated disease

## Pituitary insufficiency

• Panhypopituitarism (Cause: adenoma)
• Hypogonadism secondary to elevated PRL, GH or ACTH, cortisol.
• Short stature – GH deficiency
• TSH or ACTH deficiency is unusual and usually indicates panhypopituitarism.
• Enlarged sella turcica
• Visual field defect:
  – Bitemporal, hemianopia
  – Visual field defects
  – Visual loss
• Diabetes insipidus

## Empty sella turcica syndrome

Results from:
• Congenital incompetence of diaphragma sellae

• Pituitary surgery, radiotherapy
• Postpartum pituitary infarction (Sheehan's syndrome)
• PRL and GH- secreting pituitary adenomas may undergo sub clinical hemorrhagic infraction.

### Clinical feature

• Complaints of:
  – Systemic hypertension
  – Headache
• Skull X-ray reveals empty sella
• Anterior pituitary functions normal
• Hyperprolactinemia may be present.

### Cushing's disease

• Primary pituitary disorder
• Endocrine abnormalities include:
  – Hypersecretion of ACTH
  – Absent circadian periodicity of ACTH and cortisol secretion.
  – Absence of responsiveness of ACTH and cortisol to stress.
  – Abnormal negative feedback of ACTH secretion by glucocorticoids.

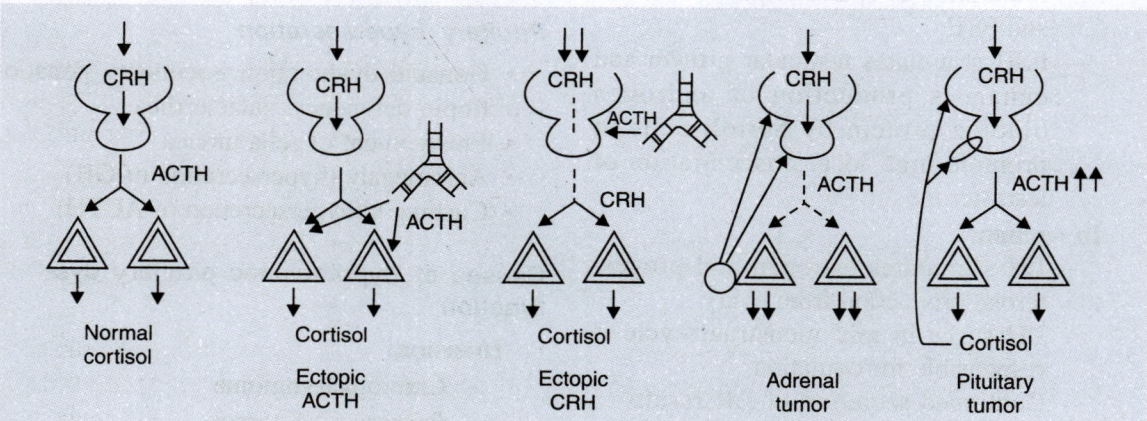

**Fig. 5.9.** Causes of Cushing's syndrome.

## Clinical features

- Signs and symptoms of hypocortisolism and adrenal androgen excess.
- Obesity: Central fat distribution
- Hypertension
  - Glucose intolerance
  - Gonadal dysfunction (amenorrhea, or impotence)
  - Moon facies, proximal muscle weakness, easy bruisability, violet straie, hirsuitism, acne, poor wound healing.

## SIADH Syndrome of inappropriate secretion of ADH

Cause:

- Malignancy: bronchogenic carcinoma
- Non-malignant: tuberculosis
- Tumor: lymphoma, sarcoma
- Trauma, infection

## Posterior pituitary

Secrete two hormones:

- ADH (vasopressin)
- Oxytocin

They are synthesized in hypothalamus and transported by nerves to posterior pituitary.

## ADH (antidiuretic hormone)

- Half life of 15-20 minutes
- Rapidly metabolized in liver and kidney.

## Renal action

- To increase permeability of luminal membrane of collecting duct via ADH sensitive water channels, aquaporin-2.
- When ADH is present, epithelial permeability increases and water is reabsorbed.
- ADH mobilizes aquaporin -2 and water permeability of luminal membrane is increased by increasing number of narrow aqueous channels at luminal surface.

## Cardiovascular action

ADH via Vi receptors in peripheral arterioles increases blood pressure.

## Diabetes Insipidus (DI)

- Results from deficient ADH secretion
- Characterized by passage of copious amount of very dilute urine.

## Types

1. Central (neurogenic) DI
2. Nephrogenic DI

## Causes DI

| Central | Nephrogenic |
|---|---|
| Hypophysectomy | Congenital |
| Surgery for hypothalamic | Familial |
| or pituitary tumor | CRF |
| Idiopathic | Sickle cell anaemia |
| Familial | Drugs: Lithium |
| Infection | Fluoride, Demeclo- |
| Infarction, infiltration | cycline |

## Oxytocin

Oxytocin primarily affects uterine smooth muscle. It increases both the frequency and duration of action potentials during uterine contractions.

Estrogen enhances action of oxytocin by reducing the membrane potential of smooth muscle cells, thus lowering the threshold of excitation.

Toward the end of pregnancy as estrogen level become higher, membrane potential of uterine muscle cells become less negative rendering uterus more sensitive to oxytocin.

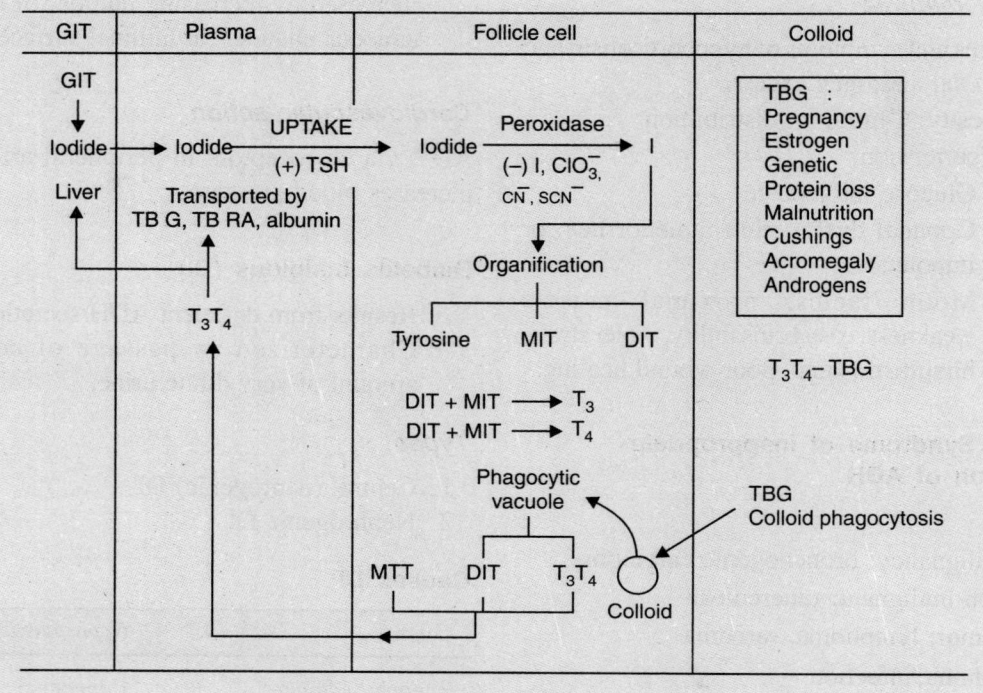

**Fig. 5.10.** Synthesis of thyroid hormones.

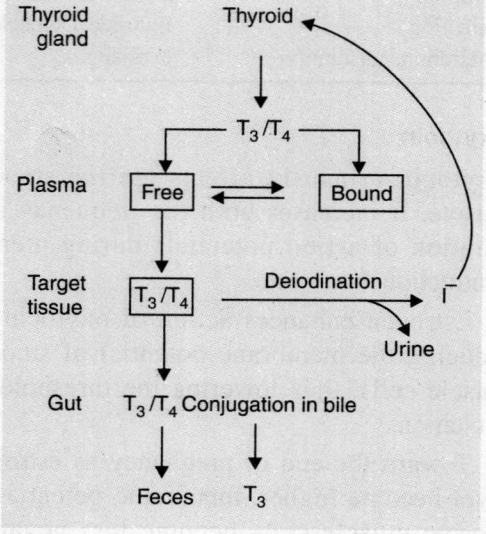

**Fig. 5.11.** Metabolism of thyroid hormone.

## (iii) Action of Specific Hormones

### Thyroid

| Hormone secreted | Cells |
|---|---|
| Thyroid $T_4$ | Follicular |
| Triiodothyronine $T_3$ | Follicular |
| Calcitonin | C-cells |

### Iodine metabolism

Iodine enters body in food or water in the form of iodine or iodate ion.

Iodate ion is converted to iodide in stomach, thyroid gland concentrates and traps iodide and synthesizes and stores thyroid hormone thyroglobuin.

WHO recommends optimal daily iodide intake:

- Adults: 150 µg
- Pregnancy and lactation: 200 µg
- $1^{st}$ year for life: 50 µg
- For 1-6 years: 90 µg
- For 7-12 years: 120 µg

For iodide intake below 50 µg/d, gland is unable to maintain adequate hormone secretion.

### Absorption

- Iodide is rapidly absorbed from GIT and distributed in extracellular fluid (ecf) and salivary, gastric and breast secretions.
- Iodide is rapidly cleared from ecf by thyroidal uptake and renal clearance.
- About 115 µg of $I^-$ per 24 hours is taken up by gland of which 75 µg $I^-$ is utilized for hormone synthesis and stored in thyroglobulin and the remainder leaks back into ecf pool.

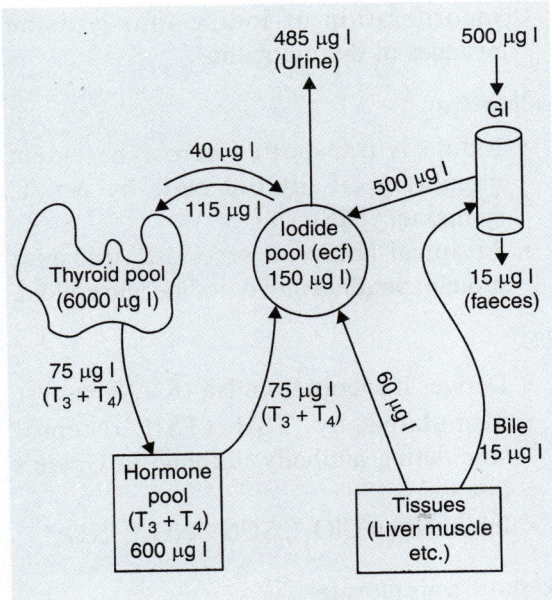

**Fig. 5.12.** Iodine metabolism

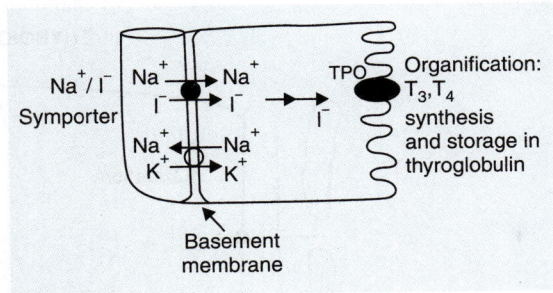

**Fig. 5.13.** Iodide transporter in thyroid cell (TPO).

- Total thyroid pool of organified iodine is 8-10 mg: store of hormone and iodinated tyrosine.
- From this pool, 75 µg of hormonal iodide is released into circulation daily.
- 600 µg of hormone $I^-$ is in circulation pool, from which 15 µg of $I^-$ as $T_3$ and $T_4$ is taken up and metabolized by tissues.
- 60 µg of $I^-$ returns to iodide pool and 15 µg of hormonal $I^-$ get glucuronated or sulfated in liver for excretion in faeces.
- Since most of dietary $I^-$ is excreted in urine, 24 hr urinary iodide excretion is excellent index of dietary intake.

### Thyroid hormone synthesis and secretion

Six major steps of synthesis:

1. Trapping of iodine: Active transport of $I^-$ across basement membrane into thyroid cell.
2. Oxidation of iodide, iodination of tyrosyl residues in thyroglobulin
3. Coupling of iodotyrosine molecule in thyroglobulin to form $T_3$ and $T_4$.
4. Proteolysis of thyroglobulin, release of free iodothyronine and iodotyrosine.
5. Deiodination of iodotyrosine and conservation and reuse of liberated I.
6. Intrathyroidal deiodination of $T_4$ to $T_3$.

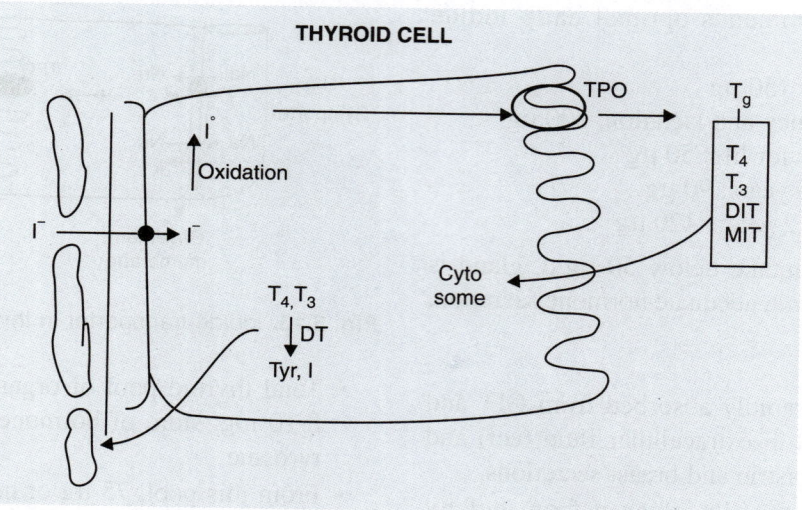

**Fig. 5.14.** Thyroid hormone.

## Thyroglobulin

- Large, glycoprolein, dimer
- Contain 0.5% iodine:
  - 5 molecules of MIT
  - 4.5 molecules of DIT
  - 2.5 molecules of $T_4$
  - 0.7 molecules of $T_3$
- Has 4 tyrosyl sites for hormogenesis, one at amino end and other three at carboxyl terminal end.
- Synthesized as prethyroglobulin monomer with 19 amino acid signal peptide by thyroglobulin gene, (Thg) on chromosome 8.
- mRNA is translated in RER, thyroglobulin chains are glycolylated in golgi apparatus and thyroglobulin dimers are incorporated into exocytic vesicles to be released into follicular lumen.
- At apical-colloid border, tyrosine within thyroglobulin are iodinated and stored in colloid.

## TPO-thyroidal peroxidase

- Membrane bound glycoprotein with heme as prosthetic group.
- Present on apical cell surface of cell.
- TPO mediates oxidation of iodide ions and incorporation of iodine into tyrosine residues of thyroglobulin.

## Iodide trap

- Iodide is transported across basement membrane of thyroid cells by $Na^+/I^-$ symporter (NIS).
- At apical border, a second $I^-$ transport protein: **pendrin** moves iodine into colloid.

## NIS

- Derives it energy from $Na^+/K^+$ ATPase
- Stimulated by TSH (TSH receptor stimulating antibody is found in Grave's disease)
- Inhibited by $ClO_4^-$, $SCN^-$, $NO_3^-$, $TcO_4^-$

## Sodium perchlorate

- Discharges nonorganified iodine from NIS

- Used to diagnose organification defects
- Used in treatment of organification induced hyperthyroidism.

## Sodium pertechnate

- Half life of 6 hours
- Give gamma emission
- Used in rapid visualization of thyroid gland for size and functioning.

## Iodination

Iodide is oxidized rapidly by $H_2O_2$ by TPO at cell-colloid interface to form active intermediate which gets incorporated into tyrosyl residues of thyroglobulin.

## Coupling

Also catalyzed by TPO, involves 3 steps:

i. Oxidation of iodotyrosyl residues to activated form by TPO

ii. Coupling of activated iodotyrosyl residue to form quinol ether intermediate.

iii. Splitting of quinol to form iodo-thyronine.

Two molecules of DIT may couple to form $T_4$. One MIT and a DIT may couple form $T_3$.

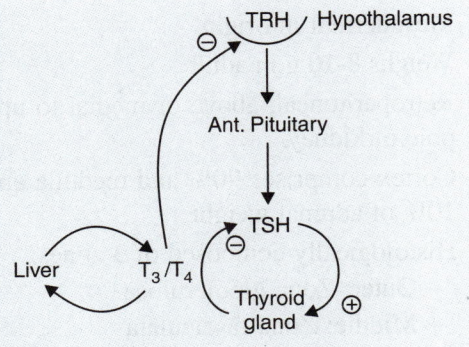

**Fig. 5.15.** Feedback regulation of thyroid hormone.

## Drugs

- Propylthiouracil, methimazole, carbimazole inhibit TPO
- Thus blocks the hormones synthesis
- Used in management of hyperthyroidism

## Proteolysis of thyroglobulin & thyroid hormone secretion

- At cell-colloid interface, colloid is engulfed into a colloid vesicle and is absorbed into thyroid cell.
- Lysosomes fuse with colloid vesicle and hydrolysis of thyroglobulin occurs to release $T_4$, $T_3$, DIT, MIT, peptide fragments and amino acids.
- $T_3$, $T_4$ are released into circulation, DIT, MIT deiodinated and $I^-$ is conserved.

**Thyroglobulin is also released in small amounts from thyroid cells:**

- Markedly increased in subacute thyroiditis, hyperthyroidism. TSH induced goiter, certain malignancies: papillary, follicular thyroid cancer
- Used as marker for metastasis.
- Thyroglobulin proteolysis is inhibited by excess iodide, lithium (lithium carbonate is used in bipolar disorders).

## Intrathyroidal deiodination

- Deiodinase, NADPH-dependent enzyme acts on DIT and MIT to release iodide which is reutilized in hormone synthesis mainly and small part of this iodide leaks into body pool.
- Deiodinase does not act on $T_3$, $T_4$ in thyroid cells
- 5'-deiodinase that converts $T_4$ to $T_3$ in peripheral tissues is also found in thyroid gland. Activity of this enzyme may increase in iodide deficiency to increase $T_3$ secretion

from thyroid gland and thus increasing metabolic efficiency of hormone synthesis.

### Inherited metabolic defects

- May involve any phase of hormonal biosynthesis resulting in impaired hormonal synthesis or dyshormogenesis.
- Features:
  - Thyroid enlargement or goiter
  - Mild to severe hyperthyroidism
  - Low serum $T_3$ and $T_4$
  - Elevated serum TSH

### Iodine deficiency & hormone synthesis

Diet low in iodine:

- Reduces intrathyroidal iodine content.
- Increases MIT/DIT ratio
- Increases $T_3/T_4$ ratio
- Decreases secretion of $T_4$
- Increases TSH.

This results in goiter with hypothyroidism.

### Thyroid hormone transport

Thyroid hormones are transported in serum bound to carrier proteins:

- TBG (thyroxine binding globulin)
- TBPA (Thyroxine binding prealbumin or transthyretin)
- Albumin

### TBG

- Polypeptide
- Synthesized in liver
- Pregnancy or estrogen therapy increases its sialic content resulting in decreased metabolic clearance and elevated levels of TBG in serum.

- Each molecule of TBG has a single binding site for $T_4$ or $T_3$.
- Androgens and glucocorticoids lower TBG
- Drugs like salicylates, phenytoin, phenylbutazone and diazepam bind to TBG, displacing $T_4$ and $T_3$.

**TBPA:**

- Polypeptide
- Binds 10% of circulating $T_4$, affinity for $T_3$ is lower.

**Albumin:**

- Has one strong binding site for $T_4$ and $T_3$
- Carries 15% of $T_4$ and $T_3$.

### Metabolism thyroid hormones

Daily  100 nmol $T_4$
  5 mmol $T_3$
  5 nmol $rT_3$ are secreted from normal thyroid gland

Plasma pool of $T_3$ is derived from 5' deiodination of $T_4$.

$rT_3$ (3, 5', 3' triiodothyronine) is metabolically inert.

### ADRENAL CORTEX

### Fact file

- Mesodermal in origin
- Weighs 8-10 g in adult
- Retroperitoneal, above or medial to upper pole of kidney.
- Cortex comprises 90% and medulla about 10% of adrenal weight
- Histologically composed of 3 zones:
  - Outer: Zona glomerulosa
  - Middle: Zona fasciculata
  - Inner: Zona reticularis

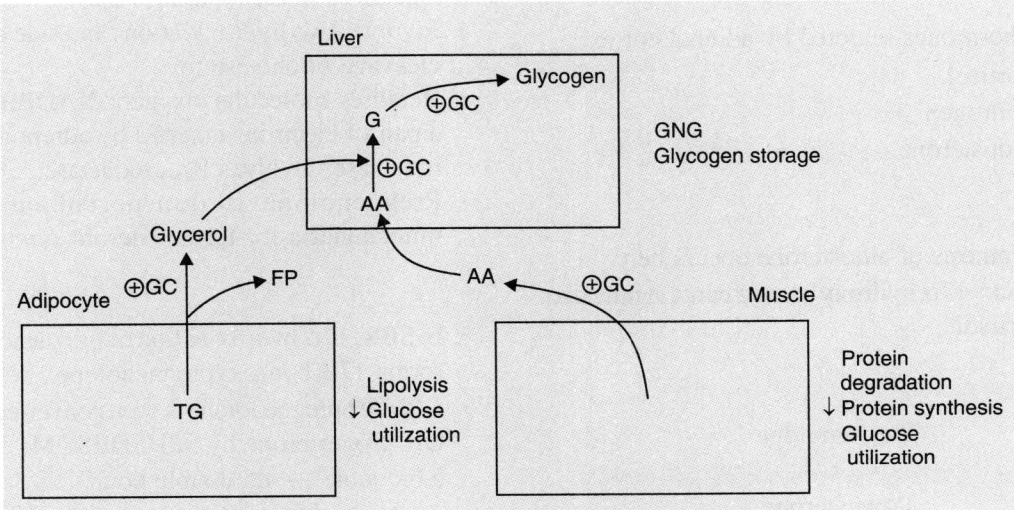

**Fig. 5.16.** Effect of GC on fuel metabolism.

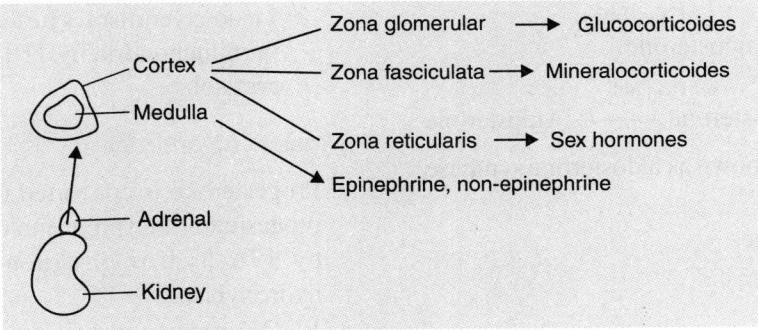

**Fig. 5.17.** Hormones secreted by adrenals

## Aldosterone

| Function | Mechanism |
|---|---|
| Conserve sodium | Facilititate Na reabsorption<br>$K^+$, $H^+$ secretion in DCT via renin-angiotensin |
| Regulate blood pressure | Renin released in response to falling blood volume and loss of $Na^+$, via renin-angiotensin system. |
| Aldosteronism | Cause: Adenoma (Conn's syndrome)<br>Idiopathic<br>Primary hyperplasia<br>Glucocorticoid suppressible<br>All responsive<br>Carcinoma |
| Symptoms | Tiredness, muscle weakness, thirst, polyuria, |
| Diagnosis | Renin activity, plasma aldosterone, low plasma K |

## Biosynthesis of hormones

Major hormones secreted by adrenal cortex:

- Cortisol
- Androgen
- Aldosterone

## Zona glomerulosa

- Synthesis of aldosterone occurs here
- Lacks $17\alpha$ hydroxylase, so can't synthesize cortisol.

## Cholesterol

Pregnenolone
↓
Progesterone
↓
11-deoxycorticosterone
↓ $P_{450}$ ald
Corticosterone
↓ $P_{450}$ ald
1δ-hydroxy corticosterone ⟶ Aldosterone

$P_{450}$ ald: Also known as aldosterone synthase mediates:

11β-hydroxylases
18 hydroxylation
18 oxidation

## Cholesterol uptake and synthesis

- Plasma lipoproteins (80% in LDL) are major source of adrenal cholesterol
- Also, cholesterol synthesis occurs in adrenals.
- Small pool of free cholesterol is also available in adrenal for rapid synthesis of steroid hormones following stimulation.

## Conversion of cholesterol to pregnenolone

- Rate limiting step
- Major site of action for ACTH in adrenal

- Occurs in mitochondria.
- Involves two hydroxylations and side chain cleavage of cholesterol
- Requires molecular oxygen, NADPH and a pair of electrons donated by adrenodoxin reductase, involves $P_{450}$ reductase.
- Pregnenolone is transported outside mitochondria for further steroid synthesis.

## Cortisol synthesis

- In SER, $17\alpha$ hydroxylation of pregnenolone forms $17\alpha$ hydroxypregnenolone.
- $17\alpha$-OH pregnenolone is then converted 17-OH progesterone by 3βHSD/ISOM: 5,6 double → 4,5 double bond
  - 21 hydroxylation converts 17-OH progesterone to 11-deoxy cortisol in SER.
  - 11-deoxycortisol is further hydroxylated in mitochondria by 11β hydroxylase to cortisol.

## Synthesis of androgens

- Progesterone is converted to $17\alpha$ hydroxy progesterone and pregnenolone is converted by $17\alpha$ hydroxypregnenolone by $17\alpha$ hydroxylase.
- 17 OH pregnenolone is converted to 19 carbon DHEA: two carbon side chains at C17 removed by C17, 20 desmolase.
- Androstenedione is produced from DHEA by CYP17 (having 17 a hydroxylase and 17, 20 lyase activity).
- Androstenedione is also produced from progesterone via $17\alpha$-hydroxyprogesterone by CYP 17.
- Androstenedione can be converted to testosterone in minimal amount.
- Peripheral conversion of androstenedione to testosterone and dihydrotestosterone occurs.

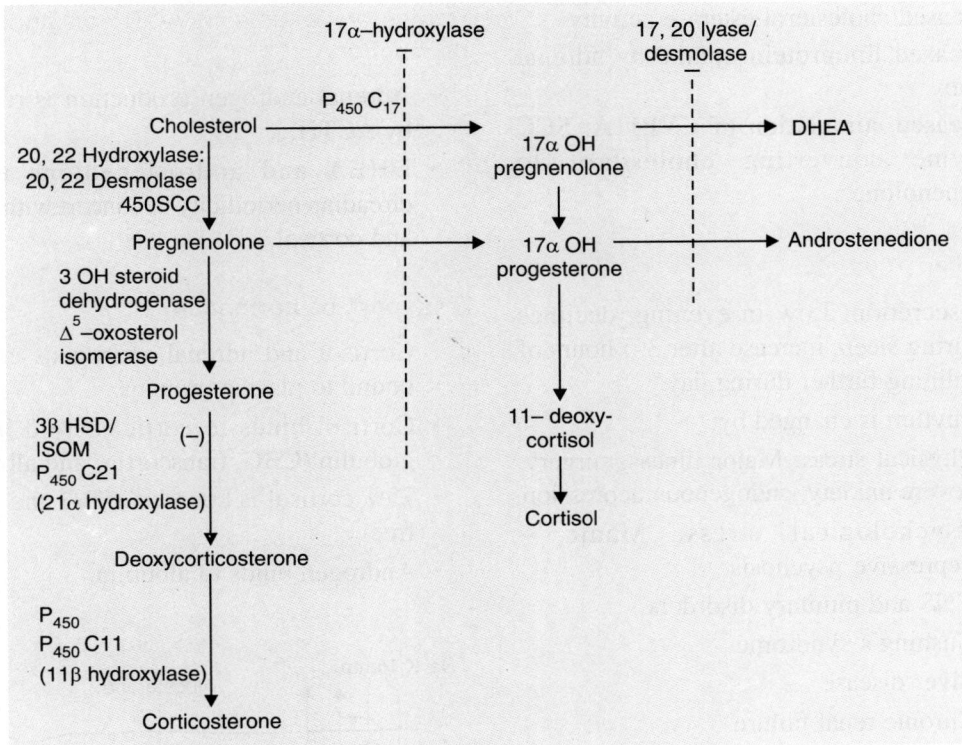

**Fig. 5.18.** Synthesis of adrenal cortex hormones.

- DHEA and DHEA sulfate are secreted in greater quantities and get rapidly converted to **testosterone** in periphery.

## Regulation of secretion of ACTH, CRH

### ACTH:

- Trophic hormone of zona fasciculate and reticularis
- Major regulator of cortisol and androgen production
- ACTH regulated by hypothalamus and CNS via:
  CRH (corticotrophin releasing hormone), AVP (arginine vasopressin)
- Binds to plasma membrane receptors via cAMP and protein kinase.

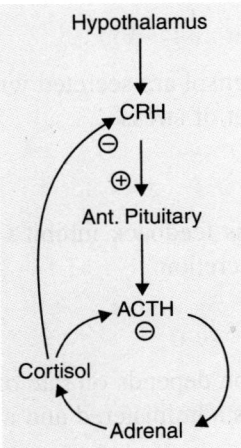

**Fig. 5.19.** Regulation of cortisol secretion.

ACTH results in free cholesterol formation by:

- Increased cholesterol esterase activity
- Increased lipoprotein uptake by adrenal cortex
- Increased stimulation of CYP11A: SCC enzyme converting cholesterol to pregnenolone.

## 1. Circadian rhythm

Cortisol secretion: Low in evening, declines further during sleep, increase after 3-5 hours of sleep, declining further during day.

This rhythm is changed by:

1. Physical stress: Major illness, surgery, severe anxiety, endogenous depression
2. Psychological stress: Manic – depressive psychosis
3. CNS and pituitary disorders
4. Cushing's syndrome
5. Liver disease
6. Chronic renal failure
7. Alcoholism
8. Cyproheptadine: antiserotonergic drug

## 2. Stress responsiveness

ACTH and cortisol are secreted within minutes following onset of stress

## 3. Feed back (F.B.) Inhibition

Glucocorticoids feedback inhibit CRH, ACTH and cortisol secretion.

## Fast F.B. Inhibition

ACTH secretion depends on rate of increase of glucocorticoids administered and not the dose.

## Delayed F.B. inhibition

Depend on both time and dose of glucocortoid administration.

## Regulatory effects of ACTH on androgen production

- Adrenal androgen production is regulated by ACTH.
- DHEA and androstenedione exhibit circadian periodicity in concert with ACTH and cortisol.

## Transport of hormones

- Cortisol and adrenal androgens circulate bound to plasma proteins.
- Cortisol binds to corticosteroid binding globulin (CBG, transcortin) and albumin.
- 75% cortisol is bound to CBG and 10% is free
- Androgen binds to albumin.

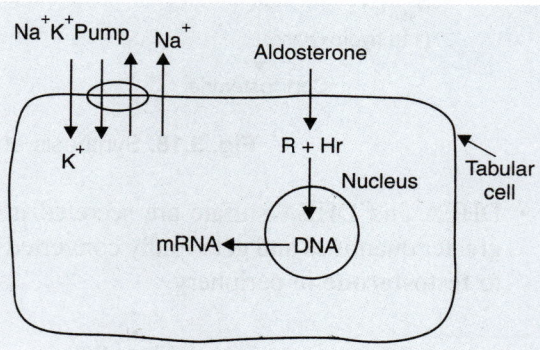

**Fig. 5.20.** Aldosterone action.

## Metabolism

Steroid hormones are conjugated in with glucuronide or sulfate. 90% of these are excreted through kidney

## Aim of metabolizing hormone

- To render them inactive
- To increase their water solubility
- To facilitate their excretion by kidney

## Biologic effects of glucocorticoids

| Target system | Specific target | Physiologic function |
| --- | --- | --- |
| Metabolism | Liver | Increase expression of GNG enzyme: PEP carboxy kinase G-6-Pase F1, 6 biPase |
| | Adipose tissue | Elevated FFA via lipolysis (to provide fuel for GNG) |
| | Skeletal muscle | Proteolysis by activating ubiquitin pathway (to provide substrate (for GNG) |
| | Blood glucose | Maintain blood glucose during fasting, increases blood glucose level. |
| Calcium | Kidney | Decrease reabsorption of calcium |
| | Bone, cartilage | Inhibit collagen synthesis, bone deposition |
| | GIT | Inhibit calcium, magnesium and phosphate absorption |
| Other endocrine | Hypothalamus, pituitary | Decrease gonadotroph responsiveness to GnRH, stimulate GH gene expression by pituitary |
| | Pancreas | Inhibit insulin secretion |
| | Adrenal medulla | Enhance epinephrine synthesis |
| | Binding proteins | Decrease CBG, TBG, SHBG (all binding proteins) |
| Immune system | Thymus lymphocyte | Cause age-related involution of thymus |
| | Monocyte | Inhibit monocyte proliferation |
| | Granulocyte | Degranulation of neutrophils |
| | Inflammatory response | Inhibit inflammation by inhibiting $PLA_2$, inhibiting production to LT, PG suppression of COX-2 |
| Skin and CT | – | Anti proliferative for fibroblasts and keratinocytes |

## DISORDERS OF ADRENAL CORTEX

### Adreno cortical insufficiency

Deficient adrenal production of glucocorticoids or mineralocorticoids results in adrenocortical insufficiency.

### Causes

**Primary:** Cause could be destruction or dysfunction of cortex e.g. Addison's disease.

**Secondary:** Deficient ACTH secretion.

### Addison's disease

Loss of >90% of adrenal cortex results in clinical manifestation of adrenocortical insufficiency.

### Causes

- Autoimmune
- Adrenal hemorrhage
- Infection
- Adrenoleukodystrophy
- Congenital adrenal hyperplasia
- Familial glucocorticoid deficiency

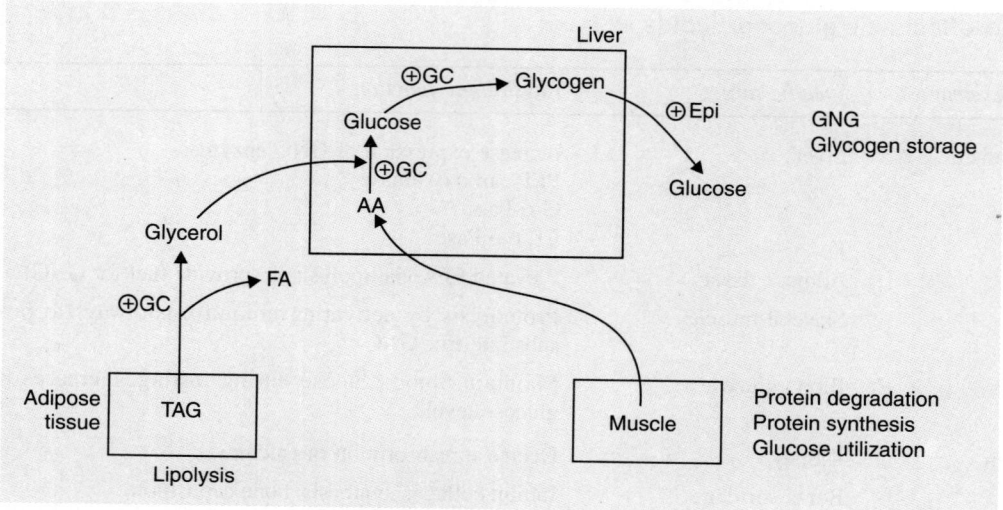

**Fig. 5.21.** Actions of glucocorticoides.

- Metastasis
- Drugs:
  - Ketoconazole
  - Metyrapone

## Cushing's syndrome

Caused by chronic glucocorticoid excess, most commonly iatrogenic

- Abnormality of pituitary or adrenal
- Consequence of ACTH or CRH secretion by non pituitary tumors:
  Ectopic ACTH, ectopic CRH

**Cushing's disease** is defined as specific type of Cushing's syndrome due to excessive pituitary ACTH secretion from a pituitary tumor.

### Classification

- ACTH- dependent
- ACTH – independent

### ACTH-dependent type of Cushing's syndrome

Ectopic ACTH syndrome and Cushing's disease are characterized by chronic ACTH hyper-secretion resulting in hyperplasia of adrenal cortex and increased secretion of cortisol, and androgen.

### ACTH-independent type of Cushing's syndrome

May be caused by a primary adrenal neoplasia.

### Clinical features

Cushing's syndrome

- Obesity:
  - Centripetal
  - Abdominal
  - Moon facies
  - Buffalo hump
- Skin: Acne due to hyperandrogenism
- Due to cortisol excess:
  - Striae
  - Bruising
  - Plethora
- Hyperandogenism:
  Hirsuitism

- Musculoskeletal:
  - Osteopenia
  - Weakness
- Neuropsychiatric:
  - Euphoria
  - Depression
  - Psychosis
- Gonadal:
  - Hyperandrogenism:
    Menstrual disorders
    Impotence
    Decreased libido
- Metabolic:
  - Hypercalciuria:
    Renal stones
  - Glucose intolerance:
    Diabetes
  - Hyperlipidemia
  - Polyuria
  - Hyperglycemia

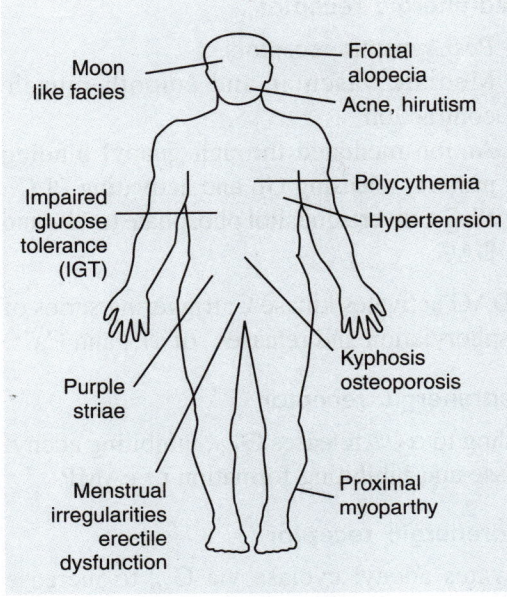

Moon like facies
Frontal alopecia
Acne, hirutism
Impaired glucose tolerance (IGT)
Polycythemia
Hypertenrsion
Purple striae
Kyphosis osteoporosis
Menstrual irregularities erectile dysfunction
Proximal myoparthy

**Fig. 5.22.** Cushing's syndrome.

**Ectopic ACTH is produced by:**
- Small cell carcinoma of lung
- Pancreatic islet cell tumors
- Carcinoid tumors (lung, thymus, gut, pancreas, ovary)
- Medullary carcinoma thyroid
- Pheochromocytoma

## ADRENAL MEDULLA

### Fact file

Part of sympathetic nervous system that secretes catecholamine
- Secretes epinephrine and nor epinephrine
- Arises from neural crest
- Constitutes $1/10^{th}$ of weight of gland
- Composed of chromaffin cells or pheochromocytes: large columnar cells arranged in clumps or cords around blood vessels

### Hormones of adrenal medulla

**Catecholamines:**
- Have a catechol nucleus with two hydroxyl side groups plus a side-chain amine
- Include: Epinephrine, norepinephrine, dopamine

### Biosynthesis

(Already discussed under protein metabolism).

### Storage

Catecholamines are stored in electron – dense granules that contain catecholamine and ATP in 4:1 ratio

### Secretion

It is mediated by release of acetylcholine from terminals of preganglionic fibers.

### Transport

Catecholamines are transported bound to albumin

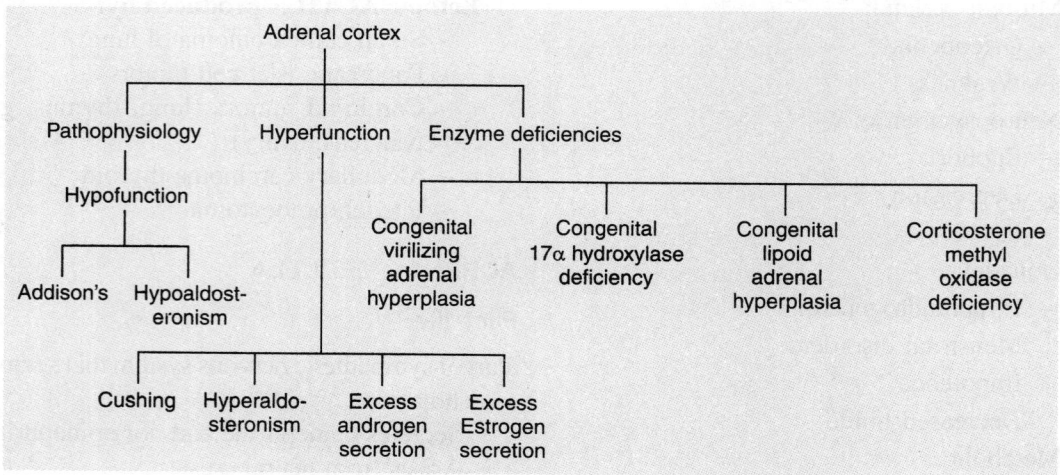

**Fig. 5.23.** Disorders of adrenal cortex.

*Metabolism*

Catecholamines are quickly metabolized into inactive compounds including metanephrine, VMA and conjugated catecholamines.

Excess intracellular norepinephrine is inactivated primarily by deamination by MAO (monoamine oxidase) forming deaminated aldehyde which get oxidized to 3,4 – dihydroxy mandelic acid (DHMA) or dihydrophenylglycol (DHPG).

Dihydrophenylglycol gets converted to VMA by enzyme catechol-O-methyl transferase (COMT), VMA is then excreted in urine.

**Adrenergic receptors**

| Receptor | Effect |
|----------|--------|
| $\alpha_1$ | ↑ 1P$_3$, DAG |
| $\alpha_2$ | ↓ cAMP, K$^+$ channels |
|  | ↓ Ca channels |
| $\beta$ | ↑ cAMP |

**Fact file: Adrenergic receptors**

• Transmembrane proteins with extracellular amino terminus and intracellular carboxyl terminus

• Has seven hydrophobic transmembrane regions

• Receptors are coupled with G-proteins

**$\alpha_1$ adrenergic receptor**

• Post synaptic receptors.

• Mediate vascular and smooth muscle contraction

• Action mediated through guanyl binding protein, releasing Gq and activating PLC.

• PLC converts inositol phosphate to 1P$_3$ and DAG.

DAG activates kinase C, triggering series of phosphorylation and release of 1P$_3$ and Ca$^{+2}$.

**$\alpha_2$ adrenergic receptor**

Binding to $\alpha_2$ ® releases $G_{1\alpha}$, inhibiting adenyl cyclase and inhibiting formation of cAMP.

**$\beta_2$-adrenergic receptor**

Activates adenyl cyclase via $G_{s\alpha}$ to increase production of cAMP which activates protein kinase A for phosphorylation of proteins.

- Mediates vascular, bronchial, uterine smooth muscle relaxation
- Regulate energy expenditure and lipolysis

### Dopaminergic receptor

Found in:

- Central nervous system
- Presynaptic adrenergic nerve terminal
- Pituitary, heart, renal and mesenteric vascular beds.

### Actions of catecholamines

**Dopamine:**

- Neurotransmitter
  - Precursor to norepinephrine
  - High serum levels cause vasodilation and increased renal flow.

**Norepinephrine:**

- Synthesized in:
  - Adrenal medulla
  - Sympathetic paraganglia
  - Brain
  - Spinal cord nerve cells ·
- Found in post ganglionic autonomic nerves in organs namely, heart, salivary gland, vascular smooth muscle, liver, spleen, kidney, muscle.

| Receptor | Action of norepinephrine |
|---|---|
| $\alpha_1$ | ↑ Ca influx |
|  | Hypertension |
|  | ↑ cardiac contraction |
|  | Dilation of pupil |
|  | Stimulation of sweating (stress, sweat) |
| $\beta_1$ | Influx of calcium |
|  | ↑ cardiac contraction and rate |
| $\alpha_2$ | Has less affinity for $\beta_2$ |
|  | Vasodilation |
|  | Hepatic glycogenolysis |

### Epinephrin

Stimulates $\alpha_1$, $\beta_1$, $\beta_2$ receptors

| Receptor | Action of epinephrine |
|---|---|
| $\alpha_1$, $\beta_1$ | Same effect as norepinephrine |
| $\beta_2$ | Vasodilation in skeletal muscle |
|  | Variable effect on blood pressure, hypertension to hypotension |

### Epinephrine stimulates

- Lipolysis
- Increase BMR

### Cardiovascular effects of catecholamines: Fact file

- $\beta_1$: Increase rate and force of contraction
- Contraction mediated by $\alpha_1$ receptor
- Vascular smooth muscle contraction regulated by $\alpha_1$, $\alpha_2$, $\beta_2$.

### Metabolic effects

- Regulate glucose and fat mobilization from storage depot

### Causes

- Glycogenolysis in liver, muscle
- Increase availability of carbohydrate for utilization
- Lipolysis release FFA and glycerol into circulation for utilization at other sites.

**Note:** All these effects are mediated by $\beta$-receptor.

### Role of catecholamines in secretion of other hormones

Norepinephrine and dopamine regulate secretion of anterior pituitary hormone.

- Dopamine – prolactin inhibiting
  - Hypothalamic releasing hormones are also under sympathetic control

- Secretion of renin by JG cells of kidney via β receptor
- β cells of pancreatic islets secrete insulin
- α cells of pancreatic islets secrete glucagon
- Release of thyroxine, calcitonin, PTH and gastrin.

## Other hormones secreted by adrenal medulla

- Opiate-like peptides: met-and leu-enkephalin
- Adrenomedullin (vasodilatory)
- Vasopressin

## DISORDERS OF ADRENALS: HYPERFUNCTIONING OF ADRENALS

### Pheochromocytoma

Rare tumor, more frequent in right adrenal, arises from chromaffin cells, patient presents with paroxysmal hypertension more often.

### Features

- 10% bilateral
- 10% familial
- 10% malignant
- 10% extramedullary

### Paraganglioma

- Extra adrenal pheochromocytoma arising from sympathetic ganglia.
- Common in juxtarenal or paraaortic region, more likely to be malignant
- Present with pain or mass.
- 10% of pheochromocytomas are hereditary and occur as a feature of certain familial syndromes: **MEN (multiple endocrine neoplasias.**

### MEN 2 – (multiple endocrine neoplasia)

- A.D
- Caused by mutation in ret protooncogene

*Symptoms*

**Paroxysms of:**
- Headache
- Sweating
- Forceful heartbeat
- Anxiety
- Tremor
- Fatigue
- Nausea, vomiting
- Abdominal, chest pain
- Visual disturbances

**Between paroxysms:**
- Increased sweating
- Cold hand and feet
- Weight loss
- Constipation

*Diagnosis*

- Increased urine VMA, metanephrine, normetanephrine.
  Pheochromocytoma develop in adrenals, patients tend to have hypertension, usually paroxysmal.
- Plasma catecholamines may be normal, metanephrine is elevated in most patients

### MEN 2a

May develop:
- Medullary thyroid carcinoma
- Hyperparathyroidism
- Pheochromocytoma
- Adrenal medullary hyperplasia

### MEN 2b

May develop:
- Aggressive medullary thyroid carcinoma
- Mucosal neuroma
- Thick corneal nerves
- Intestinal ganglioneuroma
- Marfanoid habitus

- Pheochromocytoma
- Adrenal medullary hyperplasia

## NPY (neuropeptide Y)

- Found in adrenergic granules and secreted along with norepinephrine by pheochromocytoma tumor.
- Very potent non adrenergic vasoconstrictor and vascular growth factor contributes to hypertension in most patients.

## NSE (neuron specific enolase)

- Neuroendocrine glycolytic enzyme
- Elevated in 50% of malignant pheochromocytoma.

| Hormones, peptides | Manifestation |
|---|---|
| Catecholamines | Hypertension |
| PTHrP | Hypercalcemia |
| ACTH | Cushing's syndrome |
| NPY | Hypertension |
| Erythropoietin | Erythrocytosis |
| Cytokine | Leukocytosis |
| IL-6 | Fever |

## Hormone, peptide secreted by pheochromocytoma

- Epinephrine
- Norepinephrine
- Metanephrine
- Dopamine
- ACTH
- Adrenomedullin
- Calcitonin
- Chromogranin A
- GH
- GnRH
- NPY
- Serotonin
- Somatostatin
- VIP
- 1L-6
- ANF
- Neurotensin
- Substance P
- Enkenphalin
- β-endorphin
- PTHrP
- Renin
- Cytokine

### Pheochromocytoma

| Symptoms | Cause |
|---|---|
| Paroxysmal symptoms: Headache, palpitation, anxiety, tumor, chest discomfort | Epinephrine |
| Sweating   Palm<br>            Axilla<br>            Head<br>            Shoulder | Vasoconstriction |
| Drenching sweats | Vasoconstriction |
| GIT symptoms Pain, constipation | Ischemic enterocolitis, pressure effect of tumor |
| Orthostatic hypotension and syncope | Epinephrine |
| Tachycardia followed by reflex bradycardia | Peripheral vasoconstriction |
| Facial flushing | Reflex vasodilation, following an attack |
| Fever | 1L-6 |

## Lab tests

- Plasma, urine catecholamine, metanephrine, serum chromogenin A.
- VMA and metanephrine in urine

## Factors causing misleading tests for pheochromocytoma

| Food | Reason |
| --- | --- |
| Banana | Rich in tyrosine (that gets converted to dopamine by CNS) and epinephrine and norepinephrine |
| Coffee (caffeine) | • Contains substances that are converted to catechol metabolite that causes a confusing peak in HPLC |
| | • Heavy caffeine intake causes persistent elevation in norepinephrine production. |
| Pepper | • 5 methyloxy-4-hydroxybenzylamine (MHBA) in pepper interferes with internal standard for assay for metanephrine |

## PTH (PARATHYROID HORMONE)

### Parathyroid gland

- Four glands located adjacent to thyroid gland on its posterior aspect at four poles of thyroid and exact location is variable.
- Arises from $3^{rd}$ and $4^{th}$ brachial pouches
- Composed of epithelial cells and stromal fat.

### Secretion

PTH is under exquisite control by serum concentration and there is negative feedback relationship of PTH with serum calcium concentration.

### Calcium receptor

- G-protein coupled receptor has 7 transmembrane domains; extracellular domain is involved in ion recognition.
- Intracellular loops are connected to transmembrane domain and are directly involved in coupling receptor to G-protein.

- Mutation in calcium receptor: familial benign hypocalciuric hypocalcemia
- Calcium receptors are not unique to PTH gland, and are widely distributed in brain, skin, growth plate, intestine, stomach, C-cells and other tissues.
- Thyroid C-cells secrete calcitonin in response to high extracellular calcium.
  - Increased extracellular calcium inhibits PTH secretion
- Calcium receptor couples to PLC by $G_q$, hydrolyze $P1P_2$, releasing $1P_3$ and DAG. $IP_3$ binds to receptor in ER, releases Ca which causes $\uparrow$ [Ca] and Ca influx DAG (+) protein kinase-C through channels which (–) PTH secretion. Ca influx blocks fusion of storage granule with cell membrane to release PTH.

Changes in serum calcium regulate secretion of PTH and synthesis of PTH by stabilizing prepro PTH mRNA levels and enhancing gene transcription.

Also, vitamin D regulates transcription of PTH gene.

### Synthesis and processing of PTH

PTH:

- 84 amino acid peptide
- Gene located on chromosome 11
- Gene encodes prepro PTH with 29 amino acid with extension at amino terminal: of mature PTH: 23 amino acid signal sequence (pre) and 6-residue prohormone sequence.

### Metabolism

- Half life of PTH: 2-4 minutes
- Cleared by liver and kidney
- Cleaved at 33-34 and 36-37 positions to produce:
  - Amino terminal fragment

– Carboxyl terminal fragment-cleared from blood by renal filtration.

## Actions

**PTH Lowers calcium levels:** PTH regulates serum calcium levels by its effects on three target organs:

– Bone
– Intestine
– Kidney

**In intestine:** Indirect action on intestinal absorption of calcium via vitamin D.

**In kidney:**

– Direct effect on tubular reabsorption of calcium, phosphate and bicarbonate (mainly in DCT).
– PTH inhibits reabsorption of phosphate in proximal tubule.

## PTH receptors

### PTH 1

- Binds PTH and PTH related protein (PTHrP)
- Formed in kidney and bone
- Glycoprotein
- Member of G protein receptor superfamily
- Has extracellular, 7 transmembrane and cytosolic domain
- PTH binds to sites in large extracellular domain and activates G protein.

### PTH-2

- Activated by PTH only

### PTHrP (PTH related peptide)

- Mediator of hypercalcemia of malignancy
- Strong homology to PTH, binds with equal affinity to PTH receptors
  – Secreted in abundance by malignant tumors

– Produces severe hypercalcemia and suppression of vitamin D levels
– Produced in many fetal and adult tissues
– Required for normal development as a regulator of proliferation and mineralization of chondrocytes and regulator of placental calcium transport.
– Regulate endochondral bone formation regulate growth and development in mammary gland
– Relaxation of smooth muscle and vascular smooth muscle
– Cytokine-like effect

## Calcitonin

- 32 amino acid peptide
- Secreted by parafollicular C cells of thyroid derived from neuroendocrine cells from ultimobranchial body
- Secretion under control of serum calcium levels
- C-cells use same calcium receptor as PTH cells to sense changes in calcium concentration
- C-cells increase calcitonin secretion in response to hypercalcemia

## Actions

- Inhibits osteoclastic bone resorption.
  – Morphology of osteoblast changes on exposure to calcitonin: cell withdraws its processes, shrinks in size, and retracts its ruffled border from bone surface.
- Osteoclasts and proximal tubular cells of kidney express calcitonin receptor: a serpentine receptor with 7 membrane spanning regions coupled by Gs to adenyl cyclase to generate cAMP in target cells.
- Inhibits phosphate reabsorption in kidney.

## Vitamin D

### Mechanism of action

- Main function: Regulation of calcium and phosphate homeostasis in conjunction with PTH
- Target tissue: Gut, kidney, bone
  1, 25 $(OH)_2 D_3$ is most biologically active
- **Receptor:** Vitamin D receptor (VDR)
  - 50 kDa protein
  - Has structural and functional homology to nuclear hormone receptors including steroid hormone receptors
  - Thyroid (TR), retinoic acid and retinoid X (RAR, RXR) receptors and endogenous metabolite receptors PPAR (peroxisome proliferation activation receptor), liver X (LXR) and farnesyl X receptors (FXR)
  - These are transcription factors
  - VDR forms heterodimers with RXR generally to act on vitamin D response elements (VDREs)

### Calcium absorption in intestine

Vitamin 1, 25 $DHD_3$ regulates calcium transport through intestinal epithelium at following sequence of steps:

i. Entrance into cells from lumen across brush border down a steep electrochemical gradient
ii. Passage through cytosol
iii. Removal from cell against a steep electrochemical gradient at basolateral membrane.

At brush border, 1, 25 DH $D_3$ induces change in binding of calmodulin to brush border myosin.

Also, calcium channel (CaT1) in brush border gets induced by 1, 25 $DHD_3$. Calcium transport through cytosol requires vitamin D inducible calbindin protein.

At basolateral membrane, calcium is removed from the cell by $Ca^{2+}$-ATPase, which is also induced by 1, 25 $DHD_3$.

### Actions on bone

- Vitamin D (1, 25 $DHD_3$) regulate bone formation and resorption
- 1,25 $DHD_3$ promote differentiation of osteoblasts.

### Actions on kidney

- Kidney expresses VDR and 1, 25 $DHD_3$ stimulates calbindin and $Ca^{+2}$ ATPase in distal tubule.
- Vitamin D stimulates calcium and phosphate reabsorption by kidney.

**Vitamin D response elements (VDREs) are also found in:**

  - Hematopoietic and immune system
  - Cardiac, skeletal and smooth muscle
  - Brain, liver, breast
  - Endothelium
  - Skin
  - Endocrine glands: pituitary, parathyroid, pancreatic islets, thyroid, adrenals, ovary, testis

## OSTEOPOROSIS

Condition of low bone mass and micro architectural disruption resulting in fractures with minimal trauma.

### Primary osteoporosis

Reduced bone mass and fractures in post menopausal women or older men and women.

### Secondary osteoporosis

Bone loss resulting from specific clinical disorders such as thyrotoxicosis, hyperadreno-corticism, and immobilization.

## Why bone loss occurs with estrogen deficiency

- Estrogen deprivation promotes bone remodeling by releasing constraints on osteoblastic production of skeletally active cytokines (IL-6).
- These cytokines stimulate proliferation of osteoclast precursors.
- Estradiol directly suppresses IL-6 production in human osteoblasts.

## RANKL-OPG system

- Acts as a bone regulator system
- Osteoblast signals stimulate osteoblast production
- With estrogen deficiency, OPG secretion is low, permitting a robust response of osteoclast precursors in RANKL.
- Accelerated bone turnover causes increased delivery of calcium from bone to circulation. Increased plasma calcium suppress PTH secretion, $1, 25$ DHD$_3$ production and intestinal calcium absorption.
- At menopause, loss of endogenous estrogen promotes increased daily loss of calcium (about 20-60mg/day calcium loss).
- To accommodate menopausal changes in calcium, rise in calcium intake from 1000mg to 1500mg is necessary.
- Menopausal women who receive estrogen replacement therapy show calcium balance and their rate of calcium turnover is similar to premenopausal women.

## PANCREATIC HORMONES

### Pancreas

Made up of two functionally different organs:

- Exocrine pancreas: Digestive gland
- Endocrine pancreas: Endocrine gland, source of insulin, glucagon, somatostatin, pancreatic polypeptide.

## Endocrine pancreas

- Consists of up to 1 million small endocrine glands
- Islets of Langerhans scattered in glandular substance of exocrine pancreas.
- Four cell types: A, B, D, PP (or $\alpha$, $\beta$, $\delta$, F), not distributed uniformly throughout pancreas.
- PP (or F) cells: secrete pancreatic poly peptide (PP), found in posterior lobe

In anterior portion of head of pancreas:

- B cells are predominant (80%), secrete insulin
- A cells are 20% - secrete glucagon
- D cells are 3-5% - secrete somatostatin

## HORMONES OR ENDOCRINE PANCREAS

### Insulin

- Gene located on chromosome 11
- Secreted on preproinsulin in RER, microsomal enzymes cleave preproinsulin to proinsulin immediately after synthesis.
- Proinsulin is transported to golgi apparatus and gets packed in clathrin-coated secretary granule.
- Maturation of secretary granule is associated with loss of clathrin coating and conversion of proinsulin into insulin, C-peptide by proteolytic cleavage.
- Normal mature secretary granules contain insulin and C peptide in equimolar amounts.

### Biochemistry

**Proinsulin:**

- Single chain of 36 amino acids
- Contain A and B chains of insulin with C-peptide of 35 amino acids
- Prohormone converting enzymes PC1/3 and PC2 are packaged with proinsulin

in immature secretary granules to cut and remove intervening sequences.

- Some proinsulin produced by pancreas escapes cleavage and is secreted intact into blood stream along with insulin and C-peptide. Most anti-insulin sera in immunoassay cross-react with pro-insulin.

## C-peptide:

- 31 amino acid
- Formed during cleavage of insulin from proinsulin
- No known biological activity
- Released from β-cells in equimolar amount with insulin
- Excreted by kidney

## Insulin:

- 51 amino acid
- Two peptide chain:
  - A with 21 amino acid
  - B with 30 amino acid
- Connected by two disulfide bridges.
- Half life 3-5 minutes, catabolized by insulinase in liver, kidney and placenta.

### Insulin secretion

- 40-50 units of insulin is secreted per day by normal adults.
- Basal concentration of insulin in fasting human is 10 mU/ml after standard meals; it rises above 100 mU/ml.

### Insulin release

- Glucose is the most important stimulant of insulin release.
- Glucose enters pancreatic B cells by passive diffusion (glucose transporter) and gets phosphorylated by glucokinase.
- Catabolism of glucose in B cells raises ATP/

ADP ratio which closes ATP sensitive K channels and depolarizing the cell. Calcium is required for insulin release cAMP is another modulator of insulin release.

### Factors affecting insulin release

| Stimulant | Inhibitors |
|---|---|
| Glucose, mannose | α adrenergic |
| Leucine | Somatostatin |
| Vagal stimulation | – |
| Sulfonyl urea | Drugs: Phenytoin, vinblastin, colchicine |
| Enteric hormones: gastrin, secretin,GIP (glucagon-like peptide),β-adrenergic, amino acid (arginine) | – |

## INSULIN RECEPTORS AND INSULIN ACTION

### Insulin receptor

- Member of growth factor family
- Membrane glycoprotein
- 2 protein subunits
- Encoded by a single gene
- Alpha subunit:
  - Larger
  - Reside extracellularly
  - Binds insulin
- Beta subunit:
  - Membrane spanning
  - Cytoplasmic domain-contain tyrosine kinase activity
- Alpha subunit is tethered by disulphide linkage to beta subunit.

### Action

- Insulin binds to alpha subunit; beta subunit activates itself by autophosphorylation.

- Activated beta subunit then recruits additional proteins and phosphorylates a network of intracellular substrates including insulin receptor substrate-1 (IRS-1), IRS-2 and others.
- Activated substrates recruit and activate additional kinases, phosphatases and other complex.

**Two pathways follow:**

- Mitogenic: Mediates growth effects of insulin
- Metabolic: Regulate nutrient metabolism
  - IP$_3$ kinase activated
  - Vesicle containing GLUT 4 move to cell membrane
  - Increased glycogen, lipid synthesis
  - Stimulation of other metabolic pathway

- Insulin receptor complex get internalized.

## Metabolic effect

Main function of insulin is storage of ingested nutrients in liver, muscle and adipose tissue.

## Paracrine effect

- Effect of insulin on surrounding cells is termed paracrine effect.
- Firsttly insulin reaches A cells at periphery of islet cells, reducing secretion of glucagon by A cells.
- Also, insulin acts on D cells, releasing somatostatin.
- Glucose stimulates B and D cells whose products inhibit A cells.
- Amino acids stimulate glucagon and insulin.

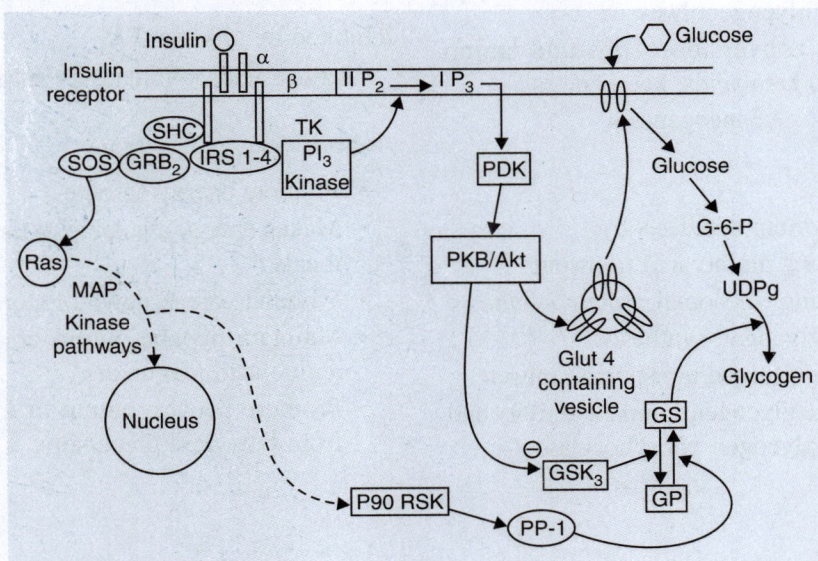

**Fig. 5.24.** Mechanism of action of insulin. (GS: Glycogen synthase; P: Phosphorylated; GSK-3: Glycogen synthase kinase 3; MAP kinase: Mitogen activated protein kinase; PDK: Phospholipid dependent kinase; PI$_3$ kinase: Phosphatidyl inositol 3 kinase; PKB: Protein kinase B; PP-1: Glycogen associated protein phosphatase-1; SOS: Son-e-sevenless related protein; TK: Tyrosine kinase)

- Higher the carbohydrate content of meal, lesser glucagon will be released.
- Predominant protein meal results in greater glucagon secretion.
- Amino acids are less effective at stimulating insulin release in absence of hypoglycemia. Amino acids are potent stimulators of A cells.

## ENDOCRINE EFFECT

### Liver

**Anabolic action:**

- Promotes glycogen synthesis and storage
- Increases protein and TAG synthesis and VLDL formation
- Inhibits gluconeogenesis
- Promotes glycolysis

**Inhibits catabolism:**

- Inhibit glycogenolysis
- Inhibit conversion of FA and amino acids to keto acids: ketogenesis
- Inhibits gluconeogenesis

### MUSCLE

- Promote protein synthesis by:
  - Increasing amino acid transport
  - Increasing ribosomal protein synthesis
- Promotes glycogen synthesis:
  - Increase glucose transport in muscle
  - Enhance glycogen synthase activity and inhibit glycogen phosphorylase

### Adipose tissue

- Increase TAG storage by:
  - Inducing lipoprotein lipase to hydrolyze TAG from lipoproteins
  - Increasing glucose transport into fat cells
  - Inhibiting hormone sensitive lipase, inhibiting intracellular lysis of fat.

### *Glucagon*

- Single polypeptide
- 29 amino acid, synthesized by A cells in islets
- Synthesized as proglucagon: 160 amino acid from which many polypeptides are released:
  - Glucagon-like peptide 1 (GLP-1)
  - GLP-2 (Glicentin related peptide)

### *Secretion*

Inhibited by glucose, FA.

Amino acids stimulate its release.

### *Action*

- Promote energy storage
- Makes energy available to tissues between meals
- Stimulate break down of stored glycogen
- Maintain hepatic output of glucose from amino acid precursors
- Promote hepatic output of ketone bodies from fatty acid precursors.

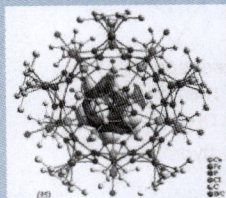

# 6

## Nutrition, Minerals and Vitamins

---

### MINERAL METABOLISM

#### CALCIUM METABOLISM

**Table 6.1.** Salient features of calcium

- Fifth most abundant element
- Most prevalent cation
- Total body calcium: 1 kg
  - 99% located in bones as hydroxyapatite
  - 1% extracellular
- Total serum calcium is maintained between 8.8-10.4 mg/dl

**Table 6.2.** Functions of calcium

- Structural component of:    Bone
                              Teeth
- Neuromuscular excitability
- Muscle contraction
- Coenzyme for coagulation factors
- Intracellular second messenger
- Release of neurotransmitters, hormones

**Calcium exists in three forms in plasma:**

- **Ionized (free) $Ca^{+2}$:** 47%, biologically active form (4.8 mg/dl); and subject to hormonal control
- **Protein bound:** 47%:80% with albumin and 20% with globulin.
  Complexed with organic acids: 6% bound to citrate, phosphate, bicarbonate, and lactate.
- Maintenance of calcium balance is dependent on efficiency of intestinal absorption along with regulation by PTH, vitamin D.

#### Dietary intake

- Daily intake of calcium should be 0.6-0.8 g/d in adults and during pregnancy and lactation it is increased to 1.2 g/d.
- Milk and dairy products, egg yolk, nuts; lentils are good sources of calcium.

287

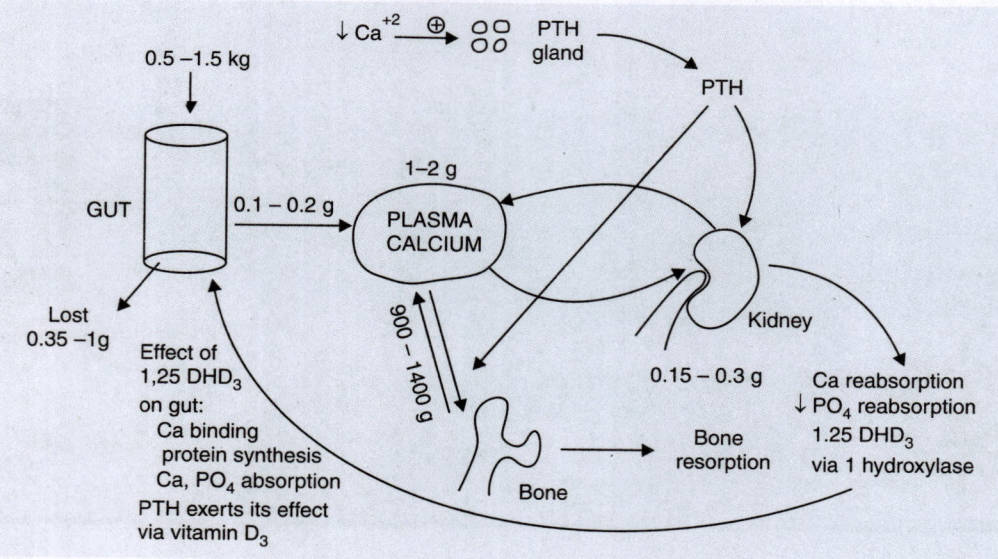

**Fig. 6.1.** Calcium homeostasis.

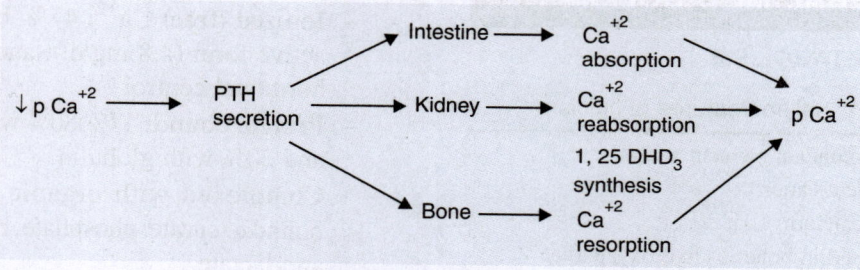

**Fig. 6.2.** Hormonal regulation of calcium.

## Site of absorption of calcium

Calcium is absorbed in upper intestine by active transport and in lower intestine by simple diffusion.

## Factors affecting calcium absorption

### Favoring

- Acidic pH
- High protein diet (lysine, arginine cause maximum absorption)

- Sugar and organic acid increase its solubility
- Citric acid

### Inhibiting

- Alkaline pH
- Oxalate
- Phytate
- Fibers
- Excess $PO_4$, Mg, Fe
- Estrogen deficiency in menopause

## Excretion of Calcium

100-400 mg/d calcium is excreted in urine.

## Regulation

Ionized calcium concentration is principal regulator of PTH secretion by negative feedback mechanism. Principal organs are bone, kidney and intestine and regulatory hormones are PTH and vitamin D.

## TETANY

### Cause

Decrease in concentration of free calcium ions in plasma causes increased neuromuscular excitability.

### Features

- Peripheral and perioral paraesthesia
- Carpopedal spasm
- Anxiety
- Seizure
- Bronchospasm, laryngospasm, Chovstek's, Trousseau's and Erb's sign
- Prolonged QT interval

  **Decrease in free calcium causes:**

  - Increased neuromuscular irritability, tetany

- Peripheral and perioral paraesthesia
- Carpal spasm
- Pedal spasm
- Anxiety, seizures, bronchospasm, laryngospasm
- Chovstek, Erb's sign
- Trousseau's sign
- Lengthening of QT interval of ECG

**Increased total calcium:**

- Anorexia, constipation, hypotonic, depression.
- Persistently/raised calcium result in: ectopic calcification of:

  Blood vessels, connective tissue, joints, gastric mucosa, cornea, renal parenchyma.

## RICKETS

**Rickets** is a disorder of defective mineralization of organic matrix of skeleton.

**Osteomalacia** is defective mineralization in adults. Since growing skeleton is involved in rickets, defective mineralization occurs both in bone and cartilagenous matrix of the growth plate.

**Table 6.3.** Calcium homeostasis

| Organ→ Hormone ↓ | Kidney | Bone | Intestine |
|---|---|---|---|
| Vitamin D | ↑ reabsorption of Ca and $PO_4$ <br> ↑ S. calcium and S.$PO_4$ | ↑Dissolution of bone <br> ↑S calcium, S $PO_4$ | ↑ absorption of Ca and $PO_4$ <br> ↑ S. Ca and S.$PO_4$: **main action** |
| PTH | **Direct most rapid change** <br> ↓ renal clearance of Ca <br> ↑ renal clearance of $PO_4$ | **Largest effect** <br> ↑ dissolution of bone <br> ↑ Ca in ecf <br> ↓ $PO_4$ in ecf | **Indirect action** <br> via Vitamin $D_3$: <br> ↑ efficiency of Ca absorption |

**Table 6.4.** Disorders of calcium balance

| *Hypocalcaemia* | *Hypercalcemia* |
|---|---|
| **Causes**<br>**PTH related:**<br>  (i) PTH absent<br>  (ii) **PTH ineffective:** CRF<br>     **Lack of active vitamin D:**<br>     MAS<br>     Type II rickets<br>  (iii) **PTH overwhelmed:**<br>     Severe hyperphosphatemia (ARF,<br>     tumor lysis, rhabdomyolysis)<br>     Osteotis fibrosa (After PTH-ectomy) | **PTH related:** Primary hypoparathyroidism<br>**Malignancy:**<br>Breast<br>Lung<br>Kidney<br>Hematology<br>**Vitamin D related:**<br>Vitamin D intoxication<br>Sarcoidosis<br><br>**High bone turnover:**<br>Hyperthyroidism<br>Immobilization<br>Thiazides<br>**Renal failure:** Secondary hyperparathyroidism, milk alkali syndrome |
| **Clinical feature:**<br>**CNS:**<br>Neuromuscular irritability<br>Numbness<br>Tingling<br>Cramps<br>Tetany | **Bone:** Ache, pain, fracture<br>**CNS:** Lethargy, depression, confusion, coma, death<br>**Neuromuscular:** Muscle weakness, Hypotonia<br>**GIT:** Constipation, nausea, vomiting, anorexia, peptic ulcer, pancreatitis<br>**Renal:**<br>Polyuria<br>Nephrocalcinosis<br>**Cardiac:** Short QT, broad-T waves, ventricular arrhythmia,<br>**Eye:** Corneal calcification |

### Cause

Vitamin D deficiency is the most common cause of rickets.

### Types of Rickets

- Type I
- Type II

**Type I:** It is inherited as autosomal recessive disorder, where there is a defect in conversion of 25 $HD_3$ to 1, 25 $DHD_3$.

**Type II:** It is also an autosomal recessive disorder due to non-functional vitamin D receptor.. Caused by single amino acid change in one of the zinc finger DNA binding domain in receptor.

### Table 6.5. Clinical features: Rickets

Skeletal deformities
    Craniotabes
    Rachitic rosary
    Harrison's groove
Susceptibility to fractures
    Weakness
    Hypotonia
Deformities of pelvis and extremities
    Bowing of:
        Tibia
        Femur
        Radius
        Ulna
Delayed dental eruptions
Enamel defects

## Vitamin D resistant (refractory) rickets

X-linked dominant disorder, seen in renal tubular disorders, rickets and osteomalacia. It develops in presence of normal intestinal functions and is not cured by vitamin D.

## PHOSPHORUS

### Table 6.6. Salient features of phosphorus

- Most abundant intracellular anion
- Major component of bone, teeth and other tissues
- Of total body phosphorus of 700 g:
  - 85% (600 g) is in bones
  - 15% is soft tissue
  - 0.1% in extracellular fluid
- In extracellular fluid, phosphorus is in a freely diffusible form
- Total serum phosphorus is maintained between 2.5-4.5 mg %.

## Phosphorus fact file

- Most abundant intracellular anion. It is critical for membrane structure and transport and energy storage

- Present in both organic and inorganic forms
- Inorganic phosphorus responsible for development of teeth and bone
- Organic phosphorus present in organic compounds such as:
  - Phosphate esters of monosaccharide (G-6-P, DHAP, F-6-P)
  - Phospholipids (lecithin)
  - Phosphoproteins lipoproteins
  - Constituent of coenzymes (NADP, TPP, PLP).

### Table 6.7. Functions of phosphorus

- Constituent of bone and teeth
- 85% of total phosphate store is in bones
- Energy transfer and storage (ATP, creatine phosphate)
- Maintenance of acid-base balance (phosphate buffer)
- Component of coenzyme (NADP, TPP, PLP)
- Constituent of phospholipids, lipoproteins, nucleic acids
- Important in intermediary metabolism: component of high energy phosphate bonds (ATP) and phosphorylated substrates

## Dietary intake

A normal adult takes about 1g phosphorus,

## Sources

Dietary phosphorus occurs in both inorganic form, in form of phosphoproteins, phosphorylated sugars and phospholipids. Dietary sources include dairy products, cereals, meat, and egg.

## Absorption

- Cow's milk phosphorus is 70% inorganic.
- Phosphorus of cereals and soft tissues of animals is combined organically
- Most phosphorus is absorbed in inorganically bound phosphorus is hydrolyzed in

small intestinal lumen and released as inorganic phosphate

- 70% is absorbed at normal intake and up to 90%, when intake is low.
- Soluble phosphates in dairy products and meat are almost completely absorbed in mid jejunum
- Insoluble phosphates in vegetables and seeds require digestion from its ligand to get absorbed

## Regulation

- Maintenance of phosphate balance is achieved largely through renal excretion.
- One third of dietary intake is excreted in feces and two third in urine.
- Phosphate levels depend on meals, PTH (parathyroid hormone) and vary widely.
- Phosphate levels are under control of mechanism by kidney with respect to PTH and vitamin D.
- Phosphorus absorption is under influence of vitamin D and its excretion is under PTH.
- Plasma inorganic phosphate is major regulator of 25 (OH) $D_3$. Rise in 1, 25 $DHD_3$ increases phosphorus absorption.

## Excretion

500 mg phosphate is excreted in urine per day. It is largely reabsorbed in proximal convoluted tubules and only 6-10% of filtered load is excreted.

## Conditions associated with increased risk of deficiency of phosphorus

- Celiac disease
- Sprue
- Alcoholism
- Hyperparathyroidism
- Insulin treatment
- Premature infant

**Table 6.8.** Disorders of phosphorus balance

| Hypophosphatemia | Hyperphosphatemia |
|---|---|
| **Cause:** | |
| Decreased intake | Hemolysis |
| Starvation | Increased intake of P |
| Malabsorption | vitamin D |
| Vomiting | |
| Increased uptake from cells: | Increased release from cells: |
| High carbohydrate diet | DM |
| Liver disease | Acidemia |
| | Starvation |
| Increased excretion: | |
| Diuretics | Bones: Malignancy |
| Hyperparathyroidism | Renal failure, Hypopara- |
| Hypomagnesaemia | thyroidism |
| | Decreased excretion: renal failure |
| | Hypoparathyroidism— Increased GH |
| Clinical features: | |
| Anorexia | |
| Dizziness | |
| Bone pain | |
| Muscle weakness | |
| Wadding gait | |
| Ectopic calcification | |

## IRON

- Iron is unique in that it operates largely as a closed system with iron stores being efficiently reutilized by the body
- Fourth most abundant element in earth crust
- Iron is one of the **most essential** trace elements in the body
- Total body iron content is 3.5 g:
  - 70% is in blood in RBCs as constituent of Hb
  - 5% in myoglobin of muscle (rest is in liver, bone marrow, muscle)
- Iron is one way substance, body converts

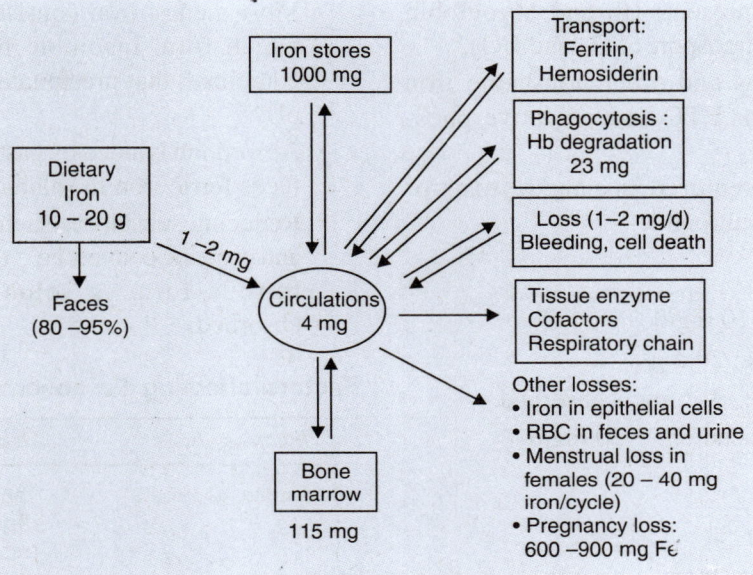

**Fig. 6.3.** Iron distribution and transport.

iron by recycling, usually iron is not excreted as it is not present in free or ionic form

- Iron is not present as free ion as it is toxic and can form free radicals
- Iron loss is by desquamation of mucosal cells

**Type of iron present in the body**

i. Essential iron (functional)
   Heme protein
   Non-heme protein
ii. Storage iron
   Ferritin
   Hemosiderin

I. **Heme protein:** Hemeprotein are protein with heme porphyrin prosthetic group attached to protein globin (Iron is present as bound to protoporphyrin).

**Classes of heme protein:** Hb, myoglobin, cytochrome, catalase, peroxidase, tryptophan pyrrolase, xanthine oxidase.

II. **Non-heme: iron:** Iron storage protein in RES (reticuloendothelial system): mobile store.

Ferritin, hemosiderin, transferrin: transport of Fe to tissues.

Fe-S flavoprotein denatured ferritin, non mobile store (transport of 'e'), ferridoxin (in plants, adrenodoxin ('e'-transport)

**Storage Iron:**
Ferritin
Hemosiderin

III. **Enzymatic iron protein**
   **Heme enzyme:** Catalase, GSH peroxidase, xanthine oxidase, tryptophan pyrrolase
   **Non heme enzyme:** Succinate dehydrogenase, glycerol phosphate dehydrogenase
IV. **Fe as cofactor:** Aconitase in Kreb's cycle uses iron as cofactor

**Biochemical function**

1. Exerts its function through compounds in

which it is present: Hb and Myoglobin required for transport of $O_2$ and $CO_2$.

2. Cytochromes and other non-heme iron necessary for ETC and oxidative phosphorylation.
3. Peroxidase required in phagocytosis of bacteria in neutrophil.

### Requirement

- Adult Male: 10 mg/d
- Adult Female: 20 mg/d
- Only 10% i.e., 1-2 mg is absorbed.
- Pregnancy, lactation: + 20 mg/d

### Sources

- Plant, animal
- Plant: Green leafy vegetable, pulses, cereals, apple
- Animal: Kidney, liver, heart, fish
- Dry fruits: Jaggery.

## ABSORPTION, TRANSPORT AND STORAGE

### Absorption

- Dietary iron is present as:
  - non heme (veg): 20-30% absorbed
  - heme iron: (non veg) 1-5% absorbed
- Bioavailability of heme iron is more compared with protoporphyrins and it is directly absorbed.
- Non-heme Iron complexes are not easily absorbed
- Non vegetarian diet has a large amount of cysteine which helps in absorption of heme iron.

### Site

- Iron absorption occurs mainly in duodenum and upper jejunum
- Only 10% of dietary iron is usually absorbed.

- Most dietary iron consists of ferric salts, which form insoluble ferric hydroxide complexes that precipitate at physiological pH.
- Absorption is aided by gastric acidity, which feeds ferric iron in soluble form.
- Reducing substances such as ascorbic acid and cysteine convert $Fe^{+3}$ to $Fe^{+2}$ (ous) form ferrous form is soluble and readily absorbed.

### Factors affecting Fe absorption

| *Increased by* | *Decreased by* |
|---|---|
| 1. Citrate, ascorbate | 1. Tannin in tea plant, Phytates, phosphates:forms tight complexes with Fe and significantly inhibit absorption |
| 2. Peptides and amino acid | 2. Ca, Cu, Zn, Pb, $PO_4$ Alkali administration MAS (malabsorption) Partial/total resection of stomach, intestine |
| 3. Acidity promote iron absorption by forming soluble complexes which readily enter upper GIT epithelium cell | |

### Non-luminal factors

i. Amount of Fe in diet e.g. presence of vitamin C, tea, coffee, GSH, phytate, oxalate, dietary fibers
ii. Form of iron – $Fe^{+2}$ more efficiently absorbed (phytate, oxalate, and phosphate)
iii. pH of intestine – parasitic infestation – ankylostoma duodenale result in iron loss.
   - Pepsin – liberates iron proteins
   - HCl, vitamin C convert $Fe^{+3} \rightarrow Fe^{+2}$

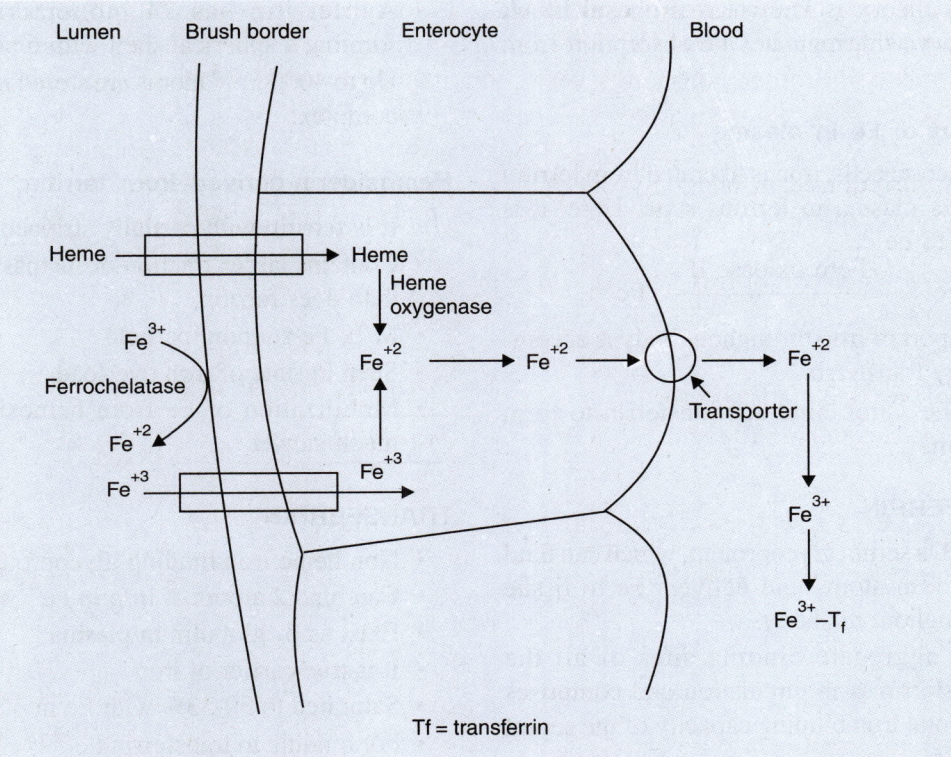

**Fig. 6.4.** Iron absorption.

- Gastric factor – gastroferrin stimulate absorption, present in gastric juice, binds iron and facilitate its uptake in duodenum and jejunum.
- Pancreatic factor inhibit absorption.

## Regulation of absorption of iron

**Unique:** homeostasis is maintained by regulation at level of absorption and not excretion

• When stores are adequate – absorption decreased
• When stores are depleted – absorption increased
• This is referred to as **"Mucosal Block theory"**.
• Iron from intestinal lumen enters mucosal cells in ferrous state

## Events in mucosal cell

1. $Fe^{+2}$ is oxidized again in mucosal cell cytoplasm to $Fe^{+3}$ by ferrooxidase I.
2. Intracellular iron carrier (IIC):
   (i) Deliver a fixed amount to mitochondria
   (ii) Transfer some $Fe^{+3}$ to apoferritin to form ferritin.
3. IIC transfers some iron across serosal cell membrane to apotransferrin to transferrin. Fe is carried in $Fe^{+3}$ form in transferrin
4. IIC holds $Fe^{+3}$ in either protein bound or chelated form which represents "carrier iron pool" in the intestinal mucosal cells which keeps IIC nearly or totally saturated and consequently reduces further Fe absorption.

This theory is known as **mucosal block theory** with regulates Fe absorption from gut.

### Transport of Fe in plasma

From mucosal cells, iron is liberated from ferritin and enters plasma in ferrous state. Here, it is oxidized to $Fe^{+3}$.

$$Fe^{+2} \xrightarrow{\text{Ferrooxidase II}} Fe^{+3}$$

Transport of iron throughout body is accomplished by transferrin.

This $Fe^{+3}$ iron bind apotransferrin to form transferrin.

### TRANSFERRIN

- 80 kDa serum glycoprotein, which can bind two iron atoms and delivers Fe to tissue throughout the body.
- The aggregate binding sites of all the transferrin is in circulation and comprises the total iron binding capacity of the serum (TIBC).
- Normally, 20-45% of iron binding sites of transferrin are filled.
- Specific receptors on plasma membrane of cells recognize transferrin leading to internalization of the protein and release of iron into the cell cytoplasm.
- Plasma transferrin concentration of 250 mg/dL can bind 400 mg iron/dl of plasma)
- Number of receptors decrease when a person is replete with iron and increase with depletion.
- Tissue having high uptake (e.g., liver) have a large number of transferrin receptors present.

### FERRITIN

- Found in bone marrow, blood, liver, spleen, intestinal mucosa

- Apoferritin has 24 monomeric units forming a spherical shell with 6 pores.
- Up to 4000 $Fe^{+3}$ atoms are stored in ferritin complex.

### Hemosiderin-derived from ferritin:

- It is ferritin with partially stripped shell.
- Contains larger fraction of its mass as iron than does ferritin
- M/E: Fe-staining particle
- Seen in state of iron overload
- Mobilization of Fe from hemosiderin is much slower

### TRANSFERRIN

- Non heme iron binding glycoprotein
- Can bind 2 atoms of iron in $Fe^{+3}$ stage
- Exist as $\beta_1$ globulin in plasma.
- It is true carrier of iron
- Saturated to 30-33% with Fe in plasma
- For binding to transferrin $Fe^{+2}$ is converted to $Fe^{+3}$ by ferrooxidase III (ceruloplasmin).
- Transport form, transports iron to RE cells, bone marrow to reach mature RBCs.

### STORAGE OF IRON

- Iron is stored in liver, spleen and bone marrow as ferritin.
- In mucosal cells ferritin is temporary storage form of iron.
- Apoferritin can take up 4000 Fe atoms/molecule.
- Ferrtin supplies iron at the time of requirement. $Fe^{+2}$ is released and FAD or FMN are formed by ferritin reductase system.
- Iron is mobilized from ferritin, firstly from RE, then mucosal and finally iron is absorbed from intestine.

# HEMOSIDERIN

- Iron storage protein, accumulates in body when supply of iron is in excess of body demands.
- Iron in ferritin is enclosed within a protein shell, apoferritin that can take up $Fe^{+2}$ and oxidize it to $Fe^{+3}$ that is deposited in the iron core.
- Iron stimulates apoferritin synthesis.
- With time, ferritin is engulfed by lysosomes and catabolized to hemosiderin: a non specific mixture of partially proteins degraded lipid and iron.
- Iron enters ferritin in a metabolically controlled fashion making it available for normal physiological function.
- While iron is trapped in hemosiderin meshwork, it returns to the metabolic mainstream of the cell in a slow and unregulated fashion.
  1 mg/L serum ferritin contains 10 mg storage iron

## HAPTOGLOBIN (Hp)

- When RBC is lysed, Hb enters circulation and will be lost in urine, but Hp takes up this Hb.
- In addition, hemopexin binds heme in circulation.

## Iron utilization

Iron is taken up by liver, bone marrow for Hb synthesis. $Fe^{+2}$ is incorporated into protoporphyrin IX by ferrochelatase for use in oxidative phosphorylation as enzyme cofactor.

## Iron turnover

- Turnover of iron in adult in 24 hours is 35-40 mg
- Plasma transferrin iron is in equilibrium with iron in storage form i.e., ferritin and hemosiderin.

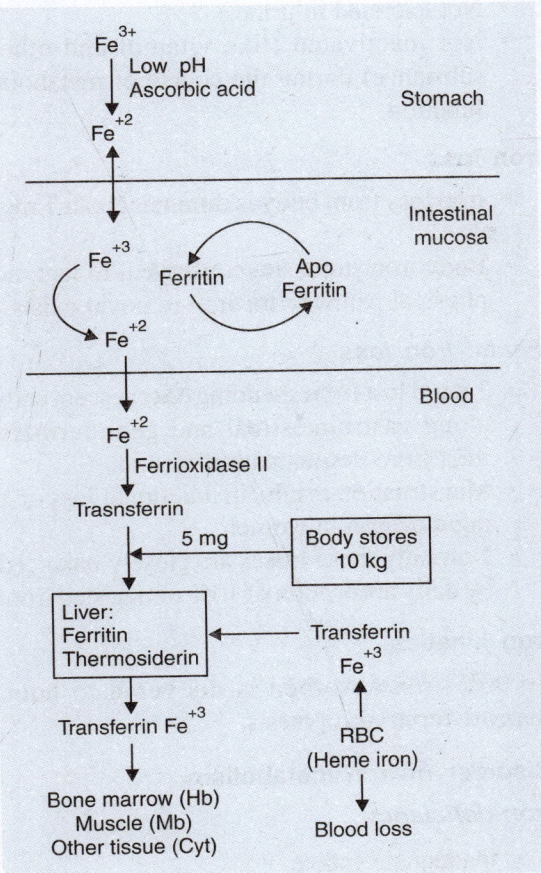

Fig. 6.5. Overview of iron metabolism.

- Small amount of iron is released each day from RBCs which are phagocytosed and released $Fe^{+2}$ is recycled into new Hb.

## Mobilization of fe from ferritin

- 1st call from RES
- 2nd call from intestinal mucosal cells
- 3rd call absorbed from intestine.

## Iron is a one-way

- It is unique, substance efficiently utilized and reutilized in the body.
- Iron losses from body are minimum.

- Not excreted in urine.
- Not inactivated (like vitamin and other substance) during the course of metabolic function.

## Iron loss

- Iron loss from body is minimal about 1 mg/d
- Body iron stores are conserved. In fact, no physical pathway for iron removal exists.

## Facts: Iron loss

- 1 mg/d lost from shedding of senescent cells along gastrointestinal and genitourinary tract from desquamation of skin.
- Menstruation results in additional loss of 1 mg/d of iron in women.
- Normally these losses are closely balanced by daily absorption of 10% of ingested iron.

## Iron kinetics

80-90% iron absorbed is delivered to bone marrow for erythropoiesis.

## Disorder of iron metabolism

### Iron-deficiency

- Inadequate Intake
- Impaired absorption, MAS, surgery excessive loss, menstrual loss, GI loss, postgastrectomy anemia.
- Ineffective erythropoiesis, kidney disease, hook worm infestation, pregnancy

## Lab findings

- Microcytic, Hypochromic anaemia
- Hb< 12 mg/dl

## Mechanism

Depletion of Fe stores
↓
Fe deficient erythropoiesis
↓
Fe deficient anaemia

## Causes of Fe-deficiency anaemia

- Hookworm infection
- Nutritional deficiency of iron
- Repeated pregnancy
- Chronic blood loss: piles, bleeding, peptic ulcer, uterine hemorrhage.
- Kidney disease - nephrosis, CRF
- Lack of absorption – gastrectomy (partial), achlorhydria
- Lead toxicity

## Signs and symptoms

Weakness, lassitude, apathy, sluggish metabolic activities, retarded growth, loss of appetite, palpitation exertional dyspnoea, koilonychia, pica.

## Treatment

Iron + folic acid.

## Iron toxicity

| Hemosiderosis | Haemochromatosis |
|---|---|
| • Iron excess<br>• Seen in subject receiving repeated blood transfusion e.g. Hemophiliacs, thalasemia, Bantu siderosis seen in African Bantu Tribe Due to habit of cooking iron in iron pots | Primary: Inherited autosomal recessive Abnormal gene on short arm of chromosome Here iron absorption is increased and transferrin levels are increased and excess iron is deposited |
| **Treatment:**<br>Phlebotomy, desferroxamine – chelating agent: chelates $Fe^{+3}$ and excreted in urine | Fe gets deposited in liver: cirrhosis<br>    Pancreas – DM<br>    Skin – discoloration |

## Magnesium (Mg)

## Fact file

- Most abundant intracellular cation
- Total body Mg 0.3 g/kg body weight

- 1% extracellular
- 31% cells
- 67% bones
- Serum magnesium: 2-3 mg/dl
- 1-4 mg/dl Mg is in unbound, diffusible form
- Ideal intake: 36-48 mg/d

Fourth most abundant cation in intracellular component:

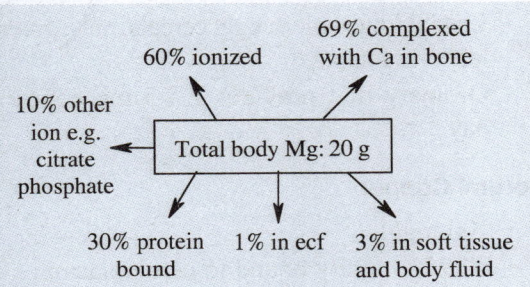

60% ionized
69% complexed with Ca in bone
10% other ion e.g. citrate phosphate
Total body Mg: 20 g
30% protein bound
1% in ecf
3% in soft tissue and body fluid

One-third of skeletal Mg is exchangeable with serum

## Function

1. Enzyme action – as cofactor (activator) of many enzymes requiring ATP e.g., H.K., GK, FK, PFK, Adenyl cyclase, ALP: cAMP dependent kinases.

   Most magnesium inside cell is bound to ATP: Mg ATP is in equilibrium with free Mg ions.

2. Neuromuscular excitability (lower muscle irritability): action similar to that of $Ca^{+2}$

3. Required for formation of bone and teeth. 70% present as apatitie in bone, dental enamel, and dentin.

## Normal Mg levels

2-3 mg%.

## RDA

350-360mg/d.

## Sources

Seed grains, nuts, peas, cereals, beans, potato, dry fruits, meat milk, fruits, fish.

## Absorption

In small intestinal cells by a specific carrier system in jejunum and ileum 30-40% is absorbed.

## Absorbed in jejunum and ileum

- 30-40% of dietary magnesium is absorbed and in case of deficiency, absorption increased to 70%
- Mg excretion: depends on GFR.
- Mg retention by kidney is very efficient
- Ecf volume expansion increase magnesium excretion, aldosterone decreases Mg reabsorption in tubules.

## Absorption

| Decreased by | Increased by |
|---|---|
| Diet | PTH |
| Calcium | Vitamin D |
| Alcohol | GH |
| Phosphate | Proteins |

**Regulation:** Occurs at following levels:
  (i) Mainly by kidney: Mg retention by kidney is very efficient.
  (ii) Absorption from GIT
  (iii) Transmembrane fluxes

When Mg intake is restricted, fecal excretion becomes negligible and urinary excretion becomes negligible.

70-80% filtered by kidney, 3-5% excreted.

Increased calcium in diet, $T_4$, GH, ADH: increase excretion in urine: PTH decrease Mg excretion.

## Deficiency

- When any of three major intracellular elements (Mg, K or $PO_4$) are deprived or lost, losses of other usually follow.
- Level below 1.7 mg, clinical features of NM irritability (hypomagnesemic tetany) appear

## Cause

Inadequate intake

GIT disorders:
- Malabsorption syndromes
- Prolonged diarrhea

Endocrine:
- Hyper/hypoparthyroidism
- Hyperthyroidism
- Diabetic ketoacidosis
- SIADH

Chronic alcoholism

Increased renal excretion:
- Alcohol ingestion
- Cisplatin therapy
- Diuretics: furosamide

Mg deficiency impairs normocalcemic response to PTH at skeletal level.

## Clinical features

- Paraesthesia, muscle cramp, irritability, confusion.
- Manifestations of associated hypocalcemia namely Trousseau, Chovek sign.

**Increased Mg levels occur in:** Renal failure, uncontrolled DM, eclampsia. Features include: nausea, sedation, decreased deep tendon reflexes, muscle, weakness, hypotension, coma, respiratory paralysis.

## COPPER

### Total Body copper
100 mg.

**Location:** Liver, muscle, brain mainly; bone: small amount.

## Plasma copper

100 mg/dl (Ceruloplasmin 25-50 mg/dl).

## Requirement

2-3 mg/d, only 10% is absorbed.

## Sources

- Liver, kidney, meat, egg, cereals, nuts, green leafy vegetable.
- Ordinary diet provides 2.5-5 mg copper/day.

## Serum Copper

- 100 mg/dl
- 90-95% tightly bound to ceruloplasmin
- 5-10% bound to albumin
- 1% bound to amino acids (histidine), transport form of copper
- Normally ceruloplasmin in serum is 25-50mg/dl, also known as ferroxidase: promotes oxidation of $Fe^{+2}$ to $Fe^{+3}$.

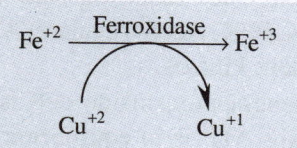

## Functions: Copper

Copper is constituent of :

1. Ceruloplasmin

   Function of ceruloplasmin (Cp):
   (i) Mobilization of iron (also known as ferroxidase I activity) and its utilization
   (ii) Acute phase protein: increased in fever and inflammation
   (iii) It is not a copper transport protein, but it binds copper tightly
   (iv) Act as a free radical scavenger.

2. **Cytochrome C oxidase**

3. **SOD (superoxide) dismutase):** dismutation of $O_2^-$ (superoxide) to $H_2O_2$

4. **Lysyl oxidase:** oxidizes four lysine residues to desmosine which makes cross linkages in collagen and elastin.

5. **Dopamine β-hydroxylase:** converts dopamine to norepinephrine.

6. **Tyrosinase:** converts tyrosine to DOPA

7. **Catalase**

8. **Others:**
   Tryptophan pyrrolase
   Uricase
   δ-aminoleuvelinic acid (δALA): Heme synthesis
   MAO (mono amine oxidase)
   Ascorbic acid oxidase

9. Phospholipid synthesis, development of bone and nervous system

## Absorption of copper

- 10% of dietary copper is absorbed in duodenum.
- Metallothionine binds in the cell and transport copper to basolateral membrane.
- Stored in liver and bone marrow
- Excreted in bile mainly
- Urine-no copper is excreted in urine
- Bound $Cu^{+2}$ get incorporated into ceruloplasmin (6-8 atoms/Cp mol) and a part is secreted by bile into feces.

## Factors affecting absorption

1. Increased by: High protein diet, citrate, phosphate, oxalate, glucuronate.
2. Decreased by: phytate, ascorbate, zinc, bile.

## DISEASES

### 1. Copper deficiency

**Causes:** MAS, nephrotic syndrome, celiac disease

**Clinical features:** weight loss, demineralization of bones, defect in collagen formation, and demyelination of nerves.

**Lab findings:** Hypochromic microcytic anaemia, fragility of blood vessels, aneurysms, hypopigmentation, myocardial fibrosis and grey hair.

### 2. Inherited disorders

**Wilson's disease** (Hepatolenticular degeneration):

- Autosomal recessive
- Copper deposited in abnormal amount in liver, lenticular nucleus of brain.
- Low level of serum copper and serum ceruloplasmin (cp) and increased excretion of copper in urine
- Copper deposition in kidney

**Cause:**

- Defect in incorporation of copper into newly synthesized apoceruloplasmin.
- Hepatic lysosomes lack normal mechanism to excrete copper into bile, the copper that has been cleaved from ceruloplasmin (cp).
- Copper excess: Inhibit formation of Cp from apo Cp and copper.
- When capacity of hepatocytes exceeds to store copper, it is released into circulation and uptake in extrahepatic sites occurs.

**Result:**

Copper gets deposited in various tissue causing:

- Hepatic cirrhosis
- CNS effects: necrosis of neurons and sclerosis
- Kidney – renal tubular absorption defects
- Eyes – **Kayser Fleischer (KF) ring** –

copper deposition in descemet's membrane: golden green ring seen on S/L (slit lamp) examination.

**Diagnosis:**
- Cp < 20 mg%
- KF ring
- Hepatic cirrhosis
- Urine copper excretion markedly increased.

### Menke's disease

- Kinky or Steel Hair Syndrome
- **X**-linked
- Affects males only
- Efflux of copper through basolateral membrane is defective.

### Clinical features

Signs of mental retardation, abnormal bone formation, anaemia, depigmentation of hair, no deposition of copper, low plasma ceruloplasmin..

### Treatment

Pencillamine – chelating agent.

### Zinc (Zn)

- Total zinc in body 1.5-3 g
- Highest in prostate, skin and ocular tissue
- Also, present in pancreas and spleen.

### Source

Liver, milk, dairy products, egg, cereals, (grains), legumes, pulses

### Requirement

10-15 mg/d, 3 mg/kg body weight.

### Absorption

- Occurs in duodenum
- Animal sources are better absorbed than vegetable sources.
- Dependent on metallothionine
- Zinc absorption appears to be proportionate to metallothionine levels in mucosal cells.
- Absorption is decreased by phytate, calcium, copper and iron.
- Increased by: peptide and amino acid
- Excretion of zinc occurs through secretion of pancreas and intestine.
- Nearly 99% of zinc is inside cells and remainder is in plasma and extracellular fluids.

### Secretion levels of zinc

Serum zinc levels are 100 mg/dL and are fairly constant: 70% is bound to albumin and proteins and is the source of metal for cellular needs.

**Zinc levels are decreased by:**
- Regional enteritis
- Nephrotic syndrome
- Liver cirrhosis
- Burns
- Trauma
- Surgery
- Hemolytic anaemia

### Function: Zinc

1. **Role in enzyme function:** Metalloenzymes (up to 300 on enzymes contain zinc):
   i. SOD
   ii. Carbonic anhydrase present in RBC and kidney.
   iii. DNA dependent DNA polymerase
   iv. DNA dependent RNA polymerase
   v. ALP (alkaline phosphatase)
   vi. Carboxypeptidase
   vii. Leucine aminopeptidase
   viii LDH
   ix. Alcohol dehydrogenase
   x. ALA synthetase.

2. **Role in vitamin A metabolism:**
   - Zinc stimulates vitamin A release from liver and increases its plasma level and its utilization in rhodopsin synthesis.
   - Retinine reductase is zinc containing metalloenzyme which participates in regeneration of rhodopsin in eye during dark adaptation.
3. **Role in Insulin secretion:** Important for synthesis and storage of insulin. Insulin in beta cell contains zinc and release of insulin.
4. **In growth and development.**
5. **In wound healing.**
6. **Role in biosynthesis of nucleotides.**

## DISEASE

### Deficiency

Causes of low serum zinc levels:

- Decreased intake or absorption – regional enteritis
- Increased Urinary loss: nephrotic, cirrhosis, hypoalbumin states
- Hypercatabolic states: trauma, burns, surgery, hemolytic anaemia, sickle disease
- Decreased with MI (myocardial infarction), infection, hepatitis, malignancy
- Severe zinc deficiency is seen in alcoholics (especially if they have cirrhosis)

### Clinical features

- Growth retardation
- Poor wound healing
- Anaemia
- Alopecia
- Tissues with a high cellular turnover are characteristically affected.
- Hyperkeratosis, dermatitis over knee, elbow.
- Skin, GIT mucosa, chondrocytes, spermatogonia, thymocytes

- Diarrhea
- Immunological dysfunction/defects of T-cell function: superinfections are common
- Gonadal atrophy
- Impaired spermatogenesis
- Congenital malformations

### Toxicity

- Inhalation of zinc fumes (welders): metal fumes, fever or brass chills
- Oral ingestion, IV administration
- Contamination of dialysis fluid with zinc from adhesive plaster

### Clinical features

- Gastric ulcer
- Pancreatitis
- Lethargy
- Anaemia
- Fever
- Nausea, vomiting
- Respiratory distress
- Pulmonary fibrosis

### Acrodermatis enterpathica

- Autosomal recessive condition
- Primary defect in zinc absorption

### Clinical features

- Acrodermatitis (lips and tips)
- Diarrhoea
- Alopecia
- GIT
- Ophthalmic, neuropsychiatric features.

### Manganese (Mn)

- Total body Mn: 15 mg
- Serum Mn: 0.001 µmol/L or 0.007 mg/dl
- Requirement: 5-6 mg/d

## Sources

Cereals, vegetables, tea, fruits.

## Absorption

- 3-4%, inhibited by iron.
- Bound to transmanganin (β-globulin) in serum and excreted in bile and pancreatic secretion.

## Function

1. **Role in enzyme action:** Mn acts as an activator of enzymes and component of metalloenzyme.

   **Co-factor for:**

   Arginase

   Glutamine synthase

   Isocitrate dehydrogenase

   Succinate dehydrogenase

   Enolase

   Hexokinase

   Phosphoglucomutase

   Lipoprotein lipase

   Metalloenzymes

   Mitochondrial SOD

   Pyruvate carboxylase

   Acetyl CoA carboxylase

   Diamine oxidase

2. Important for **synthesis** of glycoproteins and chondroitin sulfate (as it is integral part of glycosyltransferase), required for bone formation and function of nervous system.

3. **Porphyrin synthesis:** (δ ALA synthetase)

4. **Condensation of mevalonate** of squalene is manganese dependent: in cholesterol biosynthesis.

5. In antioxidant property of vitamin E

6. Required for skeletal growth

## Mn stores

Liver, kidney (mitochondria).

## Deficiency and toxicity

### Deficiency

- Rare
- Retarded growth and skeletal deformities (increase ALP)
- Bleeding disorder (increase PT time)
- Fatty liver: Decrease activity of cells of pancreas as in manganese deficiency, pancreatic hyperplasia is reported.

### Toxicity

Miners inhaling manganese dust develop: anorexia, apathy, headache, leg cramp, psychosis and pneumoconiosis.

## Fluoride (F)

Fluoride is a constituent of teeth, bone. It prevents dental caries. It is solely derived from drinking water. Mineralized tissues account for nearly 99% of total body fluoride and bone is by far the main depot.

### Requirement

1 part of F in million parts of drinking water (1 ppm) seems to serve the daily requirement of F in man, daily intake should not exceed 3 mg.

## Metabolism

### Absorption

- Inorganic fluoride is readily absorbed in the stomach and small intestine by passive diffusion and distributed almost entirely to bone and teeth.
- Fluoride enter into calcified tissue either by substituting for the hydroxyl ion or bicarbonate ion in hydroxyapatite in bone, and enamel to form fluoroapatite or by ionic exchange within the hydration shell of crystalline surface.

- Renal excretion is most important for regulation of body fluoride content with about 50% of daily intake being cleared by the kidney.

## Function

1. **Role to tooth development and dental health:**
   - Fluoride is present in human tooth in trace amounts and helps in tooth development, normal maintenance and hardening of dental enamel
   - Prevention of dental caries.
   - Cariostatic effect of fluoride is due to its entry into apatite and salts of dental enamel:
     - < 0.5 ppm fluoride in water predisposes to caries.
     - > 1.2 ppm fluoride in drinking water increase dentine:
     - may decrease calcium disposition in these tissue.
     - may cause mottling of enamel:
     - discoloration, corrosion and stratification of enamel.
2. **Role in bone development:**
   **High Fluoride intake:** Increases content of bone, stimulates osteoblasts activity.
   - Abnormal rise in calcium deposition: osteosclerosis
   - Calcification of ligaments and tendons.
   - Crippling deformities such as kyphosis, stiffness of spine, bony exostosis.

## Cobalt (Co)

Component of vitamin $B_{12}$ and deficiency symptoms are associated with symptoms of deficiency of vitamin $B_{12}$.

## RDA

- 1-2 mg of vitamin $B_{12}$.

- $B_{12}$ contains up to 0.045-0.09 mg Cobalt (i.e., 4% by weight).
- Diet contains 5-8 mg/d.
- 70-80% absorbed stored in liver.

## Source

Food from animal sources, not present in plants

## Function

1. Role in cobamide enzyme formation i.e., adenosyl cobalamin.
2. Required in methionine metabolism: enzyme transferase e.g. homocysteine methyltransferase
3. Bone marrow: development, maturation of RBCs.

## Deficiency

Anaemia ($B_{12}$ deficiency).

## Toxicity

- Prolonged administration causes polycythemia.
- Cardiomyopathy
- CHF (congestive heart failure) with pericardial effusion
- Polycythemia
- Thyroid enlargement and neurological abnormalities also have been reported as manifestation of cobalt toxicity in drinkers of beers as metal is added as foam stabilizer.

## Selenium (Se)

### Total body Se

4-10 mg.

### Principle source

Plant material.

### Requirement

50-100 mg/d.

## Absorption and execration

- Intake: 20-300 mg/d.
- Absorbed in duodenum, transported bound β-lipoproteins and excreted mainly in urine.

## Epidemiological evidence

- TPN (total parenteral nutrition)
- Kwashiorkor improves with selenium supplementation
- Incidence of GI cancer, CVS disorders, cancers show inverse relationship with Se levels.

## Function

1. Functions in metalloenzyme: GSH peroxidase (GSH Px) which destroys peroxides in cytosol i.e., plays a critical role in control of $O_2$ metabolism, particularly in breakdown of $H_2O_2$.

2. **Present as:**
   Selenomethionine
   Selenocysteine
   Selenocystine
   **Levels:**
   0.2 mg/g in blood
   In tissue: 13 mg%
   Se intake depends on nature of the soil in which crops are grown

3. Antioxidant and protects cells against FR (free radicals) – prevent lipid peroxidation

4. Sparing effect on vitamin E and reduces vitamin E requirement

5. Selenocysteine is component of GSH Px

6. Binds heavy metals: Cd, Hg and Ag and protects from their toxic effects 5' deiodinase is Se containing enzyme.

7. Necessary for normal development of spermatozoa

8. Protects animals from carcinogenic chemicals, its role in man is not established.

## Deficiency

Cardiomyopathy, CHF, Muscle degeneration.

## Toxicity

- Alopecia
- Abnormal nails, emotional lability, lassitude.

## Keshan's disease

Multifocal myocardial necrosis and decreased serum Se content due to deficiency of Se in soil and diet in Keshan province (China).

## Clinical features

- Arrhythmia, carcinogenic shock, peripheral myopathy.
- Young women and children are particularly susceptible.

## Acute poisoning

Infestation of water containing large amount of metal result in diarrhea, tetanic spasm, respiratory failure.

## Chronic poisoning

- Anorexia, hair loss, myocardial atrophy and liver necrosis in animals.
- Se is present in metal polishes and antirust compound. In human, chronic dermatitis, alopecia, brittle nails, garlicky breath (because of dimethyl selenide) is seen in occupational exposure to electronics, glass and paint industries.

## Iodine

## Total body iodine

- 25-30 mg
- 80% stored in thyroid gland, for synthesis of $T_3$ and $T_4$.

- Muscle, salivary glands, ovaries also contain some Iodine.

### Biochemistry

- **Function:** Synthesis of thyroid Hormone: $T_3$, $T_4$
- **Dietary requirement:** 100-150 µg/d in pregnancy + 50 µg/d
- **Source:** Sea food, drinking water, vegetable. High altitudes are deficient in iodine and iodine content in water, soil is low.
- **Absorption, storage, excretion:** Absorbed as iodide from small intestine: 30% intake is absorbed, 80% stored in organic form as iodothyroglobulin, Excreted in kidney mainly.

### Serum iodine levels

- 4-10 mg/dl
- Only biological role is formation of thyroid hormone and disorder of iodine metabolism causes goiter.

### Molybdenum (Mo)

Constituents of enzyme: xanthine oxidase, aldehyde oxidase.

### Requirement

- 100 µg/d
- Present in cereals, dry, fruits, legumes
- Absorbed from intestine

### Function

**Enzyme action:**
- Xanthine oxidase
- Helps in utilization of copper
- Aldehyde oxidase

**Molybdenosis:** Occurs because of increased intake.

### Clinical features

- Growth retardation, anaemia, diarrhea
- Copper, cysteine is effective in removing molybdenum from body and decreasing toxicity.

### Chromium (Cr)

- Total body chromium: 6 mg
- Serum chromium: 20 mg/dl

### Function

1. Functions primarily as component of glucose tolerance factor and chief symptoms of chromium deficiency is impaired glucose tolerance test.
2. Prevents dental caries.
3. Required for bone development.

### Requirement

50-200 mg/day.

### Sources

Grain, cereals, cheese, meat.

### Toxicity

- Occupational exposure to chromium in tanning industry:
  - Renal and hepatic failure
  - Lung damage, cancer
- Tobacco is rich in chromium
- Stainless steel utensils also provide chromium to food.

### Nickel (Ni)

- Enzyme: Urease, arginase, acetyl CoA synthetase contain nickel.
- Required for growth and reproduction.

### Deficiency symptoms

Unknown.

### Toxicity

Non toxic.

### Occupation hazard

Respiratory and dermatitis.

# NUTRITION

## ENERGY CONTENT OF FOOD

### (1) Calorific value of food

Caloric value (energy content) of a food is calculated from the heat released by the total combustion of food in a calorimeter.

### Definition

- **Caloric value** is defined as amount of heat energy obtained by burning 1g of food stuff completely in the presence of $O_2$.
- **Calorie** is unit of heat.
  One calorie represents the amount of heat required to raise the temperature of 1g of water by I°C (i.e., from 15°C to 16° C). Since calorie is a very small unit in nutrition, it is conveniently expressed as kilocalories Kcal or Cal.
- **Joule:** 1 Cal – 4.18 KJ or 4.2 KJ

### Calorie value of food

The energy values of the three principal food stuffs – carbohydrates fat and protein are measured either directly by measuring the output in a calorimeter, or by indirect method.

### (i) Direct calorimeter:

**Bomb calorimeter:** A weighed amount of sample is burnt in an atmosphere of $O_2$ by electrically heated platinum wire. The heat evolved is absorbed in a weighed amount of water which surrounds the burning chamber and rise in temperature is measured and heat evolved

is calculated. This method is accurate, easy in theory, though difficult in practice. Under most conditions, 1L of $O_2$ consumed accounts for approximately 4.83 kcal of energy expended.

### (ii) Indirect calorimetry

Technically simple. Quantity of heat produced by body as a result of combustion of food is calculated from the quantity of $O_2$ consumed. 1L of $O_2$ consumed accounts for 4.82 K cal of energy expended.

**Facts:**

- The carbohydrates and fats are completely oxidized (to $CO_2$ and $H_2O$) in the body; thence their fuel values measured in bomb calorimeter or directly in the body are almost the same.
- Proteins, however, are not burnt in the body as they are converted to products such as urea, creatinine and ammonia and excreted. Due to this reason, calorific value of protein in body is less than that obtained in a bomb calorimeter.

| Table. 6.9. Calorific value | | |
|---|---|---|
| | *Bomb calorimeter (cal/g)* | *In body E (cal/g)* |
| Carbohydrate | 4.1 | 4 |
| Fat | 9.4 | 9 |
| Protein | 5.4 | 4 |

Vitamins and minerals have no calorific value although they are involved in several important body functions including generation of energy from carbohydrates, fats and proteins.

### (2) Respiratory Quotient of food stuffs (RQ)

**Definition:** RQ is ratio of the volume of $CO_2$ produced to the volume of $O_2$ consumed (utilized in the oxidation of food stuffs).

Carbohydrates have RQ of 1, fats 0.7

$$C_6H_{12}O_6 + 6O_2 \rightarrow 6CO_2 + 6H_2O$$

$$RQ = \frac{CO_2}{O_2} = \frac{6}{6} = 1$$

Fats have RQ of 0.7

tristearin

$$2C_{157}H_{111}O_6 + 163O_2 \rightarrow 114\ CO_2 + H_2O$$

$$RQ = \frac{CO_2}{O_2} = \frac{114}{163} = 0.7$$

Protein: RQ is 0.8.

$$C_3H_7O_2N + 6O_2 \rightarrow 5CO_2 + NH_2 + CO_2$$

(Alanine)

$$RQ = \frac{CO_2}{O_2} = \frac{5}{6} = 0.8$$

RQ of a mixed diet is 0.82 – 0.85.

## Factors affecting RQ

1. **Role of diet:**
   Carbohydrate
   Fat
   Protein
   Mixed
2. **Interconversion as in DM:** As carbohydrate utilization decreases and fat utilization increases, thus RQ lowers.
3. **Exercise:** Moderate, unaltered.
   **Increased inviolent exercise:** Following exercise, lactate enters blood and stimulates pulmonary ventilation and washing out carbon dioxide and hence raising RQ.
4. **Acidosis:** RQ increased
   **Alkalosis:** RQ decreased
5. **Fever:** Increased breathing and $CO_2$ washout raises RQ.
6. **Uncontrolled diabetes:** RQ falls, carbohydrate utilization decreases and energy is supplied by fat breakdown.

## Significance

- Helpful in determining metabolic rate
- Help in diagnosis of conditions - acidosis, alkalosis.
- Acts as a guide to the type of food burning or synthesis in body as well as in organ.

## Utilization of energy in man

Man consumes energy to meet the fuel demands of the four ongoing processes in the body:

Maintenance of:

1. Basal metabolic rate (BMR)
2. Specific dynamic action (SDA) of food or thermogenic effect of food.
3. Physical activity: extra energy expenditure for physical activities.
4. Environmental temperature

In other words, while considering the energy requirement, we have to consider energy required for: BMR, SDA and extra energy expended, physical activity plus additional energy supply needed under special conditions: growth, pregnancy, lactation.

## 1. BMR

### Definition

Minimum amount of 'E' required by the body to maintain life at complete physical and mental rest in the post-absorptive state (i.e. 12 hours after the last meal).

Under basal condition, although body appears to be at total rest, several functions within the body continuously occur which include: working of heart and other organs, conduction of nerve impulse, reabsorption by renal tubules, GI (gastrointestinal) motility and ion transport across membranes ($Na^+$ - $K^+$ pump consumes about 50% of basal energy).

BMR is 'E' (energy) expenditure to maintain

basic physiological function under standard conditions BMR is proportional to lean body weight and to surface area. High in male, fever, hyperthyroidism. Low in female, starvation, and hypothyroidism.

## Measurement of BMR

Preparation of subject:
- Should be awake
- At complete physical and mental rest
- In post absorptive state (12 hr)
- In comfortable surrounding at 25°C.

### Apparatus

1. Benedict and Roth (closed circuit device)
2. Douglas Bag method (open circuit device):

Volume of $O_2$ consumed by the subject for 2-6 min period under basal conditions is determined (by recording or a graph paper using spirometry). Standard Calorific value for 1L of $O_2$ consumed is 4.825 Cal.

Heat produced in one hour
$$= 4.825 \times O_2 \times 10$$
Unit: $Cal/m^2/hr$

Body surface area is calculated by DuBois formula.

$A = H^{0.725} \times W^{0.425} \times 71.84 \times 1000$

A = Surface area in $cm^2$
H = height in cm
W = weight in kg

And dividing above by 10,000 gives $m^2$.

**Nomograms of body surface area** (in $m^2$) from height and weight are readily available in literature.

## Normal values: BMR

- Adult man 35–38 Cal/sqm/hr
- Women 32–35 Cal/sqm/hr
- A BMR value between 15% and + 20% is

considered normal. Some authors give values as 1600 cal/d in males and 1400 cal/d in females

**Read's formula** gives rough estimate of BMR

- BMR = 0.75 (PR + 0.74 × PP) – 72
- Obtained as 10%
- Range of normal ± 10%.

PR = pulse rate
PP = pulse pressure

## Factors affecting BMR

Age, sex, surface area, activity, hormone, environment, starvation, body temperature, race, disease, drug.

1. **Surface area:**
   - BMR is directly proportional to surface area (SA)
   - Lean person have greater S.A and higher BMR as compared to obese.

2. **Age:**
   - High in actively growing children
   - In adults, with growing age BMR decreases at a rate of 2% per decade.

3. **Sex:** Men have marginally higher BMR due to higher proportion of lean muscle mass.

4. **Physical activity:** High in persons with regular exercise (increased body S.A.)

5. **Hormone:** Thyroid hormone stimulates BMR. So, BMR is increased in hyperthyroidism, and decreased in hypothyroidism.

**Hormone increasing BMR:**
   - Epinephrine
   - GH
   - Cortisol
   - Sex Hormones

6. **Environment:** In cold climate, BMR is high.

7. **Starvation:** Lowered in starvation, wasting disease, malnutrition

8. **Body temperature:**
   - With 1°C rise in temperature, BMR increases by 12%
   - Fever causes rise in BMR.

9. **Diseases:**
   - Leukemia, polycythemia, infection, Cushing's raise BMR.
   - Addison's lower BMR marginally.

10. **Racial variations:** BMR of Eskimos is higher.

11. **Drugs:**
    - Caffeine, epinephrine, nicotine, alcohol increase BMR.
    - Anaesthetics lower BMR.

### Significance of BMR

**BMR is important:**

1. To calculate calorie requirement of an individual and planning of diets.
2. BMR was used in assessment of thyroid function in hypothyroidism, low thyroid hormone (when hormone assay and isotope labs were not available). Starvation influences BMR.
3. To note the effect of food and drugs on BMR.

For an adult man of 70 kg, S.A $1.7m^2$ and basal requirement will the 40 cal/m$^2$/hr

$$1.7 \times 40 \times 24 = 1632 \text{ Cal}$$

BMR of an adult male is 24 kcal/kg/hr

**SDA also known as diet induced thermogenesis:** Thermogenic effect of food is equivalent to 5-10% of total energy expenditure is attributed to expenditure due to carbohydrate to any stimulus of metabolism caused by influx of new substrate.

### SDA

- Refers to extra heat production by the body over and above the calculated caloric value, when a given food is metabolized by the body.
- Also, known as **thermogenic or calorigenic action of food**.
- This is believed to be due to expenditure of energy for digestion and absorption of food. This 'E' is trapped from the previously available energy, so that the actual energy from food is lesser than that of theoretical calculation.
- SDA can be considered as the activation energy required for a chemical reaction

### SDA for different foods

- Proteins 30%
- Lipids 15%
- Carbohydrates 5%,
  i.e. out of every 100g of proteins consumed, the 'E' available for doing useful work is 30% less than the calculated value.
  - Hence, for a mixed diet, an extra 10% calories should be provided to account for the loss of 'E' as SDA.
  - Presence of fats and carbohydrates reduce SDA of proteins.
  - Fats are more efficient in reducing SDA of food stuffs.

### Significance of SDA

For utilization of food by the body, certain amount of 'E' is consumed from the body stores. This is actually the 'E' expended by the body for utilization of food stuffs.

- 10% extra/additional calories should be added to total energy needs of body towards SDA.
- High SDA for protein implies that protein is not a good source of 'E'.

## Mechanism of SDA

- Not known exactly.
- Believed to be due to 'E' required for digestion, absorption, transport, metabolism and storage of food in the body
  1. IV administration of amino acid or oral digestion of proteins gives same SDA, showing SDA is not due to digestion and absorption
  2. Hepatectomy abolishes SDA indicating SDA is closely related to metabolic function of liver.
- SDA of protein is to meet 'E' requirement for deamination, urea synthesis, biosynthesis of proteins, synthesis of TAG (from C skeleton of amino acids).
- SDA of carbohydrate is attributed to 'E' expended for conversion of glucose to glycogen.
- SDA of fat may be due to its storage, mobilization and oxidation.

Thus, for a 70 kg man with BMR of 1600 Cal, another 80-160 Cal (96 Cal) have to be added on this account.

## Physical activity, of the body

It can be divided into:
Sedentary + 30% BMR
Moderate + 40% BMR
Heavy + 50% BMR

**Influence of mental work:**
3-4%.
Brain has basal metabolism 1/10th of entire body.

**Influence of sleep:** Low, 10% below BMR.
Additional calories are to be added for each.

## Metabolism in children

- High BMR – physical activity of children is greater, despite the fact that their period of sleep is longer than that of an adult, up

to 2month – 120 C/kg, 2-6 month – 110 C/kg.
- Energy requirement will depend upon occupation, physical activity, and life style of the individual. Requirement for pregnancy is +300 Kcal/d and lactation is +500 kcal/d.

**Table 6.10.** Energy requirement

| Physical Activity | E-requirement cal/hr |
|---|---|
| Sitting | 25 |
| Standing | 30 |
| Writing/reading/eating | 30 |
| Car driving | 60 |

**Table 6.11.** Energy expenditure

| Activity | Expenditure |
|---|---|
| House hold work | 80 |
| Cycling | 150 |
| Running moderate | 500 |
| Swimming | 600 |
| Walking upstairs | 800 |

## Energy requirement of man

Since BMR, SDA, physical activity determines the energy needed by the body.

In an individual with light work
- About 60% cal. are spent towards BMR
- About 30% cal. are spent towards physical activity
- About 10% cal. are spent towards SDA

| | |
|---|---|
| Light work | 2200-2500 cal/d |
| Moderate | 2500-2900 cal/d |
| Heavy | 2900-3500 cal/d |
| Very Heavy work | 3500-4000 cal/d |

**Calculation for 'E' requirement for a 55 kg person doing moderate work:**

1. BMR = 2.4 × 55 kg = 1320 kcal [BMR

of an adult is fixed at 24 kcal/kg body weight/day] + for activity = 40% of BMR + 528 kcal.

2. For SDA 1848 × 10%  = 184 kcal
   +
   2032 kcal
   Total ~ 2050kcal

**Table 6.12.** Total Calories required for different category of workers

| Category | Basal | SDA | For activity | Total |
|---|---|---|---|---|
| **Males** | | | | |
| Sedentary | 1600 | 160 | 800 (30%) | 2560 |
| Moderate | 1600 | 160 | 1200 (40%) | 2960 |
| Heavy | 1600 | 160 | 2400 (50%) | 4160 |
| **Females** | | | | |
| Sedentary | 1400 | 140 | 500 | 2040 |
| Moderate | 1400 | 140 | 800 | 2340 |
| Heavy | 1400 | 140 | 1600 | 3140 |

**Table 6.13.** 'E' requirement and occupation

| Type | Occupation |
|---|---|
| Light | Office work, lawyers, accountant, doctors, teachers, architects, shopkeeper |
| Moderate | Students, industry workers, housewives, fisherman and farmer |
| Very active | Agricultural worker, miners, untilled laborers, athletes, factory workers |
| Heavy | Black smith, construction workers. |

## COMPOSITION OF DAILY DIET

### Dietary carbohydrates

- Dietary carbohydrates are the chief source of energy
- Contribute to 60-70% of total caloric requirement of body.

- Required 55-65% of calorie should come from carbohydrates, e.g. for moderately active man requiring 3000 Cal/day should take 450 g carbohydrate daily.

**Dietary goal:** Carbohydrate should provide 58% of most of which should be complex carbohydrates.

Most abundant dietary constituents from nutritional point of view, can be grouped as:

(i) **Carbohydrate utilized in body (available, digestible):** Starch, glycogen, sucrose, lactose, glucose, fructose

(ii) **Carbohydrate not utilized in body (not digested unavailable):** cellulose, hemicellulose pectin, gum.

- Among carbohydrate utilized by the body, starch is most abundant and glucose is the major source of fuel for most organs and tissues.
- Sucrose (table sugar) is mainly used as sweetening agent.

### Dietary fiber

They improve bowel motility, prevent constipation, lower cholesterol absorption and improve glucose tolerance

### Requirement

**Source of dietary carbohydrates:** Table sugar, cereals, pulses, root and tubers, bread at least 40% of caloric needs should be from carbohydrates.

### Dietary fiber or fiber in nutrition

The unavailable indigestible carbohydrate in diet is called dietary fiber. They include: cellulose, hemicellulose, pectin, lignin, gum and mucilage, pentosans (Colonic fermentation produces gases: $CO_2$, $H_2$ and $CH_4$).

### Beneficial effects of fiber

1. Decrease constipation and pile formation, soften stools
2. Increase bowel motility: decreases exposure of gut to carcinogens.
3. Lower blood cholesterol
4. Eliminate bacterial toxins by adsorbing large quantity of water and toxic compounds produced by intestinal bacteria.
5. Decrease incidence of diverticulosis, GIT cancers e.g., Carcinoma colon and rectum – incidence lower in vegetarians, common in developed countries
6. Hypoglycemic action: improve glucose tolerance: by decreasing rate of glucose absorption from GIT.
7. Lower plasma cholesterol levels (hypolipidemic) by decreasing absorption of dietary cholesterol and bile acids, decrease enterohepatic circulation of bile salts and increase degradation of cholesterol to bile salts.
8. Satiety value-dietary fiber significantly adds to the weight of food stuff ingested and gives sensation of stomach-fullness.
9. They also lower incidence of diabetes mellitus and cardiovascular disease.

### Source

Fruit, leafy vegetables, vegetables, whole wheat, legumes, rice brain.

**Effects:** Cellulose and lignin in wheat bran are beneficial with regard to colonic function. More soluble fibers in legume and fruit e.g., gum and pectins decrease cholesterol possibly by binding with bile acids and dietary cholesterol.

### Requirement

**Dietary goal:** 30% fats should be provided in diet of which 30% each of saturated, mono-unsaturated and PUFA should be present. EFA required for membrane structure and fluidity and eicosanoid synthesis. Diet should include 2% calorie as linoleic acid, cholesterol consumption should be <300 mg/day.

Soluble fibers also slow gastric emptying and delay and attenuate the postprandial rise of blood glucose and consequent decrease in insulin secretion. This effect is beneficial for dieters and diabetes because it decreases rebound fall in blood glucose that stimulates appetite.

Inclusion of fiber rich food in weight reducing diets is helpful since it provides a feeling of fullness without consumption of excess calories.

### Lipids

TAG (fats and oils) are dietary source of fuel.
- Contribute 15-50% of body requirement.
- Provide twice the energy supplied by carbohydrates or proteins per unit weight (9 Kcal/g $vs$ 4 kcal/g of carbohydrates and proteins)
- Reduce bulk, improve palatability and produce satiety.

### Types of dietary fat

1. Visible fat: fat consumed as butter, ghee or oil
2. Invisible fat: fat present as part of food items, e.g., egg, fish, meat, cereals, legume, nut and oil seeds. More than half of essential FA in Indian diet is in the form of invisible fat.

**Recommended daily intake:**
- Visible fat: 10% of cal or 20 g/d, in pregnancy, 30g/d, in lactation 45 g/d.
- Dietary lipids apart from increasing palatability of food and satiety, act as dietary vehicle for lipid-soluble vitamin

and supply essential PUFA that body is unable to synthesize.

## Nutritional functions of lipids

1. Supply TAG – concentrated source of fuel to body
2. Provide essential fatty acids and fat soluble vitamin (A, D, E and K)

**Recommended daily intake:** 15-20% of total cal of which 25-30% may be PUFA

**Essential FA intake**

SFA: MUFA: PUFA 1: 1: 1,

Cholesterol intake should be <250 mg/d).

Unsaturated FA which the body cannot synthesize and therefore must be consumed in the diet are referred to as essential FA (EFA) e.g., Linoleic Acid, Linolenic Acid

Arachidonic acid can be synthesized in body from linoleic acid, but; should be present in small amount in diet.

## Deficiency features

- Impairment of growth and reproduction
- Scaly dermatitis
- Poor wound healing and hair loss.

## Excess

- Feature may lead to production of FR (free radicals) which may be injurious to the cell.
- PUFA should not be more than 30% of total fat.
- High fat consumption is also associated with cancer of breast and colon.

## Cholesterol

- Elevated cholesterol levels increase risk of atherosclerosis and coronary heart disease.
- Cholesterol synthesis continuously occurs in the body which is under feedback regulation.
- Excess cholesterol can also form a biliary stones causing obstructive jaundice
- Cholesterol is found only in foods of animal origins e.g. yolk.

## Protein

Human beings have no dietary requirement for protein *per se*, rather proteins in diet provide body's requirement for essential amino acid nitrogen and specific amino acids.

Proteins have been traditionally regarded as body building foods 10-15% of total body energy is derived from proteins. When enough carbohydrates are present, amino acids are not used for yielding energy; this is known as **protein sparing effect of carbohydrates**.

**Essential amino acids:** Amino acids that are not synthesized in the body. Nutritional importance of proteins is based on content of essential amino acids.

## Nitrogen balance

- Comparison between intake of N and excretion of N maintained by dietary intake.
- Dietary protein is almost an exclusive source of nitrogen to the body. Therefore, term N balance truly represents the protein (16% of which is nitrogen) utilization and its loss from the body.
- N is lost in urine feces, desquamated skin, hair and nails
- N-balance is determined by comparing intake of N and excretion of N (undigested proteins in feces, urea and ammonia in urine).

$$I = U + F + S$$

where I = Intake

F = Fecal loss

U = Urine loss

S = Sweat loss

- Individual is said to be in nitrogen balance if the intake and output of N are the same.
- Pregnancy, lactation, tissue repair, injury, recovery from serious illnesses and physical activity all require more dietary proteins.

### Positive N balance

(i) Intake higher than output. Some amount of N is retained in the body causing increase in body protein

(ii) Observed in growing children, pregnancy, recovery from serious illness

### Negative balance

- N output is higher than input, result is some amount of N is lost from body, depleting body protein.
- Seen in inadequate intake of protein; increased demands, malnutrition, physical stress e.g., burns, trauma, illness, surgery.

### Factors affecting N balance

1. Growth: during growth, state of positive N balance exists
2. Hormone: GH and insulin cause positive N balance; corticosteroids cause negative N balance
3. Pregnancy: positive N balance
4. Convalescence: positive N balance
5. Acute illness: negative N balance
6. Chronic illness, malignancy, uncontrolled diabetes: negative balance
7. Protein deficiency, prolonged starvation cause negative N balance.

Efficiency with which protein is used determines the total quality of protein required.

Three factors: 1. protein quality, 2. 'E' intake: sparing action 3. physical activity: increase nitrogen retention in body.

### Maintenance of N-balance

(i) Need for N intake are: obligatory N loss is 3.5 g of N/day for 65 kg person which is equivalent to 22 g/d protein of which 6-25 g should be essential amino acids.

(ii) Requirement for protein turnover: 0.7 g/kg/d.

(iii) Protein required for growth in infant, children, pregnancy, lactation.

### Biological value (BV) of protein

It is a measure of quality of protein i.e., its ability to provide essential amino acids required for tissue maintenance. Biologic values are measured on a relative scale with whole egg protein or egg albumin at 100 score.

**Protein from animal source:** Meat, poultry, milk, fish have high biologic value because they contain all essential amino acids.

**Protein from plant source:** Protein from wheat, corn, rice and beans have low biological value than animal proteins. Wheat (lysine, deficient), methionine-rich may be combined with pulses (methionine poor, lysine rich) to produce a complete proteins of improved biologic value.

Thus, eating food with different limiting amino acids at the same meal can result in a dietary combination with higher value than either of the component proteins. Animal protein can also complement the B.V. of protein such as cereal and milk.

### Importance in younger children

1. Wherever possible include eggs and milk in diet: both are good source of calorie and protein.
2. Include liberal amount of those vegetarian food with high-caloric density in diet e.g. nut, grain, dried beans and dry fruits.
3. Include liberal amount of high protein

vegetarian food which have complementary pattern.

## Nutritive value of proteins: Assessment

Quality of proteins depends on composition of essential amino acids.

Several lab methods are: PER. BV, NUP, chemical score.

1. **PER: Protein efficiency ratio:** Represented by gain in weight of albino rats per g of protein ingested: egg 4.5, milk-3, rice-2.2

2. **BV. Biological value of proteins:** Defined as % of absorbed nitrogen retained i.e., ratio of amount of N retained and absorbed.

$$B.V. = \frac{N \text{ retained}}{N \text{ absorved}} \times 100$$

**Biological value food:**

- Egg 100
- Fish 87
- Milk 85
- Soybean 67
- Potato 67
- Whole wheat bread 30

**Factors influencing BV of protein:**

- Amount and proportion of essential nutritional availability: rate of liberation of amino acid, rate of GIT absorption: both are affected by method of processing or cooking.
- Provides reasonably good index for the nutritive value of proteins
- It cannot take into account the 'N' that might be lost during the digestion process.

3. **NPU: Net protein utilization:** This is a better nutritional index than BV.

$$NPU = \frac{'N' \text{ retained}}{'N' \text{ digested}} \times 100$$

Takes into account the digestibility factor.

4. **Chemical score:** It is based on chemical analysis of the protein for the composition of essential amino acids which is then compared with a reference protein usually egg albumin.

$$\text{Chemical score} = \frac{\text{mg of limiting amino acid/g protein}}{\text{mg of same amino acid/g egg protein}} \times 10$$

**Table 6.14.**

| | |
|---|---|
| Milk | 65 |
| Fish | 60 |
| Meat | 70 |
| Soybean | 55 |
| Wheat | 42 |

Chemical score of egg protein is taken as 100 and rest of proteins are compared.

## Quality of protein:

- Higher (Ist class) /complete: animal protein, e.g., egg, meat, milk, fish, poultry.
- Lower (incomplete): plant protein, e.g., cereals, legume, nuts.

## Limiting amino acids and supplementation

Certain protein are deficient in one or more essential amino acids e.g., rice and wheat proteins are limiting in lysine and threonine and rich in methionine; and pulses are deficient in methionine and rich in lysine.

A combination of pulses plus cereal will help to overcome the deficiency of certain amino acid in one food by being supplemented from the other. This is known as **mutual supplementation**. The effect of mutual supplementation in proteins is being observed with the same meal.

## Protein turnover

Rate of turnover of body protein, half life in man is = 58 days. Liver protein $t_{1/2}$ = 10-20 days. In man, approximately half the body protein is turned over 5-6 months. Body possesses a type of amino acid pool in dynamic equilibrium with amino acids formed from degradation of body proteins and with those taken in diet. Also, there is a steady loss from the pool even when no amino acids are ingested in diet.

## 3 patterns

- Group A: Proteins rapidly synthesized, have a finite life and are degraded rapidly e.g., Hb in RBC is stable for 120 days.
- Group B: rapidly synthesized and are rapidly degraded, half life very short e.g., plasma proteins, regulate enzymes of metabolic pathway which are present at low concentration in cells and their concentration fluctuate in response to stimuli.
- Group C: turnover very slowly, e.g., brain and bone.

## Required protein goal

- 12% calorie should come from proteins. Adults: 0.8 -1 g protein/kg body weight, in pregnancy + 10 g/d, lactation + 20 g proteins.

## Dietary sources

- Cereal (6-12%), pulse (18-22%), meat (18-25%), egg 10-14%, leafy vegetable 1-2%.
- Dietary animal proteins are superior to vegetable proteins.

## RDA (Recommended dietary allowance)

RDA represents the quantities of the nutrients to be provided in the diet daily for maintaining good health and physical efficiency of the body.

## Consumption of excess proteins

- Has no physiological advantage
- Will be deaminated and resulting carbon skeleton is metabolized to provide 'E' or acetyl CoA for fat synthesis.

## Factors

1. **Sex:** Dietary allowances in men are 20% higher except iron in women. In pregnancy and lactation, additional requirements (20-30% above normal) are needed. Adult require 0.8 g/kg protein and instant need over 2g/kg body weight.
2. **Age**.
3. **Others:** RDA increases in pregnancy, lactation, illness, injury. In adults 1g/kg body weight nearly double in children.

**Table 6.15.** RDA of adult of 70 kg

|  | RDA |  | RDA |
|---|---|---|---|
| Carbohydrate | 400g | Vit. A | 1000 mg |
| Fats | 70g | D | 5 mg |
| Proteins | 56 g | E | 10 mg |
| Essential FA | 4g | K | 70 mg |
| Ca | 800 mg | C | 60 mg |
| P | 800 mg |  | 1.5 mg |
| Iron | 10g | Riboflavin | 2 mg |
|  |  | Niacin | 20 mg |
|  |  | Pyridoxine | 2 mg |
|  |  | Folic Acid | 150 mg |
|  |  | Cobalamin | 2 mg |

## Dietary principles

- Ideal body weight should be achieved and maintained
- Total fat: decrease saturated fat intake.

## Balanced diet

Defined as the diet that contains different types

| Table 6.16. | |
|---|---|
| Complex carbohydrates | 50-60% |
| Simple carbohydrates | Decrease |
| Fiber | 20-30g |
| Cholesterol | <250 mg/d |
| Salt decrease | 3-8g/d or 400-300 mg Na/day |
| Alcohol | limit |

**Table 6.17.** Caloric requirement

| Light work | 2200-2500cal/d |
|---|---|
| Moderate | 2500-2900 cal/d |
| Heavy | 2900-3500 cal/d |
| Very heavy | 3500-4000 cal/d |

**Table 6.18.** Adult men

| Pregnancy/ Lactation | Food stuff | Moderate work vegetarian g/d | Woman /non veg |
|---|---|---|---|
| +50/ + 100 | Cereals | 475 | 350 |
| +10 | Pulses | 80 | 70/55 |
| + 25/ +25 | Green leafy vegetable | 125 | 125 |
| | Other vegetable | 75 | 75 |
| | Root and tuber | 100 | 75 |
| | Fruit | 30 | 30 |
| +125/ + 125 | Milk | 200 | 200/100 |
| +15 | Fats and oil | 40 | Meat 30 |
| | | | Egg 30 |
| +10/ + 20 | Sugar and jaggery | 30 | 30 |

of foods, possessing the nutrients: carbohydrates, fats, proteins, vitamins and minerals in a proportion to meet the requirements of the body. It should be based on locally available foods and food habits within economic means of people, easily digestible and palatable and contains enough roughage.

## Planning of balanced diet

Consider age, sex, calorie requirement, and economic status and food groups.

**Rule of Thumb:** Calorie requirement is 30-35 kcal/kg body weight, in sedentary: 30, moderate: 35 kcal/kg body weight.

## Ideal body weight

- Male: 48kg for 153 cm plus or minus 1.25 kg for every cm
- Adult female: 48 kg for 153 plus or minus 1 kg or every cm

## Protein required

- 1g/kg body weight
- Balanced diet should contain calorie from

carbohydrates, protein and fat in ratio 60:20.20.

## Causes of malnutrition

| *Primary Deficiency* | *Secondary deficiency* |
|---|---|
| Inadequate dietary intake | Low absorption Decreased utilization Increased excretion or Destruction |

## Mechanism

Gradual tissue depletion of nutrient
↓
Biochemical lesions
↓
Anatomic lesion, deficiency signs e.g.: Kwashiorkor, scurvy

## Nutritional Disorders

Protein energy malnutrition encompasses a range of disorders of starvation and nutrition that nutrients such as vitamins in addition to proteins, carbohydrates and fats.

**Table 6.19.**

| Essential feature | Marasmus | Kwashiorkor |
|---|---|---|
| 1. Edema | None | Lower legs, sometimes face or generalized |
| 2. Wasting | Gross loss of subcutaneous fat "all skin and bone" | Less obvious sometimes fat |
| 3. Muscle wasting | Severe | Less than in marasmus |
| 4. Growth retardation in terms of weight | Severe | Usually present |
| 5. Mental changes | Usually none | Much less |
| 6. Hormone response to starvation (cortisol) | Increase protein catabolism | Low |
| 7. Cause | Early weaning | Late weaning |
| 8. S. albumin | Normal or slight increase | Low |
| 9. U. urea/g of creatinine | Normal or decrease | Low |
| 10. S. free amino acid ratio | Normal/decrease | Low |
| 11. Anemia | May be present | Iron or folate deficiency may be associated |
| 12. Liver biopsy | Normal or atrophic | Fatty infiltration |
| 13. U. hydroxyproline | Low | Low |

## PEM (Protein energy malnutrition)

It is most common nutritional disorder of the developing countries. PEM is widely prevalent in infants and pre-school children. Kwashiorkor and Marasmus are two extremes of PEM.

**Kwashiorkor** means sickness the elder child gets when the next child is born.

**Occurrence:** predominant between 1-5 year of age due to insufficient intake of proteins, since diet of a weaning child mainly consists of carbohydrates.

## Kwashiorkor: Clinical features

### Clinical features

Stunted growth, edema (legs and hand), diarrhea, discoloration of hair and skin (flag sign), anaemia, apathy.

### Biochemical features

Low p. albumin <2g%, Fatty liver in some cases, Hypokalaemia due to dehydration, seen with diarrhoea, total body weight water content increases (upto 60%)

### Treatment

Ingestion of protein rich diet (3-4 g protein kg body weight), monitor treatment by measuring plasma proteins levels.

## Marasmus (Means to waste)

- Usually occurs in children under 1 year of age principally seen in developing countries. It can be seen in developed world: (old age: not able to cook), in deprived individuals, anorexia nervosa (deficiency of both energy and protein).
- Predominately due to deficiency of calories seen in children given watery gruels (of cereals) to supplement breast milk, prolonged breast feeding with inadequate supplementation of other foods.

## Clinical features

Growth retardation muscle wasting, anaemia, weakness, no edema, Diarrhea is almost always present

## Treatment

Complete balanced diet with high calorie around 200 cal/kg or more may be required.

## Deficiency and excess to diet

| Deficiency | Food constituents | Excess |
|---|---|---|
| Marasmus | Energy | Obesity |
| - | Sucrose | Obesity + dental caries |
| Essential FA def | Fat | Obesity + heart disease |
| Wasting | Protein | Gout |
| Anaemia | Iron | Siderosis |
| Rickets | Calcitriol | Hypercalcemia |

## Other nutrition disorders

- Obesity
- Atherosclerosis
- Those associated with vitamins, minerals

## Obesity

- Physical state in which excess fat is accumulated in the body.
- Body weight over 20% above mean ideal weight.
- Obesity index = $W/H^2$ (W = Weight, H = Height)
- Can occur as result of ingestion of food in excess of body's needs.
- Genetic predisposition has also been suggested.

**Metabolic/endocrine factor:** Decreased $T_4$, Hyperthyroidism, hypopituitarism, hypogonadism, Cushing's, pregnancy, menopause.

**Ill effects:** Hyperlipidemia, increased incidence, decreased life span

## Treatment

- Decrease calorie intake
- Weight monitoring
- Controlled exercise

In developed countries, deprived individuals or those suffering from anorexia nervosa: malnutrition can occur.

## Special diets

1. **Diabetic:**
   - Carbohydrate 60-70%, fats 15-25%, protein 15-20% avoid sugars, refined carbohydrate.
   - Increase leafy vegetables, restrict tubers.
   - 1/3 fat should be PUFA, frequent small meals, dietary control for cholesterol: Increase PUFA intake, decrease cholesterol intake increase fibre content in diet.
2. **CRF (Chronic renal failure): and hepatic cirrhosis:** low protein, high carbohydrate.
3. **CHF (Congestive heart failure): and HT (hypertension):** salt restriction.

## Special diets

- Pregnancy 2nd trimester and 3rd :
  + 200 cal/day
  - Calcium + 500 mg/d
  - Protein + 10g day
- Lactation + 700 Cal/day
  - +20 g protein/d
  - + 500 mg/d calcium
  - + 3.6 mg/d iron extra

## Low protein diets and renal disease:

Chronic renal failure (CRF) is characterized by buildup of end products of catabolism of proteins mainly urea. Maintain these proteins with 40 g/d protein, if diet is calorically sufficient. Provide a minimum of protein with high BV. Provide calorie from carbohydrates and fats.

**Goal:** To provide just enough amino acids so as to maintain positive N balance plus monitor, plasma, protein.

## VITAMINS

- Vitamins are organic nutrients in diet that are involved in fundamental functions of body such as growth and metabolism.
- Vitamins are required in small quantities for performing specific biological functions.
- Vitamins cannot be synthesized by the body and have to be obtained from diet.

### Classification

- Lipid soluble: A, D, E, K.
- Water soluble: B, C.

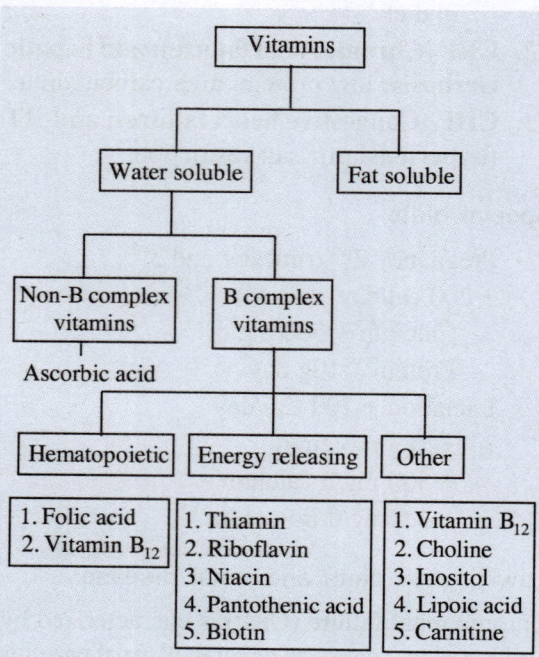

Water soluble vitamins function as enzyme cofactors.

## LIPID-SOLUBLE VITAMINS

### Vitamin A

#### Physiological functions

1. Vision: Vision in dark
2. Somatic functions: growth and differentiation
3. Reproduction: spermatogenesis, oogenesis, placental development and embryonic growth
4. Antioxidant: quenches free radicals and oxidants
5. Regulation of gene expression: Retinoic acid binds to nuclear receptors that bind to response elements on DNA to regulate transcription of specific genes.
6. Integrity of immune system

**Table 6.20.** Chemistry: Vitamin A

Precursor of 20-carbon polyphenol called retinol

Represent structurally related forms:
Retinol*
Retinal*
Retinoic acid⁺
β-carotene (provitamin A)

β-carotene:
Found in plants
Cleaved to yield retinal (2 moles) by enzyme carotene dioxygenase
Possess one sixth of vitamin A activity
6 μg β-carotene is equivalent to 1 mg of pre-formed retinal
Transported in circulation by plasma retinol binding protein (RBP)

\* Retinol, retinal are interconvertible

⁺ Once formed from retinal, retinoic acid cannot be converted back to retinol or retinal.

## Table 6.21. Vitamin A: deficiency symptoms

Defective night vision or night blindness
Keratinization of epithelium:
    Cornea
    Lungs
    Conjunctiva
    GIT
Gentiourinary tract
Bitot's spots
Xerophthalmia
Blindness
Increased susceptibility to infection (negative acute phase protein).

There is extensive recycling of retinol among plasma, liver and extrahepatic tissues.

## Table 6.22. Vitamin A: salient features

Stored in liver parenchyma cells as retinol palmitate [Mainly, 85-90% of retinol stored in perisinusoidal cells (named stellate cells)]
Transported by:
  * RBPs: SRBP (serum)
          CRPB (cytosolic)
  * Albumin
  * RABP (retinoic acid binding protein)
Hypervitaminosis occurs after capacity of RBP has been exceeded and cells are exposed to unbound retinol

* Retinol binding protein.

## Table 6.23. Vitamin A: toxicity*

Hair loss
Dermatitis
Bone pain (thickening of long bones)
Hypercalcemia and calcification of soft tissues
Hepatosplenomegaly
Nausea
Vomiting
Diarrhea
Double vision
Headache

* Teratogenic, should be avoided during pregnancy

## Table 6.24. Visual pigments

Retinaldehyde is prosthetic group of opsin protein
**Opsin proteins**
**1. Rhodopsin:**
    Occurs in rods cells of retina
    Responsible for vision in poor light
**2. Iodopsin:**
    Occurs in cones
    Responsible for colour vision
    Cone cell contains only one type of opsin and is sensitive to one colour only.

## Table 6.25. Main steps in visual cycle

11-cis retinal $\rightarrow$ all/trans retinal
Activation of rhodopsin on exposure to light
    $\downarrow$ cGMP
    Blockage of $Na^+$ entry
    Hyperpolarization of rod cell
    Release of glutamate
    Action potential generation: depolarization of bipolar cell
    Depolarization of ganglion, neuron

**11-cis retinal** is specifically bound to visual protein opsin to form rhodopsin. On exposure to light, rhodopsin undergoes conformational change and dissociates into opsin and all trans retinal (rhodopsin) bleaches and induces change in membrane permeability to generate a nerve impulse (via guanine amplification cascade).

$$\text{All-trans retinal} \xrightarrow[\text{Isomerase}]{\text{Retinal}} \text{11-cis retinal}$$

11-trans retinal and 11 cis retinal are functional form of vitamin A in visual process.

## Table 6.26. Vitamin A: Source, RDA

| | |
|---|---|
| Animal source | Liver, egg yolk, butter, milk |
| Plant source | Dark green and yellow vegetables (carotene) |
| RDA | Adult: 1000 RE, children : 400-700 RE |

## Visual cycle

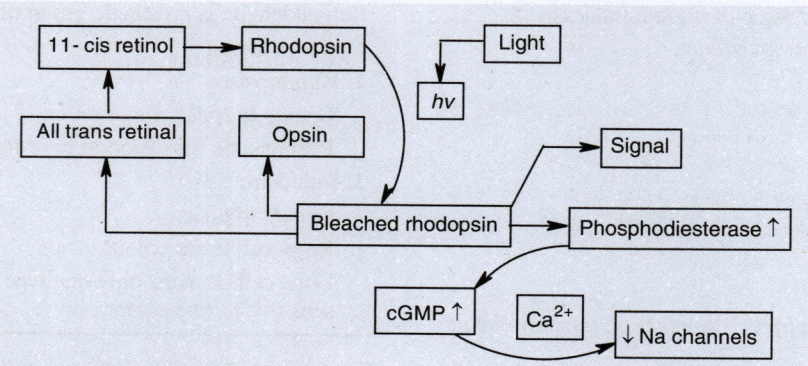

**Fig. 6.6.** Visual cycle.

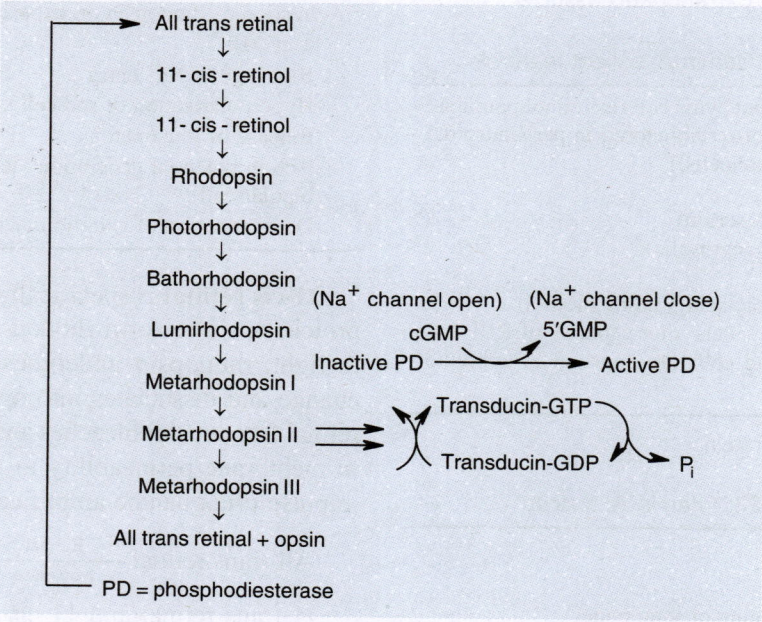

**Fig. 6.7.** Visual cycle; Steps

## Digestion, absorption and transport of vitamin a

Carotenes and retinoid esters are often complexed with proteins in food and released through the action of pepsin in stomach and proteolytic enzymes in small intestine. Released carotenoids and retinyl esters are solubilized in micelle; esterases hydrolyze retinyl esters and carotenoid esters. The micelle solutions diffuse into glycoprotein layer surrounding microvilli of duodenum and jejunum and then are absorbed and incorporated into chylomicrons.

**Table 6.27.** Antioxidant functions of vitamin A: retinoids and carotenoids

* Normal epithelial cell growth and differentiation depends on retinoid
* Inverse relationship between dietary vitamin A content and risk of cancer.
* β-carotene is an antioxidant
* Vitamin A may be protective against cancer and cardiovascular disease

## Vitamin D

**Table 6.28.** Functions of vitamin D

* Regulates calcium and phosphate metabolism
* Cell differentiation and proliferation
* Immune function
* Secretion of hormones
  Insulin
  Thyroid
  Parathyroid
* Acts like a steroid hormone and enhance gene expression

**Table 6.29.** Chemistry

* Steroid hormone
* Group of closely related sterols produced by action of Uv light on provitamins: ergosterol in plants and 7-dehydrocholesterol animal to produce:
  Ergocalciferol (plant), $D_2$
  Cholecalciferol (animal), $D_3$
  Both, $D_2$, $D_3$ are of equal potency

### Dietary sources of vitamin D

Animal: Egg, liver, butter, fatty fish, fortified milk, migarine

### Absorption and transport of vitamin D

Vitamin D can be absorbed into body from skin and digestive tract. Dietary vitamin D is stable, not prone to losses during cooking, storage and processing.

Vitamin D is absorbed in intestine in association with fat, aided by bile salts and get incorporated in chylomicrons. Absorption is fastest in duodenum followed by jejunum.

### Metabolism

$$\text{Vitamin D}_3 \leftarrow 25 \text{ hydroxylase} \rightarrow 25 \text{ OH D}_3$$

$$\xrightleftharpoons{1\alpha\text{-hydroxylase}} 1,25(OH)_2D_3 \xrightarrow{24 \text{ hydroxylase}}$$

$$1,24,25(OH)_3 D_3 \rightarrow 1,25(OH)_2 \rightarrow \text{Target tissues}$$

**Table 6.30.** Functions of 1, $25(OH)_2D_3$

**Function of 1, $25(OH)_2 D_3$:** Increase absorption of calcium and phosphorus

**Mechanism:**

Via selective DNA transcription to synthesize proteins and transporters necessary to generate biological response of hormone

Calbindin D is synthesized in response to action of 1, $25(OH)_2 D_3$, it is a Ca- binding protein

**Table 6.31.** Target tissues for vitamin D

**Target tissues for vitamin D**
Intestine
Bone
Kidney
Skin
Bone marrow
Breast
Thymus
Brain
Endocrine glands

### Excretion of vitain d

When sufficient amounts of metabolites are present, activity of 1α hydroxylase in kidney decreases significantly. 24 hydroxylase in kidney is increased and 1,24,25($OH)_3 D_3$ is produced,

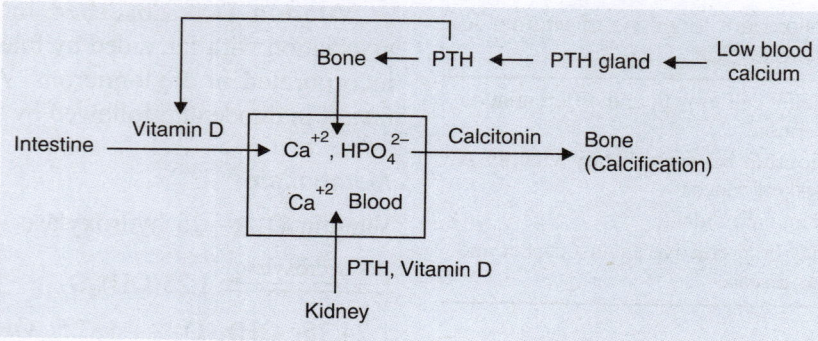

**Fig. 6.8.** Site of action of vitamin D.

| Table 6.32. Functions |
|---|
| **Action of vitamin D in bone and kidney** |
| Stimulates intracellular transport of calcium across cell membrane |
| Vitamin D plays a major role in PTH-directed: |
|     Mobilization of calcium from bones |
|     Stimulation of calcium absorption in distal renal tubule |
| Vitamin D exerts its influence on bone mineralization by super saturating plasma with calcium and phosphorus |
| Vitamin D via stimulation of osteoclast-mediated bone resorption help in remodeling of bone |

**Table 6.33.** Vitamin D (calcitriol) as a hormone

**Reasons:**
- Synthesized in skin which is a major source of vitamin
- Regulates calcium absorption and homeostasis
  Its actions are mediated by way of nuclear receptors. 1,25 DHD$_3$ belongs to super family of nuclear hormone receptors) that regulate gene expression*
- Its biologically active form is produced in kidney and is subject to feed back inhibition by itself
- Hormone receptors are present for in intestine, bone, kidney and many other tissues

\* 1, 25 DH D$_3$ binds to nuclear ®, the complex binds to specific hormone responsive elements (HRE) on DNA, resulting in mRNA and protein synthesis. Proteins include: osteocalcin, calcium binding protein CaBP (in GIT).

which get oxidized to 1,25( OH)$_2$ -24-oxo- D$_3$, that gets excreted.

## Synthesis of Vitamin D

- **Precursor:** 7-dehydrocholesterol (in humans)
- **Site:** skin, liver, kidney

| Key organ | Key Hormones |
|---|---|
| Kidney | Parathyroid |
| Intestine | Calcitonin |
| Bone | |

## Regulation

Regulation of vitamin D$_3$ metabolism is linked to parathyroid hormone (PTH). PTH secretion is stimulated by hypocalcemia. PTH stimulates 1α-hydroxylase in kidney to produce 1, 25 (OH)$_2$ D$_3$ which enters circulation and promotes calcium resorption from bone.

Calcium absorption from GIT stimulates calcium reabsorption from kidney and excretion of phosphate.

Hypercalcemia inhibits PTH release which

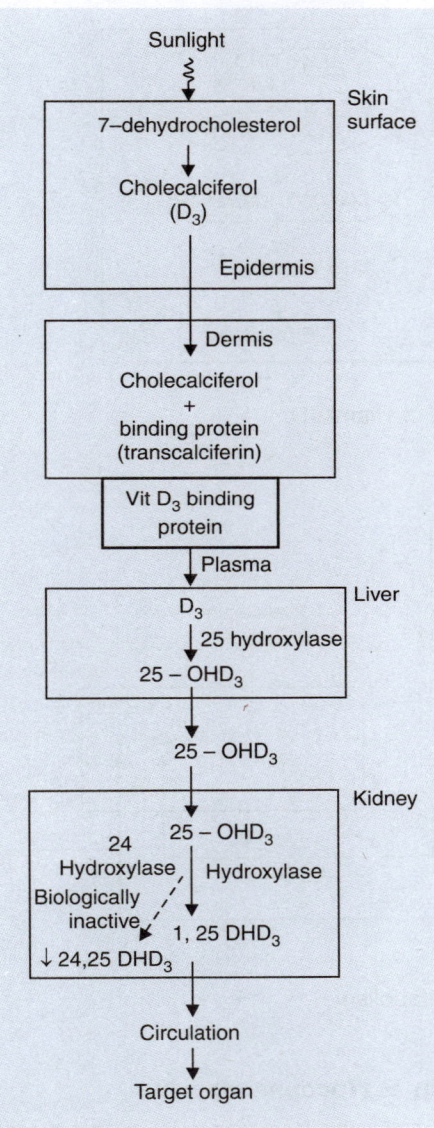

**Fig. 6.9.** Synthesis of vitamin D.

in turn inhibits 1,25 $(OH)_2$ $D_3$ synthesis and active $D_3$ is converted to inactive 24, 25 $(OH)_2$ $D_3$. Also, 1,25 $(OH)_2$ $D_3$ feedback inhibits PTH release. Synthesis of 1, 25 $(OH)_2$ $D_3$ is regulated by its own concentration, PTH hormone and phosphate levels.

---

**Table 6.34.** 25-OH $D_3$

- Major form of vitamin D in circulation
- Major storage from in liver, adipose tissue and skeletal muscle.
- Undergoes enterohepatic circulation (significant fraction)
- Hydroxylated to: 1, 25 $(OH)_2$ $D_3$ (active form) in kidney, bone and placenta; 24, 25 $(OH)_2$ $D_3$ (inactive form).

---

**Table 6.35.** Physiological role: vitamin D

| | |
|---|---|
| Bone | Stimulate calcium resorption |
| | Stimulate osteocalcin synthesis |
| GIT | Stimulates calcium and phosphate absorption (by enhancing synthesis of CaBP that transport calcium from mucosal to serosal cell of gut) |
| Kidney | Stimulate calcium reasorption |
| | Stimulate phosphate excretion |
| | [Tubules contain vitamin D and CaBP receptors] |
| Others | Immune function: maturation and proliferation of cells |

---

**Table 6.36.** Deficiency: Vitamin D

- Rickets (children)
- Osteomalacia (adults): softening of bone

---

**Table 6.37.** Conditions associated with risk for vitamin D deficiency

| |
|---|
| Alcoholism |
| Insufficient sun exposure (Muslim women) |
| Intestinal disorders: Tropical sprue, colitis, diverticulitis |
| Liver, kidney disease |
| Parathyroid disorder |
| Anticonvulsant therapy |
| Children under 6 yrs |
| Old age |

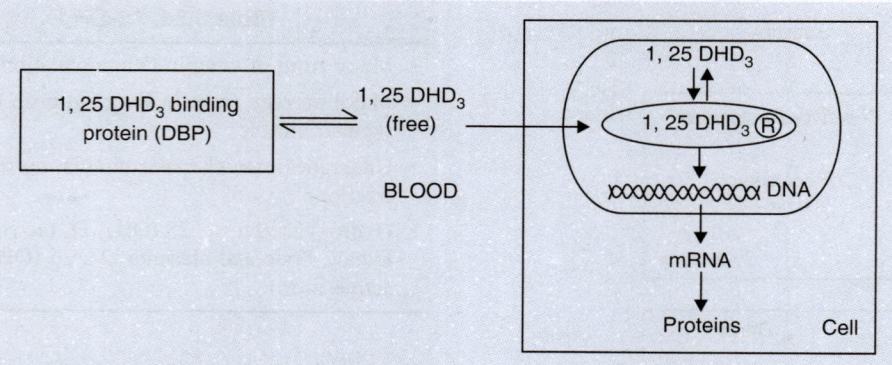

Fig. 6.10. Mechanism of action of vitamin D.

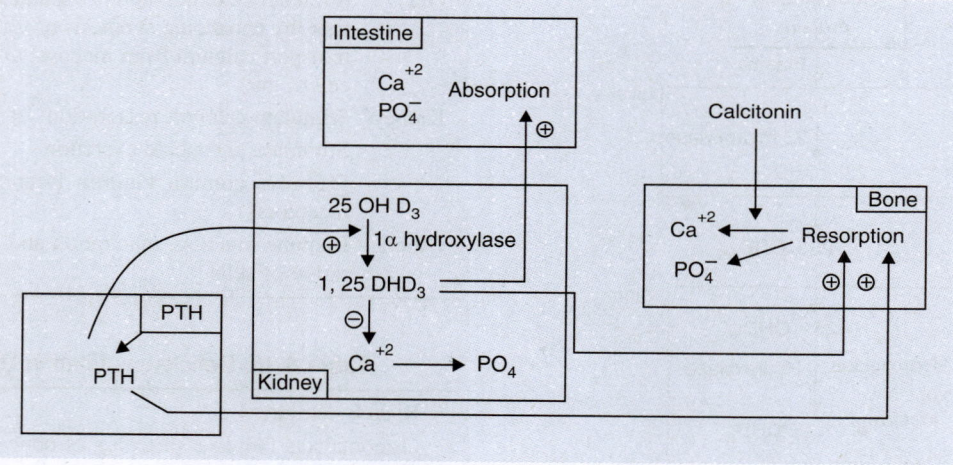

Fig. 6.11. Regulation of metabolism

**Vitamin D toxicity:** occurs in vitamin D excess leading to enhanced calcium absorption, bone resorption leading to hypercalcemia and metastatic calcium deposits. Vitamin D toxicity can occur following excessive ingestion of vitamin D. Increased oxidation of membranes and deposition of calcium in soft tissues can occur. Symptoms include: anorexia, vomiting, hypertension, renal insufficiency.

## Vitamin E (Tocopherol)

### Clinical implications of free radical and diseases

- Free radicals oxygen species may initiate disease.
- Vitamin E and other antioxidant nutrients (vitamin A, β-carotene, vitamin C) may prevent diseases such as cancer, cardiovascular and neurological diseases.

## Table 6.38. Vitamin E: Major lipid-soluble anti-oxidant

- Major antioxidant in cell membrane and lipoproteins
- Chain breaking antioxidant

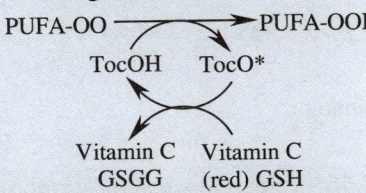

\* Act synergistically with selenium: to provide line of defense against lipid peroxidation.

## Table 6.39. Chemistry

- Comprise of two families of vitamins. Tocopherol and tocotrienol
- Isoprenoid – substituted 6-hydroxydriomane (tocol)
- Several natural forms of tocopherol exist: $\alpha$, $\beta$, $\gamma$, $\delta$.
- D-$\alpha$-tocopherol has widest natural distribution and greatest biologic activity.

## Table 6.40. Functions: Vitamin E

- No precisely defined metabolic function.
- Maintenance of intracellular membrane integrity
- Lipid-soluble antioxidant in cell membranes and lipoproteins
- Associated with reproductive function
- Front line defense against tissue damage by active oxygen
- Prevent/stop lipid peroxidation

## Table 6.41. Vitamin E deficiency

**Occurs in:** Steatorrhoea, abetalipoproteinemia, cholestatic liver disease, cystic fibrosis, intestinal resection, premature infants with inadequate reserve.

**Symptoms:** Hemolytic anemia in premature infants, sterility, degenerative changes in muscle and nerves.

\* Least toxic among fat-soluble vitamins

## Table 6.42. RDA and sources

| | |
|---|---|
| **RDA** | 8-10 mg/day: D $\alpha$-tocopherol |
| | 1meq has vitamin E activity of 1mg $\alpha$ tocopherol |
| **Source** | Vegetable oil |
| | Wheat germ |
| | Nuts |

### Absorption

- Absorbed in intestine by passive diffusion
- Absorption requires presence of bile salts and pancreatic juices
- Absorbed tocopherol is incorporated into chylomicrons, transported through lymph into circulation

### Toxicity

At high doses, muscle weakness, fatigue, nausea, diarrhea occur.

### Vitamin K

## Table 6.43. Function

**Menaquinone:**
- Essential for normal blood clotting.
- Cofactor for $\gamma$-glutamyl carboxylase enzyme that causes post-translational formation of $\gamma$-carboxy glutamyl (Gla) residues.

**Gla:**
- Bind calcium
- Calcium mediates phospholipid adsorption of Gla protein for homeostasis.

### $\gamma$-carboxylation

Factors II, VII, IX, X are synthesized by liver in inactive form and activated by carboxylation of specific glutamic acid residue by vitamin K dependent carboxylase enzyme.

Prothrombin (factor II) contains ten of these

**Fig. 6.12.** Gamma carboxylation.

| Table 6.44. Chemistry |
|---|
| Polyisoprenoid – substituted naphthoquinone include: |
| Menadione (vitamin $K_3$) |
| Menaquinone (vitamin $K_2$): in animals: synthesized by bacteria in intestine |
| Phylloquinone (vitamin $K_1$): in plants circulates as phylloquinone and its hepatic stores are in form of menaquinones |
| Menadione: 2 methyl-1, 4-naphthoquinone while other two are poly isoprenoid-substituted |

| Table 6.45. Proteins that contain γ-carboxygluta-mate |
|---|
| Factor II, VII, IX, X |
| Osteocalcin |
| Bone matrix Gla protein |

| Table 6.46. Dietary sources |
|---|
| Green leafy vegetables |
| Fruits |
| Dairy products |
| Vegetable oils |
| Cereals |
| Meat |
| **RDA:** 70-140 mg/day |

carboxylated residues (Gla) which allow chelation of calcium during coagulation.

## Role of war farin as anticoagulant

- Warfarin (Dicumarol) inhibits action of reductase that reduces epoxide form of vitamin K and mimicks vitamin K deficiency.
- Treatment of pregnant women with warfarin can lead to fetal bone abnormalities: FETAL WARFARIN SYNDROME

## Absorption of vitamin K

- Dietary vitamin K is provided as phylloquinone and menaquinone in animals. Phylloquinone is absorbed from small intestine particularly from jejunum by energy dependent process.

- Menaquinone are absorbed from distal ileum and colon by diffusion.
- Humans can absorb menaquinones synthesized by bacteria in intestine to some extent.
- Menadione, synthetic form of vitamin K is absorbed by passive diffusion in lower intestine.
- Absorption of vitamin K is enhanced by presence of bile salts and pancreatic juice.
- Absorbed vitamin K becomes part of chylomicrons, carried to liver, incorporated into VLDL and ultimately LDL.

## Metabolism

After entry into liver, vitamin K is used in

posttranslational carboxylation of proteins of homeostasis. In liver, vitamin K has very short half-life or very short term storage. It is distributed to various tissues, bone and kidney. Body pool of vitamin K is 50-100µg and is turned over once every 2.5 hours. This pool is extraordinarily very low for fat-soluble vitamin, even smaller than vitamin $B_{12}$.

Menaquinone is rapidly metabolized by conjugation (glucuronide or sulfate) and excreted in urine or in feces. Phylloquinone is degraded more slowly than menadione and get converted to 2,3 epoxide and 3-hydroxyquinone and finally excreted as glucuronides in urine and feces via bile.

## Conditions associated with increased risk of vitamin K

- Biliary fistula
- Obstructive jaundice
- Chronic diarrhea
- Chronic pancreatitis
- Liver disease
- Prolonged sulfa and antibiotic treatment in new borns.

## Vitamin K cycle

Vitamin K-dependent carboxylase reaction occurs in endoplasmic reticulum of many tissues

**Table 6.47.** Deficiency: Vitamin K

**Symptoms:**
Bleeding disorders
Hemorrhagic disease of newborn
**Cause:**
Fat malabsorption
Pancreatic dysfunction
Biliary disease
Atrophy of intestinal mucosa
Steatorrhoea of any cause
Sterilization of large intestine by antibiotics
Protein infant (inefficient placental transfer)

**Table 6.48.** Inhibitors of vitamin K action

**Use:** Serve as antithrombotic agent used in treatment of thrombosis-related disease; deep vein thrombosis pulmonary thromboembolism, patient at risk of thrombosis. e.g., atrial fibrillation
**Drugs:** dicumarin group (e.g. Warfarin)
**Site of action:** 2, 3 epoxide reductase inhibition, antidote of dicumarol-type drugs
**Metabolism of vitamin K:**
Warfarin is metabolized by $P_{450}$ enzyme, which is induced by phenobarbitone or chronic alcohol consumption causing enhanced metabolism of Warfarin (patient requires larger dose for anticoagulation). Stoppage of phenobarbitone or alcohol intake can cause over anticoagulation

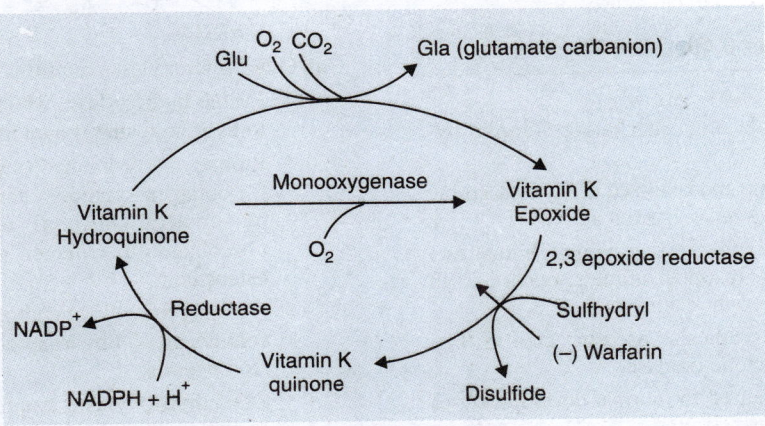

**Fig. 6.13.** Vitamin K cycle.

and requires molecular oxygen, carbon dioxide and hydroquinone.

Initially, hydroquinone is oxidized to epoxide, which activates γ-carboxylation of glutamate. 2, 3 epoxide is reduced to quinine by epoxide reductase (which can be either warfarin-sensitive reductase or warfarin-insensitive reductase) to form hydroxyquinone.

## Water soluble vitamins

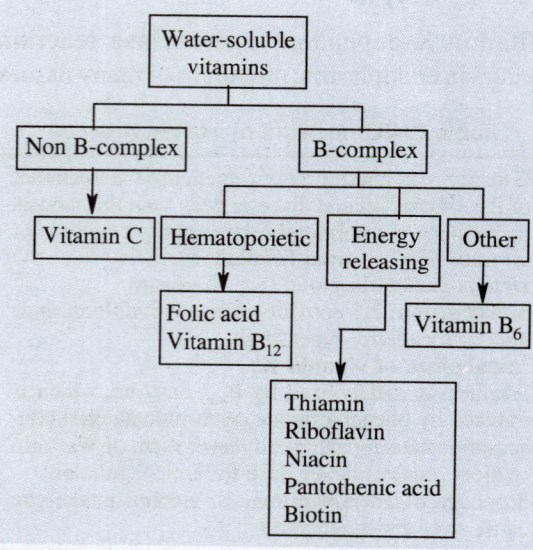

## Vitamin C

### Table 6.49. Chemistry

- Six carbon derivative
- Closely resemble monosaccharides (enolic hydroxyl)
- Exist as ascorbate and oxidized (dehydroascorbic acid) forms [both have vitamin activity]
- Vitamin for only some species namely, human and primates, fishes. In other animals, occurs as an intermediate in uronic pathway
- Human cannot synthesize ascorbic acid as they lack L-gulonolactone oxidase
- Vitamin C is required for normal development of cartilage, bone and dentine.

## Absorption of vitamin C

- Occurs via active transport system, simple diffusion in distal portion of small intestine absorption. Absorption rate vary and average rate is 90%

### Table 6.50. Vitamin C: Functions

**Coenzyme for hydroxylases**

(i) Cu-containing hydroxylase. e.g., Dopamine hydroxylase (synthesizes dopamine, catecholamines)

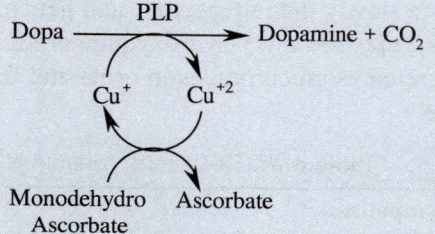

p-hydroxy phenyl pyruvate hydroxylase catalyzed reaction:

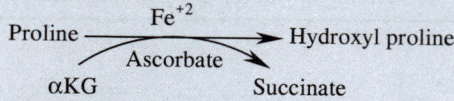

(ii) α-keto glutarate linked iron-containing hydroxylases, e.g., prolyl hydroxylase (mixed function oxygenase)

$$\text{Proline} \xrightarrow[\substack{\text{Ascorbate} \\ \alpha KG}]{Fe^{+2}} \text{Hydroxyl proline} \quad \text{Succinate}$$

(iii) Other hydroxylases requiring vitamin C:

- Lysine hydroxylase, which converts lysine to hydroxylysine is analogous to proline.
- Proline and lysine hydroxylase are required for collagen synthesis, and bone formation by posttranslational modification of procollagen to collagen and formation of osteocalcin.
- Hydroxylation in metabolism of tyrosine: conversion of 4 hydroxy phenyl pyruvate to Homogentisate
- Other hydroxylases requiring vitamin C: dopamine hydroxylase

- Transported in blood as free anion and equilibrates with body pool
- Tissues with high vitamin C concentration:
  Highest in:
  - Adrenal cortex
  - Pituitary
  - Retina
  Intermediate:
  - Liver, lung, pancreas, WBC
  Low:
  - Kidney, muscle, RBC

## 2. Reducing agent

Participates in synthesis of collagen, catecholamines, dopamine, steroidogenesis, degradation of tyrosine, bile acid formation, absorption of iron, bone metabolism, blood coagulation, and carnitine.

## 3. Antioxidant

Vitamin C is an important first line of defense against free radicals in aqueous phase. In addition, it regenerates tocopherol and gets reduced to dehydroascorbate. It has been suggested that vitamin C may play an important role in prevention of atherosclerosis and cancer.

## 4. Immune function:

Enhances synthesis of antibodies, required for normal leukocyte function.

## RDA

Daily requirements:
  30-35 mg: infants
  40-60mg: children
  60 mg: adult
  70 mg: pregnancy
  90 mg: lactation

## Metabolism

Ascorbate is oxidized into L-hydroascorbate which is oxidized to 2,3- diketogulonic acid and finally oxalic acid, threonic acid which gets metabolized and excreted as $CO_2$ and water.

## Conditions associated with deficiency of vitamin C:

- Alcoholism
- Dietary inadequacy
- Smoking
- Surgery
- Cancer
- Old age
- Stress
- Thyrotoxicosis

**Vitamin C deficiency causes scurvy.**

| Table 6.51. Scurvy | |
| --- | --- |
| Symptoms | Skin changes<br>Subcutaneous hemorrhage<br>Muscle weakness<br>Soft, swollen and bleeding gums<br>Osteoporosis, fractures<br>Poor wound healing<br>Anemia |
| Mechanism | Defective collagen synthesis<br>Osteoporosis due to inability to maintain bone matrix in association with demineralization<br>Capillary fragility increased; causing easy bruising and petechiae |

**Table 6.52.** Proposed functions of vitamin C

**Probable functions**
Proline and lysine hydroxylation
Carnitine synthesis
Dopamine hydroxylation
Peptide amidation
**Functions that may be aided or affected by vitamin C at levels of intake exceeding physiologic requirement:**
Iron absorption, distribution and storage, folate reduction (THF formation)
Lymphocytes and neutrophil function (immune function)
Protection against toxicity of heavy metals.
Sulphation (proteoglycan synthesis)

## Vitamin B complex

B complex vitamins acts as coenzymes in many metabolic pathways and often multiple deficiencies occur and single B vitamin deficiency is rare.

## Thiamin (B₁)

| Table 6.53. Function |
|---|

1. Energy transformation: TDP is coenzyme involved in oxidative decarboxylation of α-keto acid

   • Pyruvate $\xrightarrow{\text{PDH}}$ Acetyl CoA

   $\downarrow$ Pyruvate decarboxylase

   Acetaldehyde

   • α Keto glutarate $\xrightarrow{\alpha \text{ KGDH}}$ Succinyl CoA
   α carbon of keto acid becomes covalently attached to thiamin pyrophosphate (TPP).
   TPP is formed from ATP and vitamin thiamin.
   • Oxidative decarboxylation of a keto acids of: leucine, isoleucine, valine, threonine, serine.
   • Transketolase

   Xylulose 5P + ribose 5P → Sedoheptulose-T.P + glyceraldeyde -3P

2. Synthesis of NADPH and pentoses (HMP shunt: transketolase)

3. Membrane and nerve conduction: electrical stimulation of membrane results in a fall in membrane triphosphate and release of free thiamin

Aberrations in nerve function may be due to:
- Lack of energy
- Decreased amount of AcH synthesis which requires TDP
- Reduced nerve impulse transmission (regulates it).

## Deficiency

- Peripheral neuritis
- Beriberi
- Wernicke's encephalopathy

## Chemical Structure

- Only natural compound with a thiazole ring.
- Contains pyrimidine ring and thiazole ring held by a methylene bridge.
- Esterified to coenzyme diphosphate (TDP).

## Sources, RDA

- Cereals
- Pulses
- Oil seeds
- Nuts
- RDA: 0.5 mg/1000 kcal (adults)

Greater the caloric intake, larger is the requirement for B vitamins!

## Conditions associated with increased risk for a deficiency of thiamin

- Alcoholism
- Fever
- Excess glucose infusion
- Diet composed of refined carbohydrates (e.g., polished rice)
- Mg, Ca, B₆, B₁₂ deficiencies
- Folate deficiency (results in malabsorption of thiamin)
- Elderly

## Mechanism of symptomatology of thiamin deficiency

Thiamin deficiency can lead to disturbances in carbohydrate metabolism and decreased transketolase activity. Clinically, thiamin deficiency affects nervous system and heart:

(i) **"Dry" beriberi:** (dry: without fluid retention) develops due to chronic deficiency of thiamin in diet. Symptoms include peripheral neuropathy.

(ii) **"Wet" beriberi:** (Wet: associated with cardiac failure with edema) develops when deficiency is more severe. In addition to neurological symptoms, cardiovascular symptoms are more apparent namely, right-sided enlargement, tachycardia, cardiac failure; edema and anorexia are characteristics.

(iii) **Wernicke-Korsakoff syndrome:** (Wernicke's encephalopathy and Korasakoff psychosis) develop in most acute deficiencies and seen primarily in alcoholics. Raw fish contain heat labile enzyme (thiaminase) that destroys thiamin.

**Alcoholics are prone to thiamin deficiency** because:

1. Decreased intake of vitamin due to decreased food consumption.
2. Decreased absorption
3. Increased requirement in case of liver damage.

## Riboflavin

Riboflavin is associated with oxidoreductases

### Flavoproteins

- FMN and FAD function as cofactors for oxidative enzyme termed as FLAVO PROTEINS
- Flavoprotein enzymes are tightly bound to their apoproteins
- May contain metals: Mo, Fe and are known as **metalloflavoproteins**
- Wide spread in nature and represented by oxidoreductases

### Chemistry

- Heterocyclic isoalloxazine ring attached to sugar alcohol: ribitol
- Exhibit redox potential
- Colored, fluorescent, heat stable, decomposes in presence of visible light.
- Active riboflavin is FMN, FAD

### Flavoprotein oxidoreductases

- $\alpha$-amino acid oxidase ($\alpha$ amino acid)

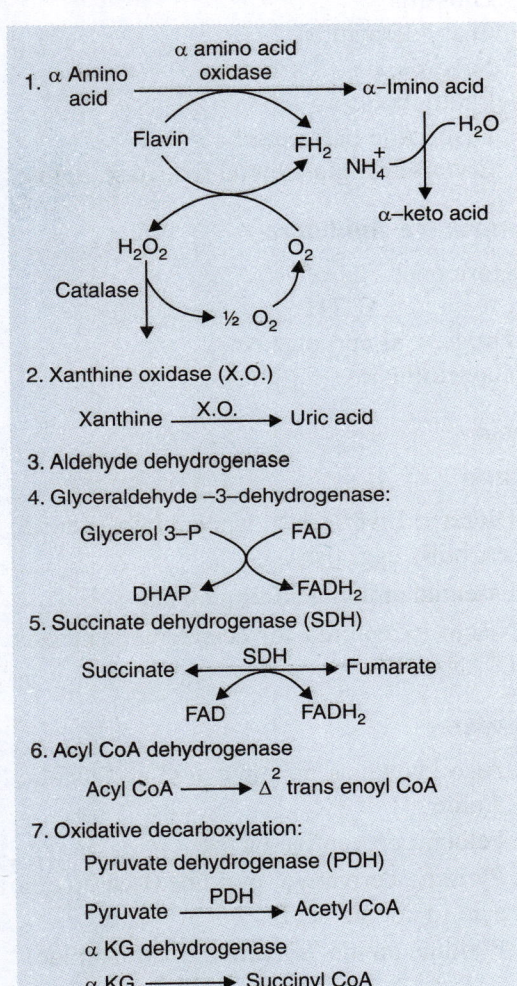

1. Xanthine oxidase (X.O.)

   Xanthine $\xrightarrow{\text{X.O.}}$ Uric acid

3. Aldehyde dehydrogenase
4. Glyceraldehyde –3–dehydrogenase:

5. Succinate dehydrogenase (SDH)

6. Acyl CoA dehydrogenase

   Acyl CoA $\longrightarrow \Delta^2$ trans enoyl CoA

7. Oxidative decarboxylation:

   Pyruvate dehydrogenase (PDH)

   Pyruvate $\xrightarrow{\text{PDH}}$ Acetyl CoA

   $\alpha$ KG dehydrogenase

   $\alpha$ KG $\longrightarrow$ Succinyl CoA

**Fig. 6.14.** Flavoprotein oxidases

### RDA

1.2-1.7 mg/d (adults).

### Sources

**Dairy:** Milk, milk products.

**Poultry:** Egg, meat, liver, kidney, fish, cereals, fruits, vegetables

### Deficiency symptoms

- Angular stomatitis, cheilosis
- Glossitis
- Scaly dermatitis
- Seborrhea
- Photophobia
- Diagnostic parameter:
  Erythrocyte glutathione reductase status

### Competitive inhibitors

Hormone: Thyroid
          ACTH
Drugs: Chlorpromazine
Galactoflavin

## Niacin

### Source

**Dietary:** Liver, yeast, whole grains, cereals, pulses, milk, egg, fish

Essential amino acid tryptophan

Niacin is required for coenzyme synthesis: $NAD^+$, $NADP^+$

### Chemistry

- Also known as nicotinic acid and nicotin-amide
  Pellagra preventive factor
- Pyridine derivative, pyridine 3-carboxylic acid (nicotinic acid)
- Pyridine amide derivative (nicotinamide).

### Facts about Tryptophan → Niacin → NAD (P)*

- 60 mg of tryptophan generate 1mg equivalent of niacin
- Requires: Vitamins:
  Thiamin
  Pyridoxine
  Riboflavin
  – Energy (ATP)

- Amino acid:
  Tryptophan
  Glutamine
- Phosphoribosyl pyrophosphate cannot supply sufficient amounts of niacin
- Niacin generates coenzymes which are involved in a variety of oxidation-reduction reaction.

### Coenzyme function: served by $NAD^+$, $NADP^+$

$NAD^+$ : catalyze oxidation reduction reaction in oxidative pathway (e.g., citric acid)

### Dehydrogenases

Cytosol: LDH (lactate dehydrogenase)
        PDH (pyruvate dehydrogenase)
Mitochondria:
        MDH (Malate dehydrogenase)
$NADP^+$: Catalyze pathways concerned with reductive synthesis (e.g., pentose phosphate pathway, PPP).

### Mechanism of oxidoreduction

It involves reversible addition of hydride ion ($H^-$) to pyridine ring and generation of free hydrogen ion ($H^+$)

$$NAD^+ + AH_2 \longleftrightarrow NADH + H^+ + A$$

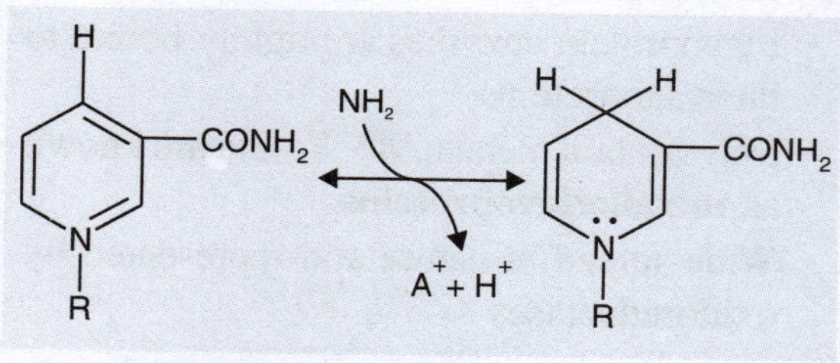

Fig. 6.15. Mechanism of oxido-reduction.

### Deficiency symptoms

Pellagra:

- Diarrhea
- Dermatitis
- Dementia

## Enzymes requiring NAD (P)/ NAD (P) H

| NAD$^+$ | NADP$^+$ |
| --- | --- |
| **Carbohydrate** | |
| Citric acid cycle | PPP pathway: |
| Lactate dehydrogenase (LDH) | Glucose -6-phosphate dehydrogenase (G6PD) |
| Pyruvate dehydrogenase (PDH) | Malic enzyme |
| Isocitrate dehydrogenase (ICD) | |
| Succinate dehydrogenase (SDH) | |
| **Lipid metabolism** | |
| β-OH acyl CoA dehydrogenase | 3-ketocyl reductase |
| Alcohol dehydrogenase | Enoyl reductase |
| Glycerol-3-phosphate dehydrogenase | HMG CoA reductase |
| | 7-α hydroxylase |
| **Protein metabolism** | |
| Branch chain a-keto dehydrogenase | Glutamate dehydrogenase |
| Glutamate dehydrogenase | Phenylalanine hydroxylase |
| Respiratory chain: NADH dehydrogenase | Dihydrofolate reductase |

### Therapeutic use

To lower plasma cholesterol by inhibiting flux of FFA from adipose tissue, leading to decreased formation of VLDL, LDL, IDL lipoproteins.

### Niacin deficiency: Causes

- Dietary deficiency
- Can occur in population where maize is staple diet: in maize niacin is present in bound unavailable from niacytin.
- Excess dietary leucine: causes niacin deficiency by inhibiting quinolinate phosphoribosyl transferase (key enzyme in tryptophan to niacin conversion)
- Pyridoxal phosphate deficiency (required as cofactor in NAD$^+$ synthesis)
- Drugs: isoniazid

- Malignant carcinoid syndrome (tryptophan diverted to form serotonin)
- Hartnup disease (impaired absorption of tryptophan)

## Pantothenic acid

Pantothenic exerts its functions through CoA, ACP (acetyl carrier protein).

### Functions

- Carrier of activated acyl or acetyl groups
- **Reactions requiring CoA:**
- Citric acid cycle:
  PDH
  α-ketoglutarate dehydrogenase
  **Fatty acid synthesis* and oxidation:**
  Acetyl CoA carboxylase
  Acyl CoA synthetase
  **Drug acetylation**
  **Cholesterol synthesis**

* Also requires ACP.

### Chemistry

Composed of Pantenoic acid and β-alanine.

### Active pantothenic acid

Coenzyme A and acyl carrier protein (ACP).

### Coenzyme A

Adenine nucleotide synthesized from phosphopantothenate with addition of cysteine and removal of carboxylic group (forming 4′ phosphopantotheinate) followed by adenylation by ATP to form dephospho-CoA. Dephospho CoA is phosphorylated to generate CoA.

### ACP

Synthesized from 4 phosphopantotheinate.

### RDA

- Not clear
- Recommended: 5-10 mg/d (adults)

### Source

Egg, liver, meat, yeast, milk, whole grain, cereals, legumes.

### Deficiency

- Rare
- Burning foot syndrome

### Vitamin B$_6$

Active vitamin B$_6$ is pyridoxal phosphate, which is a major coenzyme of metabolic pathways.

### Chemical composition

Consist of three closely related pyridine derivatives:

- Pyridoxine (alcohol)
- Pyridoxal (aldehyde)
- Pyridoxamine (amine) and their phosphate forms.

They are interconvertible, have equal vitamin activity and absorbed from intestine.

### Pyridoxal phosphate (PLP)

- Transport form in plasma
- Formed by phosphorylation by pyridoxal kinase (present in most tissues).

### Reactions catalyzed by PLP

i. Major role in amino acid metabolism:
   Transamination
   Decarboxylation (dopamine decarboxylase)
   (Tryptophan decarboxylase)
   Threonine aldose
   Glycine synthase

ii. Carbohydrate metabolism: Glycogen phosphorylase

iii. Heme synthesis: ALA synthase

### Facts

- **RDA:** 15-20 mg/day
- **Source:** Liver, avocado, banana, meat, vegetables, eggs.

### Deficiency

Common in:

- Alcoholics
- Drugs:
  Isoniazid (INH): binds to pyridoxine
  Oral contraceptive (OC) (OC increase synthesis of enzymes requiring pyridoxine vitamin).

### Symptoms

Neurological:

- Depression
- Irritability
- Confusion
- Convulsion
- Peripheral neuritis.

### Biotin

- Biotin is widely distributed in nature and normally synthesized by intestinal flora. It serves as a carrier of $CO_2$ in carboxylation reaction.
- Consumption of raw egg can cause biotin deficiency: Egg white protein avidin combines with biotin, preventing its absorption.

### Chemistry

- Imidazole derivative:
- Heterocyclic sulfur containing mono carboxylic acid
  Covalently bound to ε-amino group of lysine to form biocytin
- Contains cobalt in corrin ring

## Biotin is involved in carboxylation reactions:

1. Carbohydrate metabolism:
   Gluconeogenesis and citric acid cycle
   Pyruvate carboxylase:
   Pyruvate $\rightarrow$ OAA
   Acetyl CoA carboxylase:
   Acetyl CoA $\rightarrow$ malonyl CoA
   Propionyl CoA carboxylase:
   Propionyl CoA $\rightarrow$ methylmalonyl CoA
2. Lipid metabolism:
   Acetyl CoA carboxylase
   Propionyl CoA carboxylase
3. Protein metabolism
   $\beta$-methycrotonyl CoA carboxylase

### Biotin deficiency

- Deficiency is uncommon
- Seen in case of raw-egg consumption, multiple carboxylase deficiency

### Symptoms

- Depression
- Hallucination
- Muscle pain
- Dermatitis

### Facts

- Majority of requirement is by synthesis by intestinal bacteria
- RDA: 100-300 mg
- Source: liver, kidney, egg yolk, milk, tomatoes, grain

## Vitamin B$_{12}$

Also known as cobalamin, anti-pernicious anemia.

### Chemistry

**Empirical formula: Cyanocobalamin**: a complex ring structure: corrin ring with a central cobalt atom (similar to porphyrin ring)

### Two coenzyme forms:

- Methylcobalamin (methyl group replaces cyanide forming carbon cobalt bond)
- Produced by microorganisms. Animals obtain vitamin B$_{12}$ from intestinal flora and not plants.

### Absorption

- Mediated by intrinsic factor IF: secreted by parietal cells of gastric mucosa
- Cobalamin-IF complex travels through gut and absorbed by binding to receptor on surface of ileal mucosa
- After absorption cobalamin binds to transcobalamin (TCI, TC II)
- It is stored in liver (unique for a water-soluble vitamin) bound to TCI.
- It is secreted in bile and undergoes enterohepatic circulation (EHC) and disturbances of EHC can have major effect on vitamin B$_{12}$ status
- Methyl cobalamin and deoxyadenosyl cobalamin: active B$_{12}$ coenzymes

### IF (Intrinsic factor)

- Produced by gastric parietal cells
- Highly specific glycoprotein
- Required for absorption of vitamin B$_{12}$
- Lack of IF (or gastrectomy) causes pernicious anemia.

### Biochemical Functions

**Methylcobalamin:**

i. Homocysteine methyl transferase:

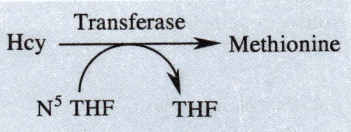

ii. Deoxyadenosyl cobalamin:

**Isomerase:** Converts methylmalonyl CoA to succinyl CoA

Occurs in odd chain fatty acid oxidation
Branch chain amino acids and pyrimidines (thymine and uracil) produce succinyl CoA directly or via propionyl CoA.

### RDA

- RDA: 3 mg/day
- Source: liver, kidney, milk, egg, fish

### Deficiency: Vitamin B$_{12}$

Occurs in:
- IF deficiency
- Vegan diet
- Ileal dysfunction

### Symptoms

- Pernicious anemia (IF deficiency)
- Megaloblastic anemia
- Neurological manifestations

### Cause of anemia in B$_{12}$ deficiency

Impaired DNA synthesis prevents cell division and formation of nucleus of new erythrocyte, resulting in accumulation of megaloblasts in bone marrow and circulation.

### Folate Trap

Vitamin B$_{12}$ deficiency leads to inhibition of both

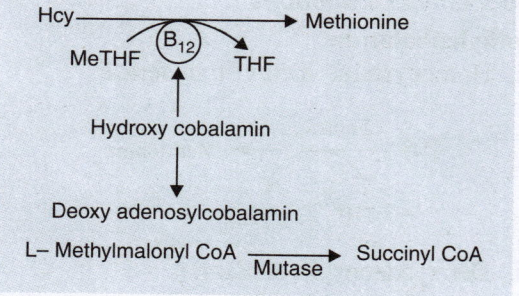

**Fig. 6.16.** Interrelationship between folate and vitamin B$_{12}$.

methylmalonyl CoA mutase and methionine synthase activity leading to:
- Methylmalonyl aciduria
- Homocystinuria
- Trapping of folate as methyl H$_4$ folate (folate trap)

**Interrelationship between folate and vitamin B$_{12}$:** Vitamin B$_{12}$ must be supplemented when folate treatment is given for megaloblastic anemia. If folate is given alone in case of vitamin B$_{12}$ deficiency, it aggravates neuropathy (refer to Fig. 6.16).

### Folic acid

Folic acid is abundant in given leafy vegetables and liver and is easily destroyed by cooking.

### Absorption

Intestinal enzymes (glutamyl hydrolase, conjugase) cleave dietary folate to monoglutamyl folate for absorption.

### Chemistry

**Pteroyl glutamic acid (PGA):** Consists of pteridine ring attached to PABA (p-amino benzoic acid) and glutamic acid.

**Plants:** Polyglutamate conjugate (seven residues) of folate

**In liver:** Pentaglutamate conjugate of folate

### Active form of folic acid: THF

Folic acid is physiologically inactive until reduced to:
- Dihydrofolate
- Tetrahydrofolate (THF)
- 5-methyl THF (N$^5$ MeTHF)
- N$^{10}$ formyl THF
- Functional form is THF-polyglutamate

## Functions: folate

Folate coenzyme (THF) acts as carriers of
1-carbon units:

**One-carbon units:**

- Methyl
- Methylene
- Methenylene
- Formyl
- Formimino
  (They are interconvertible)

**Reactions catalyzed:**

- Purine synthesis – $C_2$ and $C_8$
- Pyrimidine synthesis – dTMP

- Production of glycine, serine, ethanol-amine
- Protein synthesis – formyl methionine
- Methylation of homocysteine to methionine

**Note:** Refer to Section on 1-C metabolism in protein metabolism.

## Folate deficiency

**Cause:**

- Inadequate intake
- Impaired absorption
- Impaired metabolism

**Table. 6.54.** Water soluble vitamin: Function and deficiencies

| Vitamin | Biochemical function | Features of deficiency |
|---|---|---|
| Thiamine ($B_1$) | Cofactor for pyruvate and $\alpha$-ketoglutarate dehydrogenase | Beriberi, heart failure (wet beriberi)Wernicks–Korasakoff syndrome: ataxia, ophthalmoplegia, confusion, seen in chronic alcoholics |
| Riboflavin ($B_2$) | Precursor to coenzyme: FMN and FAD | Glossitis (atrophy of tongue,) cheilosis (fissures at corner of mouth), dermatitis, corneal ulceration. |
| Niacin ($B_3$) | Required for production of $NAD^+$ and $NADP^+$ as well as numerous dehydrogenase | Pellagra: diarrhea, dementia, dermatitis. Deficiency can occur as a result of antitubercular drug isoniazid, Hartnup's disease, carcinoid syndrome |
| Pyridoxine ($B_5$) | Required for transaminases and decarboxylation reactions | Required for GABA synthesis, so deficiency results in seizures. Deficiency can be associated with isoniazid or pencillamine use |
| Biotin | Required for carboxylation reaction | Synthesized by GIT bacteria, deficiency associated with long-term antibiotic use, consumption of raw egg (which contains avidin that binds & inhibits absorption of biotin) |
| Cobalamin ($B_{12}$) | Required by methylmalonyl CoA mutase and methionine synthase | Deficiency associated with lack of intrinsic factor megaloblastic anaemia, sub acute combined degeneration of spinal cord. |
| Folate | Reduced by DHF reductase to THF which functions as one carbon donor | Lack of folate results in impaired dTMP synthesis, hence megaloblastic anaemia folate supplementation is given in pregnant women for preventing neural tube defects |
| Vitamin C | Hydroxylation of proline in collagen, aid in iron absorption | Deficiency results in scurvy |

- Increased demand (pregnancy, lactation)

**Symptoms:**
- Megaloblastic anemia
- Neurological symptoms
- Increased erythrocyte fragility

## Antifolates

**Methotrexate:** Inhibitor of dihydrofolate reductase in human used as anticancer agent.

**Trimethoprim:** Inhibitor of folate reductase in gram-negative bacteria [Used as antibiotics].

## Facts: Folic acid

**RDA:** 100 mg/d.

**Source:** Green leafy vegetables, whole grains, cereals, liver, kidney, yeast, eggs.

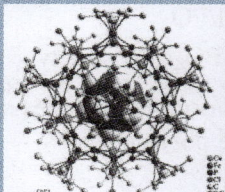

# CHAPTER 7

# Molecular Biology

## (I) NUCLEIC ACID STRUCTURE

### NUCLEIC ACID: STRUCTURE AND FUNCTION

### Nucleic acids: fact file

Exist in two forms:
- DNA (10%)
- RNA (90%)

Exist as polymers called *polynucleotides*. Each monomer is called *nucleotide*.

### Nitrogenous bases in DNA

They form hydrogen bonds in complementary fashion.

Basic pairing:
A with T only       A = T
C with G only       C ≡ G

### DNA and chromosomes

**Bacteria:**
- Single circular DNA

- E. coli chromosome has 4 million base pairs and 2000 genes.

**Eukaryotes:** Typically have several linear chromosomes inside nucleus. Humans have 46 chromosomes, 3 billion base pairs that code for up to 1lac different genes.

### Biological Importance: nucleic acid

1. **Nucleic acid:** store and transmit hereditary information
2. **DNA:** chemical basis of heredity, organized into genes.
3. **Genes:** are fundamental units of genetic information:
   - They control synthesis of DNA.
   - Genes do not function autonomously.
   - Their replication and function are controlled by various gene products.
4. **Knowledge** of nucleic acid helps in understanding genetic, molecular aspects of

disease and defining molecular level, normal cellular physiology and patho-physiology of disease.

## Gene function and regulation

Following are the important aspects of gene function that will be discussed in subsequent chapters:

- DNA structure
- Transcription
- Translation
- Protein synthesis
- Mutations
- Human genome
- Biotechnology

## Central dogma

- DNA contains the genetic information, stays in the nucleus.
- Transcription copies DNA into RNA and translation converts RNA into amino acid sequences.

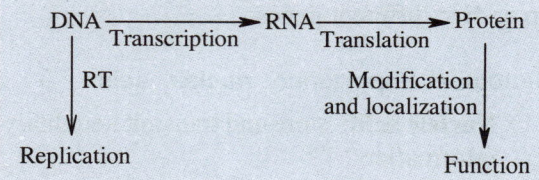

## RT: Reverse transcription

- Produces DNA copies of RNA
- More commonly associated with virus life cycle
- Also occurs in human to amplify certain highly repetitive sequences in DNA.

## DNA contains genetic information

DNA contains 4 deoxynucleotides:

- Deoxy adenylate
- Deoxy guanylate
- Deoxy cytidylate
- Thymidylate
- Monomeric limits are held in polymorphic form by 3′-5′ phosphodiesterase bridges.
- The information content of DNA resides in sequence where purine and pyrimidine deoxyribonucleotides are ordered.

  **Polarity of polymer is:**
  – One end has 5'-OH/$PO_4$
  – Other end has 3' – $PO_4$/OH moiety.

**Importance:** genetic information resides as monomeric units within the polymers.

## Chargaff's rule

In DNA molecules, [A] = [T], [G] = [C]

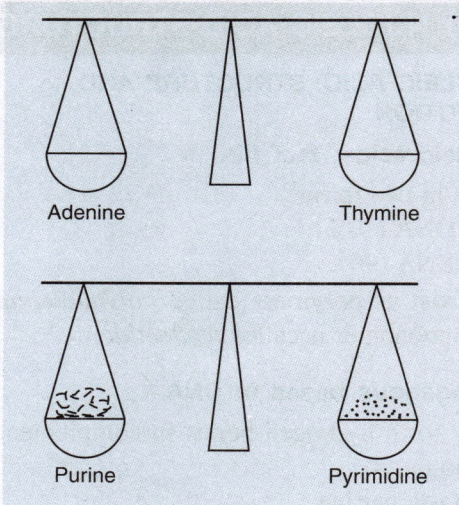

Fig. 7.1. Chargaff's rule.

This led Watson crick and Wilkins to propose double stranded structure of DNA molecule. i.e.,

%A = %T (%U)

%G = %C

% purine = % pyrimidine

## Exercise

A sample of DNA has 10% G, what is the %T:

10% G + 10% C = 20%

%A + %T = 100 − 20 = 80%

So, 40% A, 40% T

**Answer** = 40% T

## DNA double helix

- DNA molecule is composed of two poly-nucleotide chains joined by hydrogen bonds between the bases: double stranded molecule.
- Adenine on one chain base pairs with thymine on the other. Guanine base pairs with cytosine
- Base pairing on the two strands are complementary, adenine on one strand base pairs with thymine on other strand and guanine on one strand base pairs to cytosine.
- The chain runs in 5′ to 3′ direction and other in 3′ to 5′ i.e., chains are antiparallel.
- Also, double stranded molecule is twisted to form helix with major and minor grooves.
- In the interior of molecule base pairs of strands are stacked (like spiral stair case) and phosphate groups are on outer side of double helix.

## 3-D structure of DNA

- Deoxy ribosyl phosphate backbones of two strands are slightly offset from centre of helix. This result in grooves of two sizes: major groove, minor groove.
- **Right handed helix with antiparallel polarity.**

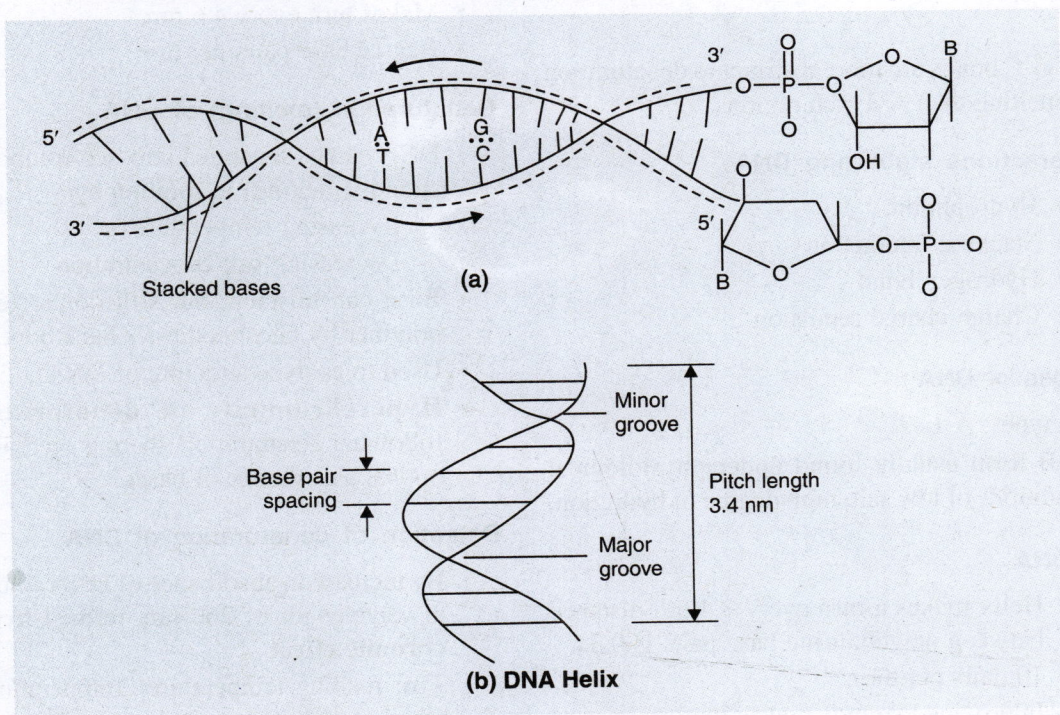

**Fig. 7.2.** (a) Structure of DNA. (b) DNA helix.

- One strand in 5'-3'
- Other strand in 3'-5' direction
- Genetic information resides in sequence of nucleotide in double-stranded DNA:
  - Template (noncoding) strand – that is copied during nucleic acid synthesis.
  - Coding strand – matches RNA transcript that encodes protein
- Base pairs are planar, oriented nearly perpendicular to axis of helix.
  'G' forms three H – bonds with 'C':
  $G \equiv C$
  'A' forms two H-bonds with 'T':
  $A = T$

There is specificity of interaction between purine and pyrimidine or opposite strands and opposing strands are termed **complementary**.

$$5' \longrightarrow 3'$$
$$3' \longleftarrow 5'$$

G-C bonds are more resistant to denaturation or melting than A-T rich regions.

### Interactions stabilizing DNA

- Hydrophobic
- Stacking interaction
- Hydrogen bond
- Charge-charge repulsion

### Types of DNA

Six types: A-E, Z.

B form usually found under physiological conditions of low salt, high degree of hydration.

### B-DNA

- Helix makes a turn every 3.4 nm distance between neighbouring base pairs is 0.34.
- 10 pairs per turn.
- Intertwined strands makes two grooves of different widths:

Major groove: Wide, and open
Minor groove: Shallow

- Strands are antiparallel, complementary
- When a solution of high salt concentration or alcohol is added, DNA structure may change to A form

### A-DNA

- Right handed
- Makes a turn every 2.3 nm, has 11 base pairs per turn

### Z-DNA

DNA molecule with alternating G-C sequences, in alcohol or high salt solutions tend to form Z form.

- Named so, because bases seem to zigzag.
- Left handed.
- Makes turn every 4.6 nm.
- Has 12 base pairs per turn.

### Denaturation (melting) of DNA

- DNA can be separated into two component strands (melting) in solution by:
  - Increasing temperature
  - Decreasing salt concentration
- Base can unstack, but still connected in polymer by phosphodiester back bone.
- Used to analyze structure of DNA.
- **Hyperchromicity of denaturation:** following denaturation, there is increase in optical absorbance of bases.

### Detection of denaturation of DNA

- By increase in absorbance of DNA solution at wavelength of 260 nm, termed **hyperchromic effect**
- **Tm:** melting temperature: Temperature at which molecule is half denatured
- Represents point at which enough heat

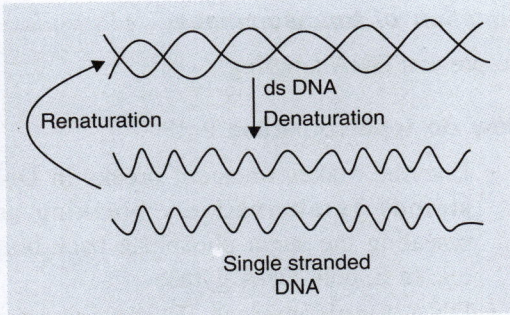

**Fig. 7.3.** DNA denaturation.

energy is present to break half the hydrogen bonds bonding two strands together.

- DNA sample with high G-C content will have high Tm due to three hydrogen bonds, while A-T has two H bonds.

**Tm** = Melting temperature: Strands of a given DNA molecule separate over a temperature range

   Tm influenced by:
   - Base composition
   - Salt concentration of solution.
   - Double stranded DNA molecule exhibit property of rigid rod and is viscous in solution.
   - Upon denaturation, it loses its viscosity.

## DNA stability

- DNA stability is provided by hydropholic stacking.
- Stability is increased by:
   - Decreased temperature
   - Increased G-C contest (3H-bond).
- Intercalating agents stack between bases.

   **Remember:**
   - Melting is denaturation
   - Annealing is renaturation

## Renaturation of DNA

- Denaturation is reversible

- Denatured strands of DNA can reform a duplex DNA structure: RENATURATION OR ANNEALING
- Following renaturation, absorbance of duplex DNA at 260 nm decreases

### Factors affecting reassociation

- Temperature: should be below Tm
- Concentration of complementary strand
- Salt conditions

   **COT analysis:** Measures dependence of DNA renaturation on low initial concentration (Co) of denatured DNA with time (t).

### Application of renaturation

- Southern blot (DNA/cDNA)
- Northern blot (DNA/RNA)
- Allow specific identification of hybrids from mixtures of DNA or RNA

### Organization of DNA

Large DNA needs to be packaged in such a way that they fit inside the cell and are still functional.

### Fact file: human genome

- Haploid genome has $3 \times 10^9$ bp, $1.7 \times 10^7$ nucleosomes
- Each of 23 chromatids in human haploid genome contains $1.3 \times 10^8$ nucleotides in one double stranded DNA molecule
- So, each DNA molecule must be compressed 8000 fold to form condensed metaphase chromosome.
- DNA in single human cell when stretched to its full length forms 1.74 m.
- Supercoiling helps to package DNA in nucleus.
- Supercoils are introduced when a closed circle to twist around its own axis or a linear piece of duplex DNA whose ends are fixed is twisted.

- Supercoiling is energy-requiring process.
- It puts molecule under torsional stress.
- Supercoiled DNA is a preferred form in biological system
- DNA exist in relaxed and super coiled form

## Supercoiling

DNA can be supercoiled:
- Positively
- Negatively

## Negative supercoiling

- Required for most biologic reactions
- Formed if DNA is wound more loosely than in Watson-Crick DNA.
- In B-DNA, it is twisted in direction opposite from clockwise turns of right-handed helix.

## Positive supercoiling

Formed if DNA is wound more tightly than in Watson Crick DNA

**Remember:** Supercoiling have higher free energy than non supercoiled relaxed DNA.

In bacteria, bacteriophage and DNA containing viruses and mitochondria:
- Ends of DNA molecules are joined to create a closed circle
- This does not destroy polarity of molecule only free 3′ and 5′ hydroxyl and phosphoryl groups are eliminated
- These closed circles can exist in released or supercoiled forms

## Topoisomerases

- Topoisomerase can relax or insert super-coils.
- During replication, unwinding of DNA may cause the formation of tangling structure such as supercoil. Without topoisomerases, DNA cannot replicate normally.

## Function of topoisomerase

To prevent DNA tangling.

## How do topoisomerase act?

- Enzyme makes transient breaks in DNA strands by alternatively breaking and resealing the sugar-phosphate back bone, e.g. In E. coli, DNA gyrase
- DNA topoisomerase II: can introduce negative supercoiling into DNA
- DNA topoisomerase I: can relax the supercoils

## Topoisomerase inhibitors

Used as anticancer drugs to stop the proliferation of malignant cells. However, these inhibitors may also stop division of normal cells.

## Genetic information is stored in nucleotide sequence of DNA

It serves two purposes:
1. Source of information for synthesis of all protein molecules of the cell and organism.
2. Provide information inherited by daughter cells or offspring.

## Comparison

| Gene expression | DNA replication |
|---|---|
| Produces all proteins in an organism | Duplicates chromosome before division |
| Transcription of DNA: RNA copy Average size of human gene: $10^4$-$10^5$ ntd pairs | DNA copy of entire chromosome $10^8$ ntd pairs |
| Translation of RNA: | |
| Protein synthesis occurs throughout interphase | Protein synthesis occurs during S-phase |
| Transcription in nucleus | Replication in nucleus |
| Translation in cytoplasm | |

# (II) DNA ORGANIZATION, REPLICATION, REPAIR

## Fact file

- Genetic information is contained in DNA of a chromosome.
- This information can be transmitted by:
  - Exact replication
  - Exchanged by a number of processes: crossing over, recombination, transposition and conversion.
- These processes provide a means of ensuring adaptability and diversity.
- If these processes go awry, diseases can result
- Mutations occur in one in every $10^6$ cell divisions
- Mutations can occur due to change in base sequence of DNA
- Viruses, chemicals, ultraviolet light and ionizing radiation increase rate of mutation
- Mutation in somatic cells are passed to same organism
- Mutation in germ line is transmitted to offspring.
- Number of diseases and most cancers are result of mutations.

## Chromatin

Chromatin consists of:

- Basic histone proteins
- Non-histone protein: acidic
- Very long DNA molecule
- Small amount of RNA

Non-histone proteins include:

  - DNA topoisomerase
  - RNA polymerase complex

## Composition

Thread-like strands of DNA wound around histone, arranged as nucleosomes: condensed, bodies of chromosomes

## Histones

Small family of closely related proteins

**Four types:**

  - $H_1$ – least tightly bound to chromatin, can be easily removed with salt solution
  - H2A
  - H2B
  - H3

## Modifications of histones occur covalently

- Acetylation
- Methylation
- Phosphorylation
- ADP-ribosylation
- Monoubiquitylation
- Sumoylation

## Role of modified histone

| Modification | Function |
| --- | --- |
| Acetylation | Chromosomal assembly during replication |
| Phosphorylation of $H_1$ | Condensation of chromosome during replication |
| ADP ribosylation | DNA repair |
| Methylation | Activation and repression of gene transcription |
| Monoubiquitylation | Gene activation, repression and heterochromatic gene silencing |

## Interaction of modified histones with each other

- $H_3$, $H_4$ form a tetramer of $(H_3/H_4)_2$
- $H_2A$ and $H_2B$ form dimer $(H_2A-H_2B)$

These histone oligomers associate to form histone octamer: $(H_3/H_4)_2 – (H_2A-H_2B)_2$

- $H_2A - H_2B$:
  - stabilize primary particle
  - firmly bind two additional half turns of DNA previously
  - loosely bound to $(H_3/H_4)_2$ tetramer
- 1.75 superhelical turns of DNA are wrapped around surface of histone octamer, forming nucleosome core particle, around 200 nucleotides of DNA wrap around core of histone
- Core particles are separated by 30 bp linker region of DNA giving beads-on-a-string appearance
- Each nucleosome interacts with one molecule of histone $H_1$ causing bead on a string structure to coil into a solenoid structure with a diameter of 30nm.
- Bending of DNA in a nucleosome

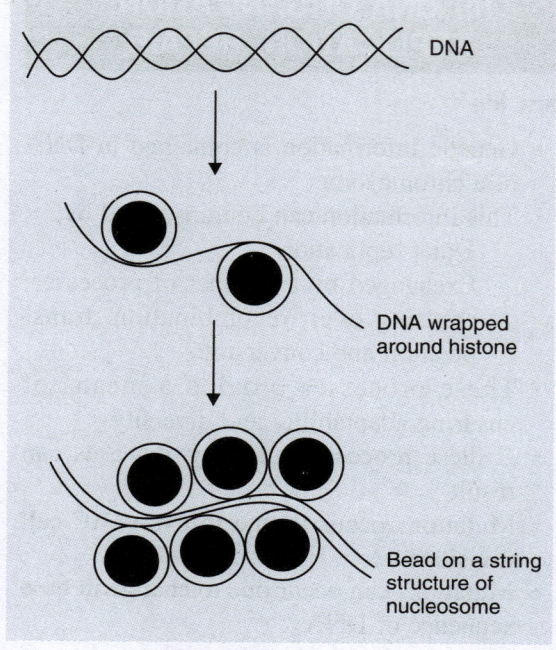

**Fig. 7.4.** Nucleosome.

### Nucleosome

- Contains histone and DNA
- DNA is supercoiled a left-handed helix over the surface of disk-shaped histone octamer
- Core histone proteins interact with DNA on the inside of supercoil.
- Amino terminal tails of all histones protrude outside this structure and undergo regulatory covalent modifications.

**Remember:**

Open chromatin: transcriptionally active

Closed or condensed chromatin: silenced.

### Active and inactive regions of chromatin

DNA in active chromatin contains:

- Large 100,000 bp long regions – sensitive to digestion by nuclease, e.g. DNase I
- Small stretches of 100-300 nucleotides that are more sensitive to DNase I

**Inactive chromatin or heterochromatin:** Densely packed chromatin in interphase

**Euchromatin:**

- Transcriptionally active chromatin
- Stains less densely
- Replicate earlier than heterochromatin in cell cycle.

### Chromosome

- Chromosomes pack DNA into final structure measuring 5 μm × 1 μm
- At metaphase, mammalian chromosomes posses 2-fold symmetry with identical duplicated sister chromatids connected at centromere

### Centromere

- AT-rich region, 102-106 in size

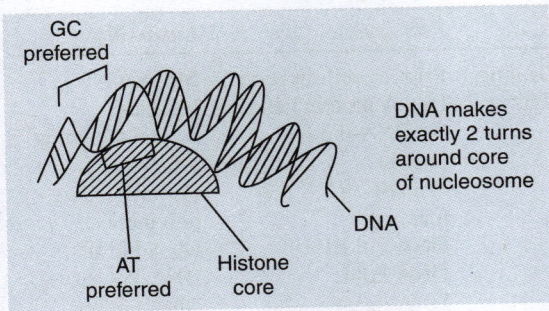

**Fig. 7.5.** Binding of DNA in a nucleosome.

- Binds several proteins with high affinity to form kinetochore.
- Kinetochore is anchor for mitotic spindle.

## Telomere

- The ends of each chromosome contain structures called telomeres
- Consists of short TG rich sequence repeats 5'-TTAGGG-3' repeats can extend several kb.

## Telomerase

- Multi subunit RNA containing complex related to reverse transcriptase
- Enzyme responsible for telomere synthesis
- Maintain length of telomere.

## Replication

Double helical model of DNA suggested that strands can separate and act as templates for formation of new complementary strand.

**Semiconservative replication:** After replication, each daughter cell receive parental DNA strand and one newly synthesized complementary strand.

DNA can make copies of itself: Replication

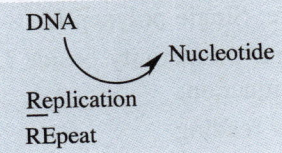

DNA
→ Nucleotide
<u>R</u>eplication
<u>RE</u>peat

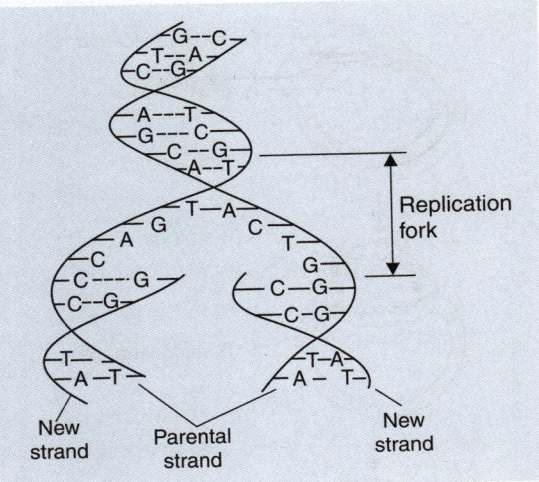

**Fig. 7.6.** Replication of DNA.

## Basic requirements for DNA synthesis

- **Substrates:**
  dNTPs: dATP, dGTP, dCTP, dTTP
- **'E':** cleavage of high energy phosphate bond between α and β phosphate
- **Template:** each strand of parental DNA serves as a template
- **Primer:** prepares template strand for addition of nucleotide
- **Enzyme:** DNA-dependent DNA polymerase

| Comparison | | |
|---|---|---|
| | *DNA polymerase* | *RNA polymerase* |
| Nucleic acid synthesized (5'→3') | DNA | RNA |
| Template | DNA | DNA |
| Substrate | dATP, dGTP, dCTP, **dTTP** | ATP, GTP, CTP, **UTP** |
| Primer | RNA (or DNA) | None |
| Proof reading activity | Yes (have 3'-5' exonuclease activity) | No |

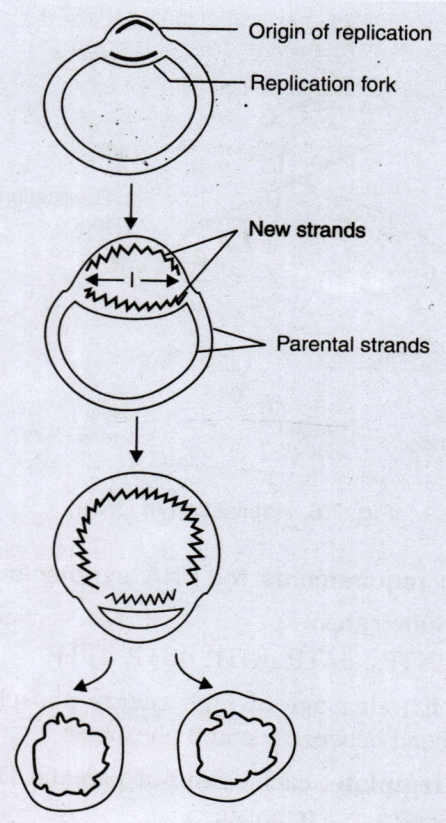

**Fig. 7.7.** Replication of circular chromosome.

### Similarities of DNA and RNA polymerases

- Newly synthesized strand is made in 5'→3' direction
- Template strand is scanned in 3'→5' direction
- Newly synthesized strand is complementary and antiparallel to template strand.
- Each new nucleotide is added when 3' OH group of growing strand reacts with a nucleoside triphosphate, which is base-paired with template strand and PPi is rebased.

| | Prokaryotic | Eukaryotic |
|---|---|---|
| Timing | Prior to cell division | S-phase |
| Enzyme | Dna A protein helicase | Helicase |
| | Sa DNA-binding protein | Sa DNA binding protein |
| | Primase (RNA polymerase) | Primase (RNA polymerase) |
| | DNA Pol III | DNA Pol θ |
| | DNA Pol I | DNA Pol ex |
| | DNA ligase | DNA ligase |
| | DNA gyrase (topo II) | DNA topo II |
| | | Telomerase |

### DNA polymerases

- E. coli: 3 types: I, II, III
- Pol I: Used to fill gap between DNA fragments of lagging strand major enzyme for gap-filling during DNA repair
- Pol II: Encoded by Pol B gene, involved in SOS response to DNA damage
- Pol III: Carries out DNA replication

### Prokaryotic DNA polymerase

| | I | II | III |
|---|---|---|---|
| 5'→3' exonuclease | + | − | − |
| 3'→5' exonuclease | − | − | − |
| Synthesis rate (ntd/min) | 600 | 30 | 30,000 |
| Molecules/cell | 400 | ? | 10 |
| Replication | + | − | + |
| Repair | + | + | − |

### DNA polymerase

- Function:
  - Replication of DNA
  - Repair of damaged DNA
- Structure: Single polypeptide
- Other enzyme activity beside DNA polymerase function:
  - Proof reading

– Excision-repair
– Nick translation

## Proof reading

- $3' \rightarrow 5'$ exonuclease activity which removes mismatched ntd.
- Assures high level of fidelity

## Excision repair

- Pol I has $5' \rightarrow 3'$ exonuclease activity
- Can hydrolytically remove a DNA segment from 5' end of strand of duplex DNA: 1-10 ntd can be removed simultaneous
- Essential for removal of primers.

## Nick translation

- Nick is break in phosphodiester bond of one strand of DNA in a double helix.
- Nick leaves a free $3' - OH$ group and a free $5'$-phosphate group.
- Pol I can function as an exonuclease and polymerase at the same time.

## POL II

- Minor polymerase of E. coli.
- Single polypeptide
- Involved in DNA repair
- Has proof reading function (3'-5')
- Lacks excision repair activity.

## POL III

- Involved in cellular replication
- Catalyzes leading and lagging strand synthesis.

## Structure

- Core complex: 3 polypeptide
- Pol I holoenzyme: 10 subunit polypeptide
- Subunits organized into asymmetric dimer with two catalytic centres.

- 2 ∈ subunits: Exonuclease activity
- 2 β subunits: Dimer: Circles DNA
- $\beta_2$ clamp: Enables Pol III holoenzyme to stay bound to DNA and facilitates high rate of replication.
- Has proof-reading 3'-5' action
- No excision repair activity.

## Remember

DNA polymerase can only copy a DNA template in $3' \rightarrow 5'$ direction and produce newly synthesized strand in 5' to 3' direction.

## DNA Pol

- Requires a primer
- Cannot initiate synthesis of new strands
- RNA serves as primer (about 10 ntd) formed by copying of parent strand by primase
- Adds dNTP to 3'-hydroxyl of RNA primer

## Eukaryotic DNA Pol

- DNA pol ∈ : Synthesize leading strand during replication
- DNA pol δ: Synthesize lagging strand
- DNA pol γ: Replicates mitochondrial DNA
- DNA pol σ: Primase
- DNA pol β and ∈ : Participate primarily in DNA repair
- DNA pol α: Replication of nuclear DNA

## Eukaryotic RNA Pol

| RNA pol | Location | Product | Amantin sensitivity |
|---------|----------|---------|---------------------|
| Pol I | Nucleolus | 28S, 18S, 5.8S rRNA | Insensitive |
| Pol II | Nucleoplasm | mRNA, some snRNA | Very sensitive |
| Pol III | Nucleoplasm | rRNA, 5S rRNA, rest of snRNA | Less sensitive |

| Step in DNA replication | Prokaryotes | Eukaryote |
|---|---|---|
| 1 Recognizition of origin of replication | dnaA protein | – |
| 2 Unwinding of DNA double helix | Helicase, requires ATP | Helicase, requires ATP |
| 3 Synthesis of RNA primers | Primase | Primase |
| 4 Synthesis of DNA: | | |
| Leading strand | DNA Pol III | Pol $\in$ |
| Lagging strand | Pol III | Pol $\delta$ |
| Okazaki fragment | | |
| 5 Removal of RNA primer | DNA pol I (5′→3′ exonuclease) | Unknown |
| 6 Replacement of RNA with DNA | DNA Pol I | Unknown |
| 6 Joining of Okazaki fragments | DNA ligase (require NAD) | DNA ligase(require ATP) |
| 7 Removal of positive supercoils ahead of advancing replication fork | DNA topo I (DNA gyrase) | DNA topo II |
| 8 Synthesis of telomeres | Not required | Telomerase |

## Functions RNA Pol

- $\alpha, \delta, \in$ : Replication
- $\beta$: No role in replication
- $\gamma$: Replication of mt DNA

## DNA synthesis and replication are rigidly controlled

Primary function of replication is to pass genetic information from parents to progeny.

## Precursors of DNA synthesis

Deoxyribose diphosphate, dATP, dGTP, dTTP, dCTP.

## Origin of replication

- In prokaryotes, replication starts at DNA sequence called origin: ori
  1. Ori C:
     - Single origin in E. coli
     - 240 bp sequence
     - Direct initiation of replication
  2. Dna A protein:
     - Protein in E. coli
     - Required for initiation of replication at origin
     - Binds to specific sequence within ori C in present of ATP and other components of replication
  3. Replication fork:
     - Replication, after initiation, proceeds away from origin
     - Replication proceeds bidirectionally.
- Prokaryotes have one site of origin on each chromosome
- Eukaryotes have multiple sites of origin on each chromosome.

## Replication fork

Replication forks are the sites where DNA synthesis is occurring. Parental strands separate, helix unwinds ahead of replication fork, 5SBP hold it in single strand conformation and topoisomerase prevent supercoiling.

Replication fork is unwound, parental

template DNA strands to which newly synthesized complementary DNA is paired.

## Steps in DNA replication

- Enzymes unwind double stranded DNA
- Proteins stabilize unwound DNA
- Leading strand synthesized continuously by DNA pol in 5'-3' direction.
- Lagging strand synthesized discontinuously.
- RNA polymerase make RNA primer and DNA polymerase extend it.
- Okazaki fragment: RNA-DNA fragment.
- DNA polymerase digest RNA primers and replace them with DNA
- DNA ligase joins discontinuous fragments of lagging strand.

## Error rate

- 1 out of $10^{10}$ bases is changed (mutation), DNA pol has proof reading function.
- Replication regions $O_1$, $O_2$, $O_3$ serve replicon region $R_1$, $R_2$, $R_3$.
- Unwinding of double helix occurs
- DNA pol synthesizes new strands using template.
- Replication region looks like a bubble called: replication bubble.

## DNA replication process

### In E. coli

- Movement of growing fork is 100 bp per second
- It takes about 42 minutes to duplicate the entire genomic DNA.

### Eukaryote

- Fork movement is 100 bp per second

- This is probably due to association of DNA with histones which may hinder the fork movement.

### In human

Replication of entire genome requires 8 hours.

## Basic event at replication fork

### 1. Lagging strand synthesis

**Okazaki fragments:** newly synthesized daughter strand is made discontinuously in the form of Okazaki fragment (5'→3' direction)

- Pol III catalyzes lagging strand synthesis
- Direction of new synthesis: 5'→3'
- New strands move away from replication fork.

### 2. Priming

- Primase enzyme initiate Okazaki fragment
- Primase initiate leading strand synthesis.
- Primer provide 3'-OH group to initiate DNA synthesis

### 3. Joining of okazaki fragments

After pol I has removed RNA primer and replaced it with DNA, ligase catalyzes the formation of phosphodiesterase bond between adjoining fragments.

### 4. Synthesis of DNA

DNA replication also requires helicase, single strand binding protein (SSBP).

**Helicase:** Unwinds duplex DNA

**SSB protein:** Bind both separated strands, preventing them to anneal

### Similarity

- Replication in bacteria and eukaryotes are similar.
- Eukaryotic DNA pol does not contain a

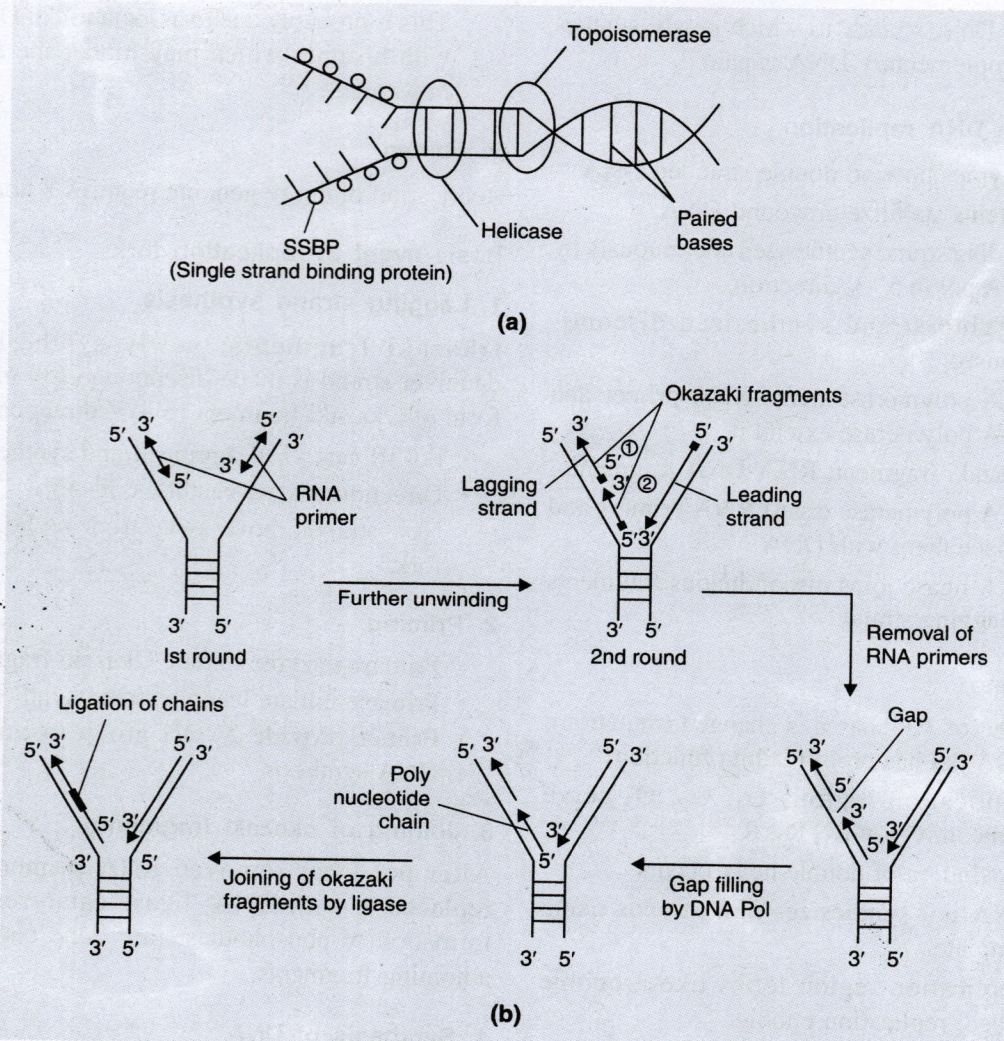

**Fig. 7.8.** (a) Separation and unwinding of parental DNA strands at replication form. (b) Replication process.

subunit similar to E. coli β subunit. They use a separate protein called proliferating cell nuclear antigen (PCNA) to clamp the DNA.

**Facts – DNA synthesis**

- DNA pol extends nucleic strands in 5'→3' direction only.

- In growing fork, direction of one strand is from 5'→3': **Leading strand:** can be synthesized continuously.

- The other strand: **Lagging strand:** its 5'→3' direction is opposite to the movement of growing fork and is synthesized disconti-nuously via Okazaki fragments.

## Factors required for propagation of replication fork

- Helicase: To unwind DNA helix
- Gyrase:
  - Topoisomerase
  - Prevents built up of replication fork
- SSBP: Enhance activity of helicase, protects ss DNA from degradation by nucleases
- Primosome: Complex of primase, hexamer of helicase, dnaB, dnaC.
  Function: primes DNA synthesis at origin
- Replisome: Termination utilization substance
- Termination:
  - Thus protein binds to termination sequence
  - Prevents helicase, dna B from unwinding of DNA, leading to termination of replication

## Eukaryotic replication

- Similar to that in prokaryotes
- Semi conservative
- Proceeds bidirectionally from many origins.

## Factors involved in eukaryotic replication

- $5' \to 3'$ exonuclease: Association with DNA pol $\beta$
- $5' \to 3'$ exonuclease: DNA pol $\delta$, $\in$ and $\gamma$ have proof-reading function
- Ligase:
  - Involved in repair and replication
  - Involved in DNA repair, synthesis
  - Uses ATP instead of NAD in prokaryotes
- Helicase
- SSBP – called replication protein (rp-A)
- Topoisomerase – relieve positive super coils.

## Topoisomerases

Topoisomerase relieve supercoils that build up in advance of replication fork.

## Types

### Topoisomerase I

- Major topoisomerase
- Relieve supercoils
- *Breaks one strand* of DNA, passing other strand through the break, then re-ligating the broken strand.

### Topoisomerase II

- Required during replication to resolve final knots that form when adjacent replication forks meet.
- Separate double helical strands of DNA by *cutting both the strands* of helices and passing other strand through the break before religating the cut helix.

### Applied aspect

Etoposide inhibits topoisomerase and is widely used in treatment of lung, ovarian, testicular and prostate cancer.

### Telomerase

In eukaryotes, the chromosome ends are called telomeres that serve two functions of telomeres:

- To prevent chromosome from fusing with each other.
- To solve end-replication problem

### Telomeres: Fact file

- Short tandem repeats of tandem sequence of TTAGGG.
- 3' end of these repeats is single stranded

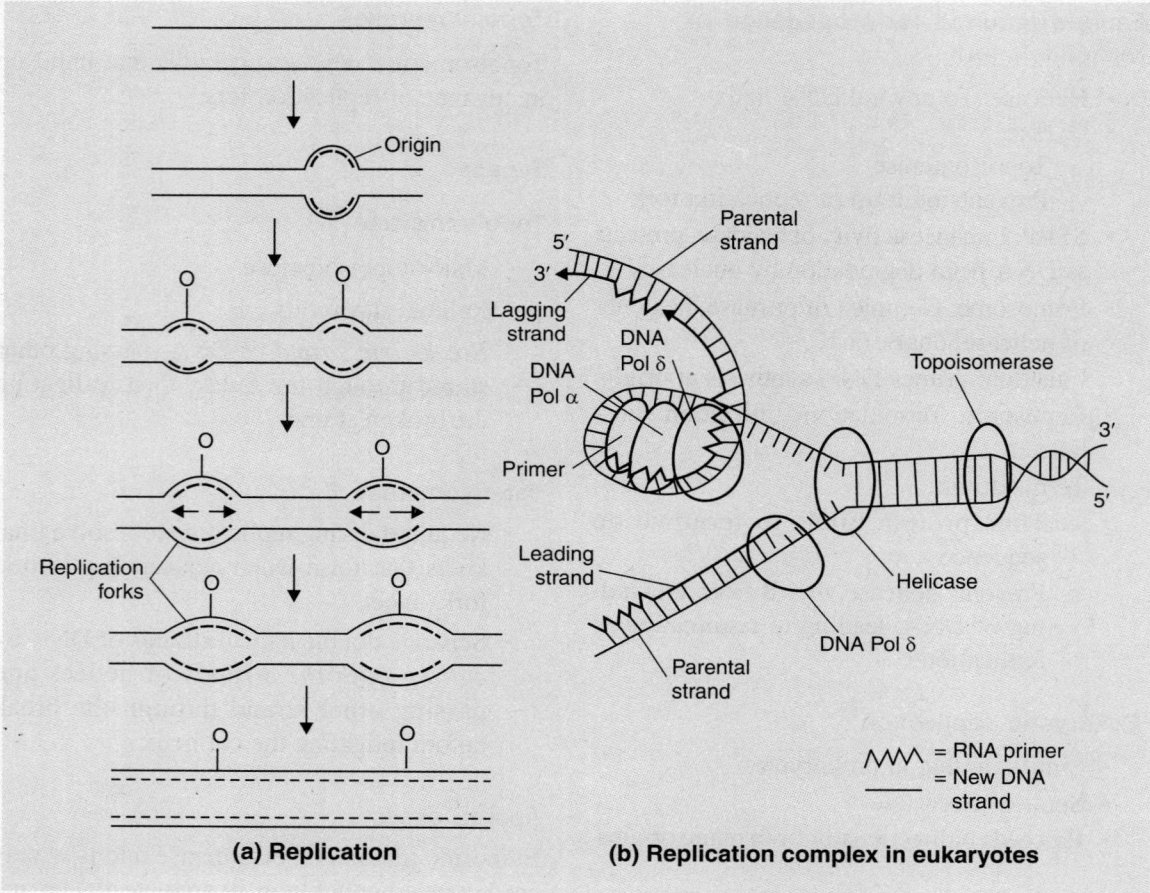

**Fig. 7.9.** (a) Replication, (b) Replication complex in eukaryotes.

- With each round of replication in most normal cells, telomeres are shortened because DNA pol cannot complete synthesis of 3′ end of each strand.

  This contributes to the *aging of cells* because telomeres become so short that chromosomes cannot function properly and cells die.

- In a human chromosome:
  - Telomere is 10-15 kb in length
  - Composed of tandem repeat sequence: TTAGGG

**Telomere extension**

- Carried out by telomerase
- Telomerase contains RNA component complementary to the telomere repeat sequence and serve as template for synthesizing DNA.
- Contain telomerase reverse transcriptase (hTRT) activity
- Through telomerase translocation, a telomere may be extended by many repeat.
- Telomerase is able to replace telomere

sequences that would be otherwise lost during replication.

## Clinical relevance: Telomerase

- Normally telomerase activity is present only in embryonic cells, germ (reproductive) cell and stem cells, but not in somatic cells.
- Cancer cells often have relatively high levels of telomerase, preventing telomeres from becoming shortened and contributing to immortality of malignant cells.
- Contributes to aging of cells.

## Telomeres

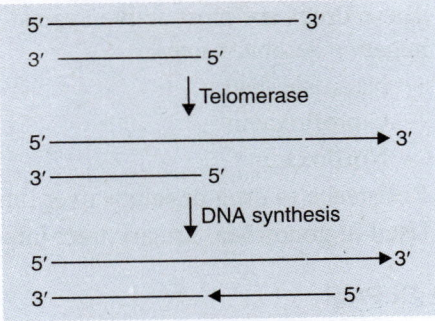

**Fig. 7.10.** Telemerases.

- To extend length of a telomere, telomerase first extends the longer strand.
- Then, using same mechanism as synthesis of lagging strand, shorter strand is extended.

## Aging

- In absence of telomerase, telomere will become shorter after each cell division.
- When it reaches a certain length, the cell may cease to divide and die.
- Synthesis of lagging strand requires a short primer which will be removed

- It is extreme end of a chromosome, there is no way to synthesize this region.
- Lagging strand is shorter than its template by atleast the length of the primer. This is so-called **End-replication problem**.

## DRUGS THAT AFFECT REPLICATION

- Antibacterial
- Antiviral
- Chemotherapeutic drugs

### 1. Antimetabolites

Inhibit/decrease product of substrate for replication (dNTP):

- 5FU-5 fluorouracil:
  - Analogue of uracil
  - Thymidylate synthase trapped in complex with F-d UMP.
- $MTX_2$:
  - Methotrexate antifolate:
  - Inhibit dihydrofolate reductase.
- 6MP, Thioguanine:
  - Analogue of purine:
    - Via HGPRT, ribonucleotidase
    - Inhibit amidotransferase

### 2. Substrate analogus: of dNTP

i. Dideoxy nucleoside analogs: Antiviral-acting on viral DNA polymerase:

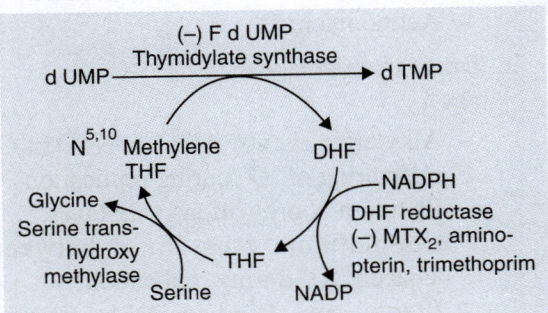

**Fig. 7.11.** Antimetabolites.

– Zidovudine (AZT)
– Didanosine (ddc)
– Zalcitabine
– Stavudine
ii. Cytarabine:
– Analogs of 2' deoxycytidine
– Slows rate of replication following its incorporation into DNA.

## Reverse transcriptase

### RNA-dependent DNA polymerase

• Requires RNA template to synthesize new DNA.
• Retroviruses (e.g. HIV), use this enzyme to replicate their genomes
• Inhibited by AZT, ddc in retroviruses
• Eukaryotic cells also contain reverse transcriptase activity:
– Associated with telomerase
– Encoded by retrotransposons: residual viral genomes permanently maintained in human. They play a role in amplifying certain repetitive sequences in DNA.

## 3. Inhibitors that intercalate directly with DNA

i. Intercalators:
– Anthracycline: dauno-/doxo-rubicin
– Actinomycin D
ii. Drugs that damage DNA:
– Alkylating agents: Alkylate NTD of G-mispairing of 'G' during replication
– Platinum-coordination complexes: Cis-platinum cross links between adjacent 'G' during replication.
– Bleomycin: Bind to DNA, causing DNA breakage.

## 4. Inhibitors of replication enzyme

• DNA pol inhibitor:
Topoisomerase inhibitor:
Quinolines, fluoroquinolines: inhibit bacterial topoisomerase, DNA gyrase
• Complexes with topoisomerase and inhibit replication:
– Etoposide
– Tenopside

## Quinolones and DNA gyrase

• Quinolines and fluoroquinolines inhibit DNA gyrase (prokaryotic topoisomerase II), preventing DNA replication and transcription.
• These drugs are most active against gram-negative aerobic bacteria:
– Nalidixic acid
– Ciprofloxacin
– Norfloxacin
• Resistance to drug develops over time.
• Used in gonorrhea, urinary tract infection.

## DNA REPAIR

### DNA damage

DNA can be damaged in number of ways:
• Through chemicals or radiation exposure
• Incorporation of incorrect base pairs during replication

### DNA repair

• Multiple repair systems have been evolved to maintain sequence stability of genomes in the cell.
• Numerous mechanisms exist in prokaryotes and eukaryotes to repair damaged DNA before mutants become fixed by replication.
• If cells are allowed to replicate using damaged template, there is risk of:

– Introducing stable mutation in new DNA

– Developing cancer if repair mechanism is defective.

• DNA repair mostly occurs in $G_1$ phase of eukaryotic cell cycle.

• Mismatch repair occurs in $G_2$ phase to correct replication errors.

## DNA repair involves 3 steps

• Removal of damaged or mismatched base filling in the gap by DNA pol

• Ligation of newly synthesized segment to rest of chain.

## DNA repair mechanisms

• Base excision
• Nucleotide excision
• Mismatch repair

| DNA repair mechanism in E. coli | |
|---|---|
| *Repair system* | *Enzyme/proteins* |
| Base excision | DNA glycosylase<br>AP endonuclease<br>DNA pol I<br>DNA ligase |
| Nucleotide excision | Uvr-A, Uvr-B, Uvr-C<br>DNA pol I<br>DNA ligase |
| Mismatch | Dam methylase<br>Exonuclease<br>Mut S, Mut L, Mut H<br>DNA helicase II<br>SSB protein<br>DNA pol III<br>DNA ligase |

## Base excision

• DNA base may be modified by deamination or alkylation

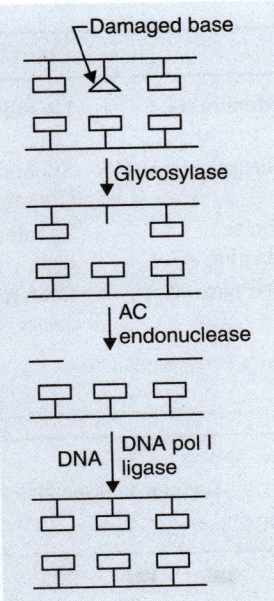

Fig. 7.12. Base excision repair.

• This position of modified (damaged) base is called ABASIC or AP SITE

• In E. Coli:

– DNA glycosylase can recognize AP site and removes its base

– Then, AP endonuclease removes AP site and neighbouring nucleotides

– Gap is filled by DNA pol I and DNA ligase.

## Nucleotide excision

**In E. coli:** UvrA, UvrB, UvrC proteins are involved in removing damaged nucleotides (e.g. thymidine dimer)

– Gap is fitted by DNA pol I and DNA ligase.

**In yeast:** Proteins similar to Uvr$_s$ are named RADxx (RAD: radiation), such as RAD$_3$, RADIO etc.

## DNA repair

| Damage | Cause | Recognition/Excision enzyme | Repair Enzyme |
|---|---|---|---|
| 1. Thymine dimers ($G_1$) | Uv radiation | Excision endonuclease (deficient in Xeroderma pigmentosum) | DNA Pol DNA ligase |
| 2. Cytosine deamination ($G_1$) | Spontaneous/ Chemicals | Uracil glycosylase, AP endonuclease | DNA pol DNA ligase |
| 3. Apurination or Apyrimidination ($G_1$) | Spontaneous/ heat | AP endonuclease | DNA pol DNA ligase |
| 4. Mismatched base ($G_2$) | DNA replication errors | Mutation on one of two genes: hMSH 2 or hMSH 1 initiates defective repair of DNA mismatches. Causes: hereditary nonpolyposis colorectal cancer (HNPCC) | DNA pol DNA ligase |

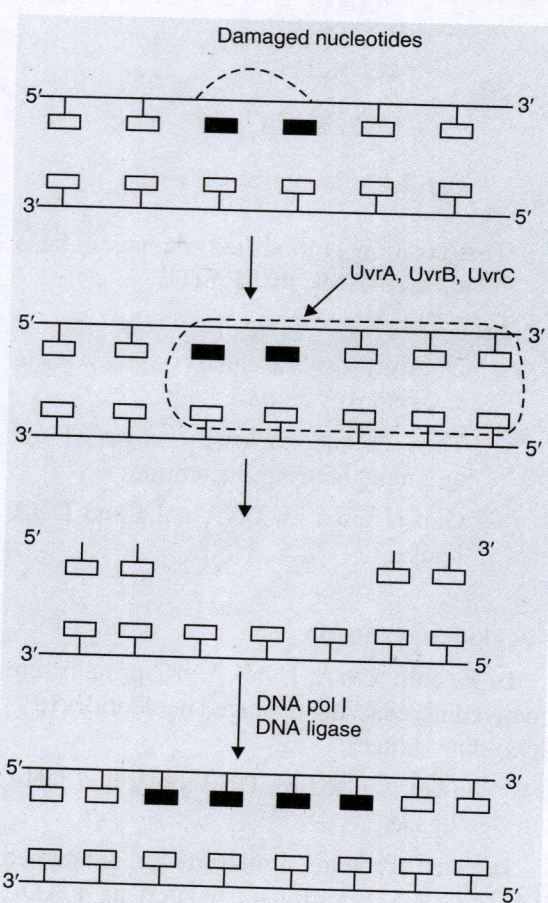

**Fig. 7.13.** Nucleotide excision repair.

### Mismatch repair

- To repair mismatched basis, system has to know which base is the correct one
- In E. coli:
  - **Dam methylase:** methylates all adenine that occur within (5') GATC sequences.
  - Immediately after DNA replication, template strand is methylated and newly synthesized strand is not methylated.
  - Thus, template and new strand can be distinguished.

### Tumor suppressor genes and DNA repair

- DNA repair may not occur properly if certain tumor suppressor genes have been inactivated by mutation or deletion
  - $p_{53}$ gene encodes a protein that prevents entry of cell with damage into S phase.
  - Inactivation or deletion is associated with Li Fraumeni syndrome and many solid tumor
- ATM gene
  - ATM gene encodes a kinase for $p_{53}$ activity.
  - ATM is inactivated in ataxia, telangiectasia.

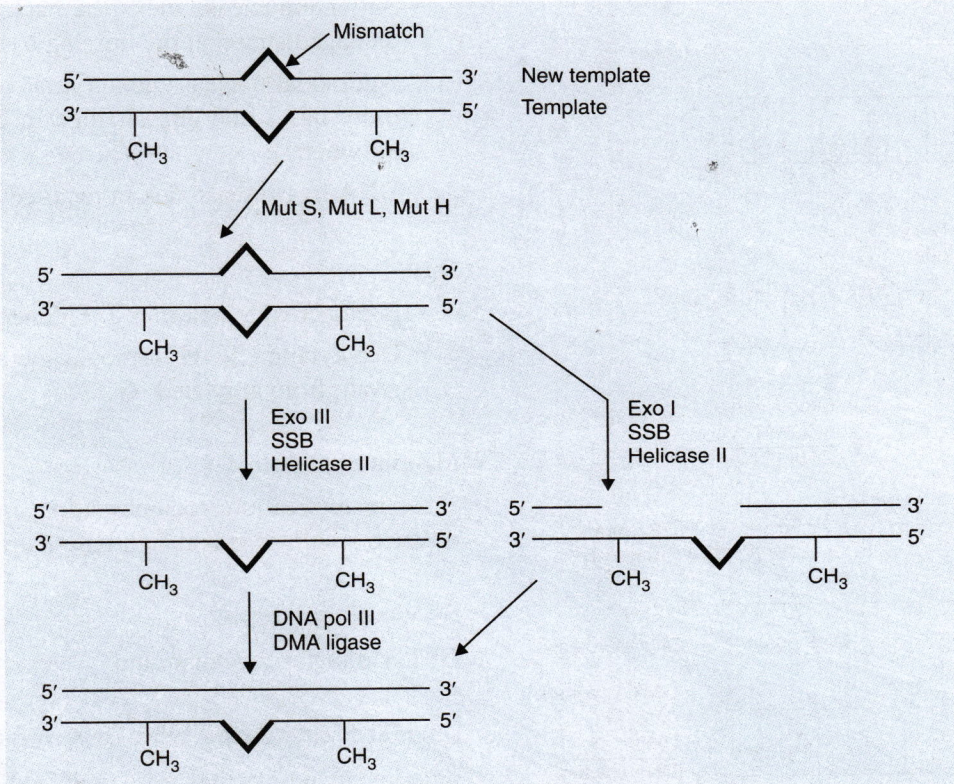

**Fig. 7.14.** Mismatch repair.

- ATM is characterized by hyper-sensitivity to X-rays, predisposition to lymphoma.
- BRCA gene: required for $p_{53}$ activity
  - BRCA-1: Breast, prostate, ovarian cancer
  - BRCA-2: Breast cancer

## Types of DNA repair

### 1. Excision repair

To recognize and excise damaged DNA
- Prokaryotes:
  - Multigene family : Uvr gene:
  - Recognizes and excises thymine dimer
- Mechanism: Uvr gene products:
  - Unwind DNA
  - Cut sugar-phosphate back bone within 7 ntd on each side of T-T dimer
- DNA pol I fills gap by synthesizing DNA in $5' \rightarrow 3'$ direction
- DNA ligases seals nick in repaired strand.

### 2. Apurenic repair

- Depurination/ depyrimidination occurs
- Repair of deaminated and missing bases occurs.
- Repair of deaminated and missing bases:
- Cytosine can become deaminated:

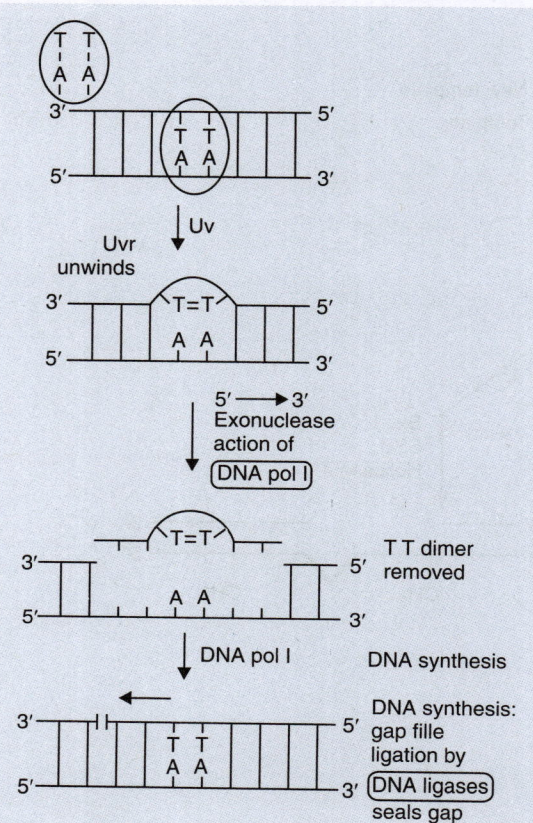

**Fig. 7.15.** Excision repair.

- Spontaneously
- By reaction with nitrous acid to form uracil
- This causes improper base pair (G-U) which is eliminated by a base excision repair mechanism.
- Failure to repair improper base pair can convert a normal G-C pair to A-T pair
- Removal of uracil: Deamination of 'C' by uracil N-glycosylase

## Base excision repair steps

- Uracil glycosylase recognizes and removes uracil base, leaving apyrimidinic (AP) site in DNA strand

- AP endonuclease nicks the back bone of damaged strand at the missing base
- Additional nuclease action removes a few more bases and gap is filled in by DNA polymerase
- DNA ligase seals nick in repaired strand.

### Direct repair

- Photoactivation cleaves T-T dimer
- Dealkylation of 'G' removes methyl/ethyl group from alkylated 'G'.

### Mismatch repair

Error in replication, recombination, insertion, deletion results in mis-match base pairing.

### Recombinant repair

Of T-T dimer, repair of strand.

### Diseases associated with DNA repair

Inherited mutations that result in defective DNA repair mechanism are associated with a predisposition to development of cancer.

**Examples:**

- Xeroderma pigmentosum
- Hereditary non polyposis colorectal cancer (HNPCC).

### Summary: DNA repair

**$G_1$ phase of eukaryotic cell cycle:**

- UV radiation: Thymine dimer: exonuclease
- Deamination (C→U): uracil glycosylase
- Loss of purine or pyrimidine: AP endonuclease

**$G_2$ phase of eukaryotic cell cycle:** Mismatch repair: hMSH1, hMSH2 (HNPCC).

# (III) TRANSCRIPTION

## Synthesis of RNA

### RNA differs from DNA:

- In RNA, sugar moiety is ribose rather than 2′ deoxyribose of DNA
- Pyrimidine component differs:
  - RNA contains A, G, C, U
  - DNA contains A, G, C, T
- RNA exists as single strand, DNA exists as double stranded helix
  Hairpin structure is possible in RNA
- RNA: Guanine content does not necessarily equal to its cytosine content, adenine content does not necessarily equal its uracil content.
- RNA can be hydrolyzed by alkali to 2′, 3′ cyclic diesters with mononucleotides, while DNA cannot be hydrolyzed due to absence of 2′ hydroxyl group.
  This alkali lability property is useful diagnostically and analytically.
- Some RNA molecules act as **catalyst** e.g. Ribozymes:
  **Ribozymes:** usually precursors of rRNA, removing internal segments of themselves and splicing the ends together.
- **Ribonuclease:** cleaving other RNA molecules (e.g. RNase pol cleaves tRNA precursors)
- **Peptidyl transferase:** contains RNA

## Transcription

DNA → RNA

Synthesis of RNA directed by a DNA template.

### How do you remember the difference?

- **R**eplication just makes a **re**peat copy of DNA
- Trans**crip**tion **rips** a new strand of **RNA**
- Trans**lat**ion starts with a new **slate** the slate of amino acids to make a protein.

### Comparison

| | DNA replication | Transcription |
|---|---|---|
| Product | DNA copy from DNA | RNA from DNA |
| Template strands | 2 | 1 |
| Primer required? | Yes | No |
| Proof reading? | Yes | No |
| Precursors | dNTPs (G, A, T, C) | NTP (G, A, U, C) |
| Main enzymes | DNA pol | RNA pol |
| Bi- or uni-directional? | Bi-directional, growing bubble | Unidirectional, moving bubble |

### RNA polymerase

- RNA polymerase initiate synthesis of new chains
- No primer required

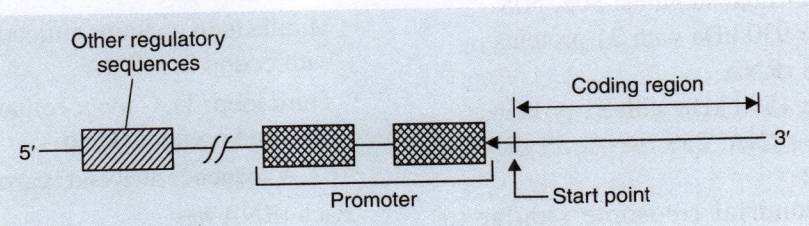

**Fig. 7.16.** Regions of a gene.

- DNA copied in 3′ to 5′ direction
- DNA copied in 3′ to 5′ direction RNA chain grows in 5′ to 3′ direction
- Ribonucleotide triphosphate: ATP, GTP, UTP, CTP serve as precursors for RNA synthesis

## Prokaryotes

RNA pol of E coli:

- Has four subunits: $\alpha_2\beta\beta'$
- Forms core enzyme and fifth subunit sigma ($\sigma$) for initiation of RNA synthesis.

## Applied aspect

**Rifampicin:**

- Inhibits $\beta$ subunit of bacterial DNA-dependent RNA pol
- Used in treatment of tuberculosis

## Ribosomes

**3 types:**
  - mRNA
  - tRNA
  - rRNA

**Site of protein synthesis:**
  - mRNA used as template
  - tRNA causes pairing with appropriate amino acids.

**Prokaryotes**, e.g. E.coli ribosome:
  - 25 nm diameter
  - 2520 kDa in mass
  - Has 2 unequal subunits: 30S, 50S
    - **30S:** 930 kDa with 21 proteins 16 S rRNA
    - **50S:** 1590 kDa with 31 proteins Two rRNA: 23S rRNA, 5S rRNA

**Eukaryotes:**
  - Mitochondrial ribosome similar to prokaryotic

  - Cytoplasmic ribosomes:
    Larger and more complex
    - 40S subunits: 30 proteins, 18 SrRNA
    - 60S subunits: 40 proteins 3S rRNA

**mRNA:** Contains a cap structure and Poly A tail

**Cap:** Methylated GTP attached to OH group on ribosome at 5′ end of mRNA

$N^7$ of guanine methylated

2′-OH group of $1^{st}$ and $2^{nd}$ ribose moiety may also be methylated.

## mRNA

- Source of coding information for protein synthesis
- Contains start and stop signals for translation
- Eukaryotic mRNA capped

## tRNA

Act as adaptors that can bind an amino acid at one end and interact with mRNA at the other.

## Structure: tRNA

- Clover leaf structure
- Contains modified nucleotides
- In eukaryotes, many nucleotides are modified: pseudouridine ($\psi$), dihydro-uridine (D), ribothymidine (T).
- First loop from 5′ end: D loop contains dihydrouridine
- Middle loop contains anticodon: base pairs with codon in mRNA
- Third loop: T$\psi$C loop: contains ribothymidine and pseudouridine
- CCA sequence at 3′ end : carries amino acid

Each tRNA has:
  - An amino acid attached to its 3′ end

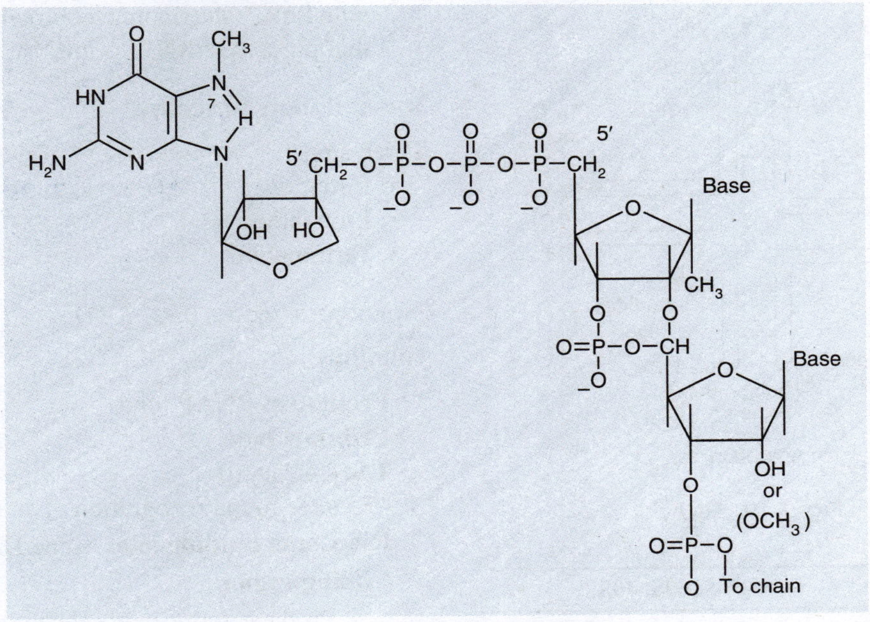

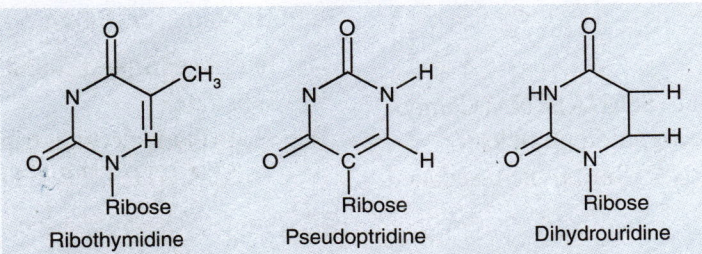

**Fig. 7.17.** Cap of mRNA

Ribothymidine     Pseudoptridine     Dihydrouridine

**Fig. 7.18.** Modified nucleotides.

– A unique anticodon which can attach to only one amino acid

– Serves to transfer amino acids to ribosome

**Comparison**

| Prokaryote | Eukaryote |
|---|---|
| Small, average size of 80 ntd | Similar |
| Modified post translationally | Similar |
| 15% of total cellular RNA | Similar |

**rRNA**

• 50% of mass of ribosome
• Structural and catalytic in function

| Prokaryote | Eukaryote |
|---|---|
| Types: Three | Four |
| Component of 50S | Components of 60S |
| 23S | 28S |
| 16S | 18S |
| 5S | 5.8S |
| | 5S |

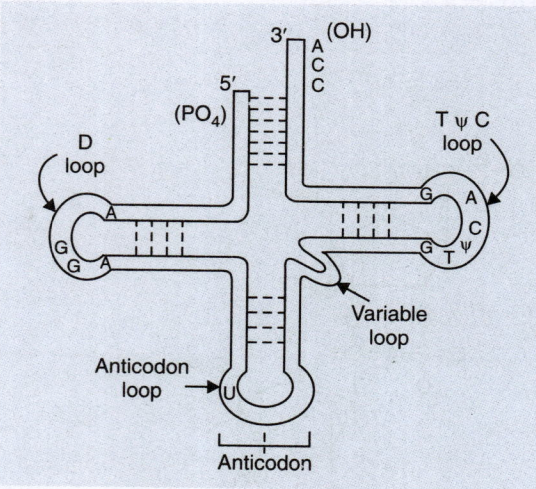

**Fig. 7.19.** tRNA.

| 70S: 50S, 30S | 80S: 60S, 40S |
|---|---|
| 80% of total cellular RNA | 4% precursor<br>71% processed rRNA |

## Small RNA

2 types:

- Small cytoplasmic (ScRNA) RNA: Component of signal recognition particles
- Small nuclear RNA (SnRNA): Associated

with SnRP (snc ribonucleoprotein) particles that process hnRNA to mRNA.

## Transcription process

Three steps:

- Initiation
- Elongation
- Termination

## Prokaryotic gene (Fig. 7.21)

## Function

**Promoter**: RNAP binds
**Pribnow box**:
TATAAT at-10
−35 site: sigma recognition
**Ribosome binding site:** Shine Dalgarno
**Coding region**:
- Produce amino acid sequence in protein
- Begins with AUG for methionine.

## Requirement for transcription

- Template: Single strand of DNA
- Substrate:
  - 4 ribonucleoside triphosphate:
  - ATP, GTP, CTP, UTP

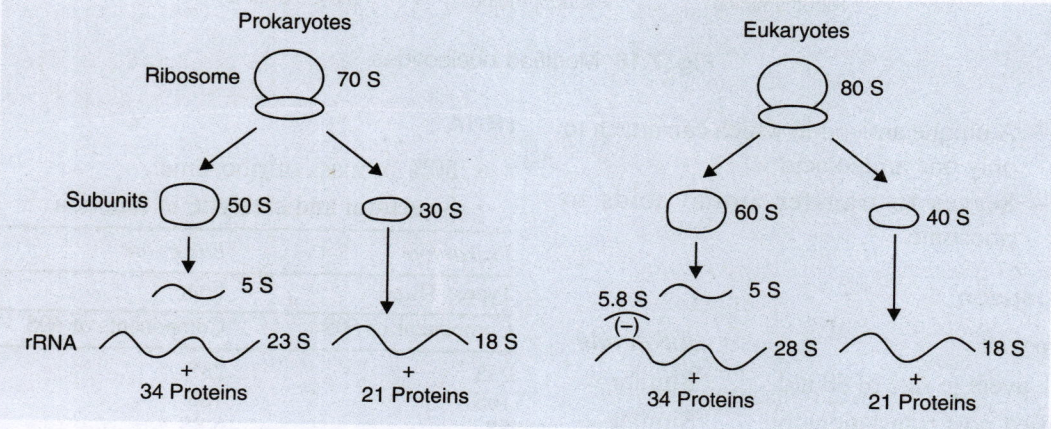

**Fig. 7.20.** Comparison of ribosomes.

| RNA pol | Location | Product | β amantin sensitivity |
|---|---|---|---|
| RNA pol I | Nucleolus | 28S, 18S, 5.8S rRNA | Insensitive |
| RNA pol II | Nucleoplasm | mRNA, SnRNA | Very sensitive |
| RNA pol III | Nucleoplasm | tRNA,ssRNA,SnRNA | Less sensitive |

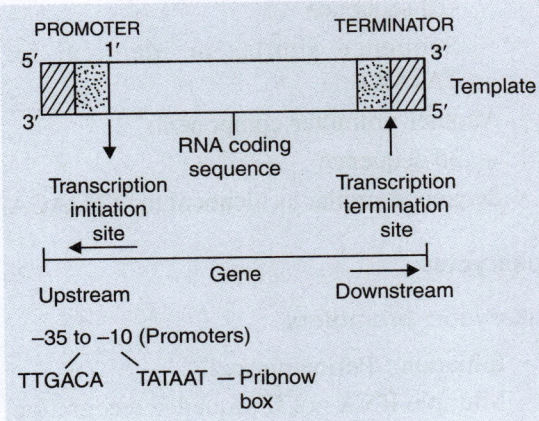

Fig. 7.21. Prokaryotic gene.

- Direction:
  - After first NTP, subsequent ntd are added to 3′ of preceding nucleotide.
  - RNA growth proceeds 5′→3′
- Enzyme: RNA pol

## RNA polymerase

### Prokaryotic RNA pol:

- Single RNA pol
- Synthesize all types of RNA in the cell
- Core polymerase ($\alpha_2$, $\beta\beta'$): responsible for making RNA
- Sigma factor ($\sigma$) required for initiation at a promoter
- After initiation of transcription, $\sigma$ factor released
- Termination of transcription requires rho ($\rho$) factor
- Inhibited by rifampin

- Actinomycin D binds to DNA, preventing transcription.

**Eukaryotic RNA pol:** Three: I, II, III

**RNA pol I:**

- Located in nucleolus
- Synthesizes 28S, 18S, 5.8S rRNA

**RNA pol II:**

- Located in nucleoplasm
- Synthesizes hnRNA/mRNA, SnRNA

**RNA pol III:**

- Located in nucleoplasm
- Synthesizes tRNA, SnRNA, ssRNA

## Comparison RNA pol (RNAP)

| Prokaryotic | Eukaryotic |
|---|---|
| Single | Three |
| Synthesize rRNA, except ssrRNA | RNAP I : rRNA except ssrRNA<br>RNAP II: hnRNA/mRNA, some SnRNA<br>RNAP III: tRNA, ssrRNA |
| Require sigma factor for initiation | No sigma factor required, require transcription factors (TF II D) which bind before RNAP |
| Sometimes require rho factor to terminate | No rho factor required |
| Inhibited by rifampin, actino-mycin D | RNAP II inhibited by amantin (mushrooms), actinomycin D |

## Prokaryotic messages are polygenic

- No processing or transport for transcript for mRNA to reach ribosomes.

- Simultaneous transcription and translation goes on.

## Eukaryotic are monogenic

Introns are present in transcript. They are required to leave nucleus to reach ribosomes where translation occurs.

## Transcription process:

### 1. Initiation

**In prokaryotes:**

- RNAP holoenzyme initiates it
- Loosely binds-35 promoter sequence
- Then tightly binds-10 promoter sequence
- RNAP untwists DNA strand by about 17 bp to create a small bubble.

## Promoter

Region before each gene in DNA that serves as an indicator to cellular mechanism that a gene is ahead.

## Start codon

- AUG (Met)
- TATA box for transcription factor.

## Promoter sequence

Transcription initiation does not require primer.

## Prokaryotic promoter

- Initiation site: Transcription for most genes always starts at the same base (positions): start point is usually a purine.
- Pribnow box:
  - 9-18 bp upstream of start point termed: -10 sequence
  - Sequence similar or identical to: TATAAT
- Another promoter component:
  - 35 sequence
- Sequence similar as identical to: TTGACA

## Eukaryotes

## Eukaryotic promoters

- Initiation : Purine normally
- Multiple RNA pol II sequence recognition elements:
  - TATA box (-25 bp upstream)
  - CAAT box (-70 bp upstream)
  - GC box region (between -40 and -110 bp upstream)
- RNA pol III promotes : 5SrRNA, tRNA
- Other sequence elements:
  - Response elements
  - Enhancers

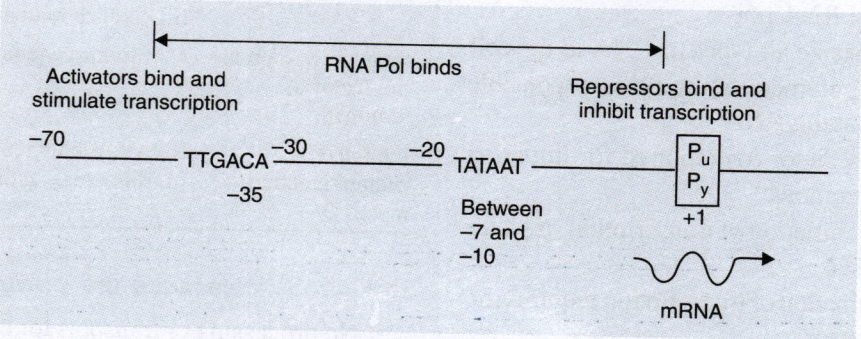

**Fig. 7.22.** Prokaryotic promoters.

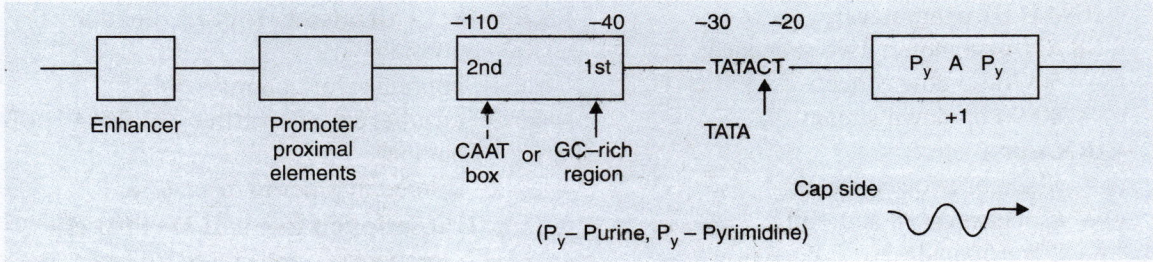

**Fig. 7.23.** Eukaryotic promoters.

**Enhancers:** Stimulate transcription rate located thousands of bp upstream or downstream

**Silencers:** Inhibit transcription

### 1. Promoter sequence in eukaryotes

- Each type of RNA pol uses different promoter

- RNA pol I and II: similar to prokaryotic promoter
- RNA pol III: Promoter used by it is unique downstream of start point
- **Initiation site:** a purine.
- **RNAP II promoter sequence:** Conserved: TATA box, CAAT box and GC box

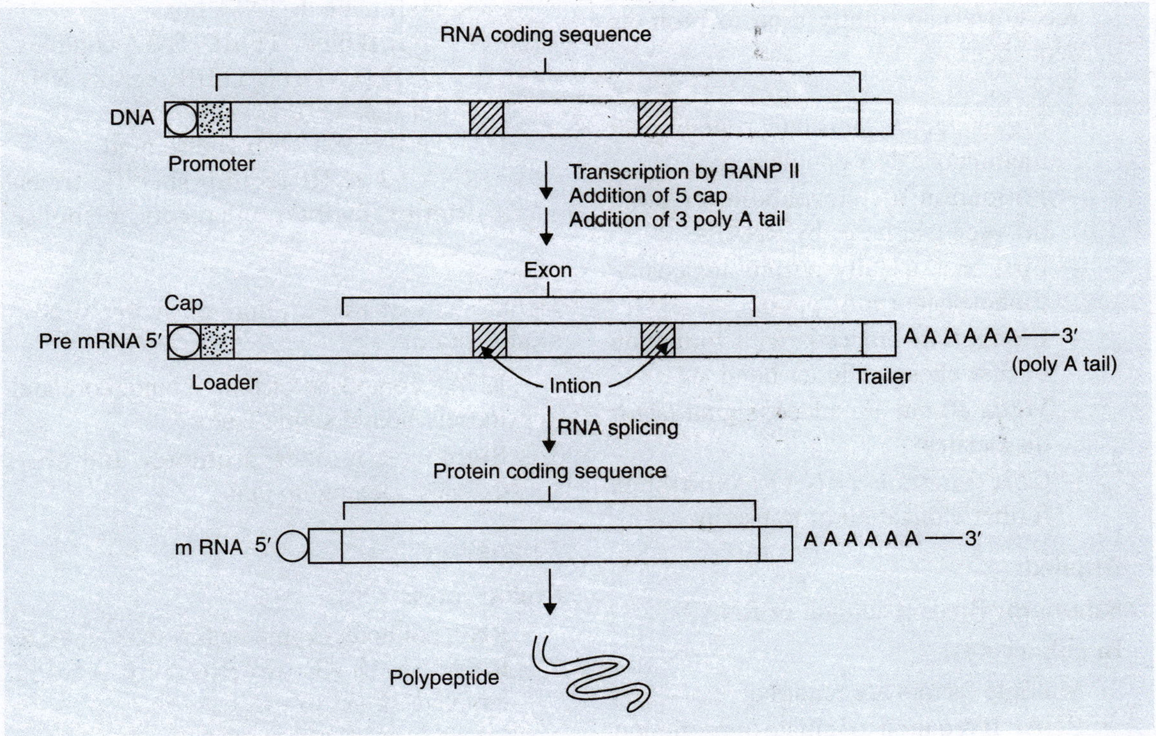

**Fig. 7.24.** mRNA formation in eukaryotes RNA coding sequence.

- **RNAP III promoters:**
- SS RNA promoter: Two sequence:
  - 50-70 bp downstream
  - 80-90 bp down stream
- tRNA promoter:
  - Made of two sequences:
  - I$^{st}$: between +8 and +30
  - 2$^{nd}$: +50 and +70
- **Other sequences:**
  - Response elements
  - Enhancers

They affect rate of initiation of transcription.

## 2. Initation factor

Required to initiate transcription

**In prokaryotes:**

- Only single factor: Sigma ($\sigma$) factor
- Function of $\sigma$ factor: Enable RNA pol to recognize and tightly bind to promote sequences.
- Process:
  - Sigma factor facilitates opening or melting of DNA double helix
  - Formation of phosphodiester bond between two bases by RNAP
  - First base usually purine nucleoside triphosphate (ppA, ppG).
  - **Elongation** proceeds with formation of first phosphodiester bond
  - When 10 ntd are added, sigma factor dissociates
  - Core enzyme (RNAP) continues further elongation of transcript

**Applied:**

**Rifampin:** Binds $\beta$-subunit of RNAP

**In eukaryotes:**

- Multiple factors are required
- RNAP II required to initiate transcription from TATA box promoters.

- **IF: Initiation factor** needed for initiation:
- important for control
- numbered according to RNA pol number
- lettered in order to discovery.
- **Transcription factor II D (TFD II):**
  - Recognizes and binds to TATA box sequences independenttly of RNAP II
  - TATA box-binding proteins (TBP): subunit of TFD II that binds to TATA box DNA sequence
  - TFD II has 8 subunits: TFD II associated proteins
- Five other transcription factors: required for inactivation of transcription by RNAP II:
  - TF II A, B, F, E, H
  - TF II D binds TATA box
  - TF II B binds TF IID-TATA complex
  - TF II D –TATA-TFIIB recruits RNA pol II & TF II F
  - TF II E and TF II H also bind.
- RNAP I & III require specific transcription factors, enhancers, response elements.

## Mechanism of recognition of promoter by sigma factor

- RNAP composed of four subunit core and loosely bound sigma factor.
- Sigma recognizes promoter and core extends opening up helix.

## Elongation

**Prokaryotes:**

- RNA pol holoenzyme begins to synthesize RNA (in 5′→3′ direction) by reading template strand (3′→5′)
- Sigma factor is released after transcript has 8-9 new RNA nucleotides

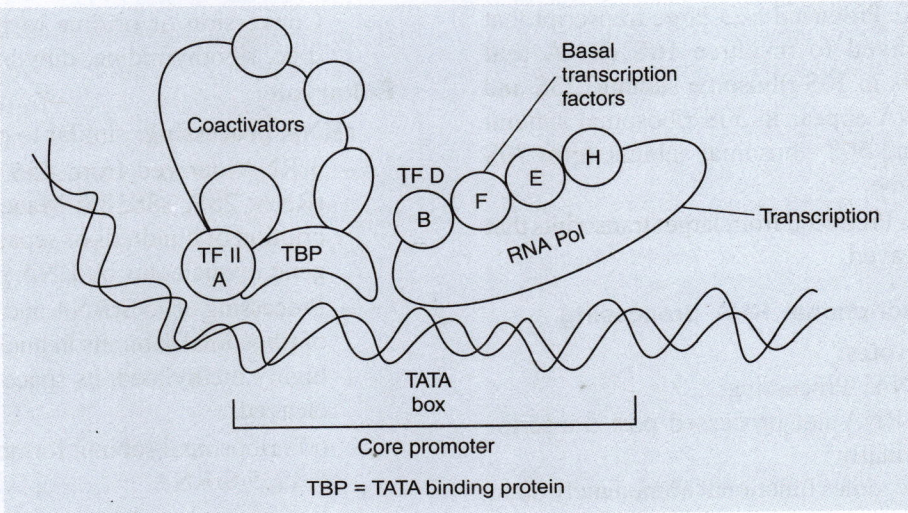

**Fig. 7.25.** Transcription apparatus. (TBP: TATA-binding protein)

- RNA pol core enzyme continues to add NTPs to growing RNA strand, transcription bubble moves downstream at 30-50 ntd/sec across the gene.

## Termination

Prokaryote and eukaryotes use identical mechanism of synthesizing RNA.

**Prokaryotes:**
- Factor dependent termination: in presence of rho factor (ρ)
- Rho factor is ATPase

**Eukaryotes:** Exact mechanism unknown.

**RNA pol I:** Terminates transcription in factor-dependent manner

**RNA pol III:** Terminates by unknown mechanism

Termination signals?

## Prokaryotic transcription termination

Two types:

**Type I: Rho-independent:**
- Consists of a palindrome that fold up on itself in a hairpin
- Followed by 4-8 $U_s$ in transcript
- Makes DNA/RNA hybrid fall apart

**Type II: Rho – dependent:**
- Do not have $U_s$
- May have hairpin region
- Protein binds ATP and RNA
- Moves along transcript to destabilizing DNA/RNA binding.

**For cell-specific gene expression, activity is modulated by:**
- Activators binding the enhancers: Located upstream: Close or far away Boost transcription rates
- Repressors binding silencers: Decrease transcription rates

## Different type of RNA

- **mRNA:** Produced as polycistronic transcript that is translated as it is being transcribed to produce several different protein. E. coli mRNA has a short half life of few minutes

- **rRNA:** Produced as a large transcript that is cleaved to produce 16S rRNA that appears in 30S ribosome subunit, 23S and 5SrRNA appear in 50S ribosomal subunit 30S and 50S ribosomal subunit form 70S ribosome.
- **tRNA:** Produced from larger transcripts that are cleaved.

## Post transcriptional RNA processing

**Prokaryotes:**

- **mRNA:** Processing:
  - mRNA not processed post transcriptionally
  - Becomes functional immediately upon synthesis
  - Its translation begins before transcription is complete
- **rRNA:**
  - A7 genes produce rRNA:
  - Each gene produces:
    30S precursor rRNA that is processed to functional rRNA:
    23S, 16S, 5S rRNA

  **Cleavage:** Upon formation of 30S rRNA precursor, nonfunctional spacers are removed by ribonuclease P and ribonuclease III.

  **Base modification:** Some bases in final rRNA get methylated to be functional.

- **tRNA: Processing:** Not formed by processing
  - tRNA genes clustered and each transcript contains sequences for 2-7 tRNA

  **Cleavage:** by ribonuclease P and D

  **Addition** of sequence CCA to 3' end by enzyme tRNA nucleotidyl transferase

  **Base modification:**
  - Methylation mainly to adopt unique functional conformation

  - Conversion of uridine to pseudouridine, ribothymidine, dihydrouridine

**Eukaryote:**

- **rRNA processing:** similar to prokaryote
  - 3rRNA derived from 45S precursor rRNA: 28S, 18S, 8S: Made by transcription of hundreds of separate rRNA gene in nucleolus by RNA pol I
  - Processing of 45 SrRNA and formation of ribosomal subunits in nucleolus 45S highly methylated, its space sequence cleaved.
  - 60S ribosomal subunit formed by 28S, 5.8S, 5 SrRNA
  - Ribosomal subunits migrate to cytoplasm where they complex with mRNA to form 80S ribosomes

- **mRNA:**
  - Formed from large precursor hnRNA
  - 5'caps
  - Poly A tail (20-200 ntd) at 3' end
  - Splicing

- **tRNA:** Similar to prokaryotes
  - **Addition of sequence CCA to 3' end**: by enzyme tRNA nucleotidyl transferase after tRNA cleaved from precursor
  - **Base modification:** by methylation
  - **Have introns:** mechanism of splicing is different from mRNA splicing

## RNA processing

Pre mRNA → mRNA

- **Capping:**
  - 5' cap of 7-methylguanosine synthesized
  - Cap protect mRNA from being degraded by enzymes
- **Splicing:** Step by step removal of introns in pre mRNA and joining of remaining exons occurs on splicosomes

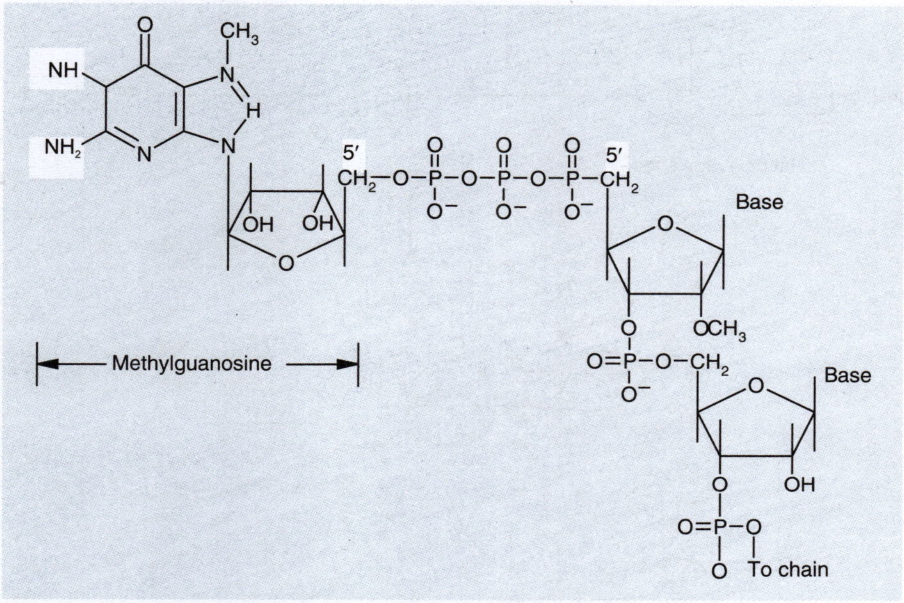

**Fig. 7.26.** Cap structure of eukaryotic mRNA.

- **Polyadenylation:** Synthesis of poly A tail by:
  - Cleavage of its 3′ end
  - Addition of 200 adenine residues to form a poly (A) tail

Thus, complete mature mRNA molecule is ready for export to cytosol for protein synthesis.

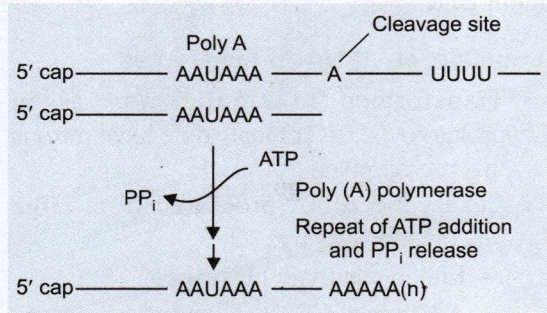

**Fig. 7.27.** Synthesis of poly (A) tail.

## Splicing

- Process of removing non coding sequences to form functional mRNA
- **Exon:**
  - **Expressed** portion of gene: transcribed portion of gene
  - Retained in processing of hnRNA to mRNA.
- **Intron: Intervening** sequences between exons.
- **Different genes have different introns:**
  - β globin gene: 2 introns
  - LDL-R gene: 17 introns
- Intron-exon junctions:
  - Conserved sequences
  - All hnRNA intron have GU sequence on 5′ border, AG sequence on 3′ border.

## Mechanism of splicing

- Multistep, catalyzed by splicesosome:
  - Splicesosome 50S-60S ribonucleotide:

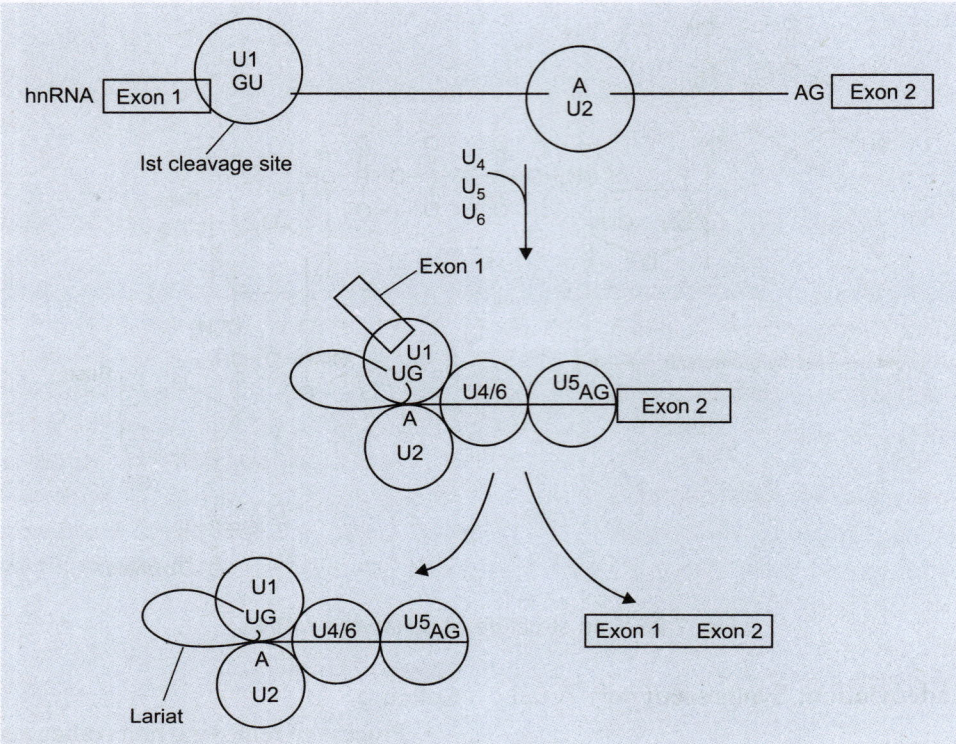

**Fig. 7.28.** Splicing process.

- Made up 5 SNRPs: U1, U2, U4, U5, U6
- Function: SnRNA responsible for:
  - Recognition of conserved sequences in introns
  - Bringing together of RNA sequences in proper alignment for splicing.
- mRNA is transported from nucleus to cytoplasm only after all the splicing is complete
- Regulation of gene expression occurs at the level of splicing

## Alternative splicing

- Common phenomenon in eukaryotes
- Produces more than one protein out of same gene

- A way of controlling gene expression in cells, e.g. 10 lac human antibodies are produced from 30,000 genes.

### Applied aspect

β Thalassemia: defects in mRNA splicing of β-globin gene

### Formation of tRNA in eukaryotes

- Transformed in similar way as in prokaryotes, except that some have introns that are removed
- Eukaryotic tRNA processed from large precursor RNAs by:
  - Endonucleolytic cleavage
  - Addition of CCA to 5' end after cleavage
  - Modification of bases of tRNA

- Some eukaryotic tRNAs have small (14-50 ntd) introns
  - Introns of different tRNA have no sequence homology
  - tRNA splicing differs from mRNA splicing

## Self splicing RNA

- Small % age of transcript from various organisms undergo splicing without protein cofactors
- Classified as:
  - **Group I:** 'G' acts as cofactors in transesterifiction reactions, release of intron without lariat formation.
  - **Group II:** Lariat formation occurs without requirement for protein
- This has led to new idea about early cellular evolution:
  - Which was originally believed to start with amino acid and protein
  - Now, it is believed that ribonucleotide and RNA may have been the most primitive biopolymers to form on earth, providing for diversity
  - That DNA and proteins may have developed later!

## Ribozyme

- RNA that act like enzymes
- Exhibit:
  - Catalytic activity
  - Substrate specificity, like proteinous enzymes!
  - Nucleotide base pairing
- Cleave 'S' RNA at a specific site and then release it without itself being consumed.
- Used as potential therapeutic agents for disease associated with inappropriate expression of RNA or expression of mutated RNA.

## (IV) TRANSLATION, GENETIC CODE

### Translation

Process by which ribosome reads genetic message in mRNA and produces a protein product according to the message's instruction.

### Process

Three phases:

- **Initiation:** Ribosome binds to mRNA and the first amino acid attaches to its tRNA
- **Chain elongation:** Ribosome adds one amino acid at a time to the growing polypeptide chain.
- **Termination:** Ribosomes release mRNA and polypeptide.

### Facts: Translation

- In eukaryotes, protein synthesis take place in cytoplasm, while transcription and RNA processing occurs in nucleus.
- All human genes except histone gene contain introns.

### Prokaryotes

- Bacteria lack nuclei, transcription and translation are coupled
- Ribosomes attach to leading end of mRNA, while transcription is still in progress: **Polygenic.**

### Eukaryotes

- Transcription occurs in nucleus and translation in cytoplasm
- Primary transcript is modified before it leaves the nucleus: RNA processing: introns removed.
- Monogenic

## Prokaryotic *vs.* Eukaryotic translation

- In eukaryotes, translation does not occur simultaneously, transcription occurs in nucleus and translation occurs in cytoplasm
- Eukaryotic start codon is AUG does not use methionine
- Eukaryotic mRNA encodes a single protein at a time, unlike bacterial mRNA which encodes many.
- Eukaryotic DNA contains introns which have to be spliced out of final mRNA transcript.

## Formation of amino acyl-transfer RNA (tRNA)

- Amino acids are activated and get attached to their corresponding tRNAs by amino acyl tRNA synthetase enzyme
- Amino acid first reacts with ATP, forming amino acyl monophosphate (AMP) which forms an ester with 2′ or 3′ OH group of tRNA specific for that amino acid, producing amino acyl tRNA and AMP.
- Once an amino acid is attached to tRNA, insertion of amino acid into a growing

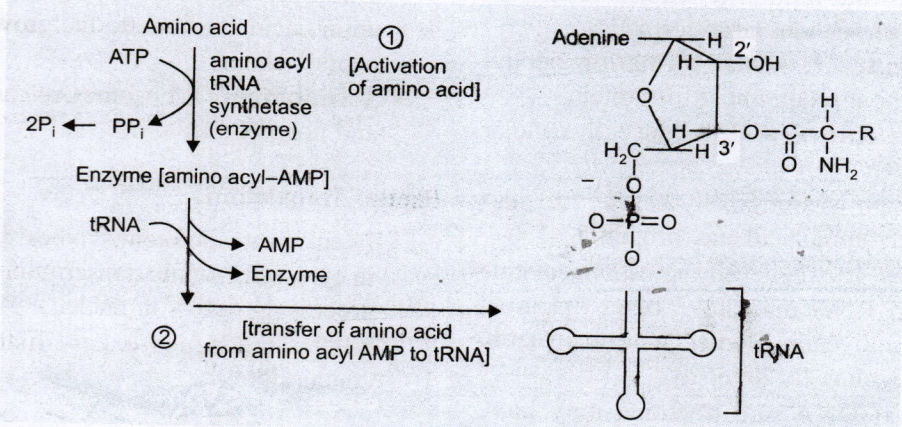

**Fig. 7.29.** Formation of amino acyl tRNA.

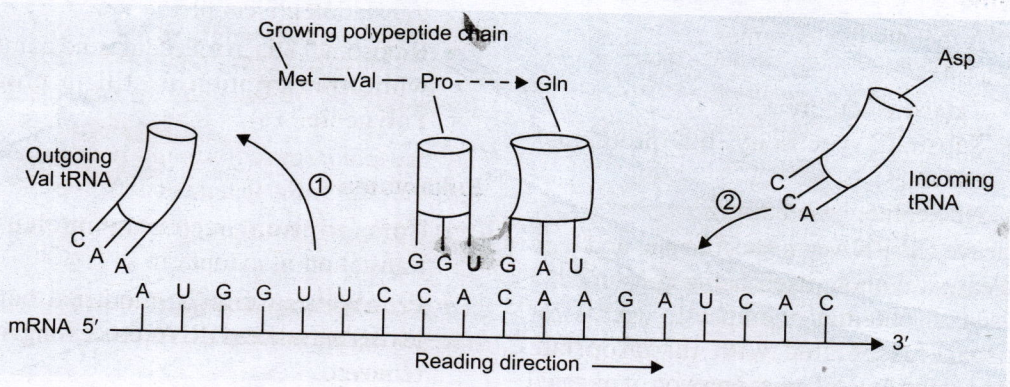

**Fig. 7.30.** Process of translation.

polypeptide chain depends on codon-anticodon interaction.

## Initiation

- mRNA attaches to 30S
- tRNA binds to mRNA where nucleotide code matches
- This triggers binding of 50S to 30S
- tRNA binds to 50S
- First t-RNA binds to start codon in P site of ribosome
- AUG is start codon of every protein
- AUG codes for amino acid methionine
- When second tRNA binds to A site, amino acid of 1st tRNA forms a peptide bond with amino acid of second tRNA.

**50S has two binding sites**:
  - A, P sites
  - First tRNA attaches to A site, then moves to P site as other tRNA approaches second tRNA and binds to A site

Peptide bonds forms between amino acid of tRNA:
  - First tRNA now gets detached from its amino acid and leaves ribosome

- Second tRNA still has two amino acids attached to it.

## Elongation

- tRNA left now moves to P site
- Ribosomes ready to accept another tRNA and continue the process
- Each tRNA adds another amino acid to growing peptide chain (thus "elongation").
- Ribosome is moving along nucleotide triplets one by one.

## Termination

- Ribosome reaches stop codon, peptide chain formation is finished.
- Last tRNA leaves ribosome, leaving behind completed peptide chain
- Ribosome separates from mRNA
- Ribosome subunits also separate and remain in this way until mRNA comes along to restart the process.

## Eukaryotic polypeptides are targeted to specific destination in cell by signal peptides

- Ribosomes are active participants in protein synthesis.

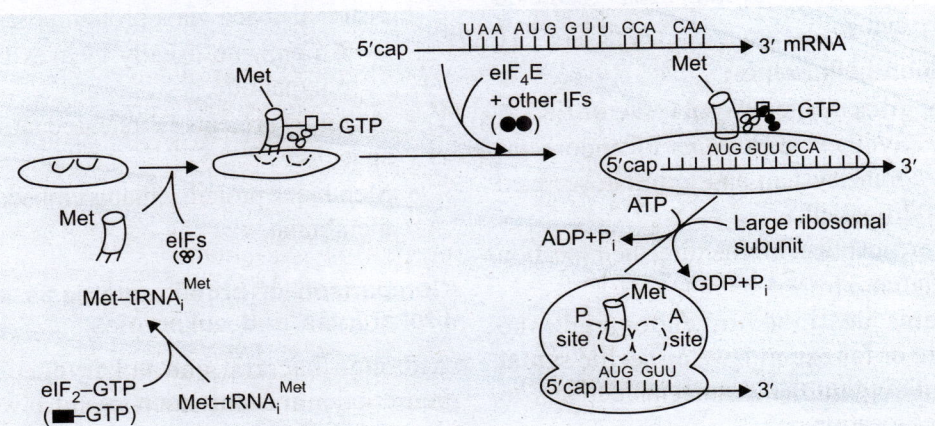

**Fig. 7.31.** Initiation of protein synthesis.

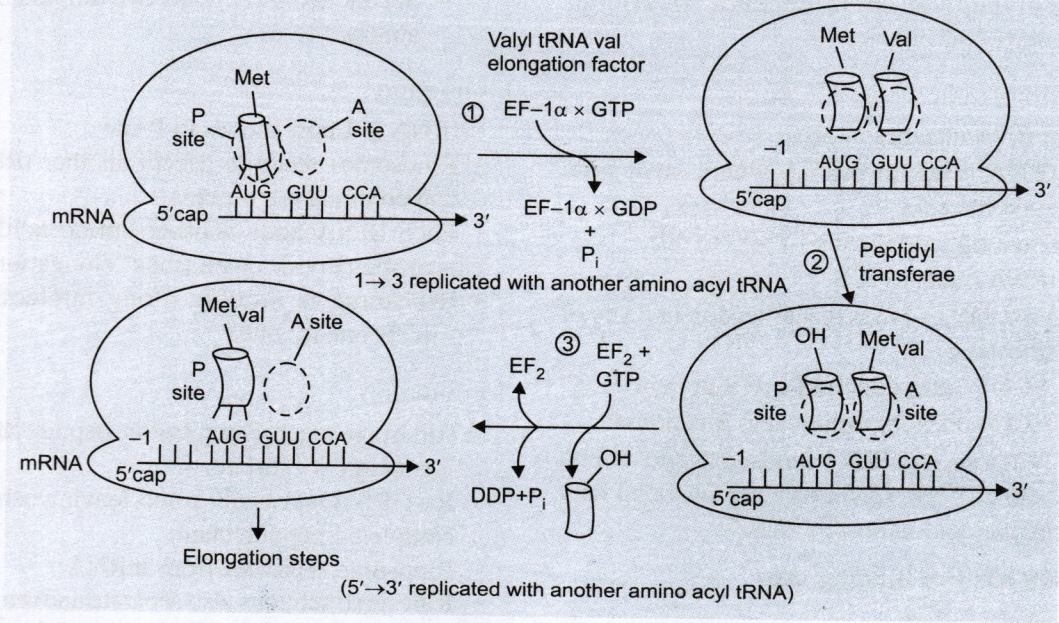

**Fig. 7.32.** Elongation.

- Ribosomes are of two types:
  Free
  Bound

  – **Free ribosomes:**
    - Suspended in cytosol
    - Synthesize proteins that reside in cytosol

  – **Bound ribosomes:**
    - Attached to cytosolic site of ER
    - Synthesize proteins of endomembrane system and protein secreted from cell.

- Both are identical in structure, their location is different.
- Proteins destined for endomembrane system or for export have a specific **signal peptide region** that ensures its delivery to correct location.
- A **signal recognition particle** (SRP) binds to signal peptide and attaches it and its ribosome to a receptor protein in ER membrane.

- After binding, SRP leaves and protein synthesis resumes with growing polypeptide sneaking across membrane into cisternal space via a protein pore.
  – An enzyme usually cleaves the signal polypeptide.

- Secretory proteins are released into cisternal space
- Membrane protein remains embedded in ER membrane.

## Comparison of protein synthesis in prokaryotes and eukaryotes

Although bacteria and eukaryotes carryout transcription and translation in similar ways, they do have differences in cellular machinery and processes:

- Different RNA polymerase and transcription factors
- Differ in termination of transcription
- Ribosomes are different
- Prokaryotes can transcribe and translate the same gene simultaneously.

## Identification initiator codon in prokaryotes

- Involves binding of initiator tRNA (N-formylmethionyl tRNA) to initiator codon (first AUG)
- 30S subunit scans mRNA for a specific sequence: **Shine – Dalgarno (SD) sequence:** at upstream of initiator codon.
- 16 SRNA involved in recognition of S-D sequence

## Initiation in prokaryotes

- Initiation complex formed by protein initiation factors:
  - IF-3 keeps ribosome subunits apart
  - IF-2 identifies and binds initiator tRNA
  - IF-2 binds GTP to bind tRNA
  - IF-1, IF-2, IF-3 bind to 30S subunit to form initiation complex.
- Once 50S subunit binds initiation complex, GTP hydrolyzed and initiator tRNA enters P site and IFs dissociate.
- Prokaryotes do not contain 5' cap on their mRNA.

## Eukaryotic initiation

- Methionyl tRNA methionine binds to small ribosomal subunit
- 5' cap of mRNA binds to small subunit
- First AUG codon base pairs with anticodon on methionyl $tRNA_i^{Met}$.
- No S-D sequence
- CAP-binding protein (CBP) binds to 5'CAP

structure of mRNA, forming *initiation complex* with initiation factor and 40S subunit.

- Methionyl $tRNA_i^{Met}$ is bound at P site, A site is unoccupied.
- Complex scans mRNA for 1$^{st}$ AUG near 5' end of mRNA.
- eIF-2 transfers tRNA to P site and GTP hydrolyzed.

## Sites

P = peptidyl
A = amino acyl

## Applied aspect:

Tetracycline: bind to 30S ribosomal subunit, blocks access of amino acyl tRNA to mRNA ribosomal complex.

## Elongation

- Correct amino acyl t-RNA occupy position at acceptor site
- Formation of peptide bond between peptidyl t-RNA at P site with amino acyl tRNA at A site.
- Translocation of peptidyl tRNA to P site
- Shifting mRNA by codon relative to ribosome
  Applied: Puromycin: analog of amino acyl tRNA inhibits translation by chain termination.

## Binding of amino acyl-tRNA to A site

- mRNA codon at A site determines which amino acyl tRNA will bind
- Codon and anticodon bind by base pairing.
- Internal methionine residues in polypeptide chain are added in response to AUG codon. They are carried by $tRNA_m^{Met}$: a second tRNA specific for methionine.

- Elongation factor and hydrolysis of GTP are required for binding.

## Formation of peptide bond

- Peptide bond forms between amino group of amino acyl tRNA at A site and carbamoyl of amino acyl group attached to tRNA at P site by peptidyl transferase.
- tRNA at P site now does not contain an amino acid is termed as: UNCHARGED
- Growing polypeptide chain is attached to tRNA in A site

## Translocation of peptidyl tRNA

- It moves from A to P site (along with attached mRNA) and uncharged tRNA released from ribosome.
- Elongation factor (EF-2/EF-G) and GTP hydrolysis required for translocation.
- Next codon in mRNA is now in A site
- Elongation and translocation steps are repeated till termination codon moves into A site.

  **Applied:** Diphtheria toxin causes ADP-ribosylation of EF-2 inhibiting translation in eukaryotes.
- EF-Tu binds to amino acyl t-RNA and delivers it to A site of ribosome
- Ef-Tu binds GTP causing conformational change, allowing it to bind to amino acyl tRNA.
- EF-Tu-tRNA complex enters ribosome and positions new tRNA at A site
- If anticodon matches the codon, GTP gets hydrolyzed, EF-Tu releases tRNA and exits ribosome

  **Applied:** Erythromycin and clindamycin inhibit protein synthesis: they bind 50S ribosomal subunit of bacteria, inhibit translocation of growing peptide.

## Analogous elongation factors in prokaryotes and eukaryotes

| Prokaryote | Eukaryotic | Function |
|---|---|---|
| EF-1a | EF-Tu | Docks tRNA in A site |
| EF-1b | EF-Ts | Recycles EF-Tu |
| EF-2 | EF-G | Involved in translocation |

## Termination

When stop codon (UGA, UAG, UAA) occupies A site, release factors cause release of polypeptide chain from ribosomes and ribosomal subunits dissociate from mRNA.

## Energetics of protein synthesis

- Protein synthesis is expensive!
- For each amino acid added to a polypeptide chain, 1 ATP and 3 GTP are hydrolyzed.

## Posttranslational modification of proteins

- Newly transcribed mRNA gene goes to cytoplasm
- mRNA on ribosomes is translated into a string of amino acids, which are directed into the lumen of ER.
- Post translation modification begins here
- Transport vesicles take proteins to golgi apparatus
- Post translational modification continues in golgi
- Proteins that will leave the cells are packaged in secretory vesicle.

## Polysomes

More than one ribosome can be attached to a single tRNA at a time in prokaryotes and this complex of mRNA with multiple ribosomes is **polysome**.

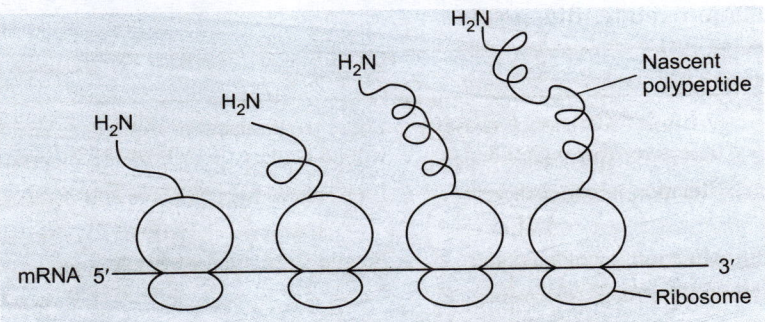

**Fig. 7.33.** A polysome.

## Co-and post translational covalent modifications

| Process | Time of occurrence |
|---------|-------------------|
| • Disulfide bond formation glycosylation | Protein folding as protein pass through ER and golgi |
| • Proteolysis | Cleavage of peptide bonds to remodel proteins and activate them |
| • Phosphorylation | Proinsulin Trypsinogen Prothrombin |
| • γ-carboxylation | Addition of phosphate by protein kinase produces $Ca^{+2}$ binding sites |
| • Prenylation | Addition of farnesyl or geranyl groups to certain membrane associated proteins |

## Examples

### Collagen

- **Prepro α chains** with signal sequence synthesized by ribosomes on RER
- Removal of signal sequence by signal peptidase in RER to form **pro α-chain**.
- **Hydroxylation** of selected proline and lysine by their respective hydroxylases:
  – Located in RER
  – Requires vitamin C

- Glycosylation of selected hydroxylation.
- Three **pro α chains assemble** to form triple helical structure (pro collagen) which is transferred to golgi where modification of oligosaccharide occurs.
- Procollagen is secreted from cell.
- Propeptides cleaved from ends of procollagen to form collagen molecules (tropo-collagen).
- Collagen molecules assemble into fibrils.
- Cross linking by lysyl hydroxylase occurs.
- Fibrils aggregate and cross-link to form collagen fibers.

## Inhibitors of protein synthesis

- **Formation of initiation complex blocked by:**
  – Streptomycin
  – Tetracycline
  Bind to rRNA of small subunit
- Introduction of amino acid tRNA and synthesis of peptide bond is inhibited by:
  – Puromycin: premature termination
  – Chloramphenicol: inhibit peptidyl transferase
- Translocation of mRNA relative to ribosome is blocked by:
  – Erythromycin
  – Fusidic acid prevent release of EF-G, GDP

## Disorders of collagen biosynthesis

| | Disease | Defect | Symptoms |
|---|---|---|---|
| 1 | Scurvy | Vitamin C deficiency causes defective hydroxylation | Loose teeth, bleeding gum, petechiae, ecchymosis, poor wound healing, poor bone development |
| 2. | Osteogenesis imperfecta | Mutation in collagen gene | Blue sclera, fractures, skeletal deformity |
| 3. | Ehlers-Danlos | Mutation in collagen and lysine hydroxylase genes | Fragile skin, hyperextensile joints, dislocations |
| 4. | Menke's disease | Copper deficiency causing deficient cross-liking | Steely hair, cerebral degeneration, arterial tortuosity, rupture. |

- Inhibit eukaryotic synthesis:
  - Diphtheria toxin: Uses NAD to inactivate eEF2 by ADP ribosylation of a modified histidine (diphthamide) in the factor.
  - Cyclohexamide inhibits chain elongation: Competitive inhibitor of peptidyl transferase.

## Genetic code

- Collection of codons that specify all amino acids found in protein
- System that enables 4 nucleotides (A, T, G, C) to code for 20 amino acid

## Base triplet

- Found in DNA molecule
- Nucleotides that code for one amino acid

## Codon

- Code for production of a specific amino acid: sequence of three bases in mRNA
- 64 possible codons ($4^3$)
- 61 codon code for amino acids
- Often 2-3 codons represent some amino acid
- Start codon: AUG
- 3 stop codon: UAG, UGA, UAA that terminate translation
- Written in 5' to 3' direction.

## Properties: Genetic code

- **Unambiguous:** each codon specifies not more than one amino acid
- **Degenerate:** more than one codon can specify a single amino acid
  - Met, Trp have more than one codon
  In this case, first bases in codon are same and base in third position varies
- **Universal:**
  - Same in all organisms
  - Some minor exceptions occur in mitochondria
- **Commaless:** There are no spaces or commas between codons on mRNA
- **Non overlapping**
- **Whobble hypothesis**
  - Third position of codon is less important than first or second
  - Correct base pairing is required at first position of codon (third of anti codon) and second position of codon (anticodon as well)
  - Third position of codon does not always need to be paired with anticodon.

# (V) CELL CYCLE

## Comparison of chromosomes

| Prokaryotes | Eukaryotes |
|---|---|
| Genome of E. coli contain $4 \times 10^6$ bp | Yeast $1.35 \times 10^7$ bp |
| >90% DNA encode protein | A small fraction of total DNA encodes protein. Many repeats of non-coding sequences |
| Lacks a membrane bound nucleus | All chromosomes are contained in a membrane bound nucleus |
| Circular DNA and supercoiled domain | DNA divided between 2 or more chromosomes |
| Histones are unknown | A set of five histones, DNA packaging and gene expression regulation |

## Cell cycle in eukaryotes

Four different phases:

**S Phase:**
- DNA synthesized
- Eukaryotes replicate only once per cell division cycle
- Lasts for 8 hrs in humans

**$G_2$ and M phase:**
- Gap phase $G_2$ occurs before mitosis and cell division (M phase)
- Variable time between two phases

**$G_1$ phase:**
- Normal cellular functions take place during this phase

**$G_0$ phase:**
- Resulting phase
- Variable time

Tumor cells do not enter $G_0$ phase.

## Cell cycle

It is a cell's life time of growth and division

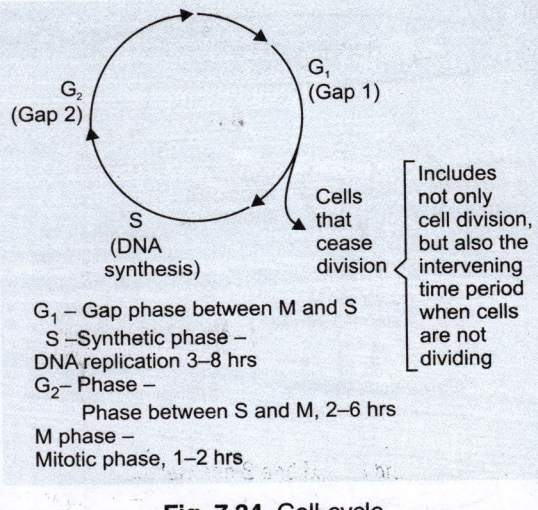

$G_1$ – Gap phase between M and S
S – Synthetic phase –
DNA replication 3–8 hrs
$G_2$ – Phase –
   Phase between S and M, 2–6 hrs
M phase –
Mitotic phase, 1–2 hrs

**Fig. 7.34.** Cell cycle.

Eukaryotic cell cycle includes:
1. Cell growth
2. Chromosome replication
3. Cell division: 2 types:
   - Mitosis
   - Meiosis

## Cell cycle phases

Interphase, cell growth and DNA replication, mitosis: nuclear and cell division.

## Cell cycle control

- Precise coordination of different phases of cell cycle is essential in all eukaryotes
- Correct order of phases is a must
- One phase must be completed before the next phase can begin
- Errors in this coordination may lead to chromosomal alterations
- Chromosomes may be lost, rearranged or distributed unequally between two daughter cells.
- This type of chromosome alteration is often seen in cancer cells.

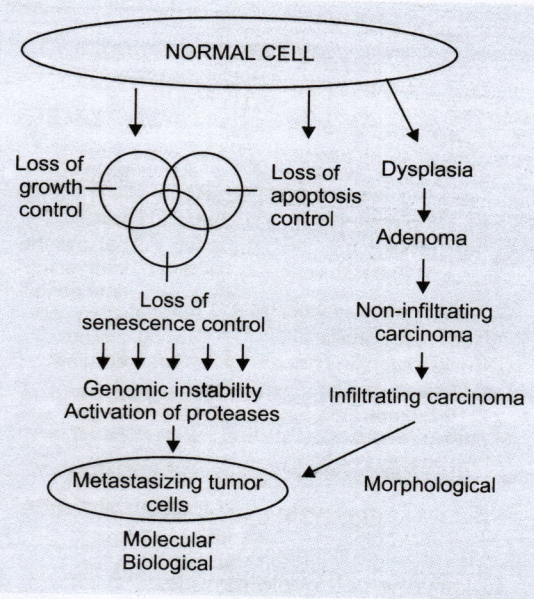

**Fig. 7.35.** Tumor progression

## Cell cycle engines

**CDKs:** Cyclin dependent kinase

## Types of cell control

Protein phosphorylation by protein kinases

**Retinoblastoma protein (Rb):**

– Regulator and tumor suppressor

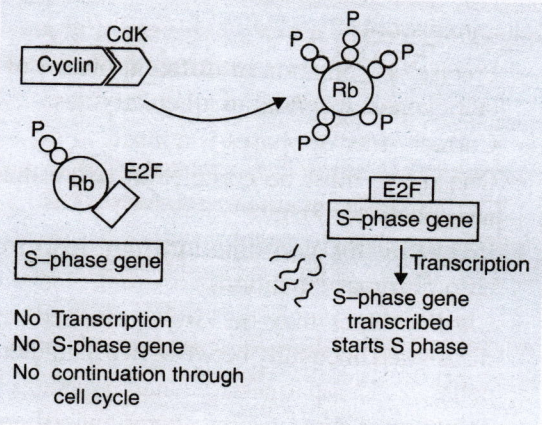

**Fig. 7.36.** Rb protein.

– Substrate for enzyme cyclin dependent kinase

– $p_{21}$ and $p_{16}$ proteins inhibit function of cells

– Thus, Rb does not get hyperphosphorylated and E2F is not able to transcribe genes and cell cycle inhibited.

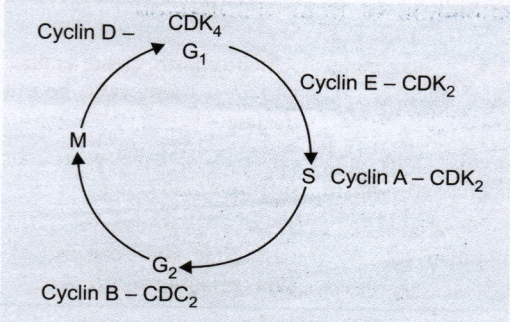

**Fig. 7.37.** CDKs.

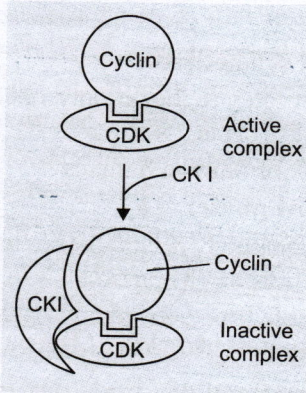

**Fig. 7.38.** Inhibition of cyclin/CDK activity

## S phase

Each chromosome replicates to form two chromatids

## $G_0$ – quiescent state

• Cells are not in process of cell division

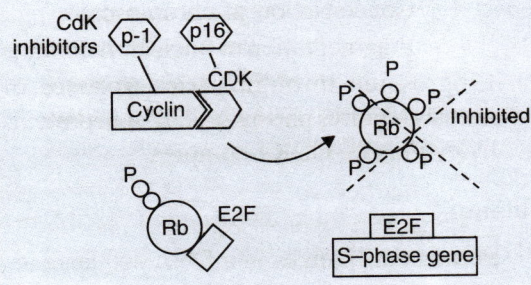

**Fig. 7.39.** Rb gene mechanism.

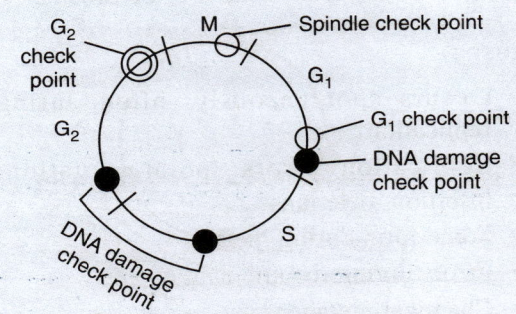

**Fig. 7.40.** Cell cycle check points.

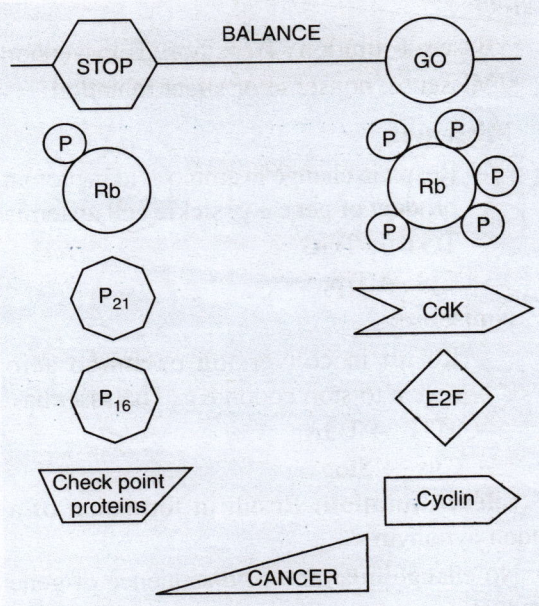

**Fig. 7.41.** Cell cycle check points and cancer.

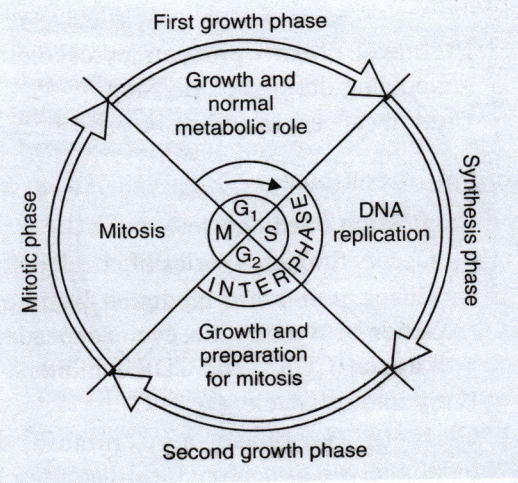

**Fig. 7.42.** Phases of cell cycle

• Cells contain diploid amount of genetic material
• Cells express proteins required for cellular housekeeping as well as proteins required to perform specialized function of cell.

## Interphase

Period between cell division

Divided into :
 – Gap 1: synthesis of DNA
 – Gap 2: growth preparation phase for mitosis

• **Gap 1:**
 – Point of entry for cells to divide and enter the cell cycle
 – Time of intense mRNA transcription for protein synthesis for proteins for resultant two daughter cells and proteins required for duplication of genome

• **S-phase:** Synthesis of DNA results in replication (semi conservative)

• **Gap 2:** Cell prepares for cell division with further protein and organelle synthesis. Also, integrity of replicated DNA is checked and assessed.

## Applied

- Paclitaxel (Taxol) prevents cytoskeleton remodeling during cell division.
- Used in cancers including breast cancer.

## Control of cell cycle

- Progression of cell cycle:
  - Occurs through a series of check point
  - Check points are mediated by interaction between cyclin, cyclin dependent kinases (CDKs) and CDK inhibitors.
- Entry into cell cycle: $G_0 \rightarrow G_1$.
- Cells in $G_0$ phase may remain so indefinitely, e.g. neuronal, cardiac muscle cells
- Or cells may enter in cell cycle, e.g. epithelial cells of GIT
- $G_0 \rightarrow G_1$ transition depends on presence of growth factors.
- $G_1 \rightarrow S$:
  - There is restriction point between $G_1$ and S phase
  - Once cell traverses this boundary, it enters S phase
  - Cyclin D levels begin to rise in late $G_1$ which bind to $CDK_4$ and $CDK_5$
  - $CDK_4$ and $CDK_5$ phosphorphorylate cyclin
  - Cyclin D-cyclin D $K_4$ or $K_6$ complex phosphorylates Rb protein, releasing the E2F bound to it.
  - E2F initiates transcription of genes
  - CDK inhibitors p21, p27, p16 block progression through cell cycle
- G2 $\rightarrow$ M:
  - Cyclin A and B accumulate in $G_2$
  - Cyclin A associates with CDK1 and $CDK_2$
  - Topoisomerase are target of CDKs, which on phosphorylation result in:
    - Condensation of chromosome
    - Fragmentation of nuclear membrane
- Progression through various phases of mitosis requires phosphorylation of proteins by cyclin B – CDK1 complex.

## Mutation

- Permanent changes in a DNA sequence.
- Creates new alleles.
- Depending on location and type, mutation can be beneficial, neutral or detrimental.

## Causes

- Occurs spontaneously, often during replication
- Replication errors: point mutation, insertion, deletions
- Some form during meiosis
- Errors during recombinant events
- Chemical mutagens
- Irradiation

## Types

- Base substitution ; Transition, Transversion
- Missense, nonsense or silent mutation

**Missense:**
- Result in change in amino acid in protein product of gene e.g. sickle cell anaemia
- TGT $\rightarrow$ TGG
- Cys $\rightarrow$ Trp,

**Nonsense:**
- Result in conversion of amino acid codon to stop codon e.g. Thalassemia
- TGT $\rightarrow$ TGA
- Cys $\rightarrow$ Stop

**Silent mutation:** Result in formation of a codon synonym

No change in amino acid sequence of gene product

- TGT → TGC
- Cys → Cys
- Deletion:
  - Deletion of one or more base pairs.
  - Frame shift mutation, producing non functional protein
- Insertion: Insertion of one or more base pairs

## Somatic mutation

- Occurs in somatic cells
- All daughter cells from mutated cells will contain the mutation

## Germ line mutation

- Heritable mutations
- Germ cell mutations are perpetuated in gametes and passed on to offspring.

## Importance of mutations

- Create new alleles
  - Allow bacteria to become antibiotic resistant, allows viruses to infect new hosts
- Induced mutations let scientists study gene function:
  - Genes with induced mutations differ in function from normal gene
  - Allows scientists to determine how a gene works:
    - Site- directed mutagenesis

## Deamination (Fig. 7.43)

## Mutation by replication errors

Replication error:
- Main source of mutations
- Occur at frequency of $10^9$-$10^{11}$.

Since cell division requires synthesis of $6 \times 10^9$ nucleotides, mutation rate is about one per cell division.

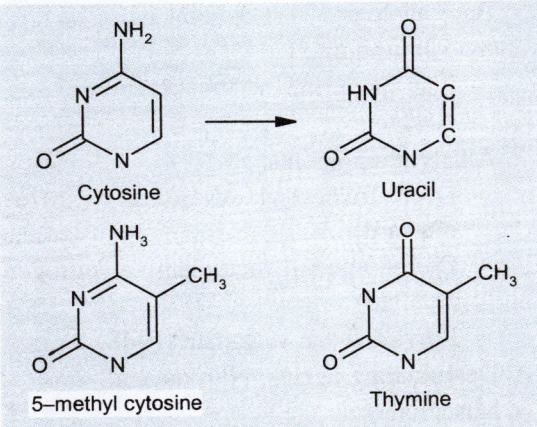

**Fig. 7.43.** Deamination.

## MUTATION BY REPLICATION ERRORS

- Commonly observed replication errors: replication slippage.
- Occurs at repetitive sequences when new strand mispairs with template strand e.g. microsatellite polymorphism.
- If mutation occurs in a coding region, it produces abnormal proteins leading to diseases e.g. Huntington's disease.

## Mutation by UV light

- UV light may cause two adjacent pyrimidine residues (cytosine or thymine) to form a dimer.
- p53 can detect this dimer in normal cells and then triggers repairing process.
- If p53 is mutated, pyrimidine dimer may lead to mutation, e.g. Cytosine dimer could cause adenine to be incorporated into new strand. Subsequent DNA replication could cause adenine to be incorporated into new strand.

## Chemical mutagens

- Chemical agents that may cause mutation.
- Most of them are also carcinogens

- Base analogs:
  - 5-bromouracil
  - 2 aminopurine
  - Acridine
- Alkalylating agents:
  - Dichyloroethyl sulphide (sulfur mustard)
  - Dichyloroethyl methylamine (nitrogen mustard)
  - Ethylmethane sulfonate (EMS)
- Deaminating agents: Nitrous acid.
- Miscellaneous
  - Hydroxylurea
  - Free radicals

## Mechanism of mutation induced by 5-bromouracil (BU)

5BU has 2 tautomeric isoforms:
- Keto (BUK) pairs with adenine
- Enol form (BUe) pairs with guanine

If in first replication, keto form gets incorporated into new DNA strand, during second replication, keto form undergoes a tautomeric shift to enol form causing: A:T to G:C mutation.

## Consequences of mutation

- Changes in base sequence of DNA can be lethal and inheritable
- **Effect of function:**
  - **Loss of functions:**
    - Complete loss of functions: Amorphic mutation
    - Occurs in recessive phenotype.
  - **Gain of function:**
    - Change in gene product such that it gains a new and abnormal function: neomorphic
    - Occurs in dominant phenotype
- Dominant negative mutation: altered gene

product causing altered molecular function, e.g. Marfan's syndrome:
  - Defective fibrillin gene product

## Xeroderma pigmentosum (XP)

- Hypersensitive to sunlight/Uv induced pyrimidine dimers
- Increased incidence of skin cancer, premature aging.

## Repair defect and breast cancer

BRCA 1 and BRCA 2: mutations confer increased risk of cancer in carriers.

## Hb structure and sickle cell disease

| Normal | Primary Structure | Sickle cell |
|---|---|---|
| Hb 1 2 3 4 5 6 7 | | Hb 1 2 3 4 5 6 7 |
| HbA | Secondary and tertiary structure | HbS |
| Molecules do not associate with one another: each carries oxygen. | Function | Molecules interact with one another to crystallize into a fiber: capacity to carry oxygen is greatly greatly reduced |
| Normal cell have normal Hb, each carrying oxygen | RBC shape | Fibers of abnormal Hb deform cell into sickle shape |

## Carcinogens

Two Types:
1. **Direct:**
   - Exist in a mutant form when they enter the body
2. **Indirect:**
   - Not mutagenic when they enter the body, but converted to mutagens on metabolism in body.

– Liver has active detoxification system that interconverts many inactive mutagens into mutagens, e.g. Cyt $P_{450}$ oxidase

# (VI) REGULATION OF GENE EXPRESSION

## Regulation is complex

- Hundreds of different enzymatic reaction happening simultaneously
- Need to respond rapidly to changes in their environment
- Complicated developmental pathways
- Enzyme can be:
  - Constitutive: needed in same amount under any growth condition
  - Inducible: not permanently needed in same amount under any growth condition.

## Regulation of gene expression

- Major mode of regulation in cell:
  - Control of enzyme activity: post translational control
  - Control of amount of enzyme present: control of transcription and translation

## Control of amount of enzyme present

- Transcriptional and translational control
- DNA binding proteins
- Protein-nucleic acid interactions
- Specific and non specific interactions, histone and sequence specific proteins
- Protein domains and interaction with inverted repeats
- Structure of DNA-binding proteins: Helix turn helix, Zinc-finger, Leucine zipper.
- Negative control of transcription repression and induction

## Inhibition of enzyme activity

- Enzyme activity can be inhibited by certain compounds in cell, e.g. Kreb's cycle inhibited by ATP, high levels of G-6-P, alanine
- Also, enzyme can be inhibited by:
  - Non covalent inhibition
  - Feedback inhibition
  - Allosteric regulation

## Post translational modification of proteins:

  - Covalent modification: reversible
  - Protein processing: irreversible
    e.g. processing of preproinsulin protein splicing.
  - Protein interaction can affect replication, transcription, translation.
  - Protein – nucleic acid interactions, e.g. non-specific interaction: histone
  - Specific interaction: sequence specific proteins

## DNA-binding proteins

## Helix-turn helix

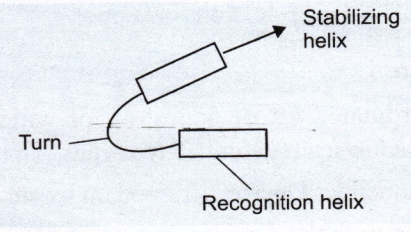

**Fig. 7.44.** Helix turn helix.

## Zinc finger structure

- Amino acid holds $Zn^{+2}$ ions
- Include 2 residues of cysteine (C) with 2 histidine (H) residues.

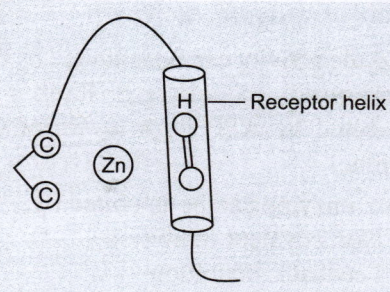

Fig. 7.45. Zinc finger structure.

## Leucine Zipper

- Leucine residues as spaced exactly every 7 amino acids
- Interaction of leucine side chains helps hold the 2 helices together.

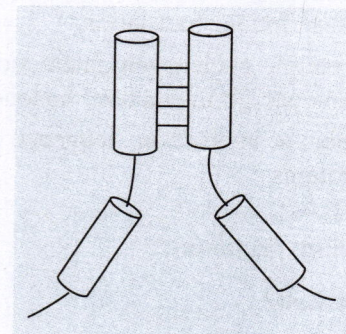

Fig. 7.46. Leucine zipper.

## Operon

A coordinated set of genes, all of which are regulated as a single unit. Two types:

- Inducible: Operon is turned on by substrate
- Repressible: Operon is turned off by the product synthesized.

**Lactose operon:** 3 segments:

**Regulator:** Gene that code for repressor.

**Control locus:** Composed of promoter and operator

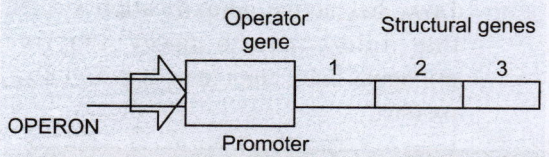

Fig. 7.47. Operon.

## Structural locus:

- Made of 3 genes, each coding for an enzyme required to catabolic lactose:
- β-Galactosidase – hydrolyze lactose
- Permerase – brings lactose across cell membrane
- β-galactosidase transacetylase-uncertain function

## Lac Operon:

**Normally off:** In absence of lactose, repressor binds operator locus and blocks transcription of downstream structural gene.

**Lactose turns operon on:**

- Binding of lactose to repressor protein changes its shape and causes it to fall off the operator.

RNA pol can bind to promoter, structural genes are transcribed

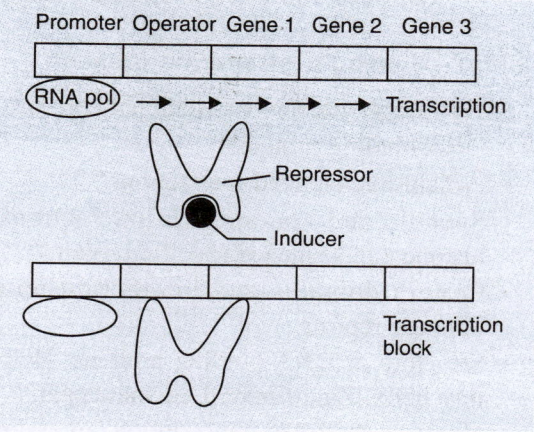

Fig. 7.48. Lac Operon.

– Lactose inhibits repressor protein

– cAMP dependent activator protein binds CAP site

– Glucose lowers cAMP, preventing activation

– Genes are expressed when lactose is present and glucose is absent.

## Prokaryotic regulation:

– Lac operon

– Histidine operon

– Tryptophan operon

## Eukaryotic gene expression

• Chromatin modifying activities:

  - Histone acetylase (favor gene expression)

  - Histone deacetylase (favor inactive chromatin)

• Scaffolding protein (condensing regions of chromatin) favor inactive chromatin

• DNA methylating enzymes (favor inactive chromatin)

• Activator proteins

• Response elements bind to DNA:

  – Upstream promoter elements

  – Enhance region

• Repressors bind silencer elements

• Activators (transcription factor):

  – Upstream promoter element

  – Enhancer response element

• Specific transcription factors:

  Steroid receptors (Zn finger)

  – cAMP – dependent activator protein, CREB (leucine zipper)

  – Homeodomain proteins:

    - pHOX, pPAX (helix-turn-helix)

## Control of eukaryotic gene expression

| Control point | Example |
|---|---|
| 1 Inactivation of chromosome or chromosomal region during development | X-chromosome in each cell in women is inactivated by condensation |
| 2. Local chromatin modifications | Acetylation of histone increases gene expression<br>Methylation of DNA silence genes |
| 3. Gene amplification | Many oncogenes are present in multiple copies, e.g. erb B amplified in breast cancer, DHF reductase gene in some tumors is amplified resulting in drug resistance |
| 4. Specific transcription factor | Steroid hormone receptor, CREB, homeodomain protein |
| 5. mRNA processing | Alternative splicing, Ab production |
| 6. Rate of translation | Heme increases initiation of $\beta$ globin translation |
| 7. Protein modification | Proinsulin $\rightarrow$ insulin |
| 8. Protein degradation | ALA synthase has half life of 1 hour |

## Regulation of protein synthesis

1. **Nutrient supply:**

   – Prokaryotes respond to changes in their supply of nutrients to obtain or conserve energy.

   Source of carbon, nitrogen are required to synthesize energy, amino acid, structural protein and enzymes

– If glucose present: enzymes of glucose utilization are made constitutively.

– If glucose absent; but other sugar is available: enzymes and proteins are produced to derive energy from that sugar. This is **induction.**

– If amino acid is present: E. coli is not required to produce that amino acid, so enzyme required for its synthesis are **repressed.**

2. **Operons:** Set of genes that are coordinately controlled that is genes are either turned on or turned off.

3. **Induction:** Inducer stimulates transcription of operon

4. **Repressor:** Corepressor inhibits transcription of an operon; it is usually an amino acid.

5. **Positive control:** Some operons are turned on by mechanisms that activate transcription

6. **Catabolite repression:** Cells prefer to use glucose when it is available and require cAMP binds to CAP which binds to site near promoter.

7. **Attenuation** occurs by mechanism by which rapid translation of nascent transcript causes termination of transcription.

8. **Factors** such as sigma factor.

## In eukaryotes

1. **Regulation** can result from changes in gene or from mechanism that affect transcription, processing and transport of mRNA, mRNA stability.

2. (i) **Changes in genes:** Genes can be lost from cells, so that functional proteins can no longer be produced, e.g. During differentiation of RBCs.

(ii) Genes can be amplified: Gene amplification is common in tumor cells e.g. neuroblastoma patient have up to 300 copies of *N-myc* genes

(iii) Segments of DNA can move from one location to another on the genome, associating with each other in various ways, so that different proteins are produced, e.g. T and B lymphocytes undergo DNA rearrangements to produce a single transcriptional unit for formation of diverse variety of antibodies.

(iv) Modification of bases in DNA affects transcriptional activity of a gene Cytosine methylated at 5 positions. Greater is methylation, less readily a gene is transcribed.

3. **Regulation of level of transcription:**

(i) Histones act as non specific repressors

(ii) Inducers (steroid hormone) enter cell to bind their receptors and activate specific genes.

4. **Regulation of mRNA processing and transport:**

– Occurs by capping, polyadenylation and splicing can alter amino acid sequence or quantity of protein produced from mRNA.

– Alternative splicing, mRNA editing and degradation is also regulated.

5. Protein synthesis is regulated at translational level during initiation or elongation reactions.

## (VII) MOLECULAR BIOLOGY TECHNIQUES: APPLICATIONS

By using molecular biology techniques (PCR, FISH, Blotting, DNA sequencing etc.) microbial diseases, genetic disorders can be diagnosed more accurately.

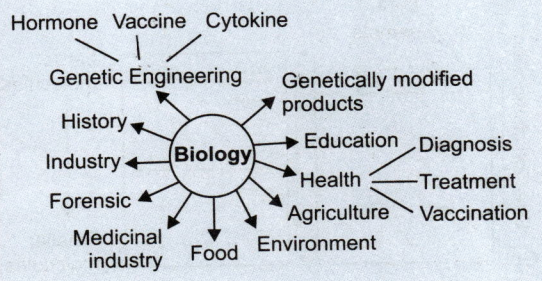

**Fig. 7.49.** Applications of molecular biology.

By using genetic and immunologic therapy, genomic structure of infectants are detected accurately and cancer can be treated.

### Recombinant DNA technology

### Fact file

A gene might be 1/1,000,000 of genome.

Three basic approaches:

- **PCR (polymerase chain reaction):** Makes many copies of a specific region of DNA
- **Cell-based molecular cloning:** Create and isolate a bacterial strain that replicates a copy of gene of interest
- **Hybridization:**
  - Make DNA single stranded.
  - Allow double-stands to reform using a labeled version of selected gene to make it easy to detect.

### PCR

- Based on DNA polymerase property of creating a second strand of DNA.
- Requirements:
  - Template DNA
  - Two primers to flank the region to be amplified
- Primers: Short (18-30 bases) DNA oligomers complementary to the ends of region being amplified
- DNA polymerase:
  - Adds new bases to 3' ends to primer to create new second strand
  - DNA polymerase from *thermus aquatics*: A bacterium that lives in nearly boiling water in Yellow stone Natural Park Hot springs
- Taq polymerase: It can withstand temperature cycle of PCR that would kill DNA pol from E. coli.

### Uses of PCR

- Diagnosis of diseases: infectious, cancer
- Forensic medicine
- Antenatal diagnosis
- Prenatal sex determination.
- Construction of useful organisms:
  - Bacteria of biological waste handling, marine spills, nitrogen fixation.
  - Detection of mutations
  - Preimplantation diagnosis of genetic diseases.
  - Paternity contesting
  - Anthropology

**Advantage of PCR:**
  - Rapid
  - Sensitive
  - Robust
  - Works even with partly degraded DNA

**Disadvantages:**
  - Only short region (up to 2kbp) can be amplified.
  - Limited amount of product is made.

### Problems in PCR

Contamination, impurities, improper sample.

**PCR cycle:** Based on cycle of three steps that occur at different temperatures

– Each cycle doubles the number of DNA molecules: 25-35 cycles produce enough DNA to be visualized on electrophoresis gel.
– Each step takes one minute to complete

**Steps:**

1. Denaturation: Makes DNA single stranded by heating to 94°C.
2. Annealing:
   - Hybridize primers to single strands
   - Temperature around 50°C
3. Extension: Build second strand with DNA pol and dNTP: 72°C.

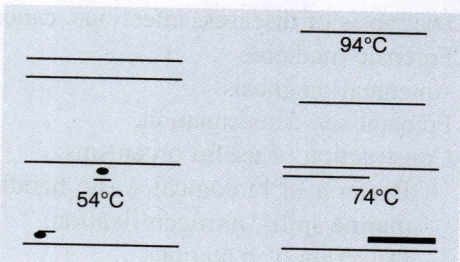

**Fig. 7.50.** PCR cycle.

## Electrophoresis

- Separation of charged molecules in electric field
- Nucleic acid have one charged phosphate (negative charged) per nucleotide
- Separation based on length: longer molecule move slower.
- Done in gel matrix to stabilize: agrose or acrylamide
- Average run: 100 volts across 10cm gel, run for 2 hours
- Stain with ethidium bromide: intercalates with DNA bases and fluoresces orange.
- Run alongside standards of known sizes to get length.

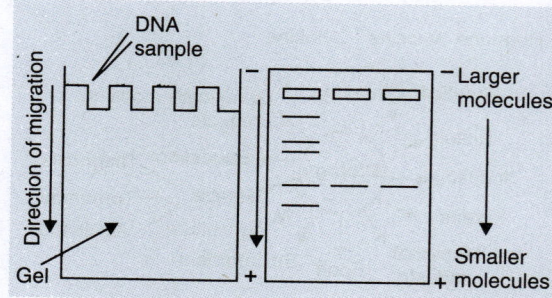

**Fig. 7.51.** Electrophoresis.

## CLONING

### Sources of DNA to done:

- Genomic DNA: Whole genome is cut into small pieces and cloned.
  **Methods:**
  - Random shear
  - Partial digestion to generate recognition site at every 256bp by restriction enzyme
- cDNA: DNA copy of mRNA, with reverse transcriptase.
- Synthetic DNA: synthesized denovo or by PCR.

## Cell based molecular cloning

### Restriction enzymes

- Cut DNA at specific sequences e.g. EcoR I
- Eco RI cut at GAATTC
- Used by bacteria to destroy invading DNA, their own DNA has been modified at corresponding sequences by a methylase

## Plasmid

- Independently replicating DNA circles (only circles replicate in bacteria)
- Foreign DNA can be inserted into a plasmid and replicated
- Plasmids for cloning carry drug resistance genes to help in selection.

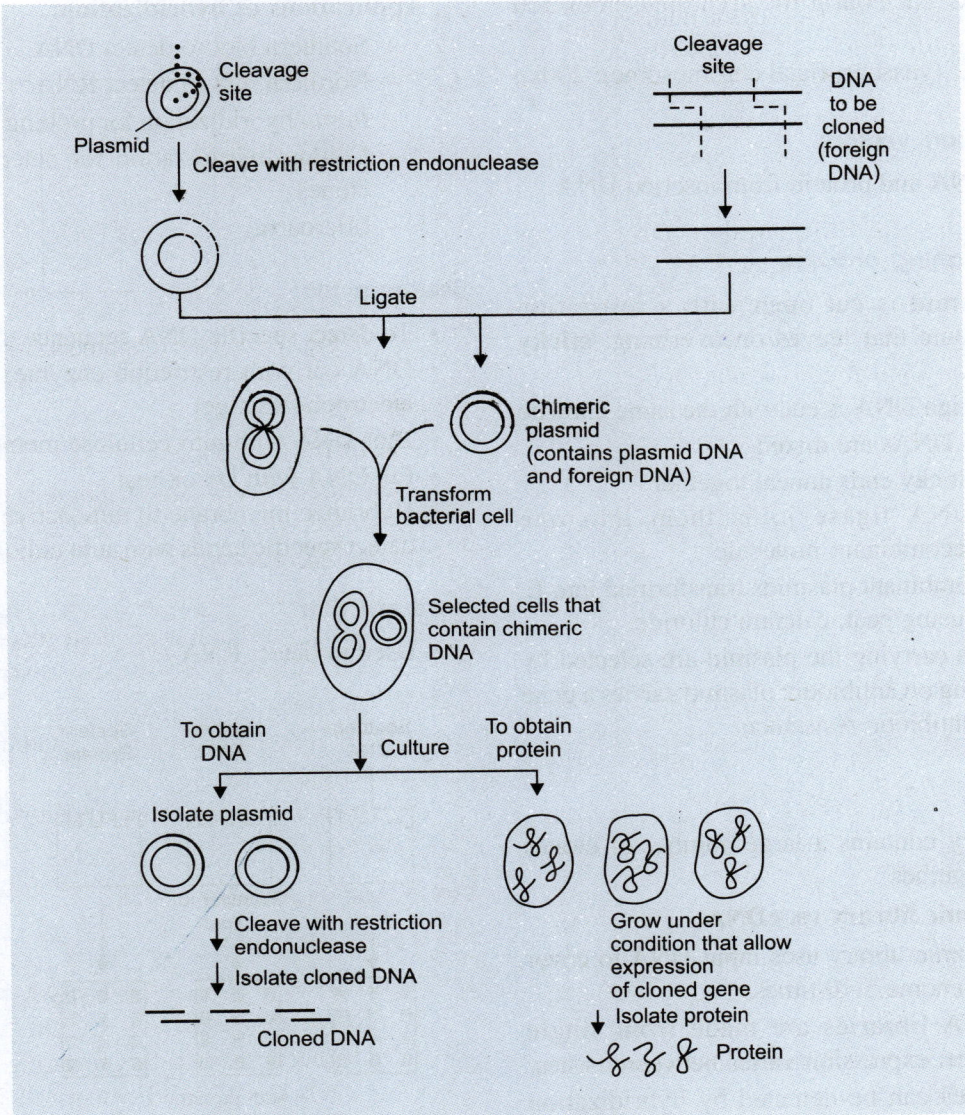

**Fig. 7.52.** Cloning of DNA in bacteria.

### DNA ligase

Attaches two pieces of DNA together.

### Transformation

- DNA manipulated in vitro can be put back into the living cells by a simple process.

- Transformed DNA replicates and expresses its genes.

### Cloning vectors

- Plasmid for up to 5kb
- Phage lambda (x): upto 50kb

- BAC (bacterial artificial chromosome): 300 kb
- YAC (yeast artificial chromosome): 200kb

## Expression vectors

Make DNA and protein from inserted DNA..

## Basic cloning process

- Plasmid is cut open with a restriction enzyme that leaves on overhang: **sticky end.**
- Foreign DNA is cut with the same enzyme
- Two DNAs are mixed
  - Sticky ends anneal together
  - DNA ligase joins them into one recombinant molecule
- Recombinant plasmids transformed into E. coli using heat, calcium chloride.
- Cells carrying the plasmid are selected by adding on antibiotic: plasmid carries a gene for antibiotic resistance

## Libraries

Library contains a large number of clones pooled together

**Genomic library vs. cDNA:**

- Genomic library uses input DNA to cover the genome 5-10 times.
- cDNA libraries are made from single tissues: expression varies between tissues.
- Clones can be detected by hybridization with labeled probes.

## Hybridization

DNA when made single stranded by melting, pairs up with another DNA or RNA with complementary sequence. If one of the DNA molecules is labeled, it can detected by hybridization.

## Applications of hybridization:

- Southern blot to detect DNA
- Northern blot to detect RNA
- *In situ* hybridization for probing a tissue
- Colony hybridization for detection of clones.
- Microarray

## Southern blot

- To detect specific DNA sequence
- DNA cut with restriction enzyme, run on electrophoresis gel
- Blot DNA with nitrocellulose membrane
- Fix DNA with Uv or heat
- Hybridize membrane to radioactive probe; detect specific bands with auto radiography.

## Northern blot

- Used to detect RNA

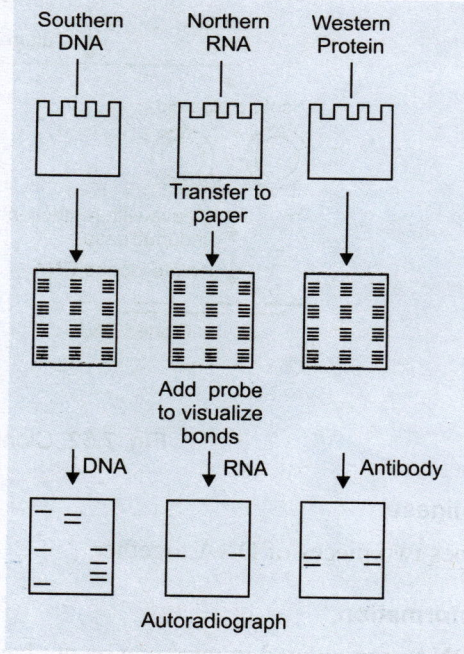

**Fig. 7.53.** Blots.

- Uses RNA instead
- RNA denatured, run on gel with formaldehyde.

## RFLP (Restriction fragment length polymorphism)

- First DNA-based genetic mapping technique
- Every individual has many variations in their DNA in terms of restriction sites
- Genomic DNA cut with restriction enzyme and Southern Blot and autoradiography is performed.

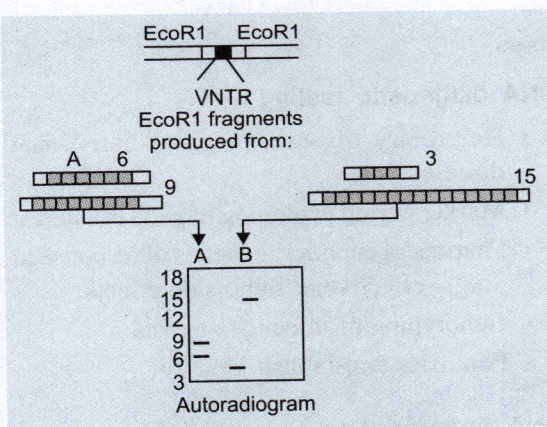

**Fig. 7.54.** RFLP produced from a gene with VNTR.

## Microarrays

- Place probes from many different genes on a glass microscopic slide and hybridize to cDNA made from mRNA isolated from a tissue. Done with 60bp long synthetic oligonucleotides using sequence information from genes.
- cDNA is fluorescently labeled
- Control and experimental conditions are compared using red and green fluorescent tags.
- Can be used to screen for DNA mutation.

## RESTRICTION DIGESTION

### Restriction enzymes

Evolved by bacteria to protect against viral DNA infection:

- Endonuclease: Cleave with in DNA strands
- Exonuclease: Digests from ends of DNA molecules

### How does it work?

Enzyme site recognition:

- Each enzyme (digests) cuts DNA at specific sequence: restriction site
- Enzyme recognizes 4-, 6- or 8- bp palindromic sequences.

| *Enzyme* | *Recognition sequence* |
|----------|------------------------|
| Ban H I  | GGATCC |
|          | CCTAGG |
| Sac I    | GAGCTC |
|          | CTCGAG |
| Sst I    | GAGCTC |
|          | CTCGAG |

Palindromic sequences
↓

5′ GAATTC 3′
3′ CTTAAG 5

↑
↓

5′ G        3′   5′ AATTC 3′
3′ CTTAA5′  3′          G 5′

Sticky ends

## EXAMPLES

↓

Pst 1        5′ CTGCAG 3′
             3′ CACGTC 5′
                    ↑

*Providencia species*
*P. stuartie*
Eco R I        GAATTC
               CTTAAG
                    ↑

Hind III
*H. influenzae*   AAGCTT
                  TTCGAA
                    ↑

## Restriction digestion

**Requirements:**
- Template DNA, uncut DNA, often phage DNA, restriction enzymes.
- Restriction buffers: NaCl, Tris
- HCl, $Mg^{+2}$, water bath.

## RELP

Restriction fragment length polymorphisms
- RF: Restriction fragment
  Fragments cut by restriction enzyme
- L: Length
  Length of restriction fragment
- P: Polymorphism

DNA variation results in RFLP:
  - SNPs: Single nucleotide polymorphisms
  - VNTRs: Tandem repeats
- AT**C**TCAATCG - person 1
- AT**A**TCAATCG - person 2
      ↑
     SNP

**SNP:** Polymorphism in sequence of bases at a single nucleotide locus

—GC—GC—GC—GC—GC—   Person 1
—.——GC—GC—GC———   Person 2

- Variable no. of tandem repeats: VNTR at a particular locus.
- VNTR alleles are highly variable regions of human DNA
- Short sequence of DNA is repeated at a specific chromosomal locus.
- Interspersed throughout human genome
- No. of repeats vary from person to person and is unique for any given individual.
- These repeats are different on paternal and maternal members of same person's chromosome pair.

Applications
- Diagnosis of genetic defects

- Study of genetic individuality
- Detection of changes in DNA sequences
- Linkage studies

## SNPs: Fact file

- Mutation that causes a single base change is known as single nucleotide polymorphisms (SNP)
- Human differ by 1bp in every 1,000 bp.
- Very common in human population
- There is average of one SNP every ~1250 bases
- <1% SNPs occur in non-coding regions

## Uses

## DNA diagnostic testing

- Hereditary disease, prenatal, late onset disease.
- Markers to aid in cloning of gene of interest
- Pharmacogenomics: genetics of response to drugs (effectiveness and side effects)
- Genotyping of infectious agents
- Forensics to establish identity

## DNA fingerprinting

- Technique to distinguish between individuals of same species by using their DNA samples.
- Variation in RFLP analysis is used, where probe hybridizes to sequence between restriction sites.

**Stages:**
1. Cells broken to release DNA
   DNA is amplified by PCR
2. DNA having hypervariable regions cut into fragments by restriction enzyme
   Each restriction enzyme cuts DNA at a specific base sequence

3. Fragments are separated according to size by gel electrophoresis
   Radioactive material added that combines with DNA fragment to produce a fluorescent image.
   Photographic copy of DNA bands is obtained.
4. Pattern of fragment distribution is then analyzed

**Uses:**

– Forensic identification: can solve crime
– Paternity testing
– Identify parentage

## Biological material for DNA fingerprinting

Blood, saliva, hair, body tissue cells, semen, vaginal cells

## DNA foot printing

- DNA bound to protein is resistant to digestion by DNase enzyme
- Sequence reaction performed
- Protected area 'Foot print' of bound protein detected.

DNA fragment
↓ DNase
DNase do not Cut DNA with protein
↓
Sample run on gel
↓
Fragment missing
↓
Foot print

## Chromosomal walking

Fragment representing one end of long piece of DNA is used to isolate another fragment that overlaps but extends the first.

Target gene identified
↓ Restriction enzyme
Original cloned fragment used as probe
↓
Each fragment tested for hybridization
↓
Overlap fragment then cloned
↓
Used as probe for second cycle of hybridization
↓
Whole chromosome mapped and cloned

## RAPD (Random amplified polymorphic DNA)

- PCR based technique, employs a single primer of arbitrary nucleotide sequence (10ntd) to amplify PCR fragments from genomic DNA.
- Primer binds many locations on template DNA
- Amplification occurs only when primer binding sites are close and oriented opposite to direction of amplified region: RAPD Locus

Genomic DNA + Taq Pol + arbitrary primer + ntd + buffer
↓
PCR
↓
Amplified products
↓
Electrophoresis → RAPD bands

## RAPD differs from PCR

- Involves one short primer (10b) instead 2 primers
- High $Mg^{+2}$ concentration

Two modifications in thermal cycle:
- Annealing temperature 36°C
- More thermal cycles: 45

**Advantage:**
- Does not require prior knowledge of DNA sequence
- Small amount of DNA required (5-20 ng).
- Easy and quick
- Generate large no. of markers
- Cost effective

**Limitation:**
- Sensitive to change in reaction condition
- Results not reproducible between labs

**Applications:**
- Measurement of:
  - Genetic diversity
  - Genetic structure of population
- Germplasm characterization
- Identification of clone
- Clarification of parentage

## Pharmacogenomics

Use of DNA sequence information to measure and predict the reaction of individuals to drugs:
- Personalized drugs
- Faster clinical trial
- Less drug side effects

## Finding disease genes

Start with DNA samples from families with inheritance of disease
↓
Use STS markers to map genes: linkage analysis
↓
Find SNPs in genetic regions that are likely candidates for involvement in that disease
↓
Get the gene from genomic subclone

- Classic genetic disease caused by mutation of single gene:
  - Huntington's
  - Cystic fibrosis
  - Tay Sachs
  - PKU
- Disease as a result of interaction of many genes:
  - Asthma
  - Heart disease
  - Cancer

## Screening of SNP

Possible with microarray technology e.g., Affymetrix Gene chips to SNP product mapping assay.

## Future of SNP

- Pharmacogenomics
  - SNP database is under preparation
  - Pharmacogenomic data is collected by pharmaceutical companies in their clinical trial
  - Genetic indications for drugs and plan to sell drugs with gene test will be the future!
- Multi locus SNP profile
  - One SNP gives information about a group of linked genes
  - There will be a few hundred to few thousand SNPs linked to medically important alleles
- A simple test to see what drug one should take
- It could provide several information about risk of cancer or heart disease of any person
- It shall serve as a number plate for a person!

## PROTEOMICS

- **Proteome** is all the proteins that are called for by genome

- Proteomics is large scale analysis of gene products involving only proteins.
  1 gene = 1 protein?
  1 gene is no longer equal to one protein
  1 gene = how many proteins

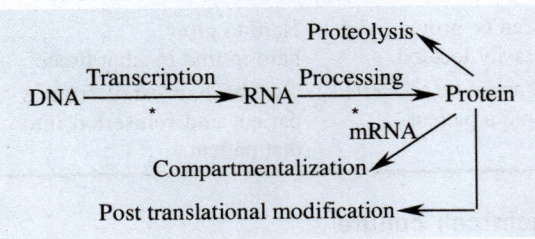

* All these steps are regulated.

## Types of proteomics

- Protein expression: Study of protein expression
- Structural proteomics: Study of 3-D structure of protein and protein complexes
- Functional proteomics: Study of functions of proteins

## Technology of proteomics

- Separation and isolation of proteins
  1D PAGE, 2D PAGE
- Edman Sequencing
- Mass spectrometry (MS) – fast, sensitive enables peptide mass and sequence to be obtained
- Database utilization

## Applications of proteomics

- Characterization of protein complexes
- Profiling of protein expression
- Yeast genomics and proteomics
- Proteome mining
- Protein arrays

## Difficulties in proteomics

- Proteins cannot be studied with speed, sensitivity and reliability that nucleic acids achieve.
- Low abundance proteins are most difficult to study with current methodologies

## Genomics

Study of DNA on a cellular scale from individual gene to entire genomic component of an organism- its genome.

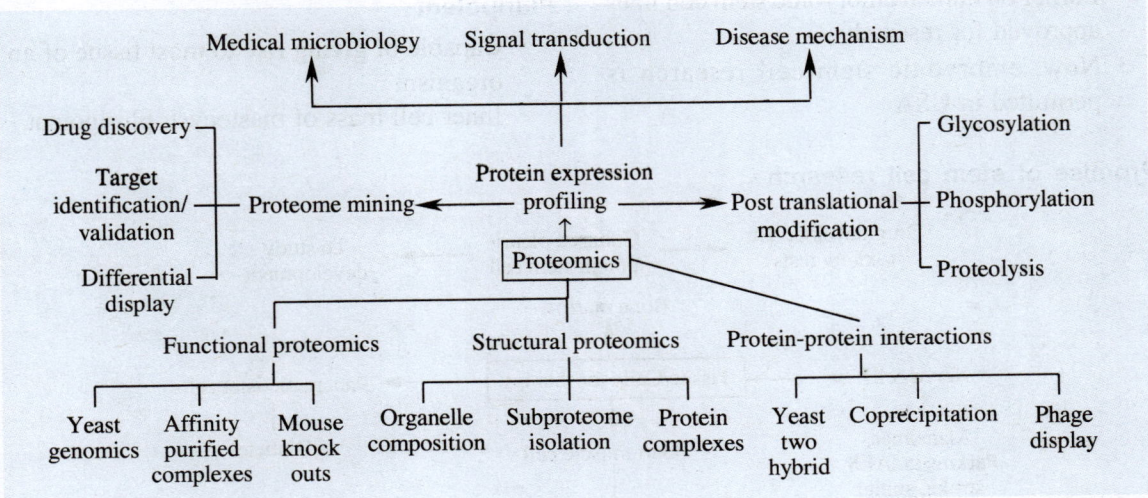

## Stem cells

- Undifferentiated cell
- Unspecialized
- Can be induced to become cells of specific function
  - Unlimited capability of dividing and renewing themselves
  - Can build tissues, specialized cell types

### Stem cell therapy is used to

- Treat disease, e.g. Parkinson's disease
- Replace damaged tissue
  - Bone marrow post-chemotherapy
  - Skin
- Understand disease
  - Cancer
  - Birth defects

## Types of stem cells

- Embryonic: Totipotent
- Adult (somatic): Pluripotent, Multipotent

## Legal and ethical issues

- Earlier 64 human embryonic stem cell lines approved for research
- Now, embryonic stem cell research is permitted in USA

## Promise of stem cell research

## Differences

| Embryonic stem cell | Adult stem cell |
| --- | --- |
| Can be induced to form any cell type | Can be induced to form only cell types found in tissue from which it is harvested |
| Can be grown in lab Easily located | Hard to grow hard to find in adult tissue |
| Cannot be reinserted into a patient | Can be harvested from a patient and reinserted into that patient |

## Stem cell culture

- Stem cells can be grown in tissue culture plastic
- Feeder layer of cells laid down first
- Fibroblasts added that secrete proteins
- Bioreactors are used to expand stem cells

## Properties of stem cell

### Totipotent

- Have unlimited capability
- Can develop to all post embryonic tissue and organs
- Embryo (fertilized egg) is totipotent

### Pluripotent

- Capable of giving rise to most tissue of an organism
- Inner cell mass of blastocyst: pluripotent

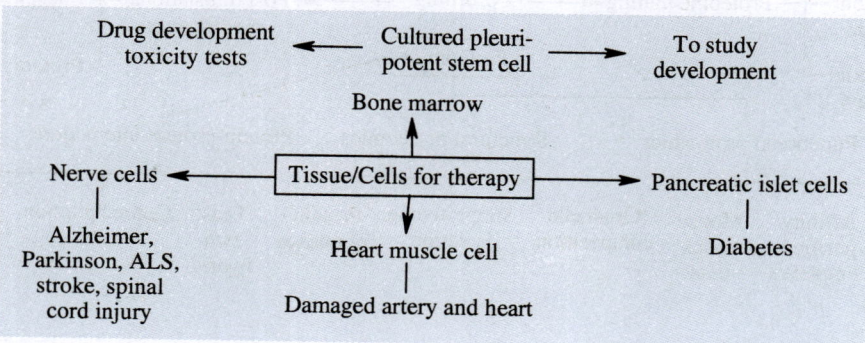

## Multipotent

Specialized to give rise to a particular type of cell, e.g. Blood stem, cells in bone marrow.

## Cord blood for stem cell cures

Umbilical cord blood contains millions of stem cells that have potential to provide therapy for many diseases and is wasted in every delivery along with placenta.

Cord blood stem cell therapy has been reported to be superior to bone marrow transplant in many reports. It has advantage of reduced incidence of graft versus host disease. Cord blood banking is available for storing umbilical cord blood for future use.

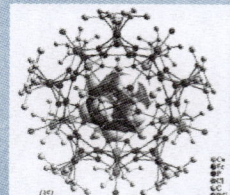

# CHAPTER 8

# Biochemistry of Cancer

## (I) INTRODUCTION

Numerous mechanisms exist to create genetic changes that result in uncontrolled cell growth. Cells proceed through multiple rounds of division during growth and maintenance of organisms. Since the cells are subjected to insults such as chemical, radiant energy or viruses, normal DNA repair mechanisms may become overwhelmed, leading to the chemical changes that result in mutations.

### BASIC PROPERTIES OF A CANCER CELL

- There are many differences in properties from one type of cancer cells.
- At cellular level, most important characteristic of a cancer cell is loss of growth control.
- Malignant cells are not responsive to those signals that cause their normal counterparts to cause growth and division.

- Cancer cells ignore inhibitory signals and continue to grow in absence of stimulatory growth signals.
- Cancer cells do not undergo aging; instead they are seemingly immortal as they continue to divide indefinitely. This property is often attributed to presence of telomerase in cancer cells and its absence in normal cells.
- Cancer cell often have highly aberrant chromosome complements termed aneuploidy.
- Cancer cells fail to elicit apoptotic response even when their chromosome content becomes highly deranged.
- Cancer cells in many cases depend on anaerobic metabolic pathways e.g. glycolysis to a much greater degree than their normal counter parts.
- Cancer cells have tendency to spread to distant sites within the body.

406

## CAUSES OF CANCER

- Diverse array of chemical, carcinogens, ionizing radiation and a variety of DNA and RNA-containing viruses have been reported to cause cancer.
- All of these agents have one property in common: they alter genome.

## GENETICS OF CANCER

### Fact file of genetics of cancer cells

- Cancer cells are found to have arisen from a single cell invariably, i.e., Cancer cell is monoclonal.
- Development of a malignant tumor is multi step process: characterized by progression of genetic alterations.
- Genes involved in carcinogenesis are those which produce products involved in control of cell cycle, intercellular adhesion and DNA repair.

## (II) GENES INVOLVED IN CARCINOGENESIS

Two types:
- Tumor suppressor gene
- Oncogenes

**Tumor suppressor genes** encode proteins that restrain cell growth and prevent cells from becoming malignant.

**Oncogenes** encode proteins that promote loss of growth control and malignancy. Oncogenes arise from protooncogenes: genes that encode proteins having a role in cell's normal activities.

Mutations that alter the protein or its expression cause oncogenes to act abnormally and promote formation of a tumor.

Most tumors contain alterations in both tumor suppressor genes and oncogenes.

## Oncogenes

- Oncogenes are derived from proto-oncogenes which are genes that encode proteins having a function in normal cell.
- Oncogenes encode proteins that promote loss of growth control and conversion of a cell to a malignant one.
- Most oncogenes play role in control of cell growth and division i.e., they act as accelerator of cell proliferation. Different oncogenes get activated in different types of tumors. Oncogenes act dominantly, single copy can cause the altered expression.

**Proto-oncogenes can be activated by:**

1. **Mutation of gene:** that alters the property of gene product
2. **Duplication of gene causing gene amplification:** produces excess of encoded protein.
3. **Chromosomal rearrangement:** cause/alter expression of gene.

| Proto-oncogene | Neoplasm | Lesion |
|---|---|---|
| ABL | Chronic myelo-genous leukemia | Translocation |
| BCL2 | B-cell lymphoma | Translocation |
| ERB B | Squamous cell carcinoma | Amplification |
| NEU/HER 2 | Adenocarcinoma breast, ovary, stomach | Amplification |
| MYC | Burkitt's lymphoma Carcinoma lung, breast, cervix | Translocation Amplification |
| H-RAS | Carcinoma colon, lung, pancreas | Point mutation |
| RET, TRK | Carcinoma thyroid | Rearrangement |

## PROTO-ONCOGENES

They are normal cellular proteins that work to regulate normal growth and development. If mutated or mis expressed, the proto-oncogenes become oncogenes and lead to aberrant cell cycle control.

Other proteins include: proteins involved in mitosis, tissue invasion and metastasis.

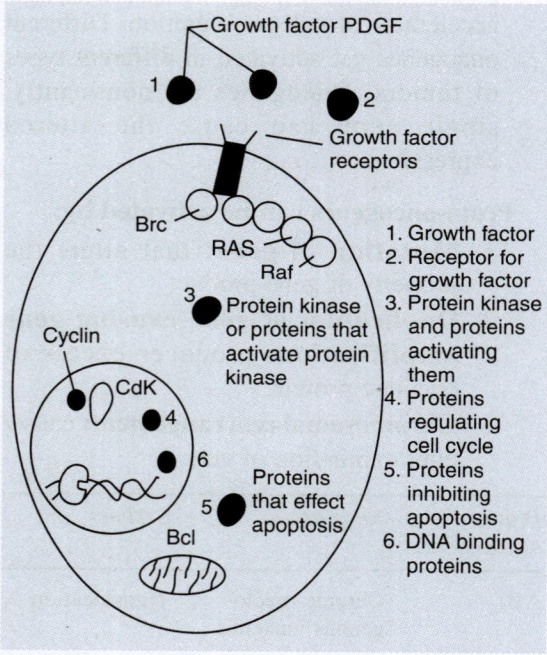

**Fig. 8.1.** Types of proteins encoded by proto-oncogenes

Aberrant expression of oncogene causes entry of cell into cell cycle with abnormal cell growth and gain of function.

Oncogenes function in growth signaling pathways.

### Growth factors

Include:

- Polypeptide growth hormones
- Fibroblast growth factors (FGF)
- Platelet derived growth factor (PDGF)

These growth factors are important for normal proliferation of cells (FGF), extracellular matrix production (PDGF).

### Growth factor receptors

- These growth factors bind to their receptors resulting in signal transduction
- Certain growth factor receptors are capable of activation even in absence of specific ligands. They have intracellular domains that function as tyrosine kinase.
- Epidermal growth factor receptors (EGFR): have three tyrosine kinase receptors: erb b-1, erb b-2, erb b-3
- If mutated, these growth factor receptors cause aberrant signaling and growth in absence of EGF.
- Over expression of Her 2/neu, also known as erb b-1 is associated with breast cancer.
- Glial cell derived neurotrophic factor (GDNF) mutation leads to autonomous growth-promoting signals in absence of ligand binding. This process is termed **rearranged during transfection** (RET). Mutation in RET are associated with MEN (multiple endocrine neoplasia) syndromes.

## SIGNAL TRANSDUCING PROTEINS

Defects occur at the level of downstream signal transduction that affects cell growth and development.

Examples:

- Ras gene
- Non-receptor tyrosine kinase proteins

### Ras gene

In inactive state, ras binds GDP, following stimulation of cell by growth factor ligand

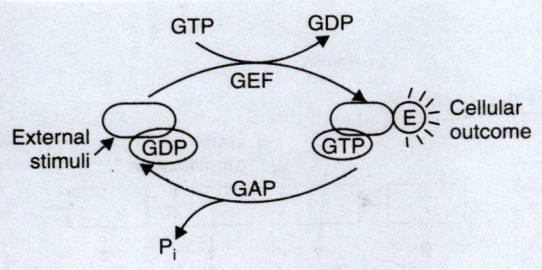

**Fig. 8.2.** Control of Ras activation.

interaction, ras exchanges GTP for GDP and activates down stream signaling events.

- Ras has intrinsic GTPase activity, terminates signal transduction events when GTP is hydrolyzed to GDP and becomes inactive.
- Ras gene is most commonly mutated oncogene and mutations are found in tumors of colon, pancreas, and thyroid.
- Non-receptor tyrosine kinase protein include: ABL, src protooncogenes
- Nuclear transcription proteins: rapidly induced when quiescent cells receive

### Ways of activating (proto-) oncogenes

| Mechanism | Oncogene | Tumor |
|---|---|---|
| 1. Amplification | ERB B2 (HER 2) | Breast, ovary, lung, lung, gastric, colon cancer |
| | NYCN | Neuroblastoma |
| 2. Point mutation | HRAS | Bladder, lung, colon cancer |
| | NIT | GIT tumor, mastocytosis |
| 3. Chromosomal rearrangement | BCR ABL 1 | Chronic myeloid leukemia |
| 4. Transduction to a region of transcriptionally active chromatin | MYC | Burkitt's lymphoma |

signals to divide and are rapidly translocated to nucleus to mediate gene transcription.

- For example: Protooncogene *myc* – that integrate divergent growth promoting pathways
- Nuclear transcription factor that bind to DNA

For example:

- WT-1 is mutated in Wilm's tumor.

### Cell cycle regulators

Cyclins, CDK, CDK inhibitors if altered, result in unchecked cell growth and CDK4 is most commonly altered gene in this class.

### Tumor suppressor genes

- Tumor suppressor genes are cellular proteins whose activity if reduced, results in uncontrolled cell growth.
- As long as a cell has its full complement of tumor-suppressor genes, it is protected against the effects of oncogenes. Transformation of a normal cell to a cancer cell is accompanied by loss of function of one or more tumor suppressor genes.
- Tumor suppressor genes are often silenced epigenetically by methylation of promoter containing CpG islands.

### Comparison of oncogene and tumor suppressor gene

| Oncogene | Tumor suppressor gene |
|---|---|
| 1. Dominant | Recessive |
| 2. Gain of function of a protein that signals cell division | Loss of function of a protein |
| 3. Mutations are somatic, not inherited | Mutations in germ cells (can be inherited) or somatic cell (not inherited) |
| 4. Some tissue preference | Strong tissue preference-e.g. RB gene in retina |

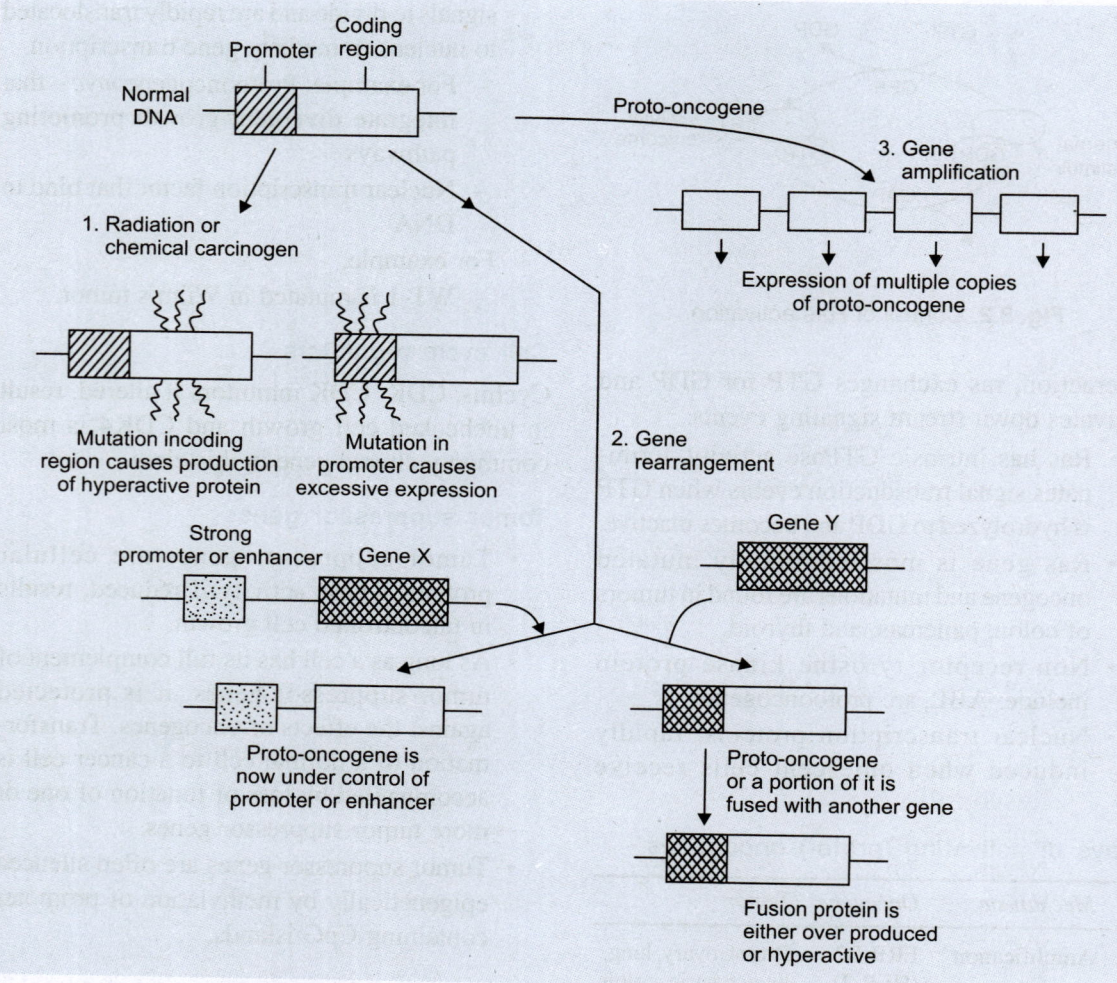

**Fig. 8.3.** Transforming mutations in proto-oncogenes.

**Table 8.1.** Genes and primary tumors

| Gene | Primary tumor | Proposed function | Inherited syndrome |
|------|---------------|-------------------|--------------------|
| APC | Colorectal | Binds β catenin, acting as transcription factor | Familial adenomatous polyposis |
| BRC A 1 | Breast | DNA repair | Familial breast cancer |
| NF 1 | Neurofibroma | Activates GTPase of Ras | Neurofibromatosis type I |
| RB | Retinal | Binds E2F | Retinoblastoma |
| WT 1 | Wilm's tumor | Transcription factor | Wilm's tumor |

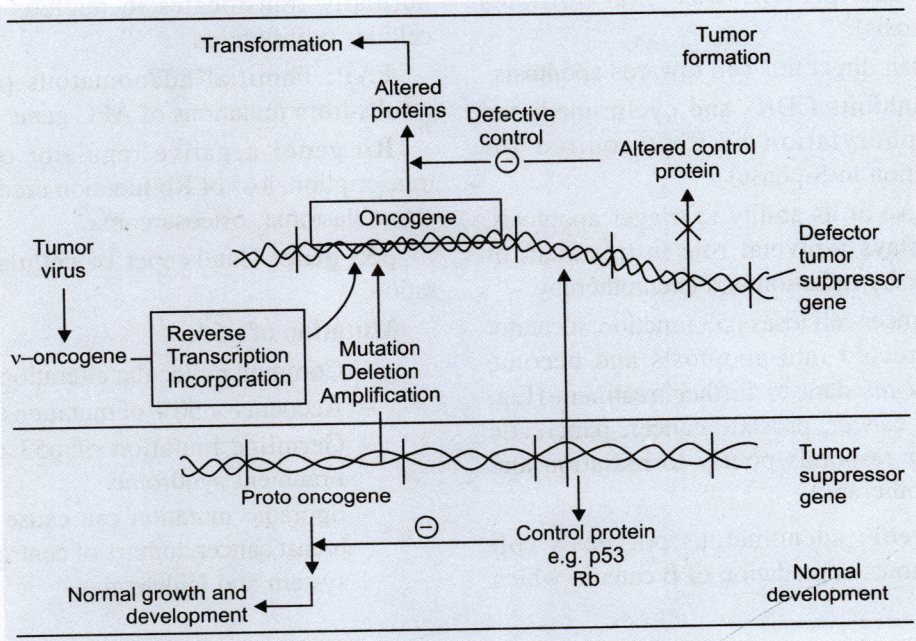

**Fig. 8.4.** Oncogene and tumor suppressor gene in tumorigenesis.

## RB gene

- Responsible for retinoblastoma – rare, familial retina tumor.
- Negative regulator of cell cycle.
- RB gene codes a protein pRb, which is involved is regulatory passage of a cell from $G_1$ to S in the cell cycle
- Dephosphorylated form of pRb interacts with certain transcription factor (E2F) preventing them from activating genes required for S phase activities
- Once pRb phosphorylated, it releases its bound transcription factor, that can activate gene expression to initiate S-phase

## Common tumor suppressor genes

- RB
- TP53
- APC
- BRCA 1 and BRCA 2

## p53 : Guardian of genome

- Induced when DNA is damaged
- Has growth inhibitory function
- Product of p53 tumor suppressor gene
- Acts as transcription factor that activates expression of p21 protein that inhibits cyclin – dependent kinase that moves a cell through cell cycle.
- p21 protein inhibits cyclin-dependent kinase that normally drives a cell through $G_1$ check point
- Damage to DNA triggers phosphorylation and stabilization of p53, leading to arrest of cell cycle, until the damage can be repaired.
- Failure to repair DNA damage leads to production of abnormal/malignant cells via activation of expression of BAX gene

(encodes protein Bax that initiates apoptosis).

- p53 can direct this cell towards apoptosis.
- p53 inhibits CDK- and cyclin-mediated phosphorylation of **Rb** (required for transition to S-phase)
- Because of its ability to trigger apoptosis, p53 plays a pivotal role in treatment of cancer by radiation and chemotherapy.
- If a cancer cell loses p53 function, it cannot be directed into apoptosis and become highly resistant to further treatment (E.g. colon cancer, prostate cancer, pancreatic cancer responds poorly to radiation and chemotherapy).

**APC gene:** adenomatous polyposis coli gene: promotes degradation of β catenin which normally translocates to nucleus to induce cellular proliferation

**FAP:** Familial adenomatous polyposis: results from mutations of APC gene.

**Rb gene:** negative regulator of nuclear transcription, loss of Rb function predisposes to retinoblastoma, osteosarcoma.

**p53 gene:** Gatekeeper of cellular proliferation.

**Mutation of p53:**

- Common molecular alteration in cancer
- Account for 50% of mutations in tumors
- Germline mutation of p53 causes Li Fraumeni syndrome
- Sporadic mutation can cause sarcoma, breast cancer, tumors of central nervous system and leukaemias.

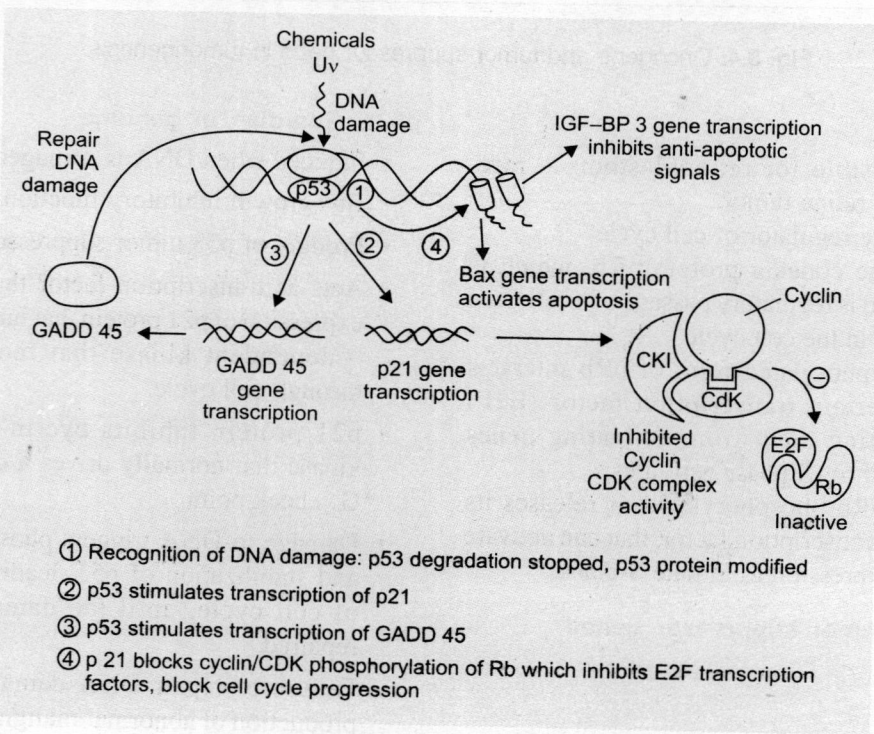

① Recognition of DNA damage: p53 degradation stopped, p53 protein modified
② p53 stimulates transcription of p21
③ p53 stimulates transcription of GADD 45
④ p 21 blocks cyclin/CDK phosphorylation of Rb which inhibits E2F transcription factors, block cell cycle progression

**Fig. 8.5.** p53 and cell cycle arrest.

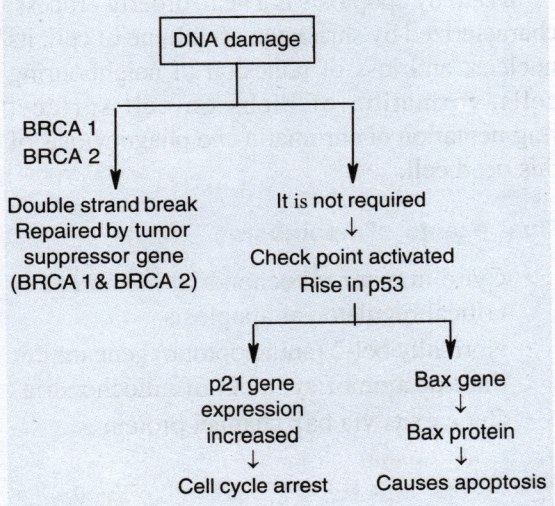

**Fig. 8.6.** Fate of DNA damage.

## Cell cycle dysregulation in cancer

- In cancer cells, all check point mechanisms are defective.
- Cells replicate despite damage, enter mitosis with unrepaired damage and become inefficient in segregating their chromosomes correctly.

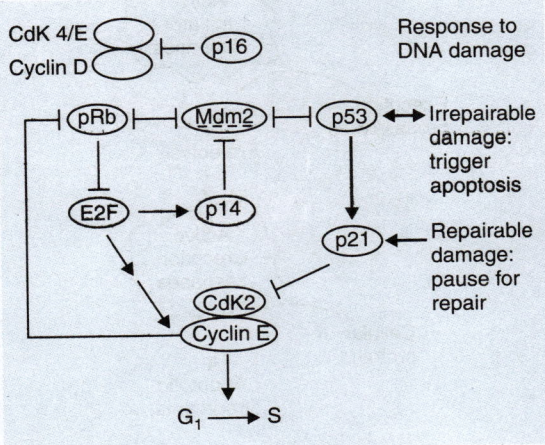

**Fig. 8.7.** Control of cell cycle progression

## Instability of genome

A universal feature of cancer cells is genomic instability.

It may be of two types:

1. **Chromosomal instability (CIN):**
   Commonest
   Tumor cells have abnormal karyotypes with extra and missing chromosomes
   Tumor cells are chromosomally unstable.

2. **Microsatellite instability (MIN):**
   DNA level instability
   Seen in certain tumors e.g. colon CA

Instability enables a cell to amass enough mutations to complete the microevolution from a normal cell (somatic) to an invasive cancer cell.

Tumors may show CIN or MIN but not both.

## Chromosomal instability and abnormal karyotypes arise in three ways:

1. Spindle check point is defective: causing numerical abnormality
2. Cells with unrepaired DNA damage progressing through cell damage: do not undergo apoptosis due to: defect apoptotic response or damaged signaling system.
3. Tumor cells replicate to the point that telomeres become too short to protect chromosome ends, leading to structural abnormalities.

## (III) APOPTOSIS

Programmed destruction of cell.

Characterized by:

- Decrease in cell volume
- Mitochondrial destabilization
- Chromatin condensation
- Nuclear fragmentation

– Cellular dispersion into fragmented apoptotic bodies.

## Programmed Cell Death (PCD)

- Very large numbers of cells of a multicellular organism are deliberately and naturally selected to die throughout its existence.
- A variety of different types of PCD are known, of these apoptosis (type I PCD) has been extensively studied and characterized by specific changes in cell structures

## Importance of PCD

| Function | Examples |
|---|---|
| 1. Killing of defective cell during development | Removal of defective, immature lymphocytes |
| 2. Killing harmful cells | Removal of harmful T cells (against self anti-gens) |
| | Removal of virally in-fected and tumor cells |
| | Removal of cells with damaged DNA |
| 3. Killing of excess, obsolete or un-necessary cells | Removal of surplus neu-rons during development Removal of interdigital cells. |

## Apoptosis results in cell death

### Mechanism

- Withdrawal of growth factor.
- Proapoptotic cytokines, tumor necrosis factor (TNF), fas ligand provide signals for apoptosis to stimulate pro apoptotic enzymes: CASPASES
- Activation of proapoptotic gene: Bax by tumor suppressor gene, p53 in case of detection of DNA mutation at $G_1/S$ checkpoint.

Death by apoptosis is a neat, orderly process, characterized by shrinkage of volume of cell, its nucleus, and loss of adhesion to neighbouring cells, formation of blebs on cell surface, fragmentation of chromatin and phagocytosis of this dead cell.

## Final events of apoptosis

- Cyt c in outer mitochondrial membrane is critical regulator of apoptosis
- Normally bcl-2 (antiapoptotic) gene inhibit translocation of cyt c out of mitochondria
- Cyt c exits via bax channel protein

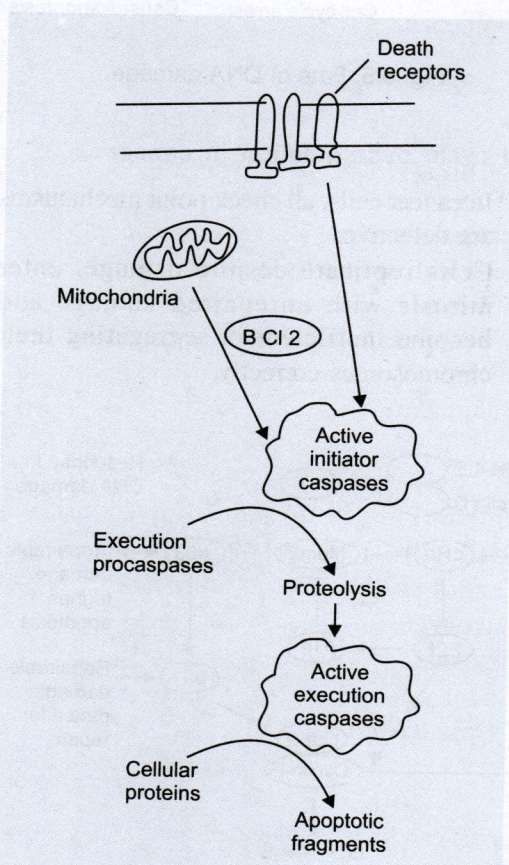

**Fig. 8.8.** Major components of apoptosis.

- Balance between bcl-2 and bax determine fate of cell, if bax predominates, cyt c is liberated to associate with proapoptotic protease activating factor (Apaf-1)
- Apaf-1 activates cascade of proteolytic events via activation of caspases.

## Caspases

- C: cysteine
  Aspase: aspartic acid protease activity
- Exist in cytoplasm as zymogen
- On stimulation apoptotic cascade begins.
- They degrade intracellular proteins and activate DNases with resultant DNA fragmentation.

## Apoptosis fact file

- Daily $10^{10}$–$10^{11}$ cells in human body die.
- During embryonic development extra neurons (that fail to find their target tissues), surplus T-cells are destroyed by apoptosis.
- Cells with irreparable genomic damage are destroyed by apoptosis normally
- Apoptosis is involved in neurodegenerative disorders (Alzheimer, Parkinson's, Huntington's)

## Targets of caspases

- Protein kinases: focal adhesion kinases (FAK), PKB, PKC, Raf1.
- Lamins in inner nuclear membrane
- Cytoskeleton proteins: intermediate filaments, action, tubulin, gelvolin
- Endonuclease termed caspase activated DNase (CAD)

## Stimuli for apoptosis

Apoptosis can be triggered both by:
- Internal stimuli (e.g. abnormality in DNA): intrinsic pathway.

- External stimuli (e.g. cytokine): Extrinsic pathway.

## Extrinsic pathway of apoptosis

- TNF produced by certain cell of immune system in response to:
  - Ionizing radiation
  - Elevated temperature
  - Viral infection
  - Toxic chemical agents (e.g. cancer chemotherapy drugs)
- TNF evokes its response by binding to its receptor TNFR 1.

## TNFR 1

- Transmembrane receptor
- Present as trimer
- Cytoplasmic domain contains death domain of 70 amino acids
- Binding of TNF to TNFR 1 causes conformational change in its death domain and binds to adaptor proteins TRADD, FADD.

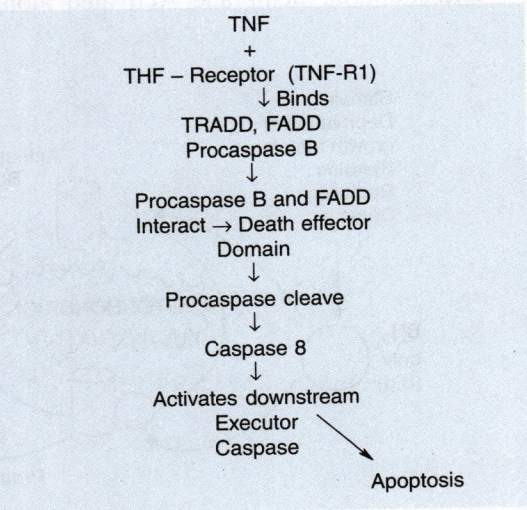

TNF
+
THF – Receptor (TNF-R1)
↓ Binds
TRADD, FADD
Procaspase B
↓
Procaspase B and FADD
Interact → Death effector
Domain
↓
Procaspase cleave
↓
Caspase 8
↓
Activates downstream
Executor
Caspase → Apoptosis

**Fig. 8.9.** Sequence of events in extrinsic pathway.

- Two procaspase-8 bind to death domain. They cleave one another to generate active caspase-8.
- Caspase-8 is **initiator** caspase and it activates downstream or **executor** caspases that carry out controlled self-destruction of cell

### Intrinsic pathway of apoptosis

- Stimuli:
  - Irreparable genetic damage
  - Lack of oxygen
  - High cytosolic $Ca^{+2}$
  - Severe oxidative stress.
- $BCl_2$: Proapoptotic family of protein Two groups:
  - Proapoptotic: Bad, Bax
  - Antiapoptotic: $Bclx_L$, Bcl-w, Bcl-2
- Following intrinsic stimuli. proapoptotic base translocates from cytosol to outer mitochondrial membrane and increases its permeability, releasing cyt c from it. Bax (and/or Bak) form channel within mitochondrial membrane. Activated along with raised cytosolic $Ca^{+2}$ (coming from ER).
- Antiapoptotic protein Bcl-2 can inhibit release of cyt c directly or indirectly.
- In cytosol, cyt c forms a complex with several procaspase 9 and the molecules called **apoptosome**.
- Procaspase get activated on joining to apoptosome complex to form caspase-9
- Caspase 9 is initiator caspase that activates downstream executioner caspases to bring about apoptosis.

### Remember

- Extrinsic (receptor-mediated) and intrinsic (mitochondria-mediated) pathways ultimately converge on same executioner caspases that cleave same cellular targets.
- Entire apoptotic program can be executed in less than an hour.
- Apoptotic cell death occurs without spilling cellular content into extracellular environment because cellular debris can trigger inflammation.

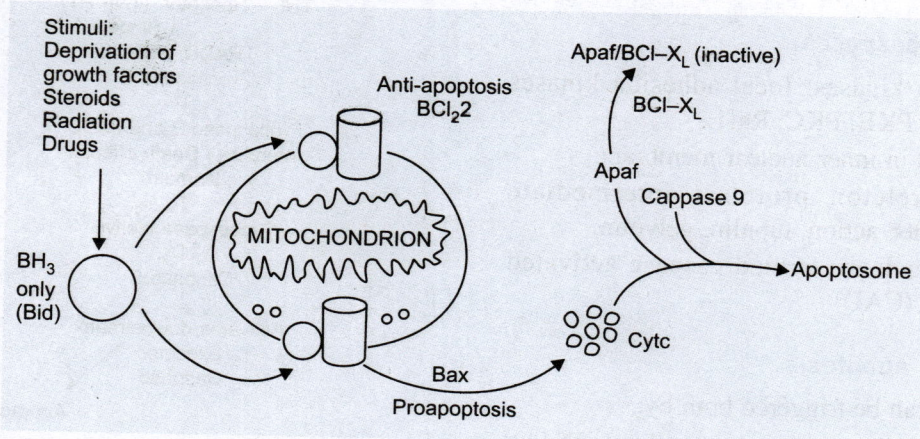

**Fig. 8.10.** $BCl_2$ and regulation of apoptosis.

Internal cellular damage

↓ Activates

Bcl 2 (e.g. Bad, Bax)

↓

Base inserted into outer mitochondrial membrane

↓ Bax forms pores

Releases cyt c in cytosol

↓

Apaf-1 and procaspose-9 bind to cyt c

↓

Apoptosome

Activated initiator

Caspase-9 complex → Procaspase 9 → caspase 9 → Apoptosis

**Fig. 8.11.** Sequence of events in intrinsic pathway.

## Sequence of events following execution of apoptotic program

- Cells lose contact with neighbors and shrink
- Cells disintegrate into apoptotic bodies
- Apoptotic bodies recognized by presence of phosphaditylserine (PS) on their surface
- Normally PS is on inner leaflet of plasma membrane, during apoptosis, phospholipids **scramblase** moves PS to outer leaflet of plasma membrane.
- This (eat me signal) is recognized by macrophages.

Thus, fate of a cell whether survival or death-depends on a delicate balance between proapoptotic and antiapoptotic signals.

# Miscellaneous

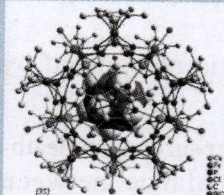

## (I) XENOBIOTICS

- *Gk. Xenos*-stranger, meaning foreign to life.
- Xenobiotics are chemical compounds, foreign to the body.
  **Examples:**
  - Drugs
  - Food additives
  - Chemical carcinogens
  - Environmental pollutants

### Why Xenobiotics hard to degrade?

- Xenobiotics are highly toxic
- Toxic byproducts often produced cytP$_{50}$ bioactivates xenobiotics in liver, causing toxicity.

### Facts file: Xenobiotics

- Xenobiotics find their way into environ- ment, e.g. insecticides, PCB (polychlori- nated bip-henyls).
- More than 2 lac manufactured environ- mental chemicals exist.
- Liver is main organ involved in their metabolism.
- Atleast thirty different enzymes catalyze reactions of xenobiotic metabolism.

### Cytochrome P$_{450}$

- Designated as CYP: Cytochrome P$_{450}$.
- >100 isoforms.
- 18 families, 41 sub families.
- Carry out metabolism of exogenous and endogenous compounds.
- Their name arise due to characteristics 450 nm peak in their absorption spectra (when reacted in their ferrous state with CO).
- They are monooxygenases.

## Xenobiotic metabolizing reactions

| Reaction type | Enzyme | Reaction |
|---|---|---|
| Hydrolysis | Epoxide hydrolase | Add water to epoxide |
| | Carboxyl esterase | Addition of water to ester bond |
| | Amidase | Addition to water to amide bond |
| Oxidation | Dehydrogenase | Oxidation of alcohol or aldehyde |
| | Monooxygenase | Oxidation of primary, secondary, tertiary amines, thioether, thiocarbamate, phosphine, nitrone |
| | Cyt $P_{450}$ | (see separate table on it) |
| Reduction | Reductase:· | |
| | • Aldehyde and ketone reductase | Reduce carbonyl group to hydroxyl group |
| | • Azoreductase | Reduce azo group to primary amines |
| | • Quinone reductase | Reduce quinine to hydroquinone |
| Conjugation | N-acetyl transferase | Add CoA to aromatic amino hydrazines |
| | Methyl transferase | Adds methyl group to compounds with groups phenol, catechol, amine, sulfihydryl |
| | GST | Conjugates carbonium ions, free radicals, epoxide |
| | UDP-glucuronyl transferase | Adds UDP-glucuronate to carboxyl, hydroxyl, amine, sulfhydroxyl, phenol group. |

## Requirement for $CYP_{450}$

- $O_2$
- NADPH
- Cyt $P_{450}$ reductase
- Sub cellular location: ER

## Cytochrome $P_{450}$

- Electron-transport heme proteins. Heme iron acts as catalytic centre
- Located in smooth endoplasmic reticulum, mitochondria
- Liver contains highest amounts, also found in small intestine, lung, and brain.
- Involved in metabolism of:
  - Endogenous compounds (e.g. steroids)
  - Phase I metabolism of xenobiotics.
- Inducible, activity altered in disease state (e.g. cirrhosis)
- Broad substrate specificity

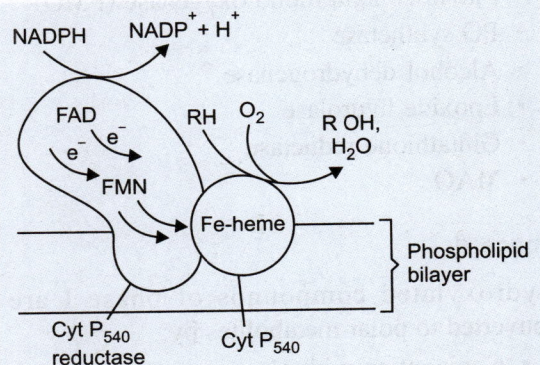

**Fig. 9.1.** Structure of $P_{450}$ enzymes. (RH = ethanol, ROH = acetaldehyde)

- Produce water soluble products, facilitating their excretion
- Their products can be carcinogenic or mutagenic at times
- Inhibited by various drugs or their metabolic products

- NADPH involved in reaction mechanism of cyt $P_{450}$, NADH not involved.
- Not involved in phase II

## Two phases of metabolism of xenobiotics

### Phase I

- Major reaction: hydroxylation
- Enzymes: monooxygenases or cyt $P_{450}$
- Hydroxylation reaction can result in: termination of action of drug.
- Also, enzyme can carry out other reactions in addition to hydroxylation namely, deamination, epoxidation, peroxygenation, reduction, nitro reduction, azo reduction.
- Limited number of enzymes with broad substrate specificity.

### Important phase I enzyme

- CYP
- Flavin-contain mono oxygenase (FMO)
- PG synthetase
- Alcohol dehydrogenase
- Epoxide hydrolase
- Glutathione reductase
- MAO

### Phase II

Hydroxylated compounds of phase I are converted to polar metabolites by:

- Conjugation with glucuronate
  - Sulfate
  - Acetate
  - Glutathione
  - Amino acids
  - Methylation

## Net outcome of two phases

- Polarity or water solubility of xenobiotics increased
  This increased water solubility facilitate their excretion from body
- Conversion of **inactive** to **biologically active** compounds, i.e., pro drugs or pro carcinogens are activated.

## Role of CYT $P_{450}$ in phase I

- Reaction catalyzed by cyt $P_{450}$:
  $$RH + O_2 + NADPH + H^+ \rightarrow R - OH + H_2O + NADP$$
- RH – xenobiotic
  Includes: drugs, carcinogens, pesticides, steroids, eicosanoids, fatty acid, retinoids, bile acid, lipid oxidation

## Inhibitors of CYP

Competitive inhibition e.g. Omeprazole: CYP2C19

## Nomenclature: Cytochrome $P_{450}$

- Abbreviated as CYP
  - Followed by Arabic number for family
  - Followed by capital letter for subfamily
  - Then, individual $P_{450}$ are assigned Arabic numerals.

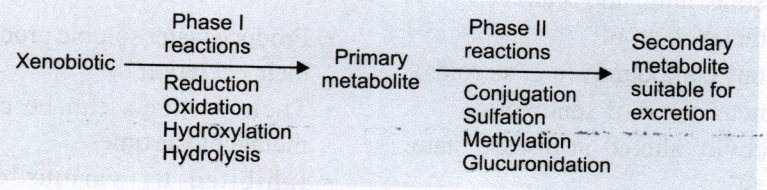

**Fig. 9.2.** General scheme of xenobiotic metabolism.

- CYP1A1: Cyt $P_{450}$ that is member of family 1, sub family A, first individual member of this sub family.
  - Nomenclature for gene is same as of CYP with addition of italics.

## Induction of CYP

- Cyt $P_{450}$ is inducible
- Inducing substance: Phenobarbital

## Mechanism of induction

- Drugs cause hypertrophy of SER with increase in amount of cyt $P_{450}$ via increased transcription of mRNA for cyt $P_{450}$. This takes 4-5 days.
- Other mechanisms include stabilization of mRNA, enzyme stabilization, effect on translation.

## Clinical implication of induction drug interaction

- Occurs when effect of one drug is altered by prior, concurrent or later administration of another, e.g. Anticoagulant Warfarin is metabolized by CYP 2 C9. If patient is given phenobarbital concomitantly it requires dosage of warfarin to be changed.
- Phenobarbital induces CYP 2 C9 and Warfarin is metabolized more quickly than before and dosage becomes inadequate increasing risk of bleeding in such patient.

## Ethanol consumption

- Ethanol induces CYP2E1.
- Tobacco smoke components are metabolized by $P_{450}$ and many are carcinogenic.
- Elevation of CYP2E1 activity by induction may increase risk of carcinogenicity from of exposure to compounds of tobacco smoke.

## PAH metabolism

- CYP1A1 metabolizes PAH (polycyclic aromatic hydrocarbons)
- PAH (procarcinogen) is inhaled by smoking and get converted to active carcinogen by CYP1A1.
- PAH can cross placenta if women is smoking

## Cyp polymorphism

- Certain cyt $P_{450}$ exist in polymorphic forms (genetic isoforms), some of which have low catalytic activity.
- This is responsible for variation in drug response among many patients.

## Therapeutic inhibition of CYP

Without an understanding of drug metabolism and drug interaction mediated by CYP, medication cannot be safely prescribed.

## Phase 2 reaction details:

### 1. Glucuronidation

- Most frequent conjugation reaction
- Glucuronyl donor: UDP – glucuronic acid
- Enzyme: glucuronsyl transferase
- Present in ER, cytosol

### Compounds glucuronidated

- 2 acetyl aminofluorene
- Phenol
- Steroids
- Morphine

Mechanism: Attachment of glucuronide to oxygen, nitrogen or sulfur of substrates.

### 2. Sulfation

- Sulfur donor:
  - PAPS
  - Adenosine 3'-phosphate 5' phospho-sulfate (active sulfur)

- Compounds sulfated:
  - Alcohol
  - Aryl amines
  - Phenols
  - Steroids
  - Glycosaminoglycans
  - Glycolipid
  - Glycoprotein

## 3. Glutathione (GSH)

$$R + GSH \rightarrow R\text{-}S\text{-}G$$

- Detoxifies electrophilic xenobiotics.
- Catalyzed by glutathione S-transferase.

### GSH-fact file

- Tripeptide
- $\gamma$-glutamyl cysteine
- Glutamic acid, cysteine, glycine
- Contains sulfhydryl groups of cysteine.
- Glutathione conjugates get further metabolized before excretion
- Glutamyl and glycinyl groups of GSH are removed and acetyl group (from acetyl CoA) gets attached to cysteinyl moiety to form mercapturic acid which is then excreted.

### Functions of GSH

- Xenobiotic metabolism
- Decomposition of hydrogen peroxide
- Important intracellular reductant: maintains SH group of enzymes in reduced state
- Transport of amino acid across membrane in kidney.
- Amino acid + GSH – GGT → Glutamyl amino acid + cysteinyl glycine.
- Example of conjugation of glutathione to cyclophosphamide.

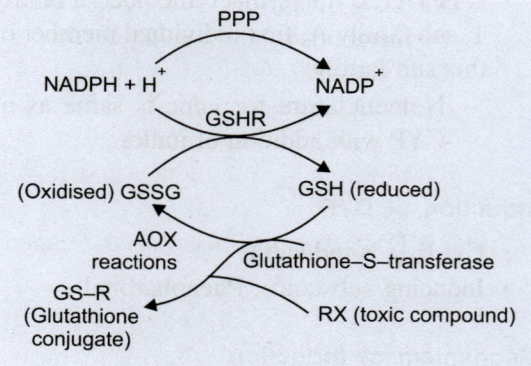

Fig. 9.3. Glutathione conjugation.

## 4. Acetylation

- Donor: Acetyl CoA (active acetate)
- Enzyme: Acetyl transferase
- Example:
  - Isoniazid: antitubercular drug is acetylated by acetyl transferase.
  - Two polymorphic forms of enzyme exist: fast, slow acetylators.
  - Slow acetylators are subjected to toxic effect of drug because it persists longer.

### Methylation

- Donor: Adenosylmethionine
- Enzyme: Methyl transferase

### EFFECTS OF XENOBIOTICS

Diverse effects are produced by drugs/ xenobiotics:

- Inactivation, activation, formation of a toxic metabolite.
- Inactivation of active form of drug to inactive form resulting in decreased bioavailability of drug.
- Activation of drug by cyt $P_{450}$ to biologically active form or toxic form.
- Cell injury (cytotoxicity) can be severe to cause cell death.

- Reactive species of xenobiotics produced by metabolism bind covalently to:
  - Cell macromolecules that can be DNA, RNA, proteins.
  - Protein, altering its antigenicity. Xenobiotic acts as a hapten and results in antibody production.
  - DNA causing chemical carcinogenesis.

## Indirect carcinogens

Certain chemicals require activation by monooxygenases in ER to become carcinogenic. Other chemicals react directly with DNA: direct carcino-genesis.

## Epoxides

Products of action of certain monooxygenases. Highly reactive, mutagenic or carcinogenic epoxide hydrolase acts on them to convert them to less reactive dihydrodiols.

## Genetically determined defects in drug reactions

| Enzyme affected | Consequence |
|---|---|
| G6PD | Hemolytic anaemia following primaquin intake |
| $Ca^{+2}$ release channel | Malignant hyperthermia |
| CYP2D6 | Slow metabolism of drugs |
| CYP2A6 | Impaired metabolism of nicotine |

## Phase I vs. Phase II metabolism

- Phase I metabolism adds or exposes a functional group on the molecule
- Results in small increase in water solubility
- Located in ER mainly
- Phase II metabolism adds an endogenous substrate to the molecule.
- Results in large increase in water solubility

CYT $P_{450}$ drug interactions

| Cyt | Drug | Effect |
|---|---|---|
| CYP2E1 | Alcohol | Induce CYP |
| | Isoniazid | Induce CYP |
| | Halothane | Metabolized to compounds that damage liver protein |
| | Enflurane | |
| | | Outcome: People with high CYP2E1 activity due to alcohol intake are at higher risk of hepatitis reaction to an anaesthetic agent |
| CYP3A4 | Rifampicin | Induce CYP |
| | Carbamazepine | Taking Rifampicin with oral contraceptives (metabolized by CYP3A4) lower efficiency of contraceptive |
| | Phenytoin | |
| | Glucocorticoid | |
| | Ketoconazole | |
| | Cyclosporins | Ketoconazole administration with Warfarin leads to excessive bleeding. |
| | Erythromycin | |

- So that it is easily excreted
- Located in cytosol mainly.

**Exceptions:** They are also present in mitochondria, nuclei and lysosomes

## Organs active in xenobiotic metabolism

- Liver
- Kidney
- GIT
- Gonads
- Adrenals
- Placenta
- Nasal epithelium

## Factors influencing $P_{450}$ metabolism:

- Specifies difference
- Individual difference
  - Genetic make up
  - Age

- Gender
- Fitness/ disease
- Diet
- Drug-drug and xenobiotic-drug interactions.

# (II) ORGAN FUNCTION TEST: LIVER, KIDNEY, GASTRIC

## LIVER

## Functions of Liver

- Liver is the 'metabolic factory' of the body.
- It has essential metabolic, synthetic and excretory functions.

## Normal liver function

**Metabolic:**
- Carbohydrate metabolism
- Lipid and lipoprotein metabolism
- Protein metabolism

**Synthetic:**
- Protein synthesis:
- Most plasma proteins: (except Ig, RhF, complement)
- Blood coagulation factors: II, V, VII, IX, XI
- Primary bile acids
- Lipoprotein
- Urea
- Bilirubin glucuronide

**Excretory:** Detoxification of:
- Xenobiotics
- Drugs
- Toxic metabolic wastes (ammonia, bilirubin

## Liver function tests

| Metabolite | ↑/↓ | Enzyme affected | Cause |
|---|---|---|---|
| Ammonia | ↑ | Ornithine transcarbamoylase | Congenital deficiency |
| | | | Cirrhosis |
| | | | Reye's syndrome |
| | | | Hepatic failure |
| **Lipids:** | | | |
| Cholesterol | ↓ | Decreased hepatic synthesis | Cirrhosis |
| **Proteins:** | | | |
| Plasma proteins | ↓ | Decreased synthesis of protein | Cirrhosis |
| | | | Chronic liver disease |
| Albumin | ↓ | Decreased synthesis of protein | Cirrhosis |
| 1g | ↓ | Decreased synthesis of protein | Hepatic failure |
| **Other:** | | | |
| α 1 AT (alpha 1 antitrypsin) | ↓ | Decreased synthesis of protein | Congenital |
| Ceruloplasmin | ↓ | Deficient hepatic copper binding apoprotein | Wilson's disease |
| Clotting factors | ↓ | Decreased synthesis | Chronic liver disease |
| **Carbohydrate:** | | | |
| Glucose | ↓ | Decreased glycogen content | Cirrhosis |
| | | | Acute liver failure |
| Bile salts | ↓ | Decreased secondary bile salts formation | Cholestasis |

## Jaundice

Jaundice is yellow discoloration of tissues due to bilirubin deposition.

| Pre-hepatic | Hepatic | Post-hepatic |
|---|---|---|
| Hemolysis | Drugs | CA pancreas, |
| Ineffective | Prematurity | CA Biliary tree |
| erythropoiesis | Hepatitis | Gallstone |
| | Inborn errors | Biliary stricture |
| | of bilirubin | |
| | metabolism | |
| | Cirrhosis | |
| | Tumors | |

### Lab findings in jaundice

| | Pre-hepatic | Hepatic | Post-hepatic |
|---|---|---|---|
| Serum bilirubin | | | |
| Unconjugated | ↑↑ | ↑↑ | ↑ |
| Conjugated | −/↓/n | ↑↑ | ↑↑↑ |
| Urine bilirubin | − | − | + |
| Fecal urobilinogen | ↑↑ | ↑ | − |
| Fecal stereobilinogen | − | ↓ | − |
| Amino transferase | ↑ | ↑↑ | ↑ |
| ALP | N | n/↑ | ↑↑ |
| Albumin | N | n/↑ | N |
| Prothrombin time | N | n/↑ | n/↑ |

## GASTRIC FUNCTION TEST

In diseasess of stomach and duodenum, alterations of gastric secretions often occur. Gastric function tests may be of value in:

- Diagnosis of gastric ulcer
- Exclusion of diagnosis of pernicious anaemia.
- Presumptive diagnosis of Zollinger Ellison syndrome
- Determination of effectiveness of surgical vagotomy.

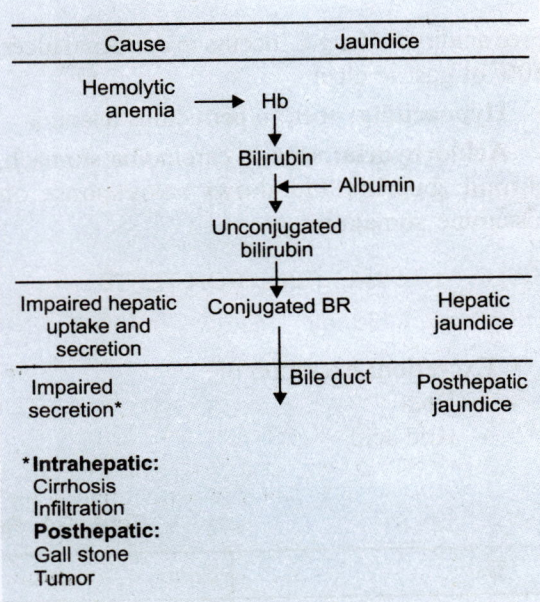

**Fig. 9.4.** Types and causes of jaundice.

## Commonly used test

1. Fractional test meal
2. Examination of gastric contents after stimulation:
   - Alcohol
   - Caffeine
   - Histamine (and augmented)
   - Insulin
   - Pentagastrin
3. Tubeless gastric analysis

**BAO:** Basal acid output (meq/L) is based on 1 hour collection of gastric secretion, normal value: 1.3-4 meq/L.

**MAO:** Maximal acid output (meq/L) amount of meq/L of acid secreted in one hour following injection of histamine/pentagastrin, normal value: 4.9-38.9 meq/L (10 times the BAO).

## Hyperacidity

Free acidity > 45mg/L, occurs in duodenal ulcer, 50% of gastric ulcer.

**Hypoacidity:** seen in pernicious anaemia

**Achlorhydria:** seen in carcinoma stomach, chronic gastritis and shows no response on histamine stimulation.

## KIDNEY (RENAL) FUNCTION TESTS

### Function of kidney

- **Excretion:** excretion of
  - Urea
  - Uric acid
  - Creatinine
  - Drugs
- **Retention of:**
  - Glucose
  - Amino acid
  - Protein
- **Drug metabolism**
- **Production of hormones:** erythropoietin, renin, 1, 25 DHD$_3$.

### Glomerular Filtration Rate (GFR)

Normal GFR is 120 ml/min approximately and is equivalent to volume of 170 L/24 h.

**Table 9.1.** Renal function test

| Test | Utility | |
|---|---|---|
| 1. Blood urea | Apart from renal function urea is dependent on factors such as protein intake, rate of tissue break down | |
| 2. Serum creatinine | Marker of decrease in (glomerular) renal function | |
| 3. Clearance (Cl) Insulin Creatinine Urea | Exogenous Endogenous | Creatinine Cl is a prognostic indicator of renal function and is nearly equal to GFR |
| 4. Cystatin C | Provide accurate assessment of moderate decrease in GFR. | |
| 5. Tubular function: Urine concentration or dilution test Urine acidification | Tubular function Tubular function | |
| 6. Urine examination | | |
| Routine: Volume pH Specific gravity Osmolality | Help to assess kidney function and diagnose disease | |
| Abnormal constituents: | | |
| Protein Blood Sugar Ketone bodies Bilirubin | Present in urine in: Renal diseases (diabetes mellitus, jaundice, hereditary defects of amino acid transport) | |

**Table 9.2.** Comparison of urea and creatinine clearance

| Urea clearance | Creatinine clearance |
|---|---|
| 1. Its value is 3/5th of GFR | 1. Values are nearly equal to GFR |
| 2. Plasma values of urea are not constant over 24 hours | 2. Its plasma values remain constant throughout the day over 24 hrs |
| 3. Urea is both secreted and reabsorbed by kidney | 3. Creatinine is neither secreted nor reabsorbed by kidney |
| 4. It is affected by rate of urine flow | 4. It does not depend on rate of urine flow |

GFR depends on:

– Rate of blood flow
– Balance between hydrostatic and oncotic forces in afferent arterioles and glomerular filter (tubular fluid).

## Clearance

It is ml of plasma cleared off a particular substance by both the kidneys per minute.

*Properties of ideal substance for clearance:*

1. It should be neither secreted nor reabsorbed by the kidney.
2. It should not be affected by rate of urine flow.
3. Its levels in blood should remain constant.
4. Its clearance should be equivalent to GFR.

## Urine osmolality

Normal values are 300 to 900 mOsm/kg in case of average fluid intake.

*Normal*:

– > 850 following 12 hrs of fluid restriction implies normal concentrating ability of kidney.
– Does not exceed 300 mOsm/kg in complete ADH deficiency.

**Table 9.3.** Tubular function tests

| 1. Proximal: | |
|---|---|
| a. Plasma: | b. Urine: |
| Urea | Volume |
| Creatinine | Specific gravity |
| Uric acid | pH |
| Bicarbonate | Glucose |
| pH | Amino acids |
| Potassium | Uric acid |
| Magnesium | Retinol binding protein |
| Phosphate | $\alpha_1$ microglobulin |
| **2. Distal:** | |
| a. Plasma: | b. Urine: |
| pH | Volume |
| Bicarbonate | pH |
| Chloride | Sodium |
| Potassium | Osmolality |

## Defects of Urinary concentration

- Diabetes insipidus
- CRF
- Hypercalcemia
- Drug toxicity, e.g. Lithium
- Renal disease

## Osmolality

$$Osmolality = 2(Na + K) + \frac{Urea}{2.8} + \frac{Glucose}{18}$$

(Osmol/kg)

Plasma osmolality is 285-295 mosmol/kg and sodium makes largest contribution.

## Regulation of water and electrolyte balance

Kidneys play a predominant role via hormones namely, aldosterone, ADH, rennin-angiotensin.

| Hormone | Action |
|---|---|
| Aldosterone | Increase Na, decrease K and $H^+$ reabsorption |
| ADH | Increase $H_2O$ reabsorption |
| Renin-angiotensin | Stimulate aldosterone secretion, constrict vascular smooth muscle |

# (III) WATER AND ELECTROLYTE BALANCE, ACID-BASE EQUILIBRIUM

## WATER AND ELECTROLYTE BALANCE
### Fluid

- 50-70% of a healthy adult body is composed of fluids
- $2/3^{rd}$ of body fluid is within cells: intracellular fluid (ICF)
- $1/3^{rd}$ of body fluid is outside cells: extra cellular fluid (ECF)

**Ecf include:** Tissue (interstitial) fluid which is found:

- Between cells
- Within tissues
- Organs of body

Plasma: fluid portion of blood lymph

**Body fluid composition of tissue varies by:**

- Tissue type: Lean tissues have higher fluid content than fat tissues
- Gender: Males have more lean tissue than females, so more body fluid

- Age: With age, lean tissue is lost and body fluid is lost with it.

## Functions of body fluid

- Dissolve and transport substances: carbohydrate, ions, amino acids, vitamins and mineral.
- Account for blood volume
- Maintain body temperature
- Protect and lubricate body tissues e.g. CSF, synovial fluid, amniotic fluid, digestive secretions
- Required for fluid and electrolyte balance and metabolic reaction.

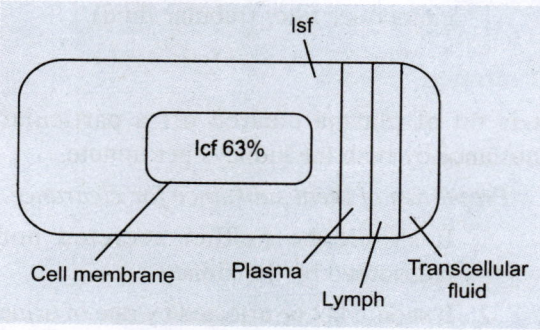

**Fig. 9.5.** Body fluid.

## Body water

- 75% of body weight in infant
- 60% in adult male
- 55% in adult female

## Body water compartments

| 2/3rd | ICF | (60%) |
|---|---|---|
| 1/3rd | ECF | (40%) |

| 15% | 3% |
|---|---|
| ISF | Plasma |

## Daily water balance

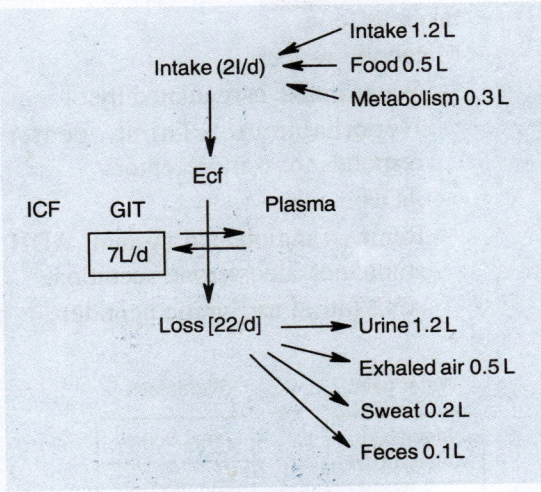

**Fig. 9.6.** Water balance.

| Drinking     2300 ml/d | Urine (1500 ml/d) |
|---|---|
| Food stuff | Feces 100 ml/d |
| Metabolic (200ml/d) | Insensible loss (300 ml/d) |
| Oxidation | Sweat (600 ml/d) |
| Polymerization | Milk |
| Body tissue | Conceptus |
| Catabolism | Plasma |

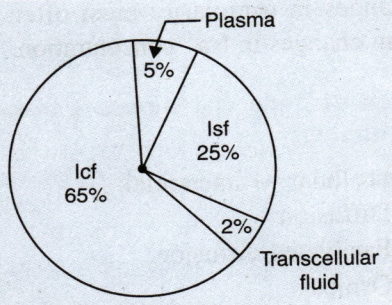

**Fig. 9.7.** Distribution of water in body fluids.

## Sources of water

- Drinking
- Food (10-15%), preformed water
- Metabolic water (5-10%)

## Metabolic water

When carbohydrates, fats and proteins are burned in body for energy using oxygen, carbon dioxide and water are produced.

| Nutrient | g of water produced/100 g |
|---|---|
| Carbohydrate | 60 |
| Fat | 108 |
| Protein | 42 |

$$Glucose + 6\,O_2 \rightarrow 6CO_2 + 6H_2O$$

$$Alanine + 3O_2 \rightarrow 2.5\,CO_2 + CO\,(NH_2)_2 + 2.5\,H_2O$$

$$Palmitic + 23O_2 \rightarrow 16CO_2 + 16\,H_2O$$

```
             Water
          ┌────┴────┐
        Input    Overflow
```

## Water balance

- Body cannot store water.
- Water lost must be replaced daily.
- Hypothalamus maintains water balance, regulation of body temperature: thirst is controlled.
- Sensation of thirst may be impaired in newborns and old age and during disease or extreme dehydration.

## Factors influencing water balance

| Intake | Loss |
|---|---|
| Social habits, climate (hot climate-thirst centre in hypothalamus controls water ingestion) | Hormonal regulation of urine production: ADH: stimulate water reabsorption in case of increased plasma osmolality |
| | Skin: Perspiration (temperature, humidity) |
| | Feces: In diarrhea |

## Body compartments

- Icf and interstitial fluid (isf) have same osmolarity and normal cells do not shrink or swell.
- Increasing osmolarity of isf draws water out of cell causing cell to shrink
- Decreasing osmolarity of isf causes cell to swell.
- Changes in osmolarity most often result from changes in $Na^+$ concentration

## Exchange of body water occurs among compartments

- Intracellular → interstitial:
  - Diffusion
  - Facilitated diffusion
  - Osmosis
  - Active transport
- Isf → lymph
- Lymph → blood plasma
- Plasma → Isf: filtration of electrolytes and nutrients from capillaries.

## Fluid balance

Maintained by:

- Replacement of water loss from body
- Water is lost through urine, sweat, exhalation, feces
- Water is gained through beverage, food and metabolic reactions.

## Maintaining fluid balance

- Loss of water:
  - Urine: most water is lost through urine
  - Kidneys control water absorption insensible water loss:
    - Skin (sweat)
    - Lungs (exhalation)
  - Diuretics: increase fluid loss via urine

## Water intake

- Most water taken as beverages some taken as food
- Metabolic water
  - Water intake is regulated by:
  - Hypothalamus: Thirst center responds to: osmoreceptors
  - ADH
  - Renin – angiotensin system: ADH stimulates aldosterone secretion.
  - ANP (atrial natriuretic peptide)

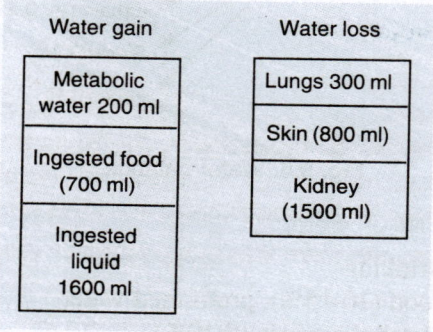

**Fig. 9.8.** Daily water gain and loss.

## Regulation of water & solute

## Water and solute loss

- Excess body water eliminated through urine
- Extent of urinary salt loss is main factor that determine urinary water loss.
- Hormone regulating $Na^+$ and $Cl^-$ reabsorption in kidney
  - AII and aldosterone: promote $Na^+$, $Cl^-$ and water reabsorption from kidney in dehydration.
  - ANP- promotes nateriuresis, excretion of $Na^+$, $Cl^-$ followed by water excretion.

## Dehydration

- CVS: Hypovolemia: decreased cardiac output, decreased BP, vasoconstriction,

Hemolysis, DIC (disseminated intra-vascular coagulation)

- Kidney: Decreased GFR, decreased renal blood flow, decreased urine flow, decreased urine specific gravity.

Decrease in volume causes increased osmolality of body fluids and stimulates thirst centre in hypothalamus, ECF volume increased.

## Causes of severe water loss

- Excessive sweating
- Inadequate consumption of water
- Repeated vomiting
- Diarrhea

## Water and solute gain:

Body water gain occurs mainly by water intake.

## ICF differs considerably from ECF

- ECF: Most abundant cation: Na, anion: Cl
- ICF: Most abundant cation: K, anion: protein phosphate ($HPO_4^{2-}$)
- ICF: $K^+$, $HPO_4$ predominant electrolyte
- ECF: $Na^+$, $Cl^-$ predominate

## Electrolytes

Blood fluid is composed of:

- Water
- Electrolyte: Na, K, Cl, P ($HPO_4^{2-}$, $PO_4^{2-}$)

## Function of electrolytes

- Regulate fluid balance: Water follows movement of electrolyte, moving by osmosis.
- Help nerves to respond to stimuli: Electrolytes (Na, Cl) generate action potential across membrane.
- Help in muscle contraction: Via movement of calcium.

## Electrolytes: Na, K, Cl

### Na

- Holds central position in fluid and electrolyte balance
- Dominant cation of ECF
- NaCl provide 90-95% of ecf osmolarity as NaCl, $NaHCO_3$
- Na in ecf remains stable

### K

- Dominant cation in ICF.

### $Cl^-$

- Prevalent anion in ECF
- Moves easily across icf and ecf via channels and transporters
- Cl is regulated by:
  - ADH: governs water loss.
  - Processes that increase or decrease in renal reabsorption of $Na^+$ affect Cl reabsorption.

## Sodium balance in ECF

- Taken up across digestive epithelium
- Excreted in urine and perspiration
- When gain exceeds losses, ecf Na rises
- When losses exceed gain, ecf Na declines
- Changes in Na concentration corrected by ADH.

## Potassium balances in ICF

- 98% potassium is in ICF
- Cells spend energy to recover K ions diffused from cytoplasm into ecf.

## Homeostasis

Ecf volume is monitored by baroreceptors at carotid sinus, aortic sinus, and right atrium

## Abnormal sodium concentration in ECF

- Hyponatremia
- Hypernatremia

## Acid-base equilibrium

- There is a large daily flux of oxygen, carbon dioxide and hydrogen ion throughout the human body along with generation of strong acids such as sulfuric acid, uric acid, lactic acid and others (all are a source of $H^+$ ion in ECF).
- The blood concentration of $H^+$ ion remains constant between 36-46 mmol/L (pH 7.36-7.46) and changes in pH have profound effects.
- Regulation of pH in a narrow range is the function of lungs, kidneys and buffers.

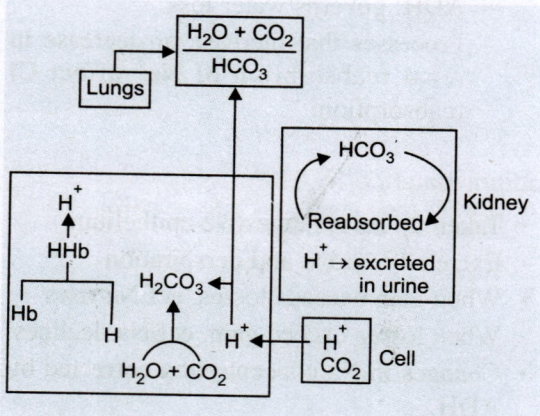

**Fig. 9.9.** Acid base balance.

## Body buffers systems include

- Bicarbonate (most important)
- Phosphate
- Proteins
- Hemoglobin
- Bone carbonate

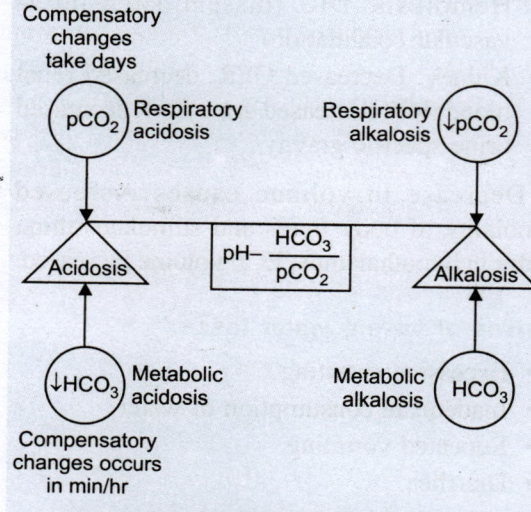

*Respiratory component stimulate metabolic compensation [via renal $HCO_3$ handling (days)]

Metabolic compensation stimulate respiratory compensation (via rate of ventilation)

**Fig. 9.10.** Primary changes in acid base disorders.

## Bicarbonate buffer system

- Unique
- Remains in equilibrium with atmospheric air
- Predominant buffer system of ECF

$$H_2CO_3 \rightleftharpoons H^+ + HCO_3$$

Henderson Hasselbach equation:

$$pH = PK + \log \frac{[HCO_3]}{pCO_2} \times 0.23$$
$$= 6.1 + \log [24/1.2] = 7.4$$
$$pH = 7.4$$

Thus, pH 7.4 is average pH of ECF at normal concentration of $HCO'_3$ and $pCO_2/CO_2$ are regulated by lungs and $HCO_3$ by kidneys]

## Facts-acid base balance

- $CO_2$ (product of carbonic acid) is removed by lungs
- Other acids are excreted by kidneys

- 1 mg/kg body weight of fixed (nonvolatile) acid produced from sulfur containing amino acids, carbohydrates and fats and this acid is also excreted by kidneys.
- Maximum acidification (pH 4.5) of urine by kidneys achieves a hydrogen ion concentration 1000 times that of blood (pH 7.4)

### Evaluation of acid-base status

- Careful history
- Arterial blood gases
- Serum electrolyte
- Urinary pH
- Urinary electrolyte

### Phosphate buffer

Sodium dihydrogen phosphate and disodium hydrogen phosphate constitute intracellular buffers.

### Protein buffers

Plasma proteins and hemoglobin are protein buffer systems of blood.

### Respiration regulation of pH

- Rapid, short term process
- Rate of respiration control rate of removal of $CO_2$. Decrease in blood pH causes hyperventilation to remove $CO_2$ and reduce $H_2CO_3$ concentration.

**Table 9.4.** Acid base disorders: classification

| Disorder | Primary change | pH | Compensatory response |
|---|---|---|---|
| Metabolic acidosis | $\downarrow HCO_3$ | $\downarrow$ | $\downarrow PCO_2$ |
| Metabolic alkalosis | $\uparrow HCO_3$ | $\uparrow$ | $\uparrow PCO_2$ |
| Respiratory acidosis | $\uparrow pCO_2$ | $\downarrow$ | $\uparrow HCO_3$ |
| Respiratory alkalosis | $\downarrow pCO_2$ | $\uparrow$ | $\downarrow HCO_3$ |
| Acidosis | pH below 7.4 Cause : metabolic, respiratory | | |
| Alkalosis | pH above 7.4 Cause : metabolic, respiratory | | |

**Table 9.5.** Clinical causes of acid-base disorders

| Metabolic | | Respiratory | |
|---|---|---|---|
| Acidosis | Alkalosis | Acidosis | Alkalosis |
| Diabetes mellitus (ketoacidosis) | Vomiting (loss of $H^+$) | COPD (chronic obstructive airway disease) | Hyperventilation (anxiety, fever) |
| Lactacidosis | Nasogastric suction (loss of $H^+$) | Cardiac arrest | Salicylate poisoning |
| Renal failure Diarrhea (loss of $HCO_3$) | Hypokalaemia | Respiratory Central depression (drugs: opiate) | Anaemia |
| Renal tubular acidosis ($HCO_3$ loss, H+ impairment) | IV $HCO_3$ administration | Airway obstruction | |

## Renal regulation of pH

- Control plasma $HCO_3$ concentration by regulating its reabsorption and synthesis.
- Highly significant.
- Urine pH lowers blood pH.
- Kidney is only route though which $H^+$ can be eliminated from the body and bicarbonate is conserved.
- $H^+$ ions combine with $NH_3$ to form $NH_4^+$ ion which are excreted into urine.

## Acid-base disorder and plasma potassium

- Because of effect of potassium on contractility of heart, both low and high potassium concentrations may be dangerous! Plasma potassium needs to be checked in case of suspected acid-base disorder.
- The body attempts to compensate for a pH in balance by adjusting the activities of lungs or kidneys.

## (IV) IMMUNOGLOBULINS

Immune system consists of tissues, cells and molecules and genes that recognize react and eliminate foreign and no self substances (antigens).

Two forms:
- Innate or nonspecific
- Adaptive or specific

Body has two types of immune response:
(i) **Humoral immunity:** Production of soluble antibodies or immunoglobulins in response to immunogen by B - lymphocytes in bone marrow.
(ii) **Cell-mediated response** is through cytotoxic or killer T cells.

## Non specific immunity

- Body's first line of defense
- Uses physiochemical barriers (mucosa of epithelium and skin) and their secretions (sweat, mucus, acid)
- Involves inflammatory response
- Mediators of inflammatory response: humoral component:
  - Polymorphs
  - Mononuclear phagocytes
  - Lymphocytes
  - Platelets
  - Endothelial cells
  - CRP
  - Complement system

## Immunoglobulins: fact file

- Produced in response to foreign substances (antigens)
- Associated with $\gamma$-globulin fraction of plasma proteins
- Unique diverse group of molecules those recognize and react with a wide range of specific antigenic structures.
- An animal can synthesize many millions of different antibodies, each with ability to interact with specific antigens: ANTIBODY DIVERSITY
- **Source of Ab diversity:**
  - Large number of variable genes
  - Somatic recombination
  - Somatic mutation
  - Deamination of $C \rightarrow U$.

As lymphocyte matures, each differentiating cell constructs particular L and H genes of virtually unique structure by recombination process.

## Structure immunoglobulins

Five major classes of immunoglobulin share a common structural form: Y-shaped molecule containing two identical units termed heavy (H) chains and two identical smaller units termed light (L) chains [Ig is a tetramer: $H_2 L_2$].

Nature of H chain determines class of immunoglobulin:

| IgG | IgA | IgM | IgD | IgE | Ig |
|-----|-----|-----|-----|-----|-----|
| $(\gamma)$ | $(\alpha)$ | $(\mu)$ | $(\delta)$ | $(\epsilon)$ | Heavy chain |

Chains can be of kappa $(\kappa)$ and lambda $(\lambda)$ type and can be found in any Ig class.

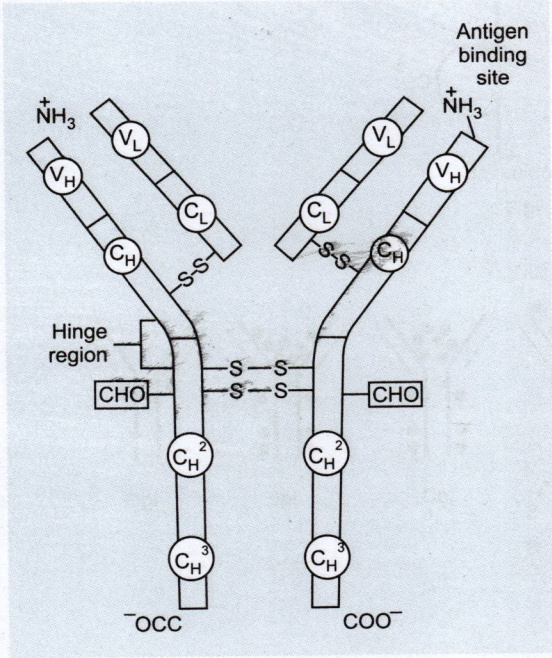

**Fig. 9.11.** Structure of immunoglobulin.

## Basic structural unit of antibody: Monomer

- Monomer, but composed of two pairs of polypeptide chains
- Ab monomer made of two identical light (L) chains and two identical heavy (H) chains.
- Each H chains is paired in same orientation: (-amino to carboxyl within L-chain)
- H and L chains held by disulphide bonds that occur:
  - Between H chains
  - Between H and L chains
  - Between L chains
- Amino portion of both L and H chains has variable structures that are adjacent to each other forming antibody binding site which binds antigen.
- Carboxyl terminal of H and L chains have a constant region which is responsible for Ig function other than epitope recognition e.g., complement activation.
- H chains, further consists of constant region (Fc) with hinge region antibody recognition region (Fab)
- Hinge region is flexible allowing movement between two antibody-binding sites
- Papain digestion splits antibody into three fragments: 2 Fab, one Fc

## IMMUNOGLOBULIN CLASSES (Fig. 9.12)

### IgG

- Most abundant
- Ig (75% of total Ab (antibody in serum)
- Composed of single Y-shaped monomer: 2H2L
- Molecular mass 160kDa
- Half life: 22 days
- Present in all extracellular fluid
- Transported across placenta provides humoral immunity to fetus activates complement.

### IgA

- Abundant in secretions protecting mucosal surfaces.

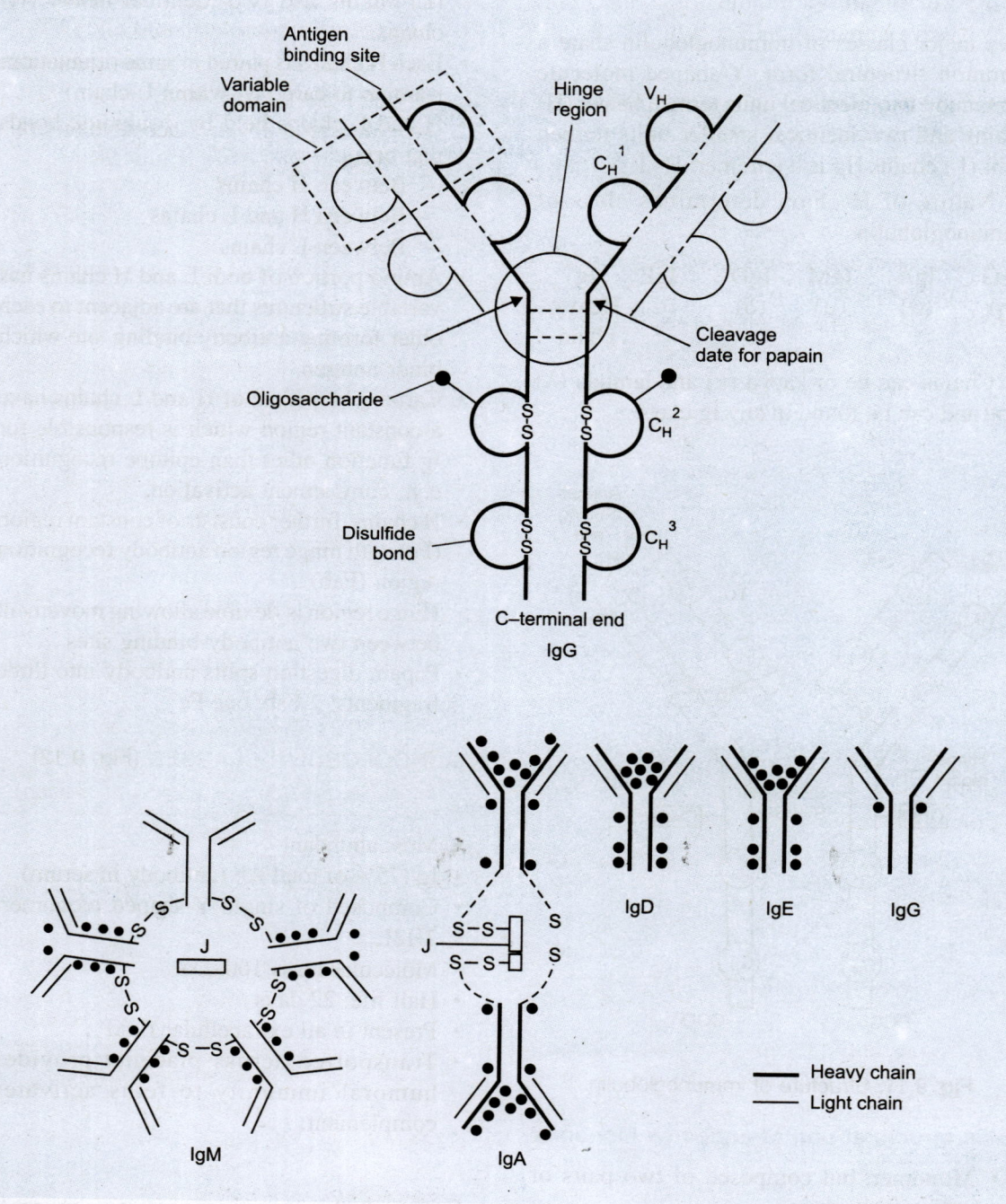

**Fig. 9.12. Classes of Ig.**

- Predominant Ig in colostrums providing passive immunity to newborn
- Half-life: 6 days
- Activate alternate complement pathway
- Exist as dimer joined by J-chain.

## IgM

- Largest immunoglobulin
- composed of 5 Y-shaped monomers held by J polypeptide
- Cannot traverse blood vessels
- Ist Ab to be produced in response to Ag
- Half life: 5 days
- Most abundant Ab produced by fetus, confined to intravascular space

## IgD

- Minor Ig
- Surface receptor for antigen in b-lymphocyte
- Monomer
- Have high carbohydrate content of numerous oligosaccharide units
- Function not clear

## Multiple myeloma

- Malignant proliferation of monoclonal plasma cells producing monoclonal antibodies with kappa or lambda light chains (Bence Jones protein) and infiltration of bone (skull, vertebrae, rib, pelvis) and organs.
- Bence Jones proteins excreted in urine and show M-band in γ-globin region on electrophoresis.

## IgE

- Present in traces
- Monomer

- Found in spleen, tonsil, adenoids and mucosal membranes of lungs and GIT
- Elicit allergic response by inducing mast cells to release histamine.
- Provide immunity in mucosal membrane and parasites.

## Monoclonal Ig

- Product of single B cell arise from benign or malignant
- Transformations of B cells
- React only with a single epitope
- May be normal or fragmented or truncated
- Produce a single band on gel electrophoresis
- Associated with myeloma, Waldenstrom's macroglobulinemia and benign monoclonal gammapathies of uncertain significance (MGUS).

## Immunologic dysfunction

Immune system's activities are mostly beneficial; however, there are several situations where they can have deleterious effects. Disorders of

**Table 9.6.** Disorders of immune regulation

| Level of response | Outcome |
|---|---|
| Decreased response | Immuno deficiency: Primary Secondary |
| Increased response | Tuberculosis Leprosy Immune complex disease Lymphoproliferative disease (monoclonal response) |
| Inappropriate response | Allergic disease: IgE |
| Increased and inappropriate response | Allergic disease Autoimmune disease (monoclonal response) |

immune regulation can be aberrations of quantity, quality or direction of response. Autoimmune diseases can arise from a malfunctioning immune system.

## Antibody deficiency disorders

Deficiency in antibody production results in agammaglobulinemia, hypogammaglobulinemia and specific immunoglobin deficiency.

1. **Infantile X-linked (Bruton's) agamma-globulinemia:** X-linked recessive trait, appears in infants older than 5-6 months after infant's supply of IgG is depleted and antibodies especially IgM are not produced.
   **Defect:** deficiency of all classes of antibodies due to failure of bone marrow, pre-B-cells to mature to circulating antibody-producing B cells.

2. **Transient hypogammaglobulinemia of infancy:** This condition also appears at 5-6 months of age.
   **Defect:** delayed production of IgG between 5-6 months of age, when maternal IgG decreases. Cause of disorder is not known.

3. **Selective Ig deficiency:** It is the most common immunodeficiency disorder where patient can be symptom-free or presents with recurrent pulmonary infections and gastrointestinal problems.
   **Defect:** failure of B cells to mature to plasma cells that produce IgG. All other classes of antibodies are normal in these patients.

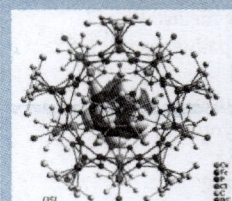

# Index